METHODS OF ANALYSIS FOR

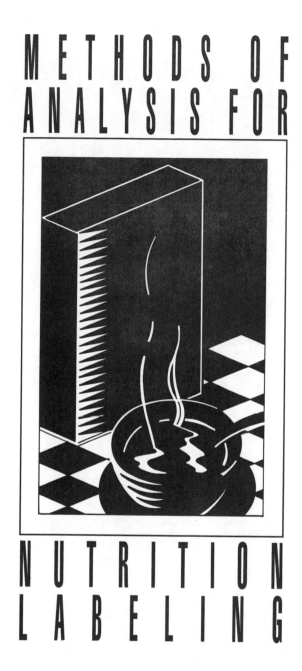

NUTRITION
LABELING

Edited By

DARRYL M. SULLIVAN

DONALD E. CARPENTER

AOAC
INTERNATIONAL

The Scientific Association Dedicated to Analytical Excellence

Printed in the United States of America
Printed on acid-free paper

ISBN No. 0-935584-52-8
Library of Congress No. 93-36961
Production Editor: Scott Hofmann-Reardon

Preface

In 1990, the Nutrition Labeling and Education Act (NLEA) mandated, for the first time, labels containing information about nutritional content of nearly all processed foods. To accomplish this task, analytical data must be generated for hundreds of thousands of foods.

To address the analytical demands of NLEA, AOAC INTERNATIONAL formed the Task Force on Methods for Nutrient Labeling Analyses, which identified and documented the availability of methods for nutritional analysis. This task force was comprised of representatives from government agencies, academia, private companies, and trade associations. The task force assessed AOAC Official Methods relative to the labeling regulations and identified and recommended further study for nutrients with inadequate methodology. This AOAC manual supports and expands the efforts of the task force and provides guidance for the proper selection of methods for nutrient labeling. Thus, the most current information available on methods for nutrition labeling is assembled in this manual.

We begin this book with a very concise abstract on the provisions of NLEA. This will assist the reader in understanding our analytical approach to nutritional analysis. The chapter by Willem de Koe provides an international approach to nutrition labeling. The details of what needs to be labeled as well as some of the specifics on how to label may differ from country to country, but the international procedures should be appropriate given the applicability for each method.

In individual chapters on carbohydrates, minerals and proximate, fat and lipids, and vitamins, information about the use of AOAC Official Methods in the food laboratory are presented. The NLEA requires approaches to nutritional analysis that have never been used before, and it is more important than ever to use the correct AOAC Official Method for the type of food being analyzed. For example, fat is now defined as the sum of fatty acids expressed as triglycerides. This compares with the now outmoded crude fat values which were defined as an ether extract. In addition, saturated fat now includes all those fatty acids without a double bond, while the older definitions cover only fatty acids with carbon chain 12-18.

In many cases, modifications to the AOAC Official Methods are required to comply with NLEA. We present the most current ideas on method adaptations and many new unofficial methods are discussed. Several AOAC Official Methods that are limited in applicability can be used with a number of different food matrices if the appropriate modifications are employed. This information is presented by some of the leading chemists in the food industry today.

When new methods are used in an analytical laboratory, or when methods are modified, the precision and accuracy of the method application must be established. Precision can usually be demonstrated with replicate assays, but accuracy requires a material or standard with a certified concentration of the analyte being measured. We have included a chapter on Standard Reference Materials to cover this vital issue. This chapter will assist the reader in locating appropriate standards for each method/matrix combination. Also included are recommendations on how to prepare your own reference materials.

Finally, all of the AOAC Official Methods acceptable for use in nutrition labeling are contained in this volume. The methods are listed in alphabetical order by nutrient. Included with most of the Official Methods are the original literature references that describe the method development studies. If the reader pays careful attention to the NLEA provisions and follows the AOAC Official Methods as described in this book, he or she will have a very thorough knowledge of how to go about testing food products for their nutritional content.

By
Darryl M. Sullivan
Donald E. Carpenter

Contents

AOAC INTERNATIONAL *Official Methods of Analysis*

Methods of Analysis for Nutrition Labeling

AOAC
INTERNATIONAL

The Scientific Association Dedicated to Analytical Excellence

Chapter 1
Provisions of the Nutrition Labeling and Education Act

Wayne Ellefson

Introduction

This chapter will concisely describe many of the provisions of the Nutrition Labeling and Education Act (NLEA) that affect the analytical laboratory. The chapter also includes label format, nutrient definitions, reference daily intakes (RDIs) and daily reference values (DRVs), nutrient claims, and serving sizes. All of these topics are necessary for proper labeling of food products.

Nutrition labeling is mandatory for processed foods (including fresh and frozen seafood packaged at the plant) and for many meat and poultry products (e.g., breaded chicken kiev). Nutrition labeling is voluntary for single ingredient raw meat and poultry and raw produce and seafood that are unpackaged or packaged at the retail establishment.

Voluntary labeling for these products will remain in effect for retail establishments, provided that 60% of the retail establishments are in compliance for at least 90% of the most frequently consumed fresh fruits and vegetables, raw fish, and major cuts of meat and poultry. These most commonly consumed items have been identified and communicated by the U.S. Food and Drug Administration (FDA) and U.S. Department of Agriculture (USDA) and need not be listed here. FDA will monitor retailers for compliance with labeling (1).

The mandatory nutrition labeling implementation date for FDA-regulated products is May 8, 1994; whereas for USDA-regulated products, it is July 6, 1994.

Nutrition Information

Label Format

The new label features a panel of "Nutrition Facts" (Figure 1) (2). The mandatory nutrients (Table 1) must be listed in the order specified (3). Voluntary nutrients (Table 1) must also be listed in the order specified. If a claim is made about any of the voluntary nutrients, nutrition information must be provided.

A simplified format (Figure 2) may be used for foods that contain insignificant amounts of seven or more of the mandatory nutrients (4). Information for the five 'core' nutrients (calories, total fat, total carbohydrate, protein, and sodium) must be listed. Other mandatory nutrients must be listed if they are present in more than insignificant amounts. Insignificant is defined as the amount that allows a declaration of zero in nutrition labeling. However, for total carbohydrate, dietary fiber, and protein, insignificant is the amount that allows a declaration of "less than 1 gram." Special provisions are made for the use of tabular, bilingual, aggregate, or linear formats (5).

Mandatory and Optional Nutrients

The quantitative requirements for each nutrient on the label vary. This information is summarized in Table 2 (6–8). NLEA defines each nutrient in the following manner:

"Serving size": Serving size must be expressed in common household units and parenthetically in metric equivalents, except for single serving containers in which the metric equivalent is part of the net content declaration.

"Servings per container": Must be expressed in half serving increments between 2–5 servings per container and in whole numbers above 5 servings per container. The terms 'approximately' or 'about' are used if the servings per container are not a whole number.

The new food label will carry an up-to-date, easier-to-use nutrition information guide, to be required on almost all packaged foods (compared to about 60 percent of products up until now). The guide will serve as a key to helping plan a healthy diet.

Serving sizes are now more consistent across product lines, stated in both household and metric measures, and reflect the amounts people actually eat.

The list of nutrients covers those most important to the health of today's consumer, most of whom need to worry about getting too much of certain items (e.g. fat) rather than too few vitamins or minerals, as in the past.

The label will now tell the number of calories per gram of fat, carbohydrate, and protein.

Nutrition Facts

Serving Size 1/2 cup (114g)
Servings Per Container 4

Amount Per Serving

Calories 90   Calories from Fat 30

	%Daily Value*
Total Fat 3g	**5%**
Saturated Fat 0g	**0%**
Cholesterol 0mg	**0%**
Sodium 300mg	**13%**
Total Carbohydrate 13g	**4%**
Dietary Fiber 3g	**12%**
Sugars 3g	
Protein 3g	

Vitamin A 80%	•	Vitamin C 60%	
Calcium 4%	•	Iron	4%

* Percent Daily Values are based on a 2,000 calorie diet. Your daily values may be higher or lower depending on your calorie needs:

		Calories:	2,000	2,500
Total Fat	Less than		65g	80g
Sat Fat	Less than		20g	25g
Cholesterol	Less than		300mg	300mg
Sodium	Less than		2,400mg	2,400mg
Total Carbohydrate			300g	375g
Dietary Fiber			25g	30g

Calories per gram:
Fat 9 • Carbohydrate 4 • Protein 4

The new title signals that the label contains the newly-required information.

Calories from fat are now shown on the label to help consumers meet dietary guidelines that recommend people get no more than 30% of their calories from fat.

% Daily Value shows how a food fits into the overall daily diet.

Daily values are also something new. Some are maximums, as with fat (65 grams *or less*); others are minimums, as with carbohydrates (300 grams *or more*). The daily values on the label are based on a daily diet of 2,000 and 2,500 calories. Individuals should adjust the values to fit their own calorie intake.

*This label is only an example. Exact specifications are in the final rules.
Source: U.S. Food and Drug Administration 1992

Figure 1. The new food label.

Table 1. Mandatory/Optional Nutrients

Calories	**Total Carbohydrate (g)**	**Vitamin A**	Folate
Calories from Fat	**Dietary Fiber (g)**	**Vitamin C**	Vitamin B$_{12}$
Calories from Saturated Fat	Soluble fiber (g)	**Calcium**	Biotin
Total Fat (g)	Insoluble fiber (g)	**Iron**	Pantothenic acid
Saturated fat (g)	**Sugars (g)**	Vitamin D	Phosphorus
Polyunsaturated fat (g)	Sugar Alcohols (g)	Vitamin E	Iodine
Monounsaturated fat (g)	**Other Carbohydrate**	Thiamin	Magnesium
Cholesterol (mg)	**Protein (g) or**	Riboflavin	Zinc
Sodium (mg)	**Corrected Protein (g)**	Niacin	Copper
Potassium (mg)		Vitamin B$_6$	

"Calories": A statement of the caloric content per serving, expressed to the nearest 5-calorie increment up to and including 50 calories, and 10-calorie increment above 50 calories, except that amounts less that 5 calories may be expressed as zero. Energy content per serving may also be expressed in kilojoule units, added in parentheses immediately following that statement of the caloric content. Caloric content may be calculated by the following means: using the general factors of 4, 4, and 9 calories per gram for protein, total carbohydrate, and total fat, respectively; using the general factors of 4, 4, and 9 calories per gram for protein, total carbohydrate less the amount of insoluble dietary fiber, and total fat, respectively; using data for specific food factors for particular foods or ingredients approved by FDA; using bomb calorimetry data and subtracting 1.25 calories per gram protein to correct for incomplete digestibility.

"Calories from fat": A statement of the caloric content derived from total fat in a serving, expressed to the nearest 5-calorie increment, up to and including 50 calories, and the nearest 10-calorie increment above 50 calories. Label declaration of "calories from fat" is not required on products that contain less than 0.5 gram of fat in a serving, and amounts less that 5 calories may be expressed as zero.

"Calories from saturated fat": A statement of the caloric content derived from saturated fat in a serving may be declared voluntarily, expressed to the nearest 5-calorie increment, up to and including 50 calories, and the nearest 10-calorie increment above 50 calories, except that amounts less than 5 calories may be expressed as zero.

"Total fat": A statement of the number of grams of total fat in a serving defined as total lipid fatty acids and expressed as triglycerides. Amounts shall be expressed to the nearest 0.5 grams increment below 5 grams and to the nearest gram increment above 5 grams. If the serving contains less than 0.5 grams, the content shall be expressed as zero.

"Saturated fat": A statement of the number of grams of saturated fat in a serving defined as the sum of all fatty acids containing no double bonds, except that label declaration of saturated fat content information is not required for products that contain less than 0.5 grams of total fat in a serving if no claims are made about fat or cholesterol content, and if "calories from saturated fat" is not declared. If a statement of the saturated fat content is not required and therefore not declared, the statement "Not a significant source of saturated fat" must be placed at the bottom of the table of nutrient values. Saturated fat content must be expressed as grams per serving to the

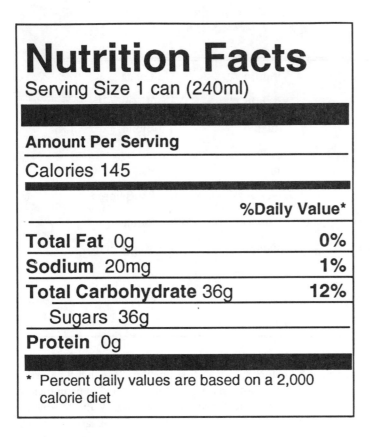

Figure 2. Nutrition facts.

nearest 0.5 grams increment below 5 grams and to the nearest gram increment above 5 grams. If the serving contains less than 0.5 grams, the content shall be expressed as zero.

"Polyunsaturated fat": A statement of the number of grams of polyunsaturated fat in a serving defined as *cis,cis*-methylene-interrupted polyunsaturated fatty acids may be declared voluntarily. When monounsaturated fat is declared or when a claim is made on the label or in labeling about fatty acids or cholesterol, label declaration of polyunsaturated fat is required. Polyunsaturated fat content must be expressed as grams per serving to the nearest 0.5 grams increment below 5 grams and to the nearest gram increment above 5 grams. If the serving contains less than 0.5 grams, the content shall be expressed as zero.

"Monounsaturated fat": A statement of the number of grams of monounsaturated fat in a serving defined as *cis*-monounsaturated fatty acids may be declared voluntarily. When polyunsaturated fat is declared or when a claim is made on the label or in labeling about fatty acids or cholesterol, label declaration of monounsaturated fat is required. Monounsaturated fat content must be expressed as grams per serving to the nearest

0.5 grams increment below 5 grams and to the nearest gram increment above 5 grams. If the serving contains less than 0.5 grams, the content shall be expressed as zero.

Table 2. Guidelines for Reporting Nutrition Label Values

Nutrient	Units	Increment	Range	"Zero" Permitted
Calories	kcal	5	0–50	<5 calories
		10	>50	
Calories from fat	kcal	5	0–50	<5 calories
		10	>50	
Calories from saturated fat	kcal	5	0–50	<5 calories
		10	>50	

Table 2. Guidelines for Reporting Nutrition Label Values

Nutrient	Units	Increment	Range	"Zero" Permitted
Total fat	g	0.5	0–5	<0.5 g
(total of lipid fatty acids and		1	>5	
expressed as triglycerides)				
Saturated fat	g	0.5	0–5	<0.5 g
(sum of all fatty acids		1	>5	
containing no double bonds)				
Polyunsaturated fat	g	0.5	0–5	<0.5 g
a (cis,cis-m-i isomers only)		1	>5	
Monounsaturated fat	g	0.5	0–5	<0.5 g
(cis isomers only)		1	>5	
Cholesterol	mg	5	all	<2 mg
Sodium	mg	0	<5	<5 mg
		5	5–140	
		10	>140	
Potassium	mg	0	<5	<5 mg
		5	5–140	
		10	>140	
Total carbohydrate	g	1	all	<0.5 g
Dietary fiber	g	1	all	<0.5 g
Soluble fiber	g	1	all	<0.5 g
Insoluble fiber	g	1	all	<0.5 g
Sugars	g	1	all	<0.5 g
Sugar alcohol	g	1	all	<0.5 g
Other carbohydrate	g	1	all	<0.5 g
Protein	g	1	all	<0.5 g

Table 2. Guidelines for Reporting Nutrition Label Values

Nutrient	Units	Increment	Range	"Zero" Permitted
Vitamin A, vitamin C,	% DV	2	0–10	<2%
calcium, and iron		5	>10–50	
		10	>50	
Other vitamins and	% DV	2	0–10	<2%
minerals with RDIs		5	>10–50	
		10	>50	

"Cholesterol": A statement of the cholesterol content in a serving expressed in milligrams to the nearest 5-milligram increment. Label declaration of cholesterol information is not required for products that contain less than 2 milligrams cholesterol in a serving and make no claim about fat, fatty acids, or cholesterol content. Such products may state the cholesterol content as zero. If cholesterol content is not required, the statement "Not a significant source of cholesterol" must be place at the bottom of the table of nutrient values. If the food contains 2 to 5 milligrams of cholesterol per serving, the content may be stated as "less than 5 milligrams."

"Sodium": A statement of the number of milligrams of sodium in a serving expressed as zero when the serving contains less than 5 milligrams of sodium, to the nearest 5-milligram increment when the serving contains 5 to 140 milligrams of sodium, and to the nearest 10-milligram increment when the serving contains greater than 140 milligrams.

"Potassium": A statement of the number of milligrams of potassium in a serving may be declared voluntarily. When a claim is made about potassium content, label declaration is required. Potassium content must be expressed as zero when the serving contains less than 5 milligrams of potassium, to the nearest 5-milligrams increment when the serving contains less than or equal to 140 milligrams of potassium, and to the nearest 10-milligram increment when the serving contains more than 140 milligrams.

"Total carbohydrate": A statement of the number of grams of total carbohydrate in a serving expressed to the nearest gram. If a serving contains less than 1 gram, the statement "Contains less than 1 gram" or "less than 1 gram" may be used. If the serving contains less than 0.5 grams, the content may be expressed as zero. Total carbohydrate content is calculated by subtraction of the sum of the crude protein, total fat, moisture, and ash from the total weight of the food.

"Dietary fiber": A statement of the number of grams of total dietary fiber in a serving expressed to the nearest gram. If a serving contains less than 1 gram, declaration of dietary fiber is not required. The statement "Contains less than 1 gram" or "less than 1 gram" may be used. If the serving contains less than 0.5 grams, the content may be expressed as zero. If dietary fiber content is not required the statement "Not a significant source of dietary fiber" shall be placed at the bottom of the table of nutrient values.

"Soluble fiber": A statement of the number of grams of soluble dietary fiber in a serving may be declared voluntarily. When a claim is made on the label about soluble fiber, declaration is required. Soluble fiber content is expressed to the nearest gram. If a serving contains less than 1 gram, the statement "Contains less than 1 gram" or "less than 1 gram" may be used. If the serving contains less than 0.5 grams the content may be expressed as zero.

"Insoluble fiber": A statement of the number of grams of insoluble dietary fiber in a serving may be declared voluntarily. "When a claim is made on the label about insoluble fiber, declaration is required. Insoluble fiber content is expressed to the nearest gram. If a serving contains less than 1 gram, the statement "Contains less than 1 gram" or "less than 1 gram" may be used. If the serving contains less than 0.5 gram, the content may be expressed as zero.

"Sugars": A statement of the number of grams of sugars in a serving declaration of sugars content is not required for products that contain less than 1 gram of sugars in a serving if no claims are made about sweeteners, sugars, or sugar alcohol content. If a statement of the sugars content is not required, the statement "Not a significant source of sugars" shall be placed at the bottom of the table of nutrient values. Sugars shall be defined as the sum of all free mono- and disaccharides (such as glucose, fructose, lactose, and sucrose). Sugars content is expressed to the nearest gram. If a serving contains less than 1 gram, the statement "Contains less then 1 gram" or "less than 1 gram" may be used. If the serving contains less than 0.5 grams, the content may be expressed as zero.

"Sugar alcohol": A statement of the number of grams of sugar alcohols in a serving may be declared voluntarily. When a claim is made on the label about sugar alcohol or sugars when sugar alcohols are present in the food, sugar alcohol content must be declared. Sugar alcohols are defined as the sum of saccharide derivatives in which a hydroxyl group replaces a ketone or aldehyde group and whose use in the food is listed by FDA (e.g., mannitol) or is generally recognized as safe (e.g., xylitol and sorbitol). In place of the term "sugar alcohol," the name of the specific sugar alcohol (e.g., "xylitol") present in the food may be used in the nutrition label provided that only one sugar alcohol is present. Sugar alcohol content shall be indented and expressed to the nearest gram. If a serving contains less than 1 gram, the statement "Contains less then 1 gram" or "less than 1 gram" may be used. If the serving contains less than 0.5 grams, the content may be expressed as zero.

"Other carbohydrate": A statement of the number of grams of other carbohydrates may be declared voluntarily. Other carbohydrates is defined as the difference between total carbohydrate and the sum of dietary fiber, sugars, and sugar alcohol. If sugar alcohol is not declared it shall be defined as the difference between total carbohydrate and the sum of dietary fiber and sugars. Other carbohydrate content is expressed to the nearest gram. If a serving contains less than 1 gram, the statement "Contains less than 1 gram" or "less than 1 gram" may be used. If the serving contains less than 0.5 gram, the content may be expressed as zero.

"Protein": A statement of the number of grams of protein in a serving, expressed to the nearest gram. If a serving contains less than 1 gram, the statement "Contains less than 1 gram" or "less than 1 gram" may be used. If the serving contains less than 0.5 grams, the content may be expressed as zero. Protein content may be calculated on the basis of the factor of 6.25 times the nitrogen content of the food except when the official procedure for a specific food required another factor.

A statement of the corrected amount of protein per serving calculated as a percentage of the DRV for protein, and expressed as Percent of Daily Value, may be placed on the label. Such a statement must be given if a protein claim is made for the products.

"Vitamins and minerals": A statement of the amount per serving of the vitamins and minerals calculated as a percent of the RDI and expressed as percent of Daily Value. The declaration of vitamins and minerals as a percent of the RDI shall include vitamin A, vitamin C, calcium, and iron, in that order, and shall include any of the other vitamins and minerals listed when they are added as a nutrient supplement, or when a claim is made about them. The declaration may also include any of the other vitamins and minerals when they are naturally occurring in food. The additional vitamins and minerals shall be listed in the order established.

The percentages for vitamins and minerals must be expressed to the nearest 2% increment up to and including the 10% level, the nearest 5% increment above 10% and up to and including the 50% level, and the nearest 10% increment above the 50% level. Amount of vitamins and minerals present at less than 2% of the RDI are not required to be declared in nutrition labeling but may be declared by a zero or by the use of an asterisk that refers to another asterisk that is placed at the bottom of the table and that is followed by the statement, "Contains less than 2 percent of the Daily Value of this nutrient," or by the statement, "Not a significant source of ___ (listing the vitamins or minerals omitted)."

The percent of vitamin A that is present as beta-carotene may be declared in the same increments as other vitamins and minerals immediately adjacent to or immediately under the nutrient name [e.g., "Vitamin A (90% as beta-carotene)"].

RDIs and DRVs

The current RDIs and DRVs are shown in Table 3 (9) and Table 4 (10). There are indications that the RDIs may be changed in the future as FDA gathers new information.

Table 3. Mandatory/voluntary RDI chart.

Nutrient	Unit	RDI
Vitamin A	International Units (IU)	5000
Vitamin C	mg	60
Calcium	g	1.0
Iron	mg	18
Vitamin D	IU	400
Vitamin E	IU	30
Thiamin	mg	1.5
Riboflavin	mg	1.7
Niacin	mg	20
Vitamin B_6	mg	2.0
Folate	mg	0.4
Vitamin B_{12}	μg	6.0
Biotin	mg	0.3
Pantothenic acid	mg	10
Phosphorus	g	1.0
Iodine	μg	150
Magnesium	mg	400
Zinc	mg	15
Copper	mg	2.0

Notes: All voluntary nutrients are required if a claim is made regarding that nutrient.

The declaration of all vitamins and minerals will be as a percent of the RDI.

Table 4. DRVs

Nutrient	2,000 calories	2,500 calories
Total fat	65 g	80 g
Saturated fat	20 g	25 g
Cholesterol	300 mg	300 mg
Sodium	2,400 mg	2,400 mg
Potassium	3,500 mg	3,500 mg
Total carbohydrate	300 g	375 g
Fiber	25 g	30 g

Nutrient Content Claims

A summary of permissible nutrient content claims is shown in Table 5 (11–14). These nutrient claims are very specific in their definitions and require appropriate and accurate analytical analysis to be verified.

Serving Sizes

FDA and USDA established reference amounts for a variety of food categories. These reference amounts are based on the amount that is customarily consumed in an eating occasion by an adult or by a child over 4 years of age. Tables 6–9 list these reference amounts (15–18). Again, the serving size must appear on the label in common household measures and the metric equivalent. A serving size that most closely approximates its reference amount will be established for each product.

More detailed information on the serving size regulations is contained in the Federal Register, **58**(3), Wednesday, January 6, 1993, beginning on page 2291.

Table 5. Relative (or Comparative) Claims

Accompanying Information

- For all relative claims, percent (or fraction) of change and identity of reference food must be declared in immediate proximity to the most prominent claim. Quantitative comparison of the amount of the nutrient in the product per labeled serving with that in the reference food must be declared on information panel.
- For Light claims: % reduction for both fat and calories must be stated but % reduction need not be specified if product is low in the nutrient.

Reference Foods

"Light" / "Lite"
(1) A food representative of the type of food bearing the claim, e.g. average value of top three brands or representative value from valid data base; (2) similar food (e.g. potato chips for potato chips); and (3) not low calorie **and** low fat (except light sodium foods which must be low calorie and low fat).

"Reduced" and "Added" (or "fortified" and "enriched")
(1) An established regular product or average representative product and (2) similar food.

"More" and "Less" (or "Fewer")
(1) An established regular product or average representative product and (2) a dissimilar food in the same product category which may be generally substituted for labeled food (e.g. potato chips for pretzels) or a similar food.

Other Nutrient Content Claims

"Lean"
On seafood or game meat that contains < 10 g total fat, < 4.5 g saturated fat and < 95 mg cholesterol/ reference serving and per 100 g (for meals and main dishes, meets criteria per 100 g and per labeled serving).

"Extra Lean"
On seafood or game meat that contains < 5 g total fat, < 2 g saturated fat and < 95 mg cholesterol per reference serving and per 100 g (for meals and main dishes, meets criteria per 100 g and per label serving).

"High", "Rich In", or "Excellent Source Of"
Contains 20% or more of the Daily Value (DV) to describe protein, vitamins, minerals, dietary fiber, or potassium per reference serving.
May be used on meals or main dishes to indicate that product contains a food that meets definition.

"Good Source Of" "Contains" or "Provides"
10-19% of the DV per reference serving.
May be used on meals or main dishes to indicate that product contains a food that meets definition.

"More"
10% more of the DV per reference serving.

"Modified"
May be used in statement of identity that bears a relative claim, e.g. "Modified Fat Cheese Cake, Contains 35% Less Fat Than Our Regular Cheese Cake."

Any fiber claim
If food is not low in total fat, must state total fat in conjunction with claim such as "More Fiber".

Table 5. (Continued) Nutrient Content Claims.

Nutrient	Free	Low	Reduced/Less	Comments
Calories § 101.60 (b)	•Synonyms for "Free": "Zero", "No", "Without", "Trivial Source of", "Negligible Source of", "Dietarily Insignificant Source of" •Definitions for "Free" for meals and main dishes are the stated values per labeled serving	•Synomms for "Low": "Little", ("Few" for Calories), "Contains a Small Amount of", "Low Source of"	•Synonyms for "Reduced"/ "Less": "Lower" ("Fewer" for calories) •"Modified" may be used in statement of identity •Definitions for meals and main dishes are same as for individual foods on a per 100 g basis	•For "Free", "Very Low", or "Low" must indicate if food meets a definition without benefit of special processing, alteration, formulation or reformulation; e.g. "broccoli, a fat-free food" or "celery, a low calorie food"
Calories § 101.60 (b)	•Less than 5 cal per reference amount •Not defined for meals or main dishes	•40 cal or less per reference amount (and per 50 g if reference amount is small) •Meals and main dishes: 120 cal or less per 100 g	•At least 25% fewer calories per reference amount than an appropriate reference food •Reference food may not be "Low Calorie" •Uses term "Fewer" rather than "Less"	•"Light" or "Lite": if 50% or more of the calories are from fat, fat must be reduced be at least 50% per reference amount. If less than 50% of calories are from fat, fat must be reduced at least 50% or calories reduced at least 1/3 per reference amount •Meal or main dish meets definition for "Low Calorie" or "Low Fat" meal and is labeled to indicate which definition is met.
Total Fat § 101.62 (b)	•Less than 0.5 g per reference amount and per serving •No ingredient that is fat or understood to contain fat except as noted below"	•3 g or less per reference amount (and per 50 g if reference amount is small) •Meals and main dishes: 3 g or less per 100 g and not more than 30% of calories from fat	•At least 25% less fat per reference amount than an appropriate reference food •Reference food may not be "Low Fat"	•"___ % Fat Free": OK if meets the requirements for "Low Fat" •"Light" - see above
Saturated Fat § 101.62 (c)	•Less than 0.5 g per reference amount and per serving •Trans fatty acids are less than 0.5 g per ref. amount and per serving •No ingredient that is understood to contain saturated fat except as noted below"	•1 g or less per reference amount and 15% or less of calories from saturated fat •Meals and main dishes: 1 g or less per 100 g and less than 10% of calories from saturated fat	•At least 25% less saturated fat per reference amount than an appropriate reference food •Reference food may not be "Low Saturated Fat"	•Next to all saturated fat claims, must declare the amount of cholesterol if 2 mg or more per reference amount; and the amount to total fat if more than 3 g per reference amount (or 0.5 g or more of total fat for "Saturated Fat Free")

Table 5. (Continued) Nutrient Content Claims.

Nutrient	Free	Low	Reduced/Less	Comments
Cholesterol § 101.62 (d)	• Less than 2 mg per reference amount. • No ingredient that contains cholesterol except as noted below* • If less than 2 mg per reference amount by special processing and total fat exceeds 13 g per reference and labeled serving, the amount of cholesterol must be "Substantially Less" (25%) than in a reference food with significant market share (5% of market)	• 20 mg or less per reference amount (and per 50 g of food if reference amount is small) • If qualifies by special processing and total fat exceeds 13 g per reference and labeled serving, the amount of cholesterol must be "Substantially Less" (25%) than in a reference food with significant market share (5% or market) • Meals and main dishes: 20 mg or less per 100 g	• At least 25% less fat per reference amount than an appropriate reference food • Reference food may not be "Low Cholesterol"	• CHOLESTEROL CLAIMS ONLY ALLOWED WHEN FOOD CONTAINS 2 G OR LESS SATURATED FAT PER REFERENCE AMOUNT, OR FOR MEALS AND MAIN DISH PRODUCTS, PER LABELED SERVING SIZE • Must declare the amount of total fat next to cholesterol claim when fat exceeds 13 g per reference amount and labeled serving (or per 50 g of food if reference amount is small)
Sodium § 101.61	• Less than 5 mg per reference amount • No ingredient that is sodium chloride or generally understood to contain sodium except as noted below*	• 140 mg or less per reference amount (and per 50 g if reference amount is small) • Meals and main dishes: 140 mg or less per 100 g	• At least 25% less sodium per reference amount than an appropriate reference food • Reference food may not be "Low Sodium"	• "Light" (for sodium reduced products): if food is "Low Calorie" and "Low Fat" and sodium is reduced by at least 50% • "Light in Sodium": if food is reduced by at least 50% per reference amount. Entire term "Light in Sodium" must be used in same type, size, color & prominence. Light in Sodium for meals = "Low in Sodium" • "Very Low Sodium": 35 mg or less per reference amount (and per 50 g if reference amount is small). For meals and main dishes: 35 mg or less per 100 g • "Salt Free" must meet criterion for "Sodium Free" • "No Salt Added" and "Unsalted" must meet conditions of use and must declare "This Is Not A Sodium Free Food" on information panel if food is not "Sodium Free" • "Lightly Salted": 50% less sodium than normally added to reference food and if not "Low Sodium", so labeled on information panel

Table 5. (Continued) Nutrient Content Claims.

Nutrient	Free	Low	Reduced/Less	Comments
Sugars § 101.60 (c)	• "Sugar Free": Less than 0.5 g sugars per reference amount • No ingredient that is a sugar or generally understood to contain sugars except as noted below* • Disclose calorie profile (e.g. "Low Calorie")	• Not Defined. No basis for a recommended intake	• At least 25% less sugars per reference amount than an appropriate reference food	• "No Added Sugars" and "Without Added Sugars" are allowed if no sugar or sugar containing ingredient is added during processing. State if food is not "Low" or "Reduced Calorie" • The terms "Unsweetened" and "No Added Sweeteners" remain as factual statements • Claims about reducing dental caries are implied health claims • Does not include sugar alcohols

Notes: *Except if the ingredient listed in the ingredient statement has an "*" that refers to footnote (e.g. "* adds a trivial amount of fat").
• "Reference Amount" = amount customarily consumed.
• "Small Reference Amount" = reference amount 30 g or less or 2 tablespoons or less (for dehydrated foods that are typically consumed when rehydrated with water only, the per 50 g refers to the prepared form).
• Statement "See _____ panel for nutrition information" must accompany all content claims. When levels exceed: 13 g **Fat**, 4 g **Saturated Fat**, 60 mg **Cholesterol**, and 480 mg **Sodium** reference amount, per labeled serving or for foods with small reference amounts per 50 g, a disclosure statement is required as part of claim (e.g. "see side panel for information on fat and other nutrients").

Implied Claims

•Claims about a food or ingredient that suggests that the nutrient or ingredient are absent or present in a certain amount or claims about a food that suggests a food may be useful in maintaining healthy dietary practices and which are made with an explicit claim (e.g. "healthy, contains 3 grams of fat") are implied claims and are prohibited unless provided for in a regulation by FDA. In addition, the Agency has devised a petition system whereby specific additional claims may be considered.

•Claims that a food contains or is made with an ingredient that is known to contain a particular nutrient may be made if product is "Low" in or a "Good Source" of the nutrient associated with the claim (e.g. "good source of oat bran").

•Equivalence claims: "contains as much [nutrient] as a [food]" may be made if both reference food and labeled food are "Good Source" of nutrient on a per serving basis.

•The following label statements are generally not considered implied claims unless they are made in a nutrition context: 1) avoidance claims for religious food intolerance or other non-nutrition related reasons (e.g. "100% milk free"); 2) statements about non-nutritive substances (e.g. "no artificial colors"); 3) added value statements (e.g. "made with real butter"); 4) statements of identity (e.g. "corn oil" or "corn oil margarine"); and 5) special dietary statements made in compliance with a specific Part 105 provision.

Terms Covered That Are Not Nutrient Content Claims

"Fresh"	A raw food that has not been frozen, heat processed, or otherwise preserved.
"Fresh Frozen"	Food was quickly frozen while still fresh.
Any fiber claim	If Food is not low in total fat, must state total fat in conjunction with claim such as "More Fiber".

Table 6. Reference amounts customarily consumed per eating occasion: infant and toddler foods

Product category	Reference amount
Cereals, dry instant	15 g
Cereals, prepared, ready-to-serve	110 g
Other cereal and grain products, dry ready-to-eat, e.g., ready-to-eat cereals, cookies, teething biscuits, and toasts	7 g for infants and 20 g for toddlers for ready-to-eat cereals, 7 g for all others
Dinners, desserts, fruits, vegetables or soups, dry mix	15 g
Dinners, desserts, fruits, vegetables or soups, ready-to-serve, junior type	110 g
Dinners, desserts, fruits, vegetables or soups, ready-to-serve, strained type	60 g
Dinners, stews or soups for toddlers, ready-to-serve	170 g
Fruits for toddlers, ready-to-serve	125 g
Vegetables for toddlers, ready-to-serve	70 g
Eggs/egg yolks, ready-to-serve	55 g
Juices, all varieties	120 mL

Table 7. Reference amounts customarily consumed per eating occasion: general food supply

Product category	Reference amount
Bakery Products	
Biscuits, croissants, bagels, tortillas, soft bread sticks, soft pretzels, corn bread, hush puppies	55 g
Breads (excluding sweet quick type), rolls	50 g
Bread sticks-*see Crackers*	
Toaster pastries-*see Coffee cakes*	
Brownies	40 g
Cakes, heavy weight	125 g
Cakes, medium weight	80 g
Cakes, light weight	55 g
Coffee cakes, crumb cakes, doughnuts, Danish, sweet rolls, sweet quick type breads, muffins, toaster pastries	55 g
Cookies	30 g
Crackers that are usually not used as snack, melba toast, hard bread sticks, ice cream cones	15 g
Crackers that are usually used as snacks	30 g

Table 7. Reference amounts customarily consumed per eating occasion: general food supply

Product category	Reference amount
Croutons	7 g
French toast, pancakes, variety mixes	110 g prepared for french toast and pancakes; 40 g dry mix for variety mixes
Grains-based bars with or without filling or coating, e.g., breakfast bars, granola bars, rice cereal bars	40 g
Ice cream cones-*see Crackers*	
Pies, cobblers, fruit crisps, turnovers, other pastries	125 g
Pie crust	1/6 of 8" crust; 1/8 of 9" crust
Pizza crust	55 g
Taco shells, hard	30 g
Waffles	85 g
Beverages	
Carbonated and noncarbonated beverages, wine coolers, water	240 mL
Coffee or tea, flavored and sweetened	240 mL prepared
Cereals and Other Grain Products	
Breakfast cereals (hot cereal type), hominy grits	1 cup prepared; 40 g plain dry cereal; 55 g flavored, sweetened cereal
Breakfast cereals, ready-to-eat, weighing less than 20 g per cup, e.g., plain puffed cereal grains	15 g
Breakfast cereals, ready-to-eat, weighing 20 g or more but less, than 43 g per cup; high fiber cereals containing 28 g or more of fiber per 100 g	30 g
Breakfast cereals, ready-to-eat, weighing 43 g or more per cup, biscuit types	55 g
Bran or wheat germ	15 g
Flours or cornmeal	30 g
Grains, e.g., rice, barley, plain	140 g prepared; 45 g dry
Pastas, plain	140 g prepared; 55 g dry
Pastas, dry, ready-to-eat, e.g., fried canned chow mein noodles	25 g
Starches, e.g., cornstarch, potato starch, tapioca	10 g
Stuffing	100 g
Dairy Products and Substitutes	
Cheese, cottage	110 g

Table 7. Reference amounts customarily consumed per eating occasion: general food supply

Product category	Reference amount
Cheese used primarily as ingredients, e.g., dry cottage cheese, ricotta cheese	55 g
Cheese, grated hard, e.g., Parmesan, Romano	5 g
Cheese, all others except those listed as separate categories, includes cream cheese and cheese spread	30 g
Cheese sauce-*see Sauce*	
Cream or cream substitutes, fluid	15 mL
Cream or cream substitutes, powder	2 g
Cream, half & half	30 mL
Eggnog	120 mL
Milk, condensed, undiluted	30 mL
Milk, evaporated, undiluted	30 mL
Milk, milk-based drinks, e.g., instant breakfast, meal replacement, cocoa	240 mL
Shakes or shake substitutes, e.g., dairy shake mixes, fruit frost mixes	240 mL
Sour cream	30 g
Yogurt	225 g
Desserts	
Ice cream, ice milk, frozen yogurt, sherbet: all types, bulk and novelties (eg, bars, sandwiches, cones)	1/2 cup-include the volume for coatings and wafers for the novelty type varieties
Frozen flavored and sweetened ice and pops, frozen fruit juices: all types, bulk and novelties (e.g., bars, cups)	85 g
Sundae	1 cup
Custards, gelatin or pudding	1/2 cup
Dessert Toppings and Fillings	
Cake frosting or icings	35 g
Other dessert toppings, eg, fruits, syrups, spreads, marshmallow cream, nuts, dairy and nondairy whipped toppings	2 tbsp
Pie fillings	85 g
Egg and Egg Substitutes	
Egg mixtures, e.g., egg foo young, scrambled eggs, omelets	110 g
Eggs (all sizes)	50 g
Egg substitutes	An amount to make 1 large (50 g) egg

Table 7. Reference amounts customarily consumed per eating occasion: general food supply

Product category	Reference amount
Fats and Oils	
Butter, margarine, oil shortening	1 tbsp
Butter replacement, powder	2 g
Dressings for salads	30 g
Mayonnaise, sandwich spreads, mayonnaise-type dressings	15 g
Spray types	0.25 g
Fish, Shellfish, Game Meats,and Meat or Poultry Substitutes	
Bacon substitutes, canned anchovies, anchovy pastes, caviar	15 g
Dried, e.g., jerky	30 g
Entrees with sauce, e.g., fish with cream sauce, shrimp with lobster sauce	140 g cooked
Entrees without sauce, e.g., plain or fried fish and shellfish, fish and shellfish cake	85 g cooked; 110 g uncooked
Fish, shellfish or game meat, canned	55 g
Substitute for luncheon meat, meat spreads,	
Canadian bacon, sausages and frankfurters	55 g
Smoked or pickled fish, shellfish, or game meat fish or shellfish spread	55 g
Substitutes for bacon bits-*see Miscellaneous*	
Fruits and Fruit Juices	
Canned or pickled	30 g
Dehydrated fruits-*see Snacks*	
Dried	40 g
Fruits for garnish or flavor, e.g., maraschino cherries	4 g
Fruit relishes, e.g., cranberry sauce, cranberry relish	70 g
Fruits used primarily as ingredients, avocado	30 g
Fruits used primarily as ingredients, others (cranberries, lemon, lime)	55 g
Watermelon	280 g
All other fruits (except those listed as separate categories), fresh, canned, or frozen	140 g
Juices, nectars, fruit drinks	240 mL
Juices used as ingredients, e.g., lemon juice, lime juice	5 mL

Table 7. Reference amounts customarily consumed per eating occasion: general food supply

Product category	Reference amount
Legumes	
Bean cake (tofu), tempeh	85 g
Beans, plain or in sauce	130 g for beans in sauce or canned in liquid; 90 g for others
Miscellaneous category	
Baking powder, baking soda, pectin	1 g
Baking decorations, e.g., colored sugars and sprinkles for cookies, cake decorations	1/4 tsp or 4 g if not measurable by teaspoon
Batter mixes, bread crumbs	30 g
Cooking wine	30 mL
Drink mixers (without alcohol)	Amount to make 240 mL drink (without ice)
Chewing gum	3 g
Meat, poultry and fish coating mixes, dry; seasoning mixes, dry, e.g., chili seasoning mixes, pasta salad seasoning mixes	Amount to make one reference amount of final dish
Salad and potato toppers, e.g., salad crunchies, salad crispins, substitutes for bacon bits	7 g
Salt, salt substitutes, seasoning salts (e.g., garlic salt)	1 g
Spices, herbs (other than dietary supplements)	1/4 tsp or 05 g if not measurable by teaspoon
Mixed Dishes	
Measurable with cup, e.g., casseroles, hash, macaroni and cheese, pot pies, spaghetti with sauce, stews	1 cup
Not measurable with cup, e.g., burritos, egg rolls, enchiladas, pizza, pizza rolls, quiche, all types of sandwiches	140 g, add 55 g for products with gravy or sauce toppings, e.g., enchilada with cheese sauce, crepe with white sauce
Nuts, seeds, and mixtures, all types; sliced, chopped, slivered, and whole	30 g
Nut and seed butters, pastes, or creams	2 tbsp
Coconut, nut and seed flours	15 g
Potatoes and Sweet Potatoes/Yams	
French fries, hash browns, skins, or pancakes	70 g prepared; 85 g for frozen unprepared french fries
Mashed, candied, stuffed, or with sauce	140 g

Table 7. Reference amounts customarily consumed per eating occasion: general food supply

Product category	Reference amount
Plain, fresh, canned, or frozen	110 g for fresh or frozen, 160 g for canned in liquid
Salads	
Gelatin Salad	120 g
Pasta or potato salad	140 g
All other salads, e.g., egg, fish, shellfish, bean, fruit, or vegetable salads	100 g
Sauces, Dips, Gravies and Condiments	
Barbecue sauce, hollandaise sauce, tartar sauce, other sauces for dipping (e.g., mustard sauce, sweet and sour sauce) all dips (e.g., bean dips, dairy-based dips, salsa)	2 tbsp
Major main entree sauces (spaghetti sauce)	125 g
Minor main entree sauces (e.g., pizza sauce, pesto sauce), other sauces used as toppings (e.g., gravy, white sauce, cheese sauce), cocktail sauce	1/4 cup
Major condiments, e.g., catsup, steak sauce, soy sauce, vinegar, teriyaki sauce, marinades	1 tbsp
Minor condiments, e.g., horseradish, hot sauces, mustards, worcestershire sauce	1 tsp
Snacks	
All varieties, chips, pretzels, popcorns, extruded snacks, fruit-based snacks (e.g., fruit chips), grain-based snack mixes	30 g
Soups	
All varieties	245 g
Sugars and Sweets	
Baking candies (e.g., chips)	15 g
Hard candies, breath mints	2 g
Hard candies, roll-ups, mini-size in dispenser packages	5 g
Hard candies, other	15 g
All other candies	40 g
Confectioner's sugar	30 g
Honey, jams, jellies, fruit butter, molasses	1 tbsp
Marshmallows	30 g
Sugar	4 g

Table 7. Reference amounts customarily consumed per eating occasion: general food supply

Product category	Reference amount
Sugar substitutes	An amount equivalent to one reference amount for sugar in sweetness
Syrups	30 mL for syrups used primarily as an ingredient (e.g., light or dark corn syrup); 60 mL for all others
Vegetables	
Vegetables primarily used for garnish or flavor, e.g., pimento, parsley	4 g
Chili pepper, green onion	30 g
All other vegetables without sauce; fresh, canned, or frozen	85 g for fresh or frozen; 95 g for vacuum canned; 130 g for canned in liquid, cream-style corn, canned or stewed tomatoes, pumpkin, or winter squash
All other vegetables with sauce: fresh, canned, or frozen	110 g
Vegetable juice	240 mL
Olives	15 g
Pickles, all types	30 g
Pickle relishes	15 g
Vegetable pastes, e.g., tomato paste	30 g
Vegetable sauces or purees, e.g., tomato sauce, tomato puree	60 g

Table 8. USDA reference amounts (meats)

Product category	Reference amount	
Infant & toddler foods		
Dinner dry mix	15 g	
Dinner, ready-to-serve, strained type	60 g	
Dinner, soups, ready-to-serve, junior type	110 g	
Dinner, stew or soup ready-to-serve, toddlers	170 g	
General food supply		
	Ready-to-serve	Ready-to-cook
Egg mixtures, (western style omelet, souffle, egg foo young)	110	n/a
Lard, margarine, shortening	1 tbsp	n/a

Table 8. USDA reference amounts (meats)

Product category	Reference amount	
Salad and potato toppers; e.g., bacon bits	7 g	n/a
Bacon (bacon, beef breakfast strips pork breakfast strips, pork rinds)	15 g	54 g = bacon; 30 g = break-fast strips
Dried; e.g., jerky, dried beef, Parma ham, sausage products with a moisture/protein ratio of less than 2:1; e.g., pepperoni	30 g	n/a
Snacks; e.g., meat snack food sticks	30 g	n/a
Luncheon meat, bologna, Canadian style bacon, pork pattie crumbles, beef pattie crumbles, blood pudding, luncheon loaf, old fashioned loaf, berlinger, bangers, minced luncheon roll, thuringer, liver sausage, mortadella, uncured sausage (franks), ham and cheese loaf, P & P loaf, scrapple souse, head cheese, pizza loaf, olive loaf, pate, deviled ham, sandwich spread, teawurst, cervelet, Lebanon bologna, potted meat food product, taco fillings, meat pie fillings	55 g	n/a
Linked meat sausage products, Vienna sausage, frankfurters, pork sausage, imitation frankfurters, bratwurst, kielbasa, Polish sausage, summer sausage, smoked or pickled meat, pickled pigs feet	55 g	n/a; 75 = uncooked sausage
Entrees without sauce, cuts of meat including marinated, tenderized, injected cuts of meat, beef patty, corn dog, bagel dog, croquettes, fritters, cured ham, dry cured ham, dry cured cappicola, corned beef, pastrami, country ham, pork shoulder picnic, meatballs, pureed adult foods	85 g	114 g
Canned meats, canned beef, canned pork	55 g	n/a
Entrees with sauce, barbecued meats in sauce	140 g	n/a
Mixed dishes NOT measurable with a cup; e.g., burrito, egg roll, enchilada, pizza, pizza roll, quiche, all types of sandwiches, cracker and meat lunch type packages, gyro, stromboli, burger on a bun, frank on a bun, calzone, taco, pockets stuffed with meat, foldovers, meat lasagna, stuffed vegetables with meat, shish kabobs, empanada	140 g (plus 55 g for products with sauce toppings)	n/a
Mixed dishes measurable with a cup; e.g. meat casserole, macaroni and cheese with meat, pot pie, spaghetti with sauce, meat chili, chili with beans, meat hash, creamed chipped beef, beef ravioli in sauce, beef stroganoff, Brunswick stew, goulash, meat stew, ragout	1 cup	n/a
Salads-pasta or potato, potato salad with bacon, macaroni and meat salad	140 g	n/a
Salads-all other meat, salads, ham salad	100 g	n/a
Soups-all varieties	245 g	n/a
Major main entree type sauce; e.g., spaghetti sauce with meat, spaghetti sauce with meatballs	125 g	n/a
Minor main entree sauce; e.g., pizza sauce with meat, gravy	1/4 cup	n/a

Table 8. USDA reference amounts (meats)

Product category		Reference amount
Seasoning mixes dry, freeze-dried, dehydrated, concentrated soup mixes, bases, extracts, dried broths, and stock/juice, freeze-dried trail mix products with meat. As reconstituted, amount to make one reference amount of the final dish:		
Gravy	1/4 cup	n/a
Major main entree type sauce	125 g	n/a
Soup	245 g	n/a
Entree measurable with a cup	1 cup	n/a

Table 9. USDA reference amounts (poultry)

Product category	Reference amount	
Infant & Toddler Foods		
Dinner dry mix	15 g	
Dinner, ready-to-serve, strained type	60 g	
Dinner, soups, ready-to-serve, junior type	110 g	
Dinner, stew or soup ready-to-serve, toddlers	170 g	
General food supply		
	Ready-to-serve	Ready-to-cook
Egg mixtures, (western style omelet, souffle, egg foo young with poultry)	110 g	n/a
Salad and potato toppers; e.g., poultry, bacon bits	7 g	n/a
Bacon; e.g., poultry breakfast strips	15 g	26 g = bacon; 18 g = break-fast strips
Dried; e.g., poultry jerky, dried poultry, poultry sausage products with a moisture/protein ratio of less than 2:1	30 g	n/a
Snacks; e.g., poultry snack food sticks	30 g	n/a
Luncheon products, poultry bologna, poultry Canadian style bacon, poultry crumbles, poultry luncheon loaf, potted poultry products, poultry taco fillings	55 g	n/a
Linked poultry sausage products, poultry franks, poultry Polish sausage, smoked or pickled poultry meat, poultry smoked sausage	55 g	n/a; 69 = uncooked sausage
Entrees without sauce, poultry cuts, ready to cook poultry cuts, including marinated, tenderized, injected cuts of poultry, poultry corn dogs, poultry bagel dogs, poultry croquettes, poultry fritters, cured poultry ham products, adult pureed poultry	85 g	114 g
Canned poultry, canned chicken, canned turkey	55 g	n/a

Table 9. USDA reference amounts (poultry)

Product category	Reference amount	
Entrees with sauce, turkey and gravy	140 g	n/a
Mixed dishes NOT measurable with a cup; e.g., poultry burrito, poultry enchiladas, poultry pizza, poultry quiche, all types of poultry sandwiches, cracker and poultry lunch-type packages, poultry gyro, poultry stromboli, poultry frank on a bun, poultry burger on a bun, poultry taco, chicken cordon bleu, poultry calzone, poultry lasagna, stuffed vegetables with poultry, poultry kabobs	140 g	n/a
Mixed dishes measurable with a cup; e.g. poultry casserole, macaroni and cheese with poultry, poultry pot pie, poultry spaghetti with sauce, poultry chili, poultry chili with beans, poultry hash, creamed dried poultry, poultry ravioli in sauce, poultry a la king, poultry stew, poultry goulash	1 cup	n/a
Salads-pasta or potato, potato salad with poultry, macaroni and poultry salad	140 g	n/a
Salads-all other, poultry salads, chicken salad, turkey salad	100 g	n/a
Soups-all varieties	245 g	n/a
Major main entree type sauce; e.g., spaghetti sauce with poultry	125 g	n/a
Minor main entree sauce; e.g., pizza sauce with poultry, gravy	1/4 cup	n/a
Seasoning mixes dry, freeze-dried, dehydrated, concentrated soup mixes, bases, extracts, dried broths, and stock/juice, freeze-dried trail mix products with poultry. As reconstituted, amount to make one reference amount of the final dish:		
Gravy	1/4 cup	n/a
Major main entree type sauce	125 g	n/a
Soup	245 g	n/a
Entree measurable with a cup	1 cup	n/a

References

(1)   *Federal Register*, U.S. Government Printing Office, Vol. 56, pp. 60888–60889
(2)   Mermelstein, N. (1993) *Food Technol.* **47**, 81–96
(3)   *Federal Register*, U.S. Government Printing Office, Vol. 58, No. 3, pp. 2175–2205; Vol. 58, No. 61, p. 17104
(4)   *Federal Register*, U.S. Government Printing Office, Vol. 58, No. 3, p. 2202
(5)   *Federal Register*, U.S. Government Printing Office, Vol. 58, No. 158, p. 44076
(6)   *Federal Register*, U.S. Government Printing Office, Vol. 58, No. 3, pp. 2175–2178
(7)   *Federal Register*, U.S. Government Printing Office, Vol. 58, No. 158, p. 44076
(8)   (personal communication) Nutrition Network, Irvine, CA
(9)   *Federal Register*, U.S. Government Printing Office, Vol. 58, No. 61, p. 17104
(10)   *Federal Register*, U.S. Government Printing Office, Vol. 58, No. 3, p. 2179

(11)   *Federal Register*, U.S. Government Printing Office, Vol. 58, No. 3, p. 2302
(12)   (personal communication) FDA/CFSAN, Office of Food Labeling and Planning Branch, Washinton, DC, February 4, 1993
(13)   (personal communication) Nutrition Network, Irvine, CA
(14)   *Federal Register*, U.S. Government Printing Office, Vol. 58, No. 158, p. 44020
(15)   *Federal Register*, U.S. Government Printing Office, Vol. 58, No. 3, p. 2294
(16)   *Federal Register*, U.S. Government Printing Office, Vol. 58, No. 3, pp. 2294–2298
(17)   *Federal Register*, U.S. Government Printing Office, Vol. 58, No. 3, p. 667
(18)   *Federal Register*, U.S. Government Printing Office, Vol. 58, No. 3, pp. 667–668

Chapter 2
International Approach to Nutrition Labeling

Willem J. de Koe

Introduction

Most countries around the world have legislation based on the general principle that prepackaged foods must not be labeled in a deceptive manner. Food labeling is regulated, and consumers have come to rely on it for accurate information about foods they are buying. Labeling requirements can differ significantly among countries. The Nutrition Labeling and Education Act (NLEA) regulates nutrition labeling on U.S. food. The analytical approaches and Official Methods of AOAC INTERNATIONAL apply to these international standards as well as to NLEA.

Codex Alimentarius

The Food and Agriculture Organization (FAO) and the World Health Organization (WHO) established the joint FAO/WHO Food Standards Programme in 1962. Its purpose is to protect the health of consumers and to ensure fair practices in food trade. This is accomplished by the development of international food standards, guidelines and codes of practice. The Codex Alimentarius Commission is responsible for administering the Food Standards Programme and for publication of Codex texts in the Codex Alimentarius.

Codex General Standard for the Labeling of Prepackaged Foods

The Codex General Standard for the Labeling of Prepackaged Foods is one of the most significant standards developed by the Commission.

The Codex Guidelines on Nutrition Labeling adopted in 1985 were developed to promote international consistency in nutrition labeling. The Codex Guidelines require that the nutrient declaration appear on the label whenever a nutrition claim is made for a food.

The mandatory information comprises the following: energy value; contents of protein, fat and digestible carbohydrate; amount of any nutrient for which a claim is made; and amount of any nutrient considered relevant for maintaining good nutritional status as required by national legislation (e.g., sodium). In addition, total sugars are to be declared when a claim is made for the type of carbohydrate in a food, and saturated and *cis*-polyunsaturated fatty acids are to be declared when a claim is made for fatty acids. Vitamins and minerals for which recommended intakes are established or which are of nutritional importance in the country concerned may be declared, provided they are present in significant amounts.

To be effective, nutrient information should be presented in a manner that consumers can understand and use. Currently, metric units are to be used, and energy, protein, vitamins and minerals may also be given as a percent of a reference standard. The basis for expression may be either per 100 g or 100 ml food and/or per serving of food, depending on the preference of the country.

Claims

In 1979, Codex adopted general guidelines on claims, which were supplemented in 1985 by the Codex guidelines on nutrition labeling. The guidelines on claims are currently being revised.

Health Claims

The claims used in this connection include general terms such as "natural," "pure," and "fresh"; quantitative terms relating to the reduced or increased presence, absence or nonaddition of certain nutrients or substances; and implicit references to the prevention of certain health risks. Claims for the role or action of essential nutrients in human health such as protein, vitamins and minerals should help to promote a better understanding of the importance of achieving adequate intakes of these nutrients.

Such claims should be restricted to those functions of the body that are necessary for the maintenance of good health, for normal growth and development, and are accepted by the experts and authorities.

Comparative Claims

Comparative claims are those that compare the nutritional properties of two or more foods. The term "reduced" is used both as an absolute claim and as a comparative claim. When it is used as an absolute claim, the degree of reduction is not quantitated on the label and the consumer is not informed either of the magnitude of the reduction, which may vary depending on the component (1/3 for energy, 75% for sodium) or on the identity of the food that is not reduced. The term "reduced" should, therefore, be treated as a comparative claim only, and the amount of the reduction and the identity of the food being compared should be shown on the label.

Claims for Nutrient Content

The IUNS Committees on Food Standards in 1985 and its successor in 1989, the Committee on the Nutritional Aspects of Food Standards, noted that foods modified to reduce components that consumers wish to avoid (fat, salt, etc.), are valuable parts of diets designed to be either preventative or therapeutic in nature, provided that the modifications are quantitatively substantive. Definitions for adjectival descriptors for "avoidance" components of foods should generally be based on the amount per stated serving coupled with the amount in 100 grams of the food.

In line with current dietary guidelines and consumer interest, descriptors are needed for the following food components: energy, fat, saturated fat, cholesterol, sodium, carbohydrates, protein, fibre, vitamins and minerals. Relevant claims are as follows: low, free, high (good source), and very high (excellent source, rich in).

Proposed definitions for "low energy" and "energy reduced" are contained in the Codex Proposed Draft Standard for the Labeling of and Claims for Prepackaged "Low Energy" and "Reduced Energy" Foods. Definitions for "low sodium" and "very low sodium" are contained in the Codex Standard for Special Dietary Foods with Low Sodium Content (including salt substitutes).

European Community Council Directive 90/496/EEC on Nutrition Labeling of Foodstuffs

On September 24, 1990, the European Community passed Council Directive 90/496/EEC on nutrition labeling of foodstuffs, which generally follows the Guidelines of the Codex Alimentarius. Nutrition labeling is optional under the Directive except in cases where a nutrition claim appears in labeling, in presentation, or in advertising other than generic advertising. A "nutrition claim" is defined as "any representation and any advertising message which states, suggests or implies that a foodstuff has particular nutrition properties due to the energy (calorific value) it provides, provides at a reduced or increased rate, or does not provide, and/or due to the nutrients it contains, contains in reduced or increased proportions, or does not contain."

The basic nutrition label under the Directive includes the following:

<u>Group One</u> ("big four")
(a)   energy value;
(b)   the amounts of protein, carbohydrate and fat.

Where a nutrition claim is made for sugars, saturates, fibre or sodium, the information provided consists of Group Two:

Group Two

(a)   energy value;

(b)   the amounts of protein, carbohydrate, sugars, fat, saturates, fibre and sodium.

Nutrition labeling may also include the amounts of one or more of the following: starch; sugar alcohols; monounsaturates; polyunsaturates; cholesterol; and any of the minerals or vitamins for which recommended daily allowances (RDA's) have been provided in the Annex to the Directive, if present in significant amounts (defined as 15% of the recommended allowance supplied by 100 g or 100 ml of the product or the amount in a single portion package), including an expression of the percentage of the RDA.

Nutrition Labeling in the Several Member States of EEC

In 1990, several countries volunteered to address mainly Codex system developments in regards to uniform nutrition labeling of food products with guaranteed reliable information. The following requirements for effective nutrition labeling were set up: the information to be provided on nutrition labels must be scientifically sound and in line with present day nutrition thinking, nutrition labels should provide the information consumers want in a form that is clearly understood, nutrition labeling should not present practical problems for the manufacturer or the retailer, and nutrition labels should be quickly and easily recognizable.

Nutrients Specified on the Nutrition Indicator

To ensure that the nutrition label is of practical use, only essential nutrients should be specified. Thus, the basic panel (see label below) should contain energy content, to be expressed in kilojoules and kilocalories, and levels of the constituents that supply energy such as carbohydrates, protein, and fat in unit weight (grams).

nutrition indicator
vanilla ice cream 100 g
730 kilojoule 175 kilocalorie

carbohydr.	protein	fat
21 g	3.5 g	8.5 g

Eat moderately and a varied diet

The information on carbohydrates could be further specified to include the proportion of sugars, expressed in grams. If required, additional information such as the amount of saturated fat (grams), linoleic acid (grams), and salt (grams) could be provided as follows:

nutrition indicator		
vanilla ice cream 100 g		
730 kilojoule 175 kilocalorie		
carbohydr.	protein	fat
21 g	3.5 g	8.5 g
		including
including		linoleic ac. 4.5 g
sugars 20 g		saturated 0.5 g
	sodium 0.1 g	
Eat moderately and a varied diet		

In a country such as The Netherlands, where the diet contains a wide variety of foods, vitamin and mineral deficiencies do not occur often. However, as consumers are aware of the value of vitamins and minerals in their daily diet, it was decided to include information on four of the more important vitamins and minerals: vitamin B_1, vitamin C, calcium and iron. The amounts contained in the food are not given on a unit basis but as a proportion of the daily recommended intake. This is indicated on the label by five circles as follows:

nutrition indicator		
vanilla ice cream 100 g		
730 kilojoule 175 kilocalorie		
carbohydr.	protein	fat
21 g	3.5 g	8.5 g
		including
including		linoleic ac 4.5 g
sugars 20 g		saturated 0.5 g
	sodium 0.1 g	
vitamin B_1 00000		calcium 00000
vitamin C 00000		iron 00000
00000 recommended daily intake		
Eat moderately and a varied diet		

For example, if a particular quantity of a food product provides one tenth of the daily requirement, then only half of one of the circles is filled. Inclusion of information on dietary cholesterol and dietary fibre was considered but was not included at present.

Even though International and U.S. food labeling approaches have many similarities, some differences exist. These differences may impede international trade unless a uniform system of labeling is developed.

Chapter 3
Report of the AOAC INTERNATIONAL Task Force
On Methods for Nutrient Labeling Analyses

Introduction

The Nutrition Labeling and Education Act of 1990 (NLEA) was signed into law on November 8, 1990. Even though many foods have been labeled voluntarily for nutritional content since 1973, this far-reaching piece of legislation made mandatory, for the first time, the labeling of nearly all foods with information about their nutritional content. NLEA required the U.S. Food and Drug Administration (FDA) to develop revised regulations that would mandate the labeling of several previously unlabeled food components (total dietary fiber, complex carbohydrates, sugars, saturated fat, and calories from fat). In November of 1991, FDA published their response to NLEA in the form of proposed regulations in the *Federal Register* (FR, November 27, 1991, pp. 60365–60891). Although not required by the NLEA, the U.S. Department of Agriculture (USDA) also proposed regulations requiring mandatory labeling of nutrients. The USDA proposal (*Federal Register*, November 27, 1991, pp. 60301–60364) was harmonized with the FDA proposal. The FDA document amounted to over 500 pages and discussed everything from methodology and serving sizes to exemptions and preemptions. The proposal not only included the list of mandatory nutrients to be labeled but also expanded the previous list of those that could be voluntarily labeled. In the proposal, FDA explicitly acknowledged concern over the availability of analytical methodology for complex carbohydrates, sugars, and protein quality. FDA also continued to acknowledge that, for compliance purposes, the known variability of appropriate analytical methods would be an important aspect in evaluating compliance. With only the single exception of the new analytical methodology proposed for protein quality, the FDA proposals looked primarily to AOAC INTERNATIONAL for appropriate methods.

AOAC Response

The analytical community was quick to recognize the immense task that lay before it. Analytical data would have to be generated for hundreds of thousands of foods that may not have been analyzed previously. As FDA had rightfully recognized, validated methodology for some of the new mandatory nutrients was not available. Without accurate and reliable analytical methods, compliance with the NLEA would be impossible, as would enforcement. To address the immediate needs required by the proposed regulations, AOAC [with participants drawn from government agencies, academia, private companies, and trade associations (Table 1)] formed the Task Force on Methods for Nutrient Labeling Analyses with the following mission/responsibilities:

1. Identify and publicize the availability of validated methods for nutrient analysis currently available through AOAC.

2. Identify needed revisions in existing AOAC Official Methods for nutrition labeling.

3. Identify additional methods for nutritional analysis in need of validation and official action by AOAC.

4.   Develop an approach or approaches that can be used by AOAC to initiate necessary studies and recruit researchers and collaborators.

5.   Identify and publicize standard reference materials available for use with current validated methods for nutritional analysis. Identify needs for additional reference materials for current validated methods. Develop an approach for incorporating reference materials as part of the methods validation process.

Task Force Actions

Identification of Available Adequate Validated Methods

The task force drew upon the resources offered by the entire AOAC membership and worked closely with other organizations. One of the first tasks undertaken by the task force was a survey of analysts working in analytical laboratories that specialized in food analysis. This was done to determine what methods were currently being used and the analyst's evaluation of the adequacy of those methods. The survey also asked about reference standards and the use of control samples. A review of the survey responses revealed that laboratories were using a great variety of AOAC methods, sometimes with modifications, and that a great many methods were being applied successfully to product matrixes for which the methods had not been explicitly validated. Assignments were undertaken by individual members of the task force to review AOAC methods for specific nutrients. Using all resources available to them, the individual members determined which methods were adequate for the purposes of nutritional labeling. The review process was carried out by nutrient and product matrix combinations. Even though the survey did indicate that many non-AOAC methods were routinely being used and that laboratories found some of these alternative methods to be acceptable, the mission of the task force was to identify AOAC Official Methods that have been accepted and validated. After the individual task force members reviewed each analyte and matrix combination, their recommendations were collectively reviewed by the entire task force with the assistance of AOAC technical staff. The result of the review process was a listing of adequate AOAC Official Methods that was published in the July 1992 issue of *The Referee*, the AOAC newsletter (Table 2, updated version). A complementary list was generated, specifying methods that needed development and validation, updating, revision, or further work to extend their applicability. This list was published in the October 1992 issue of *The Referee*.

Identification of Needed Methodology Revisions

During the review process, AOAC members raised several substantial concerns about the applicability of some AOAC methods for certain analytes. Of particular concern was the availability of multiple Official Methods for a given nutrient or food component. The task force was aware that in some instances the analytical result was a reflection of the biases of the method and not necessarily a true measure of the nutrient in the food. The method reviewers determined that the various Official Methods designated for total fat do not necessarily measure the same food components and thus may not produce equivalent results. Certain methods for total fat may include food components that do not contribute to dietary fat intake. Other methods may underestimate the total fat in the food being analyzed; therefore, they also underestimate the contribution that the food being analyzed makes to fat intake. Similarly, some moisture methods do not measure moisture *per se* but either residual solids or total volatile materials, which are not necessarily equivalent. Therefore, the task force decided that the methodology for these nutrients needed further study. Two subcommittees were formed to carefully examine these issues and to make recommendations to the task force. The task force members also felt that, because of the important role carbohydrates have in the new nutrition label (declarations for total carbohydrate, complex carbohydrates, total dietary fiber, and simple sugars) and because of concerns over the chemical definition of the various carbohydrate fractions, it was important to evaluate the adequacy of carbohydrate methods. Therefore, a subcommittee was also formed to specifically examine the suitability of methods for carbohydrates.

Subcommittee on Total Fat Methods

The Subcommittee on Total Fat Methods concluded that the lack of a single, clear, concise definition for fat as an analyte was a significant contributing factor to the issues regarding fat analysis. AOAC does not define analytes but rather validates methods for analytes as defined. Therefore, the subcommittee recommended that the regulatory agencies involved with nutrition labeling (i.e., USDA and FDA) adopt a single, clear, concise definition for fat and that AOAC INTERNATIONAL then validate methods commensurate with those definitions. The subcommittee further went on to evaluate each of the current AOAC Official Methods for fat or fat fractions and outlined and tabulated the key characteristics of each. The task force adopted the subcommittee's report, and it was published in the September 1992 issue of *The Referee* (Table 3; *see* also Chapter 5).

Subcommittee on Moisture Methods

The Subcommittee on Moisture Methods reached a conclusion similar to that of the Subcommittee on Total Fat Methods regarding the cause of discrepancies in results between methods used for moisture analysis. As in the case of fat, moisture has not been clearly defined but is a function of the methodology used for the determination. Because moisture content of foods is essential to all calorie calculations, the subcommittee recommended this issue be addressed on a regulatory basis in the future. To assist the membership of AOAC and the users of *Official Methods of Analysis*, the subcommittee compiled a listing of the AOAC Official Methods for moisture along with the methods' characteristics. The compiled list and the subcommittee report, which was accepted by the task force, was published in the January 1993 issue of *The Referee* (Table 4).

Subcommittee on Carbohydrate Methods

On the basis of the current, most widely accepted definition of dietary fiber, the Subcommittee on Carbohydrate Methods concluded that the AOAC Official Methods currently validated are adequate for the determination of total, insoluble, and soluble dietary fiber for nutrition labeling. The subcommittee also determined that reference materials are available for laboratories to use for analytical quality control. This information and the conclusions of the subcommittee were contained in a report accepted by the task force and published in the November 1992 issue of *The Referee* (Tables 5 and 6; *see* also Chapter 4). When the regulatory agencies published their final labeling regulations in early 1993, the subcommittee updated its report by reviewing methods for the analysis of mono- and disaccharides and determining where methods are needed. The subcommittee found that established liquid chromatographic methods were suitable for the determination of glucose, fructose, maltose, sucrose, and lactose. The report also suggested that the classical chemical and enzymatic procedures would have utility in certain limited applications. Even though the final labeling regulations dropped the requirement for the mandatory declaration of "complex carbohydrates," the subcommittee recommended that, as in the case of total fat and moisture, a clear, concise definition of complex carbohydrates should be developed. AOAC should then support method development and validation to meet this definition.

Addressing Methodology Needs

The response of AOAC members to the efforts of the task force has, thus far, been highly encouraging. Not only have AOAC members responded with methods for validation and offered to serve as collaborators and associate referees, but various trade associations and professional groups have recruited members from their ranks for the efforts necessary to validate additional methods that meet the needs of the new regulations. New AOAC Associate Referees have been appointed in several areas, and collaborative studies on needed methods are being pursued.

Identification of Needs for Reference Materials

The task force recognized that analytical laboratories do not have a great deal of resources to draw from for standard reference materials (SRMs), certified reference materials, or quality assurance materials for nutrient analyses. Whereas SRMs are readily available for many inorganic compounds of environmental or manufacturing interest, food-based SRMs containing labile nutrients are less available. Even though many laboratories have tried to overcome this deficiency by developing in-house reference materials, there have been no guidelines as to certification of these materials or their development and handling. Two subcommittees were formed to address reference materials and guidelines for developing in-house analytical quality assurance control materials, respectively.

Subcommittee on Reference Materials

The Task Force on Methods for Nutrient Labeling Analyses established a Subcommittee on Reference Materials to address the issues involved with identifying and publicizing reference materials available for use with current AOAC Official Methods for nutrition analysis. They also addressed the need for additional reference materials for current validated methods and developed an approach for incorporating reference materials as part of the methods validation process.

The subcommittee surveyed the reference materials currently available to laboratories doing nutrition analysis. As a result of this survey, a report on their availability, compiled by analyte and matrix, along with their sources, was published in the August 1992 issue of *The Referee* (*see* also Chapter 7) for those nutrients whose inclusion is mandatory on the nutrition label.

Recognizing the ongoing needs in the area of reference materials for method development, validation, and quality control, and further recognizing the need to define reference materials that will represent food and food matrices during methods validation work, the task force supports the formation and development of a Technical Division on Reference Materials within AOAC. Task force members have been supportive of and active in initiating such a technical division. A group of scientists, of which many task force members were a part, met at AOAC headquarters on December 8, 1992, to petition the AOAC Board of Directors to form the Technical Division. The Board of Directors approved the Technical Division on Reference Materials on March 23, 1993. This group will be charged with pursuing the following recommendations: the identifying and/or developing reference materials for quality control of methods for nutrition analysis, identifying and/or developing a set of reference materials representative of foods for use in validation studies, and facilitating the availability of reference materials to laboratories in a cost effective manner.

Subcommittee on In-House Control Materials

The Subcommittee on In-House Control Materials surveyed the AOAC membership regarding the formulation, validation, and use of in-house quality control materials. Using the survey results where possible, the subcommittee developed a set of guidelines to aid laboratories in the development of in-house quality control materials. These guidelines were published in the May 1993 issue of *The Referee* (*see* also Chapter 7).

Definition of Food Matrices

The task force selected twenty food groups to be used in evaluating the adequacy of methods for nutrition labeling. The available methods for a given nutrient were evaluated specifically for each matrix group of foods (e.g., fruits, fish and shellfish, beverages, or meats). Whereas such groupings are reasonable from a dietary perspective, the groups are neither inclusive nor exclusive from the perspective of the applicability of analytical methods. The twenty food groups selected by the task force as a basis for judging methods currently validated by AOAC have certain commonalities, and in many cases, their characteristics overlap. These matrix characteristics are as follows: fat (high or low), moisture (high or low), protein (high or low), and carbohydrate (high or low); or they are at an intermediate level in all these major components. The task force recognized that the ability to categorize foods on a more fundamental chemical basis would facilitate both the development of analytical methods and appropriate standard reference materials. A subcommittee was formed to develop a proposal for defining foods in terms of a matrix of the major food components (i.e., fat, protein, and carbohydrate).

The subcommittee determined that defining foods of a particular matrix group on the basis of fat, protein, and carbohydrate content would be both possible and advantageous. The moisture level of a sample can readily be adjusted by drying or adding water. Thus, if a method is affected by the moisture level of the matrix, this can be handled. The remaining major components of the samples and their various combinations of levels can be represented by a set of nine samples that span specific ranges of fat, protein and carbohydrate content. Deliberations within the task force and at other AOAC forums have indicated a great deal of concern about the level of effort necessary to extend the applicability of Official Methods from foods specifically studied in a collaborative study to other foods of interest. The adoption of this more systematic approach toward classifying foods should greatly simplify the collaborative study process and the process of extending the applicability of methods.

Likewise, there is a great deal of concern regarding the availability of reference materials relevant to the particular food under study. With this in mind, the task force recommends the development or selection of a series of reference samples that could be used by laboratories during the methods validation process. To encourage the incorporation of reference materials into the methods validation process, the Subcommittee on Reference Materials determined that the reference materials to be incorporated must be truly representative of food or food matrices, readily available, and available at prices that encourage their use. For reference materials to be representative of foods or food matrices, those matrices must be clearly defined, and the definitions must be accepted throughout the validation process. The reference samples would have characteristics such that the set of samples would represent all the food matrices and would allow the collaborators who have completed a collaborative study using this set to be confident of the applicability of their method. The task force recommends that this approach [outlined by the Subcommittee on Reference Materials and reported in *The Referee* (1993) **17**(7), p. 1,6–7; *see* also Chapter 7] be adopted by the Official Methods Board of AOAC INTERNATIONAL for future collaborative studies used for the methods validation process for analyses of foods for nutrition labeling purposes.

Follow-up Recommendations

On January 6, 1993, USDA and FDA issued the final regulations to be operable under NLEA (*Federal Register*, January 6, 1993, pp. 631–691 and 2065–2964, respectively). The Task Force on Methods for Nutrient Labeling Analyses, after reviewing the final regulations, again reviewed the status of AOAC Official Methods for nutrition labeling in light of changes made since the regulations were proposed. Updated reports [listing methods deemed adequate (Table 2) and also methods in need of development and validation, updating, revision, or further work to extend their applicability (Table 7)] from the review were published in the March and April 1993 issues of *The Referee*.

The final regulations, in response to concerns expressed regarding the measurement and labeling of total and saturated fats, adopted a concise definition for each analyte. Total fat is defined as the sum of the lipid fatty acids (expressed as their triglycerides), and saturated fat is defined as all lipid fatty acids containing no double bonds. The Task Force Subcommittee on Total Fat Methods reassessed the information reported in the September 1992 issue of *The Referee* on validated methods for fat in light of the adopted definition and issued an updated report in *The Referee* in February 1993.

The last meeting of the task force was held on February 8, 1993. It has completed its mission and has put into place procedures that will assure the availability of validated analytical methods for nutrients in foods. The task force thanks its individual members and the AOAC staff for their time, efforts, and devotion. The accomplishments of this task force have demonstrated the importance and value of AOAC INTERNATIONAL and the forum it provides for regulatory, academic, and industrial analytical chemists to meet and resolve issues of concern. The benefits derived are of value to the scientific and regulatory community and to the general public.

Table 1. AOAC INTERNATIONAL Task Force on Methods for Nutrient Labeling Analyses, Committee Members and Participants

J. DeVries, Chair, General Mills Inc.
S. Bailey, Lancaster Laboratories Inc.
K. Boyer, Southern Testing & Research Laboratories
M. Bueno, U.S. Food and Drug Administration
D. Carpenter, Kraft General Foods
H. Chin, National Food Processors Association
N. Craft, Southern Testing and Research Laboratories
M. Deutsch, U.S. Food and Drug Administration
D. Emery, Emery & Associates
D. Firestone, U.S. Food and Drug Administration
N. Fraley, Armour Swift Eckrich, Inc.
W. Hummer, U.S. Food and Drug Administration
W. Ikins, Silliker Laboratories Inc.
A. Kistler, Pet Inc.
S. Lee, Kellogg Co.
W. Landen, U.S. Food and Drug Administration
R. Lane, University of Alabama
J. Morawski, Waters Associates
J. Ngeh-Ngwainbi, Kellogg Co.
P. Oles, Lancaster Laboratories Inc.
L. Prosky, U.S. Food and Drug Administration
L. Reimann, Woodson Tenent Laboratories
A. Sheppard, U.S. Food and Drug Administration
D. Soderberg, U.S. Department of Agriculture
A. Soliman (deceased)
D. Sullivan, Hazleton Laboratories
J. Tanner, U.S. Food and Drug Administration
E. Waysek, Hoffman La Roche Inc.
W. Wolf, U.S. Department of Agriculture
E. Young, U.S. Food and Drug Administration

Table 2. Acceptable Official Methods for Nutrition Labeling

AOAC No.	Method	Matrixes[a]
ASH		
940.26A[b]	Ash of Fruits and Fruit Products	A, J
920.153[b]	Ash of Meat	B, L, M
925.51A[b]	Ash of Canned Vegetables	C, P, T
950.14A[b]	Ash of Nonalcoholic Beverages	D
920.100[b]	Ash in Tea	D
925.49[b]	Ash of Confectionery	E
972.15	Ash of Cocoa Products	E
945.18	Ash of Cereal Adjuncts, Direct Method	F
930.22	Ash of Bread, Direct Method	F
935.42	Ash of Cheese, Gravimetric Method	G
945.46	Ash of Milk, Gravimetric Method	H
920.117	Ash of Butter	H
930.30	Ash of Dried Milk	H
920.108	Ash of Cream, Gravimetric Method	H
945.48E	Ash of Evaporated Milk	H
920.115E[b]	Ash of Sweetened Condensed Milk	H
938.08[b]	Ash of Seafood	I, Q
986.25	Ash of Milk-Based Infant Formula, Gravimetric Method	K
950.49[b]	Ash of Nuts and Nut Products	N
923.03	Ash of Flour, Direct Method	R
935.39	Ash of Baked Products, Direct Method (without fruit)	R
941.12	Ash of Spices, Gravimetric Method	S

Table 2. Acceptable Official Methods for Nutrition Labeling

AOAC No.	Method	Matrixes[a]
BETA CAROTENE		
941.15	Carotene in Fresh Plant Materials and Silages, Spectrophotometric Method (naturally occurring carotene only)	A, C, J, P, T
CALCIUM		
968.08	Minerals in Animal Feed, AAS Method	All
975.03	Metals in Plants, AAS Method	All
980.03	Metals in Plants, Spectrographic Method	All
965.09	Minor Nutrients in Fertilizers, AAS Method	All
953.01	Metals in Plants, Emission Spectrographic Method	A, C, F, J, P, T
985.01	Metals and Other Elements in Plants, ICP Method	A, C, F, J, P, T
921.01	Ca in Plants, Micro Titrimetric Method	A, C, F, J, P, T
951.01	Ca in Plants, Nitrocreosol Method	A, C, F, J, P, T
983.19	Ca in Mechanically Separated Poultry and Beef Titrimetric Method	B, L
968.31	Ca in Canned Vegetables, Titrimetric Method	C, T
945.41	Ca in Bread, Titrimetric Method	F
944.03	Ca in Flour, Titrimetric Method	F
991.25	Ca, Mg, and P in Cheese, AAS and Colorimetric Methods	G
984.27	Ca, Cu, Fe, Mg, Mn, P, K, Na, and Zn in Infant Formula, ICP Method	K
985.35	Minerals in Ready-To-Feed Milk-Based Infant Formula, AAS Method	K
CHOLESTEROL		
976.26	Cholesterol in Multi-component Foods, GC Method (only >10 mg/100)	All

Table 2. Acceptable Official Methods for Nutrition Labeling

AOAC No.	Method	Matrixes[a]
COPPER		
985.35	Minerals in Ready-To-Feed Milk-Based Infant Formula, AAS Method	All
984.27	Ca, Cu, Fe, Mg, Mn, P, K, Na and Zn in Infant Formula, ICP Method	All
960.40	Copper in Food, Colorimetric Method	All
968.08	Minerals in Animal Feed, AAS Method	All
975.03	Metals in Plants, AAS Method	All
980.03	Metals in Plants, Spectrographic Method	All
953.01	Metals in Plants, Emission Spectrographic Method	A, C, F, J, P, T
985.01	Metals and Other Elements in Plants, ICP Method	A, C, F, J, P, T
953.03	Cu in Plants, Colorimetric Method	A, C, F, J, P, T
985.40	Cu in Liver, AAS Method	L
990.05	Cu, Fe, Ni in Edible Oils and Fats, AAS Method	O
CYANOCOBALAMINE		
960.46	Vitamin Assays, Microbiological Method with **952.20** Cobalamin (Vitamin B_{12} Activity) in Vitamin Preparations, Microbiological Method	All
986.23	Cobalamin (Vitamin B_{12} Activity) in Milk-Based Infant Formula, Turbidimetric Method	K
DIETARY FIBER-INSOLUBLE		
991.42	Insoluble Dietary Fiber in Food and Food Products, Enzymatic-Gravimetric Method	A, C–F, J, K, N, P, R–T
991.43	Total, Insoluble and Soluble Dietary Fiber in Foods, Enzymatic-Gravimetric Method	A, C–F, J, K, N, P, R–T
DIETARY FIBER-SOLUBLE		
991.42	Insoluble Dietary Fiber in Food and Food Products, Enzymatic-Gravimetric Method (by calc; direct method is under AOAC review)	A, C–F, J, K, N, P, R–T

Table 2. Acceptable Official Methods for Nutrition Labeling

AOAC No.	Method	Matrixes[a]
991.43	Total, Insoluble and Soluble Dietary Fiber in Foods, Enzymatic-Gravimetric Method	A, C–F, J, K, N, P, R–T

DIETARY FIBER-TOTAL

AOAC No.	Method	Matrixes[a]
985.29	Total Dietary Fiber in Foods, Enzymatic-Gravimetric Method	A, C–F, J, K, N, P, R–T
991.43	Total, Insoluble and Soluble Dietary Fiber in Foods, Enzymatic-Gravimetric Method	A, C–F, J, K, N, P, R–T

FAT-POLYUNSATURATED

AOAC No.	Method	Matrixes[a]
979.19	*cis,cis*-Methylene Interrupted Polyunsaturated Fatty Acids in Oils, Spectrophotometric Method (Suitable after isolation of fat.)	All
957.13	Polyunsaturated Acids in Oils and Fats, Spectrophotometric Method	O

FAT-TOTAL

Total fat has been concisely defined under NLEA as the sum of lipid fatty acids expressed as triglycerides. Currently, no AOAC Official Methods meet that definition *per se*. See the February 1993 issue of *The Referee* for the task force report on fat that contains a number of methods that approximate the definition and may be useful on an interim basis until methods can be collaboratively studied.

FOLACIN

AOAC No.	Method	Matrixes[a]
960.46	Vitamin Assays, Microbiological Method with **944.12** Folic Acid in Vitamin Preparations, Microbiol. Method (Suitable for free form only) (*L. casei* commonly preferred, but not collaboratively studied.)	All
992.05	Folic Acid in Infant Formula, LC Method	K

IRON

AOAC No.	Method	Matrixes[a]
968.08	Minerals in Animal Feed, AAS Method	All
975.03	Metals in Plants, AAS Method	All
980.03	Metals in Plants, Spectrographic Method	All
965.09	Minor Nutrients in Fertilizers, AAS Method	All
953.01	Metals in Plants, Emission Spectrographic Method	A, C, F, J, P, T
945.40	Iron in Bread, Spectrophotometric Method	F

Table 2. Acceptable Official Methods for Nutrition Labeling

AOAC No.	Method	Matrixes[a]
950.39	Iron in Macaroni Products, Spectrophotometric Method	F
944.02B	Iron in Flour, Spectrophotometric Method	F
984.27	Ca, Cu, Fe, Mg, Mn, P, K, Na and Zn in Infant Formula, ICP Method	K
985.35	Minerals in Ready-To-Feed Milk-Based Infant Formula, AAS Method	K
990.05	Cu, Fe, Ni in Edible Oils and Fats, AAS Method	O

MAGNESIUM

AOAC No.	Method	Matrixes[a]
975.03	Metals in Plants, AAS Method	All
980.03	Metals in Plants, Spectrographic Method	All
965.09	Minor Nutrients in Fertilizers, AAS Method	All
953.01	Metals in Plants, Emission Spectrographic Method	A, C, F, J, P, T
985.01	Metals and Other Elements in Plants, ICP Method	A, C, F, J, P, T
991.25	Ca, Mg, P in Cheese, AAS and Colorimetric Methods	G
984.27	Ca, Cu, Fe, Mg, Mn, P, K, Na and Zn in Infant Formula, ICP Method	K
985.35	Minerals in Ready-To- Feed Milk-Based Infant Formula, AAS Method	K

MOISTURE

See the task force report on moisture in the January 1993 issue of *The Referee*.

NIACIN

AOAC No.	Method	Matrixes[a]
960.46	Vitamin Assays, Microbiological Method with **944.13** Niacin and Niacinamide in Vitamin Preparations, Microbiological Method	All
961.14	Niacin and Niacinamide in Drugs, Foods and Feeds, Colorimetric Method	All
981.16	Niacin and Niacinamide in Foods, Drugs and Feeds, Automated Method	All

Table 2. Acceptable Official Methods for Nutrition Labeling

AOAC No.	Method	Matrixes[a]
975.41	Niacin and Niacinamide in Cereal Products, Automated Method	F
985.34	Niacin and Niacinamide in Ready-To-Feed Milk-Based Infant Formula, Microbiological-Turbidimetric Method	K
PANTOTHENIC ACID		
960.46	Vitamin Assays, Microbiological Method with **945.74** Pantothenic Acid in Vitamin Preparations, Microbiological Method (Suitable for free form only)	All
PHOSPHORUS		
958.01	Total Phosphorus in Fertilizers, Spectrophotometric Molybdovanadophosphate Method	All
957.18	Microchemical Determination of Phosphorus, Kjeldahl Digestion Method	All
964.06	Phosphorus in Animal Feed, Alk Ammonium Molybdophosphate Method	All
965.17	Phosphorus in Animal Feed, Photometric Method	All
980.03	Metals in Plants, Spectrographic Method	A, C, F, J, P, T
953.01	Metals in Plants, Emission Spectrographic Method	A, C, F, J, P, T
985.01	Metals and Other Elements in Plants, ICP Method	A, C, F, J, P, T
966.01	Phosphorus in Plants, Gravity Quinolinium Molybdophosphate Method	A, C, F, J, P, T
931.01	Phosphorus in Plants, Micro Method	A, C, F, J, P, T
970.39	Phosphorus in Fruits and Fruit Products, Spectrophotometric Molybdovanadate Method	A, J
969.31	Phosphorus in Meat, Alk Ammonium Molybdophosphate Method	B, L
972.22	Phosphorus in Meats, Automated Method	B, L
991.27	Phosphorus in Meat and Meat Products, Spectrophotometric Method	B, L
948.09	Phosphorus in Flour	F

Table 2. Acceptable Official Methods for Nutrition Labeling

AOAC No.	Method	Matrixes[a]
990.24	Total Phosphorus in Cheese and Processed Cheese, Photometric Method	G
991.25	Ca, Mg, P in Cheese, AAS and Colorimetric Methods	G
984.27	Ca, Cu, Fe, Mg, Mn, P, K, Na, and Zn in Infant Formula, ICP Method	K
986.24	Phosphorus in Milk-Based Infant Formula, Spectrophotometric Method	K
935.59	Total Phosphorus in Food Dressings, Alk Ammonium Molybdophosphate Method	O
930.35G,H,I	Phosphorus in Vinegars, Alk Ammonium Molybdophosphate Method	S
POTASSIUM		
985.35	Minerals in Ready-To-Feed Milk-Based Infant Formula, AAS Method	All
956.01	K/Na in Plants, Flame Photometric Method	A, C, F, J, P, T
953.01	Metals in Plants, Emission Spectrographic Method	A, C, F, J, P, T
985.01	Metals and Other Elements in Plants, ICP Method	A, C, F, J, P, T
975.03	Metals in Plants, AAS Method	A, C, F, J, P, T
980.03	Metals in Plants, Spectrographic Method	A, C, F, J, P, T
965.30	K in Fruits and Fruit Products, Flame Photometric Method	A, J
990.23	Na and K in Dried Milk, Flame Emission Spectrophotometric Method	H
969.23	Na and K in Seafood, Flame Photometric Method	I, Q
984.27	Ca, Cu, Fe, Mg, Mn, P, K, Na, and Zn in Infant Formula, ICP Method	K
PROTEIN		
981.10	Crude Protein in Meat, Block Digestion Method	All
955.04	Total N in Fertilizers, Kjeldahl Method	All

Table 2. Acceptable Official Methods for Nutrition Labeling

AOAC No.	Method	Matrixes[a]
977.02	Total N (Crude Protein) in Plants, Automated and Semiautomated Methods	A, C, F, J, P, T
978.04	Total N (Crude Protein) in Plants, Kjeldahl Methods	A, C, F, J, P, T
920.152	Protein in Fruit Products, Kjeldahl Method	A, J
992.15	Crude Protein in Meat and Meat Products, Combustion Method	B, L
939.02	Milk Protein in Milk Chocolate, Kjeldahl Method	E
990.03	Crude Protein in Animal Feed, Combustion Method	F
990.02	Crude Protein in Animal Feed, Semiautomated Method	F
920.87	Total Protein in Flour	F
945.18B	Protein in Cereal Adjuncts, Kjeldahl Method	F
930.25	Protein in Macaroni Products	F
950.36	Protein in Bread	F
991.20	Total Nitrogen Content of Milk, Kjeldahl Method	H
991.22	Protein Nitrogen Content of Milk, Kjeldahl Method (Direct)	H
991.23	Protein Nitrogen Content of Milk, Kjeldahl Method (Indirect)	H
930.33	Protein in Ice Cream and Frozen Desserts, Kjeldahl and Dye Binding Methods	H
930.29	Protein in Dried Milk, Kjeldahl Method	H
967.12	Protein in Milk, Dye Binding Method I	H
975.17	Protein in Milk. Dye Binding Method II	H
975.18	Protein in Milk, Mid-Infrared Spectrophotometric Method	H
972.16	Fat, Lactose, Protein, and Solids in Milk, Mid-Infrared Spectrophotometric Method	K
986.25C	Protein in Milk-Based Infant Formula, Kjeldahl Method	K
928.08	Nitrogen in Meat, Kjeldahl Method	L

Table 2. Acceptable Official Methods for Nutrition Labeling

AOAC No.	Method	Matrixes[a]
977.14	Nitrogen in Meat, Automated Kjeldahl Method	L
981.10	Nitrogen in Meat, Block Digestion Method	L
950.48	Crude Protein in Nuts and Nut Products, Kjeldahl Method	N
935.39C	Protein in Baked Products	R
PROTEIN QUALITY		
991.29	True Protein Digestibility of Foods and Food Ingredients, Rat Bioassay Method with **982.30** Protein Efficiency Ratio, Calc Method	All
960.48	Protein Efficiency Ratio, Rat Bioassay Method	All
PYRIDOXINE		
960.46	Vitamin Assays, Microbiological Method with **961.15** Vitamin B_6 in Food Extracts, Microbiological Method	All
985.32	Vitamin B_6 in Ready-To-Feed Milk-Based Infant Formula, Microbiological Method	K
RIBOFLAVIN		
960.46	Vitamin Assays, Microbiological Method with **960.33** Riboflavin (Vitamin B_2) in Vitamin Preparations, Microbiological Method	All
970.65	Riboflavin (Vitamin B_2) in Foods and Vitamin Preparations, Fluorometric Method	All
981.15	Riboflavin in Foods and Vitamin Preparations, Automated Method	All
985.31	Riboflavin in Ready-To-Feed Milk-Based Infant Formula, Fluorometric Method	K
SODIUM		
985.35	Minerals in Ready-To-Feed Milk-Based Infant Formula, AAS Method	All
956.01	K/Na in Plants, Flame Photometric Method	A, C, F, J, P, T
953.01	Metals in Plants, Emission Spectrographic Method	A, C, F, J, P, T

Table 2. Acceptable Official Methods for Nutrition Labeling

AOAC No.	Method	Matrixes[a]
980.03	Metals in Plants, Spectrographic Method	A, C, F, J, P, T
966.16	Na in Fruits and Fruit Products, Flame Spectrophotometric Method	A, J
990.23	Na and K in Dried Milk, Flame Emission Spectrophotometric Method	H
969.23	Na and K in Seafood, Flame Photometric Method	I, Q
976.25	Na in Foods for Special Dietary Use, ISE Method	K
984.27	Ca, Cu, Fe, Mg, Mn, P, K, Na and Zn in Infant Formula, ICP Method	K
THIAMINE		
942.23	Thiamine (B_1) in Foods, Fluorometric Method	All
957.17	Thiamine (B_1) in Bread, Fluorometric Method	F, R
953.17	Thiamine (B_1) in Grain Products, Fluorometric Method	F, R
986.27	Thiamine (B_1) in Milk-Based Infant Formula, Fluorometric Method	K
TRYPTOPHAN		
960.46	Vitamin Assays, Microbiological Method with **988.15** Tryptophan in Foods and Food and Feed Ingredients, Ion Exchange Chromatographic Method	All
VITAMIN A		
974.29	Vitamin A in Mixed Feeds, Premixes, and Foods, Colorimetric Method	B, G, H, I, K, L, M, Q
992.04	Vitamin A (Retinol Isomers) in Milk and Milk-Based Infant Formula, LC Method	H, K
992.06	Vitamin A (Retinol) in Milk-Based Infant Formula, LC Method	K
VITAMIN C		
984.26	Total Vitamin C in Food, Semi-automated Fluorometric Method	A, C–H, J, K, P, R, T

Table 2. Acceptable Official Methods for Nutrition Labeling

AOAC No.	Method	Matrixes[a]
967.22	Vitamin C (Ascorbic Acid) in Vitamin Preparations, Microfluorometric Method	A, C–H, J, K, P, R, T
967.21	Vitamin C (Ascorbic Acid) in Vitamin Preparations and Juices, Titrimetric Method (Colorless juices only)	D
985.33	Vitamin C (Reduced Ascorbic Acid) in Ready-To-Feed Milk-Based Infant Formula, Titrimetric Method	K
VITAMIN D		
982.29	Vitamin D in Mixed Feeds, Premixes, and Pet Foods, LC Method	All
936.14	Vitamin D in Milk, Vitamin Preparations and Feed Concentrates, Rat Bioassay Method	All
981.17	Vitamin D in Fortified Milk and Milk Powder, LC Method	G, H, K
VITAMIN E		
971.30	α-Tocopherol and α-Tocopheryl Acetate in Foods and Feeds, Colorimetric Method	All
992.03	Vitamin E Activity in Milk-Based Infant Formula, LC Method	K
ZINC		
968.08	Minerals in Animal Feed, AAS Method	All
975.03	Metals in Plants, AAS Method	All
980.03	Metals in Plants, Spectrographic Method	All
965.09	Minor Nutrients in Fertilizers, AAS Method	All
986.15	As, Cd, Pd, Se, and Zn in Food, Multielement Method	All
944.09	Zn in Food, Colorimetric Method	All
969.32	Zn in Food, AA Method	All
953.01	Metals in Plants, Emission Spectrographic Method	A, C, F, J, P, T
985.01	Metals and Other Elements in Plants, ICP Method	A, C, F, J, P, T
941.03	Zn in Plants, Mixed Color Method	A, C, F, J, P, T

Table 2. Acceptable Official Methods for Nutrition Labeling

AOAC No.	Method	Matrixes[a]
953.04	Zn in Plants, Single Color Method	A, C, F, J, P, T
984.27	Ca, Cu, Fe, Mg, Mn, P, K, Na and Zn in Infant Formula, ICP Method	K
985.35	Minerals in Ready-To-Feed Milk-Based Infant Formula, AAS Method	K

[a] Matrixes were considered representative of all food types and are as follows: A, fruit baby foods; B, meat baby foods; C, vegetable baby foods; D, beverages and juices; E, candy; F, cereals and products; G, cheese; H, dairy products; I, fish; J, fruits; K, infant formula or medical diet; L, meat (beef, pork, or fowl); M, mixed dinners (TV dinners); N, nuts; O, oils/fats (dressings); P, potatoes and products; Q, shellfish; R, sweet mixes (cake, pie, etc.); S, spices; and T, vegetables.

[b] These methods refer to **900.02A**, Ash of Sugar, in surplus status, no longer in use with sugar. Method **923.03** may be substituted.

Thanks to the efforts of M. Bueno, D. Carpenter, H. Chin, M. Deutsch, J. DeVries, N. Fraley, W. Hummer, W. Ikins, W. Landen, S. Lee, J. Morawski, P. Oles, L. Prosky, D. Soderberg, A. Soliman (deceased), D. Sullivan, J. Tanner, W. Wolf.

Table 3. Fat Analysis for Nutritional Labeling—AOAC Official Methods[a]

Method No.	Title	Brief Description	Applicable Matrixes	Comments
960.39	Crude Fat in Meat	Pet or diethyl ether extn	Baby food-meats, meats	Mono-, di-, and triglycerides and most of the sterols, glycolipids, phospholipids, and waxes
976.21	Crude Fat in Meat	Rapid Sp gr mth; tetrachloroethylene extn	Baby food-meats, meats	Mono-, di-, and triglycerides and most of the sterols, glycolipids, phospholipids, and waxes
985.15	Crude Fat in Meat & Poultry Prod	Rapid microwave-methylene chloride solv. extn	Baby food-meats, meats	Mono-, di-, and triglycerides, glycolipids phospolipids, and waxes; sterol yield may be reduced
920.39B	Crude Fat in Animal Feed	Diethyl ether extn	Cereals & prod; not adequate if heat processed, extruded, or has sugar added	Mono-, di-, and triglycerides and traces of other lipid components

Table 3. Fat Analysis for Nutritional Labeling—AOAC Official Methods[a]

Method No.	Title	Brief Description	Applicable Matrixes	Comments
920.39C	Crude Fat in Animal Feed	Diethyl ether extn; H_2O prewash if high in sugar	Cereals & prod, sweet mixes (cakes & pies); not adequate if heat processed	Mono-, di-, and triglycerides; may not quant. extract tot lipids; recommend further review or study of mth
945.18A	Fat in Cereal Adjuncts	Pet ether extn	Cereals & prod, sweet mixes (cakes and pies); **not adequate if heat processed**	Mono-, di-, and triglycerides; may not quant. extract tot lipids; recommend further review or study of mth
945.38F	Fat in Grains	Refers to **920.39C**	Cereals & prod; **adequate if not heat processed**	Mono-, di-, and triglycerides and traces of other lipid components
933.05	Fat in Cheese	Acid hydr., pet and diethyl ether extn re-extraction	Cheese	Mono-, di-, and triglycerides and traces of other lipid components; sterol yield greatly reduced
905.02	Fat in Milk	Alk treatmt, pet and diethyl ether extn re-extraction	Dairy	Mono-, di-, and triglycerides and traces of other lipid components
989.05	Fat in Milk	Alk treatmt, pet and diethyl ether extn	Dairy	Mono-, di-, and triglycerides and traces of other lipid components
938.06	Fat in Butter	Pet or diethyl ether extn	Butter	Mono-, di-, and triglycerides and traces of other lipid components
920.111A	Fat in Cream	Alk treatmt, pet and diethyl ether extn re-extraction	Dairy	Mono-, di-, and triglycerides and traces of other lipid components
920.111B	Fat in Cream	Babcock, acid hydr., vol. anal	Dairy	Mono-, di-, and triglycerides and phospholipids; sterol yield reduced
952.06	Fat in Ice Cream & Frozen Desserts	Alk treatmt, pet and diethyl ether extn re-extraction	Dairy	Mono-, di-, and triglycerides and traces of other lipid components
945.48G	Fat in Evaporated Milk	Alk treatmt, pet and diethyl ether extn re-extraction (refers to **905.02**)	Dairy	Mono-, di-, and triglycerides and traces of other lipid components

Table 3. Fat Analysis for Nutritional Labeling—AOAC Official Methods[a]

Method No.	Title	Brief Description	Applicable Matrixes	Comments
932.06	Fat in Dried Milk	Alk treatmt, pet and diethyl ether extn	Dairy	Mono-, di-, and triglycerides and traces of other lipid components
948.15	Crude Fat in Seafood	Acid hydr., pet and diethyl ether extn	Fish, shellfish	Mono-, di-, and triglycerides, fatty acid portion of phospholipids and glycolipids; in some prod with high sugar content, may overest. fat; sterol yield may be reduced **964.12**
986.25	Fat in Milk-Based Infant Formula	Alk treatmt, pet and diethyl ether extn; re-extn (refers to **945.48G**)	Infant formula/medical	Mono-, di-, and triglycerides and traces of other lipid components
925.32	Fat in Eggs	Acid hydr., pet and diethyl ether extn	Eggs/egg prod; **May not be adequate for some egg products containing sugar**	Mono-, di-, and triglycerides, fatty acid portion of phospholipids and glycolipids; sterol yield may be reduced
948.22	Crude Fat in Nuts and Nut Prod	Diethyl ether extn	Nuts; **not adequate for nuts containing sugar**	Mono-, di-, and triglycerides and traces of other lipid components
950.54	Tot Fat in Food Dressings	Acid hydr., pet and diethyl ether extn	Oils/fats (dressings)	Mono-, di-, and triglycerides, fatty acid portion of phospolipids and glycolipids
945.44	Fat in Fig Bars & Raisin Filled Cookies	Acid hydr., pet and diethyl ether extn re-extraction	Sweet mixes (cakes & pies) and baked cereal products	Mono-, di-, and triglycerides and fatty acid portion of phospholipids and glycolipids; sterol yield may be reduced; re-extn may not remove all sugars; recommend further review or study of mth
963.15	Fat in Cacao Prod	Pet ether extn	Chocolate prod	Mono-, di-, and triglycerides and traces of other lipid components
925.07	Fat in Cacao Prod	Pet and diethyl ether extn	Candy	Mono-, di-, and triglycerides and traces of other lipid components
920.177	Ether Extract of Confectionery	Pet and diethyl ether extn; re-extn	Candy	Mono-, di-, and triglycerides and traces of other lipid components

Table 3. Fat Analysis for Nutritional Labeling—AOAC Official Methods[a]

Method No.	Title	Brief Description	Applicable Matrixes	Comments
920.172	Ether Extract of Prepared Mustard	Diethyl ether extn	Mustard	Mono-, di-, and triglycerides and traces of other lipid components
963.22[b]	Methyl Esters of Fatty Acids in Oils and Fats	GC mth following prep of methyl esters (according to **969.33**)	All	Fatty acid profile; recommend further review or study of mth to make method adequate for quantitative analysis of fatty acids
979.19[b]	*cis,cis*-Methylene Interrupted Polyunsaturated Fatty Acids in Oils	Enzymatic-Spectro-photometric mth	All	

[a] This list has been prepared thanks to the efforts of S. Bailey, D. Carpenter, H. Chin, J. DeVries, N. Fraley, W. Hummer, A. Kistler, S. Lee, J. Ngeh-Ngwainbi, P. Oles, and D. Sullivan.
[b] Fatty acid methodology and *cis,cis*-methylene interrupted procedure.

Table 4. Moisture Analysis for Nutritional Labeling—AOAC Official Methods

AOAC No.	Title	Brief Description	Applicable Matrixes	Comments
925.04	Moisture in Animal Feed	Distillation with toluene	Spices	Method measures water as moisture in sample.
986.21	Moisture in Spices	Distillation with toluene or hexane	Spices	Method measures water as moisture in samples.
972.20	Moisture in Prunes and Raisins	Moisture meter method	Dried fruit	Measures conductivity and equates this to moisture.
977.10	Moisture in Cacao Products	Karl Fischer, electrochemical method	Milk chocolate & confectionery coatings	Method measures water as moisture in samples.
984.20	Moisture in Oils and Fats	Karl Fischer, electrochemical method	Oils & fats except for alk. or oxidized samples	Method measures water as moisture in samples.

Table 4. Moisture Analysis for Nutritional Labeling—AOAC Official Methods

AOAC No.	Title	Brief Description	Applicable Matrixes	Comments
920.116	Moisture in Butter	Pressure = atmospheric Temp = bp (H_2O) on sand to constant weight	Butter	Method measures all 100˚C volatile components. Residual Solids Method.
925.10	Solids (Total) and Moisture in Flour	Pressure = atmospheric Temp = 130˚C–100˚C Air oven for 3 h	Flour	Method measures all 100˚C volatile components. Residual Solids Method.
925.23	Solids (Total) in Milk	Pressure = atmospheric Temp = 98–100˚C Air oven for 3 h	Milk	Method measures all 100˚C volatile components. Residual Solids Method.
930.15	Moisture in Animal Feed	Pressure = atmospheric Temp = 135˚C for 2 h	Animal feeds	Method measures all 130˚C volatile components. Residual Solids Method.
931.04	Moisture in Cacao Products	Pressure = atmospheric Temp = 100˚C air oven to constant weight	Cacao products	Method measures all 100˚C volatile components. Residual Solids Method.
935.29	Moisture in Malt	Pressure = atmospheric Temp = 103–106˚C Air oven for 3 h	Malt	Method measures all 103–106˚C volatile components. Residual Solids Method.
941.08	Total Solids in Ice Cream and Frozen Desserts	Pressure = atmospheric Temp = 100˚C Air oven for 3.5 h	Ice cream and other frozen desserts	Method measures all 100˚C volatile components. Residual Solids Method.
948.12	Moisture in Cheese (Rapid screening method)	Pressure = atmospheric Temp = 130˚C Air oven for 1.25 h	Cheese	Method measures all 130˚C volatile components. Residual Solids Method.

Table 4. Moisture Analysis for Nutritional Labeling—AOAC Official Methods

AOAC No.	Title	Brief Description	Applicable Matrixes	Comments
952.08	Solids (Total) in Seafood	Pressure = atmospheric Temp = 100°C air oven 4 h or Temp = 100°C draft oven for 1 h	All marine products except raw oysters	Method measures all 100°C volatile components. Residual Solids Method.
984.25	Moisture (Loss of Mass on Drying) in Frozen French-Fried Potatoes	Pressure = atmospheric Temp = 103°C Air oven for 16 h	Quick-frozen french-fried potatoes	Method measures all 130°C volatile components. Residual Solids Method.
985.14	Moisture in Meat and Poultry Products	Pressure = atmospheric Temp = 130°C + Microwave oven	Meat and poultry	Method measures all 130°C volatile components. Residual Solids Method.
950.46B(a)	Moisture in Meat	Pressure = atmospheric Temp = 100–102°C air oven for 16–18 h	Meat and meat products	Method measures all 100°C volatile components. Residual Solids Method.
950.46B(b)	Moisture in Meat	Pressure = atmospheric Temp = 125°C air oven for 2–4 h	Meat and meat products	Method measures all 125°C volatile components. Residual Solids Method.
920.151	Solids (Total) in Fruits and Fruit Products	Pressure = <100 mm Hg Temp = 70°C 2 h wts to <3 mg change	Fruits and fruit products	Method measures moisture in sample.
925.40	Moisture in Nuts and Nut Products	Pressure <100 mm Hg Temp = 95–100°C Constant Weight (ca 5 h)	Nuts and nut products excluding high sugars or glycerols	Method measures moisture in samples.
926.08	Moisture in Cheese	Pressure <100 mm Hg Temp = 100°C Constant Weight (ca 4 h)	Cheese	Method measures all 100°C volatile components. Residual Solids Method.

Table 4. Moisture Analysis for Nutritional Labeling—AOAC Official Methods

AOAC No.	Title	Brief Description	Applicable Matrixes	Comments
926.12	Moisture and Volatile Matter in Oils and Fats	Pressure = <100 mm Hg Temp = bp (H_2O) + 25°C to constant weight	Fats & oils	Measures all volatile components in sample. Residual Solids Method.
927.05	Moisture in Dried Milk	Pressure = <100 mm Hg Temp = 100°C Constant Weight (ca 5 h)	Dried Milk	Method measures all 100°C volatile components. Residual Solids Method.
934.01	Moisture in Animal Feed	Pressure = <100 mm Hg Temp = 95–100°C (P=<50 T=<70 w/i sugar)	Animal feeds	Method measures moisture, better at lower T and P.
934.06	Moisture in Dried Fruits	Pressure <100 mm Hg Temp = 70°C Constant Weight (ca 6 h)	Dried fruit	Method measures moisture in samples.
920.115(d)	Sweetened Condensed Milk; Total Solids	Pressure <100 mm Hg Temp = 100°C Constant Weight (ca 6 h)	Sweetened condensed milk	Method measures all 100°C volatile components. Residual Solids Method.
925.30(b)	Solids (Total) in Eggs	Pressure <25 mm Hg Temp = 98–100°C Constant Weight (ca 5 h)	Liquid or dried eggs	Method measures all 98–100°C volatile components. Residual Solids Method.
925.09	Solids (Total) and Moisture in Flour	Pressure <25 mm Hg Temp = 98–100°C Constant Weight (ca 5 h)	Flour	Method measures moisture in samples.
945.43	Moisture in Fig Bars and Raisin-Filled Crackers.	Pressure <50 mm Hg Temp = 98-70°C 16 h with sand	Fig bars and raisin-filled crackers	Method measures moisture in samples.
964.22	Solids (Total) in Canned Vegetables	Pressure <50 mm Hg Temp = 69–71°C Multi-step steam-air oven-vacuum oven drying, final = 2 h in vacuum	Canned vegetables	Method measure moisture in samples.

Table 4. Moisture Analysis for Nutritional Labeling—AOAC Official Methods

AOAC No.	Title	Brief Description	Applicable Matrixes	Comments
925.45(a)	Moisture in Sugars-Vacuum Drying	Pressure <50 mm Hg Temp = 70˚C (preferably 60˚C) 2 h + until weight loss <2 mg	Cane and beet, raw and refined sugars	Method measures moisture in samples.
925.45(b)	Moisture in Sugar-Drying at atmospheric pressure	Pressure = atmospheric Temp = 100˚C 3 h + until weight loss <2 mg	Cane and beet, raw and refined sugar	Method measures all 100˚C volatile components. Residual Solids Method.
925.45(d)	Moisture in Sugars-Drying on Quartz Sand	Pressure <50 mm Hg Temp = 70˚C (preferably 60˚C) until wt loss <2 mg (ca 18 h)	Massecuites, molasses, and other liquid and semiliquid products	Method measure moisture in samples.
985.26	Total Solids in Processed Tomato Products by Microwave Moisture analyzer	Pressure = atmospheric Temp = 125˚C + To constant weight	Tomato products	Method measures volatile in samples.
972.16	Solids in Milk by NIR	Reflectance spectroscopic method	Milk products	Method measure moisture in samples.

Table 5. HPLC Methods for Carbohydrate Analysis

Method	Sugars	Matrix	Traction	Clean-up	Analytical Column/Detector	Mobile Phase
			Analysis on amino silica columns[a,b,c]			
982.14	glucose fructose sucrose maltose	Presweetened cereals (defatted)	50% ethanol, 85–90˚C, water bath, 25 min	centrifuge; C$_{18}$ cartridge 0.45 μm filter	Amino bonded silica 300 x 4 mm/RI	Acetonitrile H$_2$O (80:20)
980.13	fructose glucose lactose maltose sucrose	Milk chocolate (defatted)	H$_2$O, 85–90˚C water bath, 25 min	centrifuge; 0.45 μm filter	Amino bonded silica 300 x 4 mm/RI	acetonitrile; H$_2$O (80:20)

Table 5. HPLC Methods for Carbohydrate Analysis

Method	Sugars	Matrix	Traction	Clean-up	Analytical Column/Detector	Mobile Phase
984.17	fructose glucose sucrose maltose	Licorice extracts	H_2O, 0–90°, 25 min	0.45 μm filter C_{18} cartridge	Amino bonded silica 300 x 4 mm/RI	CH_3CN–H_2O (83 +17)
977.20	fructose glucose sucrose	Honey	aqueous CH_3CN	0.45 μm filter	Amino bonded silica 300 x 4 mm/RI	CH_3CN–H_2O, CH_3CN–H_2O, (83 + 17)
Analysis on ion exchange resin columns						
983.22	Minor saccharides (dextrose total DP$_2$ total DP$_3$)	Corn sugar	H_2O	5% (w/w) mixed exchange resin in sample soln.	610 x 7 mm Ion exchange Ca^{2+} 78°C	H_2O
979.23	Major saccharides (glucose fructose maltose psicose)	Corn syrup	H_2O	5% (w/w) mixed exchange resin in sample soln.	610 x 7 mm Ion exchange 50 W-x 4, Ca^{2+} 78°C	H_2O

[a] Methods **982.14** and **980.13** should have broad applicability, because samples are defatted before extraction.
[b] May need to eliminate the NaCl interference as indicated in **982.14**.
[c] Recommend collaborative study to extend to other matrixes (i.e., dairy products).

Table 6. Other Methods for Sugar Analysis

AOAC No.	Method	Brief description	Applicable matrixes
Gas chromatography			
971.18	Carbohydrates in Fruit Juices	Sample clarified with Pb acetate, deriv to TMS deriv and sep on silicone phase; det mono and disaccharides[a]	All
973.28	Sorbitol in Foods	Acetate deriv of sorbitol are detd	Fruits
Charcoal column chromatography			
954.11	Separation of Sugars in Honey	Charcoal Col Chrom followed by detn of fractions[a]	All

Table 6. Other Methods for Sugar Analysis

AOAC No.	Method	Brief description	Applicable matrixes
979.21	Separation of Sugars in Honey	Charcoal Col Chrom, followed by detn of fractions[b]	All
		Enzymatic methods	
969.39	Glucose in Corn Syrups and Sugars	Glucose oxidase mth (colorimetric detn using -dianisidine)	Corn syrups
984.15	Lactose in Milk	Hydr lactose with β-galactosidase, released galactose meas by NAD red mth (UV)	Milk
		Reducing sugar methods—copper reduction	
906.03	Invert Sugar in Sugars and Syrups	Munson-Walker mth	Sugars and syrups[b]
923.09	Invert Sugar in Sugars and Syrups	Lane-Eynon gen vol mth using Soxhlet reag (mod Fehling soln)[d]	Sugars and syrups[c,d]
929.09	Invert Sugar in Sugars and Syrups		Sugars and syrups
945.59	Invert Sugar in Sugars and Syrups[e]		Sugars and syrups[f]
945.60	Invert Sugar in Sugars and Syrups	Meissl-Hiller mth	Sugars and syrups[e]
950.56	Invert Sugar in Sugars and Syrups[e]	Quisumbing-Thomas mth	Sugars and syrups
955.36	Invert Sugar in Sugars and Syrups	Berlin Institute mth with Müller's soln	Sugars and syrups
970.58	Invert Sugar in Molasses	Lane-Eynon const vol mth	Molasses
931.07	Glucose and Sucrose in Eggs	Dissol, pptn of protein, quanti by titr	Eggs
936.06	Glucose in Cacao Products	Defat, dissolv in H_2O, prod clar with Pb acetate and quanti by mod Munson-Walker mth (using Sichert-Bleyer table for glucose)	Chocolate
938.18	Glucose in Cacao Products	Defat, dissolv in H_2O, quanti using Soxhlet reag, clar with Pb acetate, Zerban-Sattler mthd	Chocolate
938.02	Glucose in Cacao Products	Ref to **938.18** or **936.06**	
925.37	Glucose (Commercial) in Fruits and Fruit Products	Ref to **930.37**	Fruits and fruit prod
933.02	Glucose in Plants	Shaffer-Somogyi micro mth	

Table 6. Other Methods for Sugar Analysis

AOAC No.	Method	Brief description	Applicable matrixes
935.62	Glucose in Sugars and Syrups	Lane-Eynon and Munson-Walker mths	
945.67	Glucose in Corn Syrups and Sugars[e]	Steinhoff mth	
959.11	Glucose in Sugars and Syrups	Shaffer-Somogyi micro mth	
935.63	Fructose in Sugars and Syrups	Lane-Eynon and Munson-Walker mth	
932.15	Fructose in Sugars and Syrups	Jackson-Mathews, mod of Nyns Selective mth (similar to Shaffer-Somogyi)	
960.06	Fructose in Plants	Somogyi-Micro or Munson-Walker mth	
950.57	Arabinose, Galactose, and Xylose and other Sugars in Sugars and Syrups	Shaffer-Somogyi Micro and other mths	
920.139	Sucrose in Lemon, Orange, and Lime Extracts	Ref to **945.27, 925.48, 930.36**	
902.02	Sucrose in Vanilla Extract	Ref to **925.47, 925.48, 930.36**	
920.184	Sucrose in Honey	Ref to **920.183**	
920.189	Sucrose in Maple Products	Ref to **930.36**	
925.35	Sucrose in Fruits and Fruit Products	Invert with HCl or invertase then Munson-Walker mth	
925.44	Sucrose in Food Dressings	Munson-Walker % invert sugar bef/aft inversion	
930.07	Sucrose in Plants	Invert sugar by HCl or invertase, then Lane-Eynon mth	
930.36	Sucrose in Sugars and Syrups	Invert sugar with HCl or invertase, Munson-Walker mth	
950.51	Sucrose in Nuts and Nut Products	Ref to **920.40**[e]	
927.07	Lactose in Meat	Benedict Solution Mth	
930.32	Lactose in Process Cheese	Invert sugar with HCl, then Munson-Walker mth	
933.04	Lactose in Milk Chocolate		
935.65	Lactose in Sugars and Syrups	Munson-Walker or Lane-Eynon mth	
945.48	Evaporated Milk—Lactose	Ref to **896.01, 930.28**	
952.05	Lactose in Bread	Titr mth with Somogyi reag	

Table 6. Other Methods for Sugar Analysis

AOAC No.	Method	Brief description	Applicable matrixes
984.15	Lactose in Milk	Enzymatic mth	
935.64	Maltose in Sugars and Syrups	Munson-Walker or Lane Eynon mths	
906.01	Sugars (Reducing) in Plants	Munson-Walker mth	
920.190	Sugars (Reducing) in Maple Products as Invert Sugar		
920.183	Sugars (Reducing in Honey	Munson-Walker and Lane-Eynon mths	
921.03	Sugars (Reducing) in Plants[e]	Quisumbing-Thomas mth	
925.15	Sugars in Roasted Coffee	Munson-Walker or Lane-Eynon mths	
925.36	Sugars (Reducing) in Fruits and Fruit Products	Ref to **925.35**	
925.42	Sugars (Reducing) Before Inversion in Food Dressings	Munson-Walker mth	
925.43	Sugars (Reducing) After Inversion in Food Dressings	Invert sugars by HCl then Munson-Walker mth	
925.52	Sugars in Canned Vegetables	Munson-Walker mth on red sugars bef/aft inversion with HCl	
931.02	Sugars in Plants	Clar with Pb acetate or ion-exchange resins	
935.39G	Sugars in Baked Products	Ref to **975.14**	
945.29	Sugars (Total Reducing) in Brewing Sugars and Syrups	Munson-Walker or Lane-Eynon mths	
945.66	Total Reducing Sugars	Ref to **923.09** and **906.03**	
950.50	Sugars (Reducing) in Nuts and Nut Products	Munson-Walker mth	
968.28	Total Sugars in molasses as Invert Sugar	Lane-Eynon Const Vol Vol mth	
975.14	Sugars in Bread	Munson-Walker mth for red sugars, for sucrose ref to **925.05**	
		Reducing sugar methods—ferricyanide reduction	
939.03	Sugars (Reducing and Nonreducing) in Flour	Clar with Na tungstate followed by titr with ferricyanide and thiosulfate	Cereals, potatoes, sweet mixes

Table 6. Other Methods for Sugar Analysis

AOAC No.	Method	Brief description	Applicable matrixes
		Polarimetric methods	
896.01	Lactose in Milk		
896.02	Sucrose in Sugars and Syrups	Polarizing bef/aft inversion with HCl or invertase	Reducing Sugars
920.189	Sucrose in Maple Products	Direct and invert polarizations bef/aft inversion with HCl	
920.115	Sweetened Condensed Milk-Sucrose	Polarizing bef/aft inversion with HCl	
925.35	Sucrose in Fruits and Fruit Products	Polarizing bef/aft inversion with HCl	
925.47	Sucrose in Sugars and Syrups	Polarizing bef/aft inversion with invertase	
925.46	Sucrose in Sugars and Syrups	Saccharimeter reading, sample soln clar with Pb acetate or alumina cream, ICUMA mth[c]	
925.48	Sucrose in Sugars and Syrups	Polarizing bef/aft inversion with HCl	
926.13	Sucrose and Raffinose in Sugars and Syrups	Polarizing bef/aft inversion with invertase-melibiase	
926.14	Sucrose and Raffinose in Sugars and Syrups	Polarizing bef/aft inversion with HCl	
970.57	Sucrose in Molasses	Polarizing bef/aft inversion with invertase	
942.20	Sucrose in Sugar Beets	Hot H_2O digestion then polarization	
945.55	Sucrose in Gelatin	Polarizing bef/aft inversion with HCl	
950.30	Sugars (Reducing) in Nonalcoholic Beverages	Ref to **950.29**	
950.29	Sucrose in Nonalcoholic Beverages	Polarizing bef/aft inversion with HCl or invertase	
950.31	Glucose (Commercial) in Nonalcoholic Beverages	Ref to **930.37**	
930.37	Glucose (Commercial) in Sugars and Syrups		
		Infrared methods	
972.16H,I	Lactose in Milk	Mid-infrared[g]	
975.19	Lactose in Milk	Ref to **972.16H,I**	

62

Table 6. Other Methods for Sugar Analysis

AOAC No.	Method	Brief description	Applicable matrixes
		Gravimetric methods	
930.28	Lactose in Milk Gravimetric mth	Dairy prod	
920.110	Lactose in Cream	Ref to **930.28**	Dairy prod

[a] Applicable to broad range of matrixes if samples are defatted and extracted before analysis.
[b] International Commission for Uniform Methods of Sugar Analysis (ICUMSA) approved method.
[c] Lane-Eynon method may require filtration of reagents. Recommend not using asbestos as a filtering aid.
[d] Be cautious of potential interferences from oligosacch and lactic acid.
[e] Surplus mth.
[f] For low levels of invert in sucrose.
[g] Must be calibrated against a primary method.

Table 7. Matrixes Needing Methods

Recommendations	Matrixes[a]
ASH (D. Soderberg)	O
• Recommend replace references to **900.02** with **923.03**	
BETA CAROTENE (M. Deutsch)	B, D–I, K–O, Q–S
• Need method/cs[b] and source of standards	
• Need method to separate *cis* and *trans* isomers	
• Need method for encapsulated products	
BIOTIN (M. Deutsch)	All
• Need method/cs	
• Modification of **960.46** + FDA SOP 305 to use *L. plantarum* recommended	
CARBOHYDRATES-SUGAR ALCOHOLS (M. Clarke)	All
• Need method/cs	
CARBOHYDRATES-SUGARS (M. Clarke)	
• Cs of HPLC method with wide matrix applicability recommended	
CHOLESTEROL (M. Deutsch)	All < 10 mg/100
• Cs underway on direct saponification method	
COPPER (Open[c])	
• Need cs for Cu as analyte in **968.08**, **975.03**, **965.09**, **984.27**, **985.35**, **970.18**, **980.03**	

Table 7. Matrixes Needing Methods

Recommendations	Matrixes[a]
• Add note to **968.08** that Pt dishes are preferable, that losses may occur using porcelain dishes	
CYANOCOBALAMINE (M. Deutsch)	
• Cs recommended for **960.46** + **952.20** to use *L. leichmanui* for all matrixes	
DIETARY FIBER-INSOLUBLE (L. Prosky)	
• Cs recommended for sample preparation of high-fat samples.	
DIETARY FIBER-SOLUBLE (L. Prosky)	
• Cs recommended for sample preparation of high-fat samples.	
DIETARY FIBER-TOTAL (L. Prosky)	
• Cs recommended for sample preparation of high-fat samples.	
DRAINED WEIGHT (Open [c])	
• Need procedure for pickled veg., fruits, and tuna	
FAT-MONOUNSATURATED (D. Firestone)	All
• Recommend adoption of AOCS method where applicable	
FAT-POLYUNSATURATED (D. Firestone)	
• Recommend revision of extraction procedure	
FAT-SATURATED (D. Firestone)	A, C, J, T
• Recommend revision of extraction procedure	
• Modification of **969.33** to extend matrixes and quantitation of fatty acids in all foods recommended	
• Recommend cs for samples <350 mg fat content	
• Need method for C-4 to C-6 fatty acids	
FAT-TOTAL (D. Firestone)	All
• Need quantitation method for fatty acids	
FOLACIN (M. Deutsch)	
• Cs recommended for **960.46** + **944.12** + FDA SOP 315 to use *L. casei* for free form	
• Cs recommended for **960.46** + **944.12** + FDA SOP 320 to use *S. faecalei* for products containing free form	
• Cs recommended for **960.46** + FDA SOP 330 to use *K. apriculata* for bound form	

Table 7. Matrixes Needing Methods

Recommendations	Matrixes[a]
IODINE (Open[c])	All
• Need method/cs; consideration of ceric sulfate reduction recommended	
IRON (Open [c])	
• Recommend extension of applicability statements to foods for **965.09**, **968.08**, **985.35**, **975.03**, **980.03**	
MAGNESIUM (Open [c])	
• Recommend extension of applicability statements to foods for **965.09**, **985.35**, **975.03**, **985.35**, **980.03**	
• Recommend extension of applicability statement to A–C, F–H, K–M, P, Q, T for **984.27**	
MOISTURE (Open [c])	B, F, I, J, L–O, Q, R for high sugar products
• Recommend modification of **952.08** to eliminate asbestos use	
• See Moisture Report in the January 1993 issue of *The Referee*	
NIACIN (M. Deutsch)	
• Recommend extension of applicability statement to B, D, F–H, J, P for **985.24**	
• Recommend extension of applicability statement to all foods for **944.13**	
• Recommend cs on niacin in fortified foods using HPLC method in JAOAC (in press)	
• Cs recommended for **960.46** + **944.13** to use *L. plantarum* for all matrixes	
PANTOTHENIC ACID (M. Deutsch)	All
• Cs recommended for **960.46** + **945.74** to use *L. plantarum* for free form	
• Cs recommended for **960.46** + FDA SOP 350 + USDA 97 to use *L. plantarum* for total pantothenic acid for all matrixes	
• Cs recommended for **960.46** + FDA SOP 340 to use *A. suboxydaus* for panthenol	
PHOSPHORUS (Open [c])	
• Recommend extension of applicability statements to foods for **958.01**, **957.18**, **964.06**, **965.17**	
• Recommend extension of applicability statement to A, E–M, O–R, T for **986.24**	
POTASSIUM (Open[c])	
• Recommend extension of applicability statement to include food for **985.35**	
• Recommend extension of applicability statement to C, K, O for **984.27**	

Table 7. Matrixes Needing Methods

Recommendations	Matrixes[a]

PROTEIN (D. Soderberg)

• Recommend modification of Kjeldahl method to include spices

• Recommend cs of Dumas for all matrixes

PYRIDOXINE (M. Deutsch)

• Recommend cs based on JAOAC **39**, 157(1956)

• Cs recommended for **960.46** + **961.15** to use *S. uvarum* for total B_6, all matrixes

RIBOFLAVIN (M. Deutsch)

• Recommend cs for HPLC method

• Recommend extension of applicability statement to foods for **940.33**

• Recommend modification of **970.65** and **981.15** to incorporate standard addition

• Cs recommended for **960.46** + **940.33** to use *L. casei* for all matrixes

SAMPLING/SAMPLE PREP (Open [c])

• Recommend completion of AOAC book on sampling

• Recommend inclusion of sampling and sample preparation in future AOAC methods

SODIUM (Open [c])

• Recommend extension of applicability statement to food for **985.35**

• Recommend extension of applicability statement to C, K, O for **984.27**

STEARIC ACID (D. Firestone)

• Need quantitative method

THIAMINE (M. Deutsch)

• Recommend extension of applicability statement to all food for **986.27**

• Recommend extension of applicability statement to D, H–J, Q for **957.17**

• Cs recommended for simultaneous determination of B_1, B_2, and B_6 using fluorescence detection, JAOAC **75**, 561(1992)

• Cs recommended for **960.46** + FDA SOP 360 to use *L. viridescens* for all matrixes

TRYPTOPHAN (M. Deutsch)

• Cs recommended for FDA SOP 500, 501, and 502, HPLC for free form

• Cs recommended for **960.46** + FDA SOP 365 to use *L. plantarum* for bound and free forms

66

Table 7. Matrixes Needing Methods

Recommendations	Matrixes[a]
VITAMIN A (M. Deutsch)	A, C–F, J, N–P, R–T

• Cs recommended for new HPLC method based on **992.04**, for other than infant formula to apply to variety of matrixes. Modify sample size and replace ambient 18 h with high temp/short time saponification

| VITAMIN C (M. Deutsch) | B, I, L–O, Q, S |

• Need method/cs using HPLC to separate erythorbate, ascorbate, and dehydroascorbate

• Recommend modification of **984.26** to include meats, nuts, seafood, spices, and oils/fats

• Recommend adoption of ACNA HPLC method, JAOAC **75**, 887(1992), for vitamin C in variety of foods

VITAMIN D (M. Deutsch)

• Recommend extension of applicability statements to foods for **982.29 936.14**

• Recommend cs on GPC/HPLC method, NIST–Anal. Chem. **60**, 1929(1988)

• Recommend cs using HPLC method, reversed or normal phase

VITAMIN E (M. Deutsch)

• Recommend cs of HPLC method

• Recommend modification of current methods with solvent substitution for chloroform

• Need further investigation into standards, methodology, and standard conversion factors

ZINC (Open [c])

• Recommend extension of applicability statements to foods for **985.35**, **968.08**, **975.03**, **980.03**, **965.09**

• Recommend extension of applicability statement to A–F, H–M, O, P, R, T for **984.27**

[a] Those analytes for which no matrix is specified can be analyzed using AOAC Official Methods listed in the March 1993 issue of *The Referee*. The methods in that list are deemed to be adequate on the basis of collaborative studies and/or common use for the analyte/matrix combinations listed although not all analyte/matrix combinations listed have been fully collaboratively studied. *See* Appendix 2, Table 1, for matrix identification.

[b] cs, collaborative study.

[c] No current general referee (GR) for these specific analytes/topics. Contact AOAC International, Technical Services, 2200 Wilson Blvd, Suite 400, Arlington, VA 22201, +1 (703) 522-3032.

Note: GR for analytes in infant formula/medical diets is M. Bueno, FDA HFF-266, 200 C St, SW, Washington, DC 20204, +1 (202) 205-4445.

AOAC General Referees and Their Topics

■ *D. Soderberg*.—Meat, Poultry, Meat and Poultry Products—USDA/FSIS, 300 12th St, SW, Washington, DC 20205, +1 (202) 205-0039

- *M. Deutsch.*—Vitamins and Other Nutrients—FDA, HFF-264, 200 C St, SW, Washington, DC 20204, +1 (202) 205-4263
- *M. Clarke.*—Sugars and Sugar Products—Sugar Processing Research, Inc., 1100 Robert E. Lee Blvd, New Orleans, LA 70124, +1 (504) 286-4542
- *L. Prosky.*—Dietary Fiber—FDA, HFF-268, 8301 Muirkirk Rd, Laurel, MD 20708, +1 (301) 344-6005
- *D. Firestone.*—Fats & Oils—FDA, HFF-426, 200 C St, SW, Washington, DC 20204, +1 (202) 205-4381 Thanks to the efforts of M. Bueno, D. Carpenter, H. Chin, M. Deutsch, J. DeVries, N. Fraley, W. Hummer, W. Ikins, W. Landen, S. Lee, J. Morawski, P. Oles, L. Prosky, D. Soderberg, A. Soliman (deceased), D. Sullivan, J. Tanner, W. Wolf.

Chapter 4
Carbohydrates/Dietary Fiber Analysis for Nutrition Labeling

Sungsoo C. Lee, Jonathan W. DeVries, and Darryl M. Sullivan

Inroduction

A review of the AOAC INTERNATIONAL carbohydrate (sugars, dietary fiber) methods for meeting the Nutrition Labeling and Education Act (NLEA) requirements indicated a number of food matrices for which validated methods did not exist.

In this chapter, a thorough background on carbohydrates is provided to help in understanding the analytical challenges. A wide variety of AOAC methods and some insights into their areas of applicability are presented.

1. Chemical Classification of Carbohydrates

The term carbohydrates goes back to an earlier era of chemistry when it was thought that all compounds of this class were hydrates of carbon, on the basis of their empirical formula, e.g. $C_n(H_2O)_n$ (1–3). Since that time, many compounds have been identified that deviate from this general formula but retain common reactions, and thus are also classified as carbohydrates. A more useful definition of carbohydrates might be "polyhydroxy aldehydes or ketones and their derivatives." This definition encompasses sugar alcohols, deoxy and amino sugars and sugar carboxylic acids. Carbohydrates are commonly classified into monosaccharides, oligosaccharides and polysacchrides.

1.1. Monosaccharides

Monosaccharides are polyhydroxy-aldehydes or -ketones, generally with an unbranched chain of carbon atoms. The most common monosaccharides include glucose, fructose and galactose.

Sugars differing in configuration at any single chiral center other than C-1 are called epimers. Thus, D-mannose is the C-2 epimer of D-glucose, and D-galactose is the C-4 epimer of D-glucose. Actual sugar rings, as they occur in nature, are not flat as represented in the typical Haworth projections shown in text books. Many hexoses occur mainly in the fairly rigid chair form; fewer exist in the more flexible boat forms. There are other forms, such as half chairs and skew arrangements, but these are of higher energy and are less frequently encountered.

1.2. Oligosaccharides

Oligosaccharides are carbohydrates that are obtained from the condensation of monosaccharides with the elimination of water. This class of carbohydrate compounds, containing 2–9 sugar units, are water soluble. Disaccharides consist of two monosaccharide units. Best known representatives of the oligosaccharides are the disaccharides, sucrose, maltose and lactose. Disaccharides may be homogenous or heterogeneous with respect to their monomer composition. Homogeneous disaccharides from D-glucose include cellobiose and maltose. Examples of heterogeneous disaccharides are sucrose (formed from glucose and fructose) and lactose (formed from glucose and galactose).

Oligosaccharides such as maltose, cellobiose, maltotriose, and maltotetrose contain a free hemiacetal group that can react to produce a carbonyl function. Such carbohydrates are called reducing sugars because of their ability to reduce metal ions such as Cu^{2+} while the sugar is oxidized to a carboxylic acid. Sucrose does not contain a free hemiacetal function; therefore, it is not easily oxidized and is termed a nonreducing sugar.

69

Tri- and tetra-saccharides also occur in foods and may be homogeneous, heterogeneous, reducing or nonreducing. Trisaccharides include raffinose and tetrasaccharides include stachyose. Larger oligosaccharides are also present in foods, notably the maltose oligomers (degree of polymerization, DP = 4–9) in corn syrups. The cyclic alpha-D-glucopyranosyl oligomers of 6–9 units are called Schardinger dextrins.

1.3. Polysaccharides

Polysaccharides are composed of 10 or more monosaccharide units bound to each other by glycosidic linkages. These compounds are usually amorphous, colorless, almost tasteless, and vary greatly in digestibility. Most polysaccharides are large molecules composed of several hundred or even thousands of monosaccharide units. Chemical subclassification of polysaccharides has been proposed in two ways. First, the polysaccharides can be classified based on monosaccharide composition. These classes are as follows: homopolysaccharides, which are composed of many units of a single monosaccharide and include cellulose, starches and glycogen; heteropolysaccharides, which consist of two or more different monosaccharide components and include hemicelluloses, pectins, mucilages and resins; and conjugated compounds composed of saccharides plus lipids or protein. Secondly, polysaccharides can also be classified into starches and nonstarch polysaccharides based on linkage types of the monosaccharide units. Nonstarch polysaccharides can be further divided into homo- and hetero-types. Chemical classification of carbohydrates is presented in Table 1.

Table 1. Chemical Classification of Carbohydrates

Types of Carbohydrates	Representatives
Monosaccharides	glucose
	fructose
	galactose
	galacturonic acid
	glucuronic acid
Oligosaccharides	
Disaccharides	sucrose
	maltose
	lactose
Trisaccharides	raffinose
Tetra-	stachyose
DP 5-9	higher oligosaccharides
Polysaccharides	

Table 1. Chemical Classification of Carbohydrates

Types of Carbohydrates	Representatives
Method A (based on uniformity of composing monosaccharide types)	
Homopolysaccharides	cellulose
	starches
	glycogen
Heteropolysaccharides	pectins
	mucilages
	gums
Method B (based on linkage types of monosaccharides)	
Starches	amylose
	amylopectin
Nonstarch polysaccharides	
homo NSP	cellulose
hetero NSP	pectin
	hemicelluloses
	gums

2. Definition of Carbohydrates for Nutrition Labeling Purposes

Chemical classification of carbohydrates as outlined above may not be the same as the nutritional definition. For example, monosaccharides and disaccharides, components of oligosaccharides, are generally classified into a single category as simple sugars because of their shared functional and nutritional properties. Alditols, derived from mono- and disaccharides, have unique functional properties and are generally referred to as sugar alcohols. Lignin and polysaccharides, which are resistant to digestion by human alimentary enzymes, are often classified as dietary fiber. The carbohydrates definition recommended by the U.S. Food and Drug Administration (FDA) (4, see Table 2) provides more meaningful nutritional information to consumers.

Table 2. FDA Definition of Carbohydrates for Nutrition Labeling

Types of Carbohydrates	Examples
Sugars	
Monosaccharides	glucose, galactose, fructose
Disaccharides	sucrose, maltose lactose
Sugar Alcohols	
Alditol derivatives of reducing sugars	sorbitol, xylitol mannitol malitol
Dietary Fiber	
Soluble	pectins gums, mucilages hemicelluloses
Insoluble	cellulose hemicelluloses
Other Carbohydrates	
Oligosaccharides of DP 3 and up	stachyose raffinose
Available starches	dextrins (available) amylose and amylopectin

2.1 Sugars and Sugar Alcohols

Sugars are defined as the sum of mono- and disaccharides. The most commonly found sugars in foods are glucose, fructose, galactose, maltose, sucrose, and lactose. Sugar alcohols are used as sugar substitutes in food formulations to decrease water activity in intermediate moisture foods, as softeners, as crystallization inhibitors and for improving the rehydration characteristics of dehydrated food. Sorbitol is commonly found in nature in many fruits. Malitol, the reduction product of maltose, is widely used in food products.

2.2. Dietary Fiber

Dietary fiber is defined as polysaccharides and lignin that are resistant to hydrolysis by human alimentary enzymes (5, 6). Using this definition, dietary fiber includes nonstarch polysaccharides, resistant starch, and lignin. This definition has received general acceptance by professionals in the field (7). Distinction between soluble dietary fiber (SDF) and insoluble dietary fiber (IDF) is based on the solubility characteristics of dietary fiber in hot aqueous buffer solutions, as encountered in the enzymatic-gravimetric methods.

2.3. Other Carbohydrates

Other carbohydrates include higher oligosaccharides (DP 3-9) and available starches. The term "complex carbohydrates," which was first introduced in 1977 by the U.S. Senate Select Committee on Nutrition and Human Needs (8), has equivocal definitions. "Complex carbohydrates" meant available starches to the Committee when the term was first proposed. However, many professionals in the field believe that the definition of complex carbohydrates should be equal to that of polysaccharides, i.e. "the sum of available starches and nonstarch polysaccharides." In the final regulations implementing the NLEA, FDA accepts the convention that complex carbohydrates equals available starches.

Currently, no analytical methodology has been published and validated that will provide quantitation of the proposed "digestible carbohydrates having a degree of polymerization (DP) of 10 or greater." Due to lack of validated methodology, the Food Labeling Regulations finalized in January 6, 1993, do not include "complex carbohydrates" in the terminology for nutrition labeling, although the term "other carbohydrates" is. Because of emphasis placed on complex carbohydrates in dietary recommendations and guidelines, it is important that direct and indirect methodology be validated so that complex carbohydrate information can be included in the nutrition label. Technical literature and task force member experience indicate that oligosaccharides with a degree of polymerization of two to nine can be quantitated by high-pressure liquid chromatography (HPLC) techniques. The quantity of oligosaccharides obtained could be subtracted, along with sugars, sugar alcohols, and dietary fiber, from the total carbohydrate of the food to give the quantity of complex carbohydrates (available carbohydrates of DP > 10). Alternately, some starch and dietary fiber analytical procedures could be modified to quantitate complex carbohydrates. For example, the filtered enzyme digestate fractions from dietary fiber analytical procedures of sugar-free samples could be analyzed for total sugars and converted to complex carbohydrates.

Considering the importance of complex carbohydrates in the human diet (8-9), AOAC should promote the development and validation of appropriate methodology for complex carbohydrates. The availability of appropriate methodology would allow regulatory reassessment of the nutrients list that was deemed desirable for future labeling purposes. Validated methodology would allow consumers access to information on complex carbohydrates, whether defined as digestible carbohydrates of DP > 10 (proposed NLEA definition) or as the sum of available carbohydrates and dietary fiber.

As it stands now, other carbohydrates are to be estimated as the difference between total carbohydrates and the sum of dietary fiber, sugars, and sugar alcohols (when declared).

3. Analysis of Sugars

Most AOAC approved methods for sugar determinations are indirect physical, enzymatic, or semi-empirical chemical methods (10). Earlier AOAC methods depended heavily on chemical methods that are nonspecific; they detect a class of sugar such as reducing sugars rather than individual sugars. These chemical methods are based on color reactions effected by the reducing properties of the carbonyl group, the condensation of degradation products of sugars in strong mineral acids with various organic compounds or on oxidative cleavage of neighboring hydroxyl groups. The methods were improved through the years, but very few were collaboratively studied.

As analytical techniques advanced and the determination of individual carbohydrates was considered important, the specificity of saccharide testing has improved by using column chromatography. Because of their high specificity and the capability for simultaneous determination of several sugars, chromatographic methods are advantageous and have been actively developed over the past two decades. Both gas liquid chromatography (GLC) and HPLC have been used for sugar analysis. HPLC is now considered the more advantageous method for routine sugar analysis.

3.1. The Choice of Methods for the Analysis of Sugars in Foods

The choice of methods in the sugar analysis must be based on a knowledge of the composition of the mixture of sugars in the food. If a single sugar is present and there are no interfering substances, almost any analytical method may be used. Most analytical methods require the removal of interfering materials prior to analysis. The appropriate pretreatment depends on the method to be used. For example, reducing sugar methods will require the elimination of other reducing substances. Reversed-phase HPLC with refractive index (RI) detection may require removal of chloride ion.

For the many mixed diets containing various combinations of sugars, the method of choice is more limited. Reducing sugar methods alone may not accurately measure the total sugar content for samples containing any combination of glucose, fructose, sucrose, maltose, and lactose. The use of certain enzymes provides specific methodology for the analysis of the sugar mixture in some food samples. However, sequential assays must be carried out.

3.2 HPLC Methods

For nutrition labeling purposes, HPLC may be the most appropriate technique for accuracy, precision and practicality. The polar bonded normal-phase HPLC methods **982.14** and **980.13** should have broad applicability, because samples are defatted then the sugars are extracted and analyzed. These methods are most widely used for routine analysis of ordinary samples in food laboratories. When carrying out these methods, caution must be taken to test the HPLC system for interference from sodium chloride that might be present in the sample. Sodium chloride usually elutes between glucose and sucrose on the amino silica columns used in these methods, but it also occasionally coelutes with one or the other. Steps must be taken to eliminate sodium chloride, as indicated in **982.14**.

This technique began to be applied to sugar analysis in the 1970s. The separation performance of these columns and the detectors has continuously improved to achieve complete separation and quantitation of mono- and di-saccharides. HPLC often offers direct injection of a sample with little pretreatment. The interpretation of many HPLC chromatograms is simple. Underivatized sugars can be determined using a variety of chromatographic modes in conjunction with RI detection. Several extensive reviews of different techniques are in the literature (11–14).

The most common types of HPLC column packings in commercial use for separating sugars in foods are amino-bonded silica or metal loaded cation exchangers based on resin or a silica substrate. Methods **982.14**, **980.13**, **984.17**, and **977.20** are based on amino-bonded silica columns with or without guard column. Methods **979.23** and **983.22** are based on ion mediated partition, in particular cation (Ca^{2+}) exchange resin columns.

3.2.1. Amino-bonded silica

Initial research by Hurst and Martin (15), Iverson and Bueno (16), and DeVries et al. (17), included some technical work comparing different techniques. These formed the basis for collaborative study and adoption as official methods by the AOAC (**977.20**, **980.13**, **982.14** and **984.17**).

Elution orders of carbohydrates using an aminopropylsilane-bonded silica column packing and an acetonitrile–water mobile phase follow carbohydrate polarity: first monosaccharides and sugar alcohols, then disaccharides, and finally the higher oligosaccharides. The separation mechanisms have been attributed to partition of the sugars between the water-enriched stationary phase and the mobile phase (18) and to adsorption via hydrogen-bonding between the sugar hydroxyl groups and the amino functional groups (19). Increased water content of the mobile phase reduces carbohydrate retention. The acetonitrile:water ratio in the mobile phase is typically 80:20. Amono-bonded column facilitate the separation of fructose, glucose, sucrose, maltose, and lactose. Xylitol coelutes with fructose and sorbitol and mannitol coelute with glucose.

The presence of salt in the sample extract interferes with the analysis because chloride ions elute closely after glucose. Wills et al. (20) eliminated the interference by adding the ion-pairing reagent tetrabutylammonium phosphate to the acetonitrile–water mobile phase in order to increase the retention of the sugars and reduce the retention of chloride. DeVries et al. (21) minimized NaCl interference by washing the column for 2 h at 1.5 mL/min with a solution of 0.1% TEPA (pH approximately 7 with HOAc) in acetonitrile–water (80 + 20). The column was finally washed with 100 mL normal mobile phase. For column testing purposes, a test solution (approximately 2 mg NaCl/mL) in the same injection solvent as that used for the sugar standards was prepared and injected immediately after the sugar standards and before the sample solutions. The recommendations of DeVries et al. to eliminate NaCl interference have been incorporated into method **982.14**.

Other than the food matrices which have been collaboratively evaluated for applicability under the auspices of AOAC, a variety of food matrices have also been analyzed for sugar by methods employing amino silica columns. Examples include beverages, processed fruits, dairy products, cakes and snacks (22), soft drinks (23), honey (24), cream, beverages and cereals (16), diet composite reference material (25), defatted soya flour (26), potatoes (27), vegetables (28) and infant foods, cakes and snacks (29).

3.2.2 Cation exchange resin columns

Resin-based cation exchangers are loaded with a metal counter-ion, usually calcium, lead, or silver, which remains ionically bound to the polymer under the appropriate operating conditions. Columns packed with such resins are designed to be operated at 80°C with distilled water as the mobile phase, but up to 30% by volume of acetonitrile can be added to the eluent as an organic modifier. The addition of 1mM triethylamine (TEA) to the water eluent improves the chromatography of sugars on Ca^{2+}-form resins and allows a column temperature below 80°C to be used. The TEA will gradually displace the calcium from the resin, thus periodic column regeneration is recommended (30). AOAC methods **979.23** and **983.22** are based on calcium-loaded exchange resins with water as eluent. Operating temperature of the column is 78°C.

The presence of sucrose in the dairy products may cause a problem because it is poorly resolved from lactose using a Ca^{2+}-form resin. The presence of sodium chloride may not interfere with the analysis as it elutes before the sugars of interest (31).

3.2.3. Related method: anion-exchange columns

The combination of anion-exchange separations with pulsed amperometric detection (PAD) provides a versatile system for carbohydrate analysis (32–34). Carbohydrates are weak acids (pK 12–14), and they can be separated by direct anion-exchange using high pH eluents on an anion-exchange column of moderate capacity.

Because carbohydrates are electro-active in alkaline solutions, electrochemical detection combines well with anion separations that use sodium hydroxide as eluent. The advent of PAD, now commonly used with high performance anion-exchange chromatography (HPAEC), greatly improved the detection sensitivity limit. With this detector, carbohydrates, even those without reducing groups, can be measured with high sensitivity without requiring pre- or postcolumn derivatization.

Despite its high detection sensitivity, this method may not be the most cost-effective approach for routine sugar analysis for ordinary food samples in quality control (QC) laboratories, where multitudes of samples are analyzed daily. It can be more time consuming, and the operating system is more demanding, when compared to methods **982.14** and **980.13**. Also, required alkaline conditions for chromatography have the potential for epimerization and degradation, well known for reducing sugars. However, this problem may not be serious with routine food samples. With PAD, not only sugars but also amino acids, peptides or organic acids can yield a positive response. PAD does not yield a uniform molar response for different oligosaccharides. Thus, the exact molar responses for each oligosaccharide must be obtained for quantitation.

Application of this method to carbohydrate analyses will continue to grow. At present, this method is the most suitable for carbohydrate analysis of complex samples, such as glycoprotein, oligosaccharides, and sugar components in dietary fiber residues. The method needs to be collaboratively studied to evaluate the method performance for AOAC consideration.

3.3. GLC Methods

The application of GLC to sugar analysis has been slower than the application to other classes of compounds. The major problem is the lack of volatility of the polar carbohydrate compounds. The most popular means of pretreating sugars for GLC analysis is to prepare their trimethylsilyl (TMS) derivatives (14) as in AOAC methods for sugars, **971.18**, and for sorbitol, **973.28**. The use of pyridine tends to produce tailing peaks. Other usual sugar derivatives are alditol acetates, oxime-TMS ethers, acetyl-TMS, or Alditol-TMS.

Flame ionization detectors (FID) used in GLC are generally more sensitive than RI detectors used in HPLC. The sugar content of complex samples such as dietary fiber residues after acid hydrolysis can be successfully determined by GLC techniques. However, for routine analysis of ordinary sugar samples, GLC may not be the most cost-effective approach, unless only small amounts of samples are available or the sugar content of samples is very low.

3.4. Colorimetric Methods

These methods are based on reducing properties of the aldehyde or keto group of sugar molecules (35–36). This is probably the most important chemical property to be used in sugar analysis prior to the advent of HPLC. The reactive aldehyde or keto groups reduce alkaline solutions of metallic salts to the metallic oxides or the free metals. These methods can be successfully used when a known sugar is present in the sample extract. For the sample with a mixture of sugars, these approaches alone may not give an accurate estimation of total sugar content. These methods are considered semi-empirical because of the nonspecificity of reducing sugars and compounds containing reducing properties. Sugar mixtures may be analyzed if standards with a composition similar to that of the test sample are used.

Colorimetric reducing sugar methods are generally categorized into copper reduction, ferricyanide reduction, dinitrosalicylate reduction, and para-hydroxy benzoic acid reduction methods and condensation reactions. Most AOAC approved colorimetric sugar methods are based on the reduction of copper. A ferricyanide method is also available.

3.4.1. Copper reduction method

Many variations of the original Fehling's reagent have been used because they have special merits for particular food stuffs. The principal aim of most of these modifications has been to improve the precision of this reduction method and to remove the cause of the major variations in the yield of cuprous oxide. Of these, the alkalinity of the reagent, the rate and time of heating, and the concentration of the sugar in the sample appear to be important. The Lane-Eynon volumetric method and Munson-Walker titrimetric methods are the most frequently used AOAC methods.

In the Lane-Eynon method, the sugar solution is titrated against the hot Soxhlet reagent, which is a modified Fehling reagent, in two stages: the bulk of the solution required to effect almost complete reduction and then dropwise to an endpoint with methylene blue. This method is widely used for determination of glucose, lactose, and invert sugars in various food matrices. In the Munson and Walker method, a fixed volume of solution is heated under standard conditions with the Fehling's reagent and the cupric oxide formed is filtered off. Cupric oxide precipitate is either weighed directly, measured volumetrically by titration with permanganate or thiosulphate, or measured electrolytically. These methods have been extensively studied and detailed calibration data are available.

3.4.2. Ferricyanide reduction

The reaction takes place in alkaline solution, and the reduction can be measured either by iodometric procedures or colorimetrically. Method **939.03**, sugars in flour, is based on this principle. The stability of alkaline ferricyanide reagent and less demanding experimental conditions compared to copper reduction have made this procedure a method of choice in many automated reducing sugar analyses.

3.5. Enzymatic Methods

This approach provides specific procedures for some mono- and disaccharides. These methods can be used successfully when known types of carbohydrate samples are analyzed. The methods will not provide a complete profile of mono- and disaccharides.

These enzymatic methods can be classified into 2 categories: colorimetric and UV (35, 37). The colorimetric methods involve the use of specific enzymes to react with sugar to produce a compound that reacts with a chromogen. The intensity of color reaction is measured spectrophotometrically. Method **969.39**, a glucose oxidase method for determination of glucose in corn syrups and sugars, falls into this category. The UV methods involve the coupling of a biochemical reaction and the reduction of nucleotides. These methods may require prehydrolysis of disaccharides with specific carbohydrases. Method **984.15**, determination of lactose in milk, belongs to this category. Several other UV methods are available in kit form from Boeringer Mannheim (37). These kits include methods for glucose, glucose/fructose, glucose/fructose/sorbitol, lactose/galactose and glycerol. These UV method kits have a potential for reliable determinations of specific sugars of interest. These UV methods need to be collaboratively studied in order to evaluate their method performance.

4. Analysis of Dietary Fiber
4.1. The Choice of Methods

There have been continuous improvements in dietary fiber methodology over the last century. Even at present, there is no universal method that can meet the analytical demands of all purposes. The method selected is based on the individual chemist's needs. For the choice of method, each chemist or laboratory should evaluate several factors, such as the nature of questions they are attempting to answer, accuracy, precision, job efficiency, cost effectiveness, personnel requirements, and regulations.

Currently, dietary fiber methodology can be classified into the following three major categories:
(1) Enzymatic-gravimetric,
(2) Nonenzymatic-gravimetric, and
(3) Enzymatic-chemical methods, which include
        a. enzymatic-colorimetric,
        b. enzymatic-GLC, and
        c. enzymatic-HPLC.

Recently, technical details of DF analysis have been thoroughly reviewed by Asp et al. (6) and Lee and Prosky (38).

4.2. Enzymatic-Gravimetric Methods

The main advantages of the methods are that they are relatively accurate and precise compared to other approaches and are in agreement with the definition of dietary fiber that has been accepted by most researchers in the field. Moreover, these methods are simple, inexpensive, and easy to perform and do not require highly trained personnel and high capital investments, particularly when compared to more sophisticated methods using GLC or HPLC techniques. However, they do not provide detailed information on the components of dietary fiber. Overall, the methods are considered the most suitable for routine analysis for fiber labeling and QC research purposes.

Methods **985.29** (TDF), **991.43** (TDF, SDF, and IDF), and **991.42** (IDF) should have broad applicability because the sample is defatted and/or desugared. Methods **985.29** and **991.43** will give comparable values for TDF, and the methods **991.43** and **991.42** will give comparable values for SDF and IDF. With method **991.43**, total dietary fiber can be measured independently or calculated as the sum of SDF and IDF. Defatting is recommended for samples containing higher than 10% fat, and desugaring is recommended for those containing more than 50% sugars on dry weight basis. Drying is recommended for samples containing high moisture, typically the sample difficult to grind. Thus, the methods are valid for high-fat, high-sugar, and high-moisture samples. The methods specify the drying conditions as well as defatting and desugaring procedures. If any pretreatment is a part of the analysis, analytical results must incorporate the loss on drying, defatting, or desugaring to obtain dietary fiber content of the "as received" product.

FDA's and the U.S. Department of Agriculture's (USDA) final food labeling regulations, which were published in the January 6, 1993, issue of the Federal Register (4), have recognized the AOAC methods **985.29** (TDF) and **991.43** (TDF, SDF/IDF) as suitable methodology for the analysis of dietary fiber for nutrition labeling purposes. In addition, the most recent International Survey on Dietary Fiber Definition, Analysis, and Reference Materials (7) indicates that the professionals in the dietary fiber research field strongly support the enzymatic-gravimetric technique as the most appropriate approach for nutrition labeling and QC purposes.

The principle of methods **985.29**, **991.42**, and **991.43** as outlined by Prosky et al. (39–42), Schweizer et al. (43), and Lee et al. (44) is as follows. Duplicate samples of dried foods, fat-extracted if containing >10% fat, undergo sequential enzymatic digestion by heat stable alpha-amylase, protease, and amyloglucosidase to remove starch and protein. For total dietary fiber, enzyme digestate is treated with 4 volumes of 95% ethanol (final ethanol conc., 78% v/v), filtered, washed with acetone, dried, and weighed. For IDF, enzyme digestate is filtered, and the residue is washed with warm water, dried, and weighed. For SDF, the filtrate and washes are combined, the SDF is precipitated with ethanol, filtered, dried and weighed. The TDF, SDF, and IDF residue values are corrected for protein, ash, and blank.

Method **991.43** is essentially the same as methods **985.29** and **991.42**, with minor modifications. In Method **991.43**, a buffer solution containing MES (morpholinoethane sulfonic acid) and TRIS (trishydroxymethyl aminomethane) is used to minimize co-precipitation of buffer reagents in 78% ethanol. In contrast to the inorganic phosphates used in methods **985.29** and **991.42**, this buffer is not sensitive to changes in ethanol concentration nor the final pH of the enzymatic digestate, making the DF determination procedure more rugged.

Method **985.29** has been the basis of the total dietary fiber tables listed in USDA Handbook No.8. Methods **991.42** and **991.43** have been chosen by USDA for the construction of soluble and insoluble dietary fiber tables. Methods **985.29** and **991.42**, with minor modifications, have been the basis of the Japanese dietary fiber tables established in 1990 and 1992 (45; Nishimune, personal communication). Method **991.43** has been used for constructing the total, soluble, and insoluble dietary fiber tables for 200 Mexican foods (Rosado, personal written communication).

Recently, another gravimetric method, method **992.16**, has been made official for the purpose of routine TDF analysis. The method uses the neutral detergent fiber (NDF) procedure and combines it with a separate determination of autoclave induced, hot water-soluble DF to derive TDF values (46). The values for NDF plus autoclave-induced, hot water-soluble DF are in good agreement with the TDF values measured by methods **985.29** and **991.43**. This method was approved by AOAC for TDF determinations only, not for SDF and IDF determinations. Separate analyses of IDF and autoclave-induced, water-soluble DF are necessary for TDF analysis.

Limitations of the current AOAC dietary fiber methods

1. Viscous samples such as desugared fruits and mucilagenous products usually encounter filtration problems. For these samples, a smaller sample size would alleviate the slow filtration process. For desugared fruit samples, the sample size can be reduced to 0.3–0.5 g, and 0.1–0.2 g for psyllium and flaxseed. The difficulty of separating soluble and insoluble fractions of these samples is not unique to the gravimetric method; similar treatments are required for separation by centrifugation, a technique that is often used in enzymatic-chemical procedures.

2. Current enzymatic-gravimetric methods, as with other current DF analytical approaches, require a drying and/or a defatting step prior to determining DF for a number of food matrices. These matrices include frozen desserts, TV dinners, mayonnaise, and fiber drinks, which may have been formulated to contain dietary fiber. Drying the sample and defatting with petroleum ether or other solvents may introduce additional sources of error. These preparatory steps are also labor intensive (47).

3. Complete removal of protein on most samples is not usually achieved during the protease incubation step. The correction factor, 6.25 × Kjeldahl nitrogen value, is somewhat arbitrary, because the exact conversion factor may vary depending on the type of protein in the sample residue (6, 47).

4.3. Nonenzymatic/Gravimetric Methods

Nonenzymatic/gravimetric methods include crude fiber (CF), acid detergent fiber (ADF), and neutral detergent fiber (NDF) techniques. These are useful methods but cannot be used for nutrition labeling. Recently, a nonenzymatic/gravimetric method was developed for analysis of TDF in low-starch products such as fruits and vegetables (48). This method has been collaboratively studied under the auspices of AOAC. For most human diets containing starch, this method will overestimate the TDF content.

4.3.1. Crude Fiber

The crude fiber method measures fiber as a sum of lignin and cellulose. The crude fiber method received official approval by AOAC for flour (**920.86**) and animal feed (**962.09**) in 1920 and 1962, respectively.

The method is highly empirical, although it used the most advanced techniques at the time the method was developed. It should also be noted that the method is still being used for nutritional labeling purposes in some countries where Western diseases are not of major health concerns.

4.4. Enzymatic-Chemical Methods

In the enzymatic-chemical procedures, isolated DF residues undergo acid hydrolysis. The resulting sugars are determined by various chemical means. In the chromatographic methods, monosaccharides only are detected by using either GLC or HPLC, and uronic acids are determined colorimetrically or by a decarboxylation method. Thus, the resultant DF values are calculated as the sum of these two analyses (i.e., the sum of monosaccharides and uronic acids with correction factors). In the colorimetric methods, sugars, both mono- and oligosaccharides, and uronic acids are determined mostly by reducing sugar methods.

During the acid hydrolysis procedure, conversion of polysaccharides to monosaccharides takes place at different rates depending on the types of DF residues and acid hydrolysis conditions. Whereas some polysaccharides are still converted into monosaccharides, some sugars released at the earlier stage of acid hydrolysis are being degraded. Acid hydrolysis conditions as well as conversion factors to compensate acid hydrolyzed loss of individual sugars need further optimization (49).

4.4.1 Uppsala GLC Method - The 1992 AOAC Study

GLC methods seemingly have an advantage over other methods in characterizing the saccharide profile of dietary fiber, which includes neutral sugars and uronic acids. These methods are generally considered accurate and precise for dietary fiber determinations. At present, only the Uppsala GLC method has been proven reliable for reproducibility when measuring neutral sugars (glucose, fructose, arabinose, and xylose) and uronic acids among various laboratories.

Acid hydrolysis conditions and acid hydrolysis loss factors used in the calculation critically affect the final values for dietary fiber and its components. In addition, these methods are time-consuming, expensive, and require highly trained personnel and high capital investments. Presently, the methods described above do not provide the food industry with enough justifications to use the methods for nutrition labeling or QC purposes. Research should be continued to further improve the accuracy, precision, and ruggedness of this type of methodology.

Currently, the Uppsala method is collaboratively being studied for TDF determination under the auspices of AOAC. The principle of the method is as follows. Desugared, defatted food sample undergoes Termamyl (Novo-Nordisk) treatment at 96°C for 30 min (50, personal communication). The suspension is cooled to 60°C and treated with amyloglucosidase overnight. Enzyme digestates are precipitated in 80% ethanol and centrifuged. After drying, residues are subjected to acid hydrolysis for liberation of neutral sugars and uronic acids. Neutral sugars are determined as alditol acetate derivatives by GLC, and uronic acids are determined by colorimetric methods.

An important point to note is that this method does not use any protein digestion step. A protein digestion step may critically affect the solubility of DF, because more DF is liberated into the incubation medium as protein is released from the sample (51).

5. Related Dietary Fiber Methods

5.1. Colorimetric Methods

The colorimetric determination of DF is faster, less expensive, and easier to perform when compared to other enzymatic-chemical approaches. In addition, its potential for automation is the highest among all fiber techniques, although automation techniques have not been developed in this area. The main disadvantage of the approach is that the method depends on nonspecific color reactions of reducing sugars, whose reactivities with a chromogen vary depending upon the types of sugars or uronic acids. Thus, it requires calibration against a reference method that gives detailed profiles of DF components. In this approach, it is assumed that the composition of any sample is very similar to that of a standard sugar mixture, and that correction factors for acid hydrolysis loss of individual DF components in the sample are similar to those of a standard solution during the acid hydrolysis step. Any deviations from these assumption may result in errors of varying degrees. Thus, for unknown samples, the method is considered unreliable. It does not provide detailed information on DF components. The method is still useful in a laboratory where known types of samples are analyzed routinely. More meaningful data interpretation of colorimetric results can be achieved by calibration against the values obtained by reference methods involving GLC or HPLC techniques.

5.1.1. Unavailable carbohydrate method of Southgate (1969)

Southgate (52) first obtained more purified DF residues from samples by precipitating enzymatic digestate in 80% ethanol after starch removal by takadiastase. This has been the basis of most current DF techniques using 80% ethanol as a precipitant of DF in enzymatic digestates. Southgate also fractionated food DF into its components, soluble and insoluble noncellulosic polysaccharides (NCP), cellulose, and lignin.

This method was used in constructing fiber tables since the 1970s in the United Kingdom. The method was a breakthrough technique at that time, although it was criticized for nonspecific color reactions for quantifying sugars.

5.1.2. Dimitrosalicylate (DNS) reduction method for nonstarch polysaccharides (NSP)

This method (53, 54) is based on the principle that DNS reagent is reduced to 3-amino-5-nitrosalicylic acid, and the reducing end of sugars or uronic acid is oxidized to show the color reaction. The degree of reactivity and the resulting color intensities are unique among monosaccharides, disaccharides, and uronic acids (55, 56). The NSP measured by this technique would be influenced by the presence of certain types of oligosaccharides, Maillard reaction products, tannins, furfurals, hydroxymethyl-furfural, and other interfering materials (57–60).

5.2. The GLC Method for Nonstarch Polysaccharides

Since its inception, the method has gone through several modifications without explanations on the chemical basis (61–64). Several different versions of the method have been acclaimed for their chemical accuracy. However, Mongeau and Brassard (65) found that these method changes critically affected the ratio of xylose/glucose present in NSP. Clarification is required on how all the method changes affected the NSP values and individual sugar components and should include explanations on a chemical basis. Information on reproducibility of individual sugar component values is required for scientific evaluation of this GLC method performance.

An important point to note is that soluble NSP content is calculated as the difference between total and insoluble dietary fiber in this method. Englyst et al. (personal communication) suggest that incomplete precipitation of soluble NSP can be avoided by calculating soluble NSP as the difference between total and insoluble NSP. However, Wolters et al. (66) reported that an overestimation of the measured amount of soluble NSP could be the reason why soluble NSP was calculated as the difference between total and insoluble NSP.

The effect of DMSO, which is used in this method to solubilize starch, should be further investigated, because it has also been recognized as a solvent for hemicelluloses (67–69).

5.3. HPLC Methods for TDF

Within the past several years, HPLC methods based on anion-exchange columns with PAD detectors were reported to characterize the monosaccharide composition of DF residues (70). Previous HPLC method development efforts have not been successful when using amino-bonded silica columns with RI detection because of insensitivity of the system and poor resolution of various monosaccharides (e.g., glucose, fructose, galactose, xylose, mannose, arabinose, and rhamnose). With the availability of PAD detectors, HP anion-exchange chromatography has allowed the quantitation of monosaccharides in hydrolyzed DF residues. Although this method seems promising, its precision needs to be evaluataed in a collaborative study.

References

(1)   Belitz, H.D., & Grosch, W. (1987) *Food Chemistry*, Springer Verlaj, Heidelberg, Germany

(2)   Hui, Y.H. (1992) *Enclyclopedia of Food Science and Technology*, Vol. 1, John Wiley & Sons, Inc., New York, NY

(3)   Aurand, L.W., Wood, A.E., & Wells, M.R. (1987) *Food Composition and Analysis*, Van Nostrand Reinhold Co., New York, NY

(4)   Food and Drug Administration (1993) "Food Labeling," *Fed. Register* **58**, 2302–2964

(5)   Trowell, H., Southgate, D.A.T., Wolever, T.M., Leeds, A.R., Gassull, M.A., & Jenkins, D.J.A. (1976) *Lancet* **i**, 967

(6)   Asp, N.G., Schweizer, T.F., Southgate, D.A.T., & Theander, O. (1992) in *Dietary Fiber - A Compenent of Food: Nutritional Function in Health and Disease*, T.F. Schweizer and C.A. Edwards (Eds), Springer-Verlag, London, UK, pp 57–101

(7)   Lee, S.C., Prosky, L., & Tanner, J.T. (1993) in *Quality Assurance for Analytical Laboratories*, M. Parkany (Ed.), Royal Society of Chemistry, London, UK, in press

(7)   Lee, S.C., Prosky, L., & Tanner, J.T. (1993) in *Quality Assurance for Analytical Laboratories*, M. Parkany (Ed.), Royal Society of Chemistry, London, UK, in press

(8)   U.S. Senate Select Committee on Nutrition and Human Needs (1977) *Deitary Goals for the United States*, U.S. Government Printing Office, Washington, DC

(9)   U.K. Department of Health (1991) *Dietary Reference Values for Food Energy and Nutrients for the United Kingdom*, Report of the Panel on Dietary Reference Values of the Committee on Medical Aspects of Food Policy, HMSO, London, UK

(10)   *Official Method of Analysis* (1990) 15th Ed., AOAC International, Arlington, VA

(11)   Scott, F.U. (1992) in *Food Analysis by HPLC*, L.M.L. Nellet (Ed.) Marcel Dekker, Inc., New York, NY, pp 259–274

(12)   Shaw, P.E. (1988) *Handbook of Sugar Separations in Foods by HPLC*, CRC Press, Inc., Boca Raton, FL

(13)   Ball, G.F.M. (1990) *Food Chem.* **35**, 117–152

(14)   Robards, K., & Whitelaw, M. (1986) *J. Chromatogr.* **373**, 81–110

(15)   Hurst, W.J., & Martin, R.A. Jr (1977) *J. Food Sci.* **44**, 892–895

(16)   Iverson, J.L., & Bueno, M.P. (1981) *J. Assoc. Off. Anal. Chem.* **64**, 139–143

(17)   DeVries, J.W., Heroff, J.C., & Egberg, D.C. (1979) *J. Assoc. Off. Anal. Chem.* **62**, 1292–1296

(18)   Verhaar, L.A.Th., & Kuster, B.F.M. (1982) *J. Chromatogr.* **234**, 57–64

(19)   D'Ambiose, M., Noel, D., & Hanai, T. (1980) *Carbohydr. Res.* **79**, 1–10

(20)   Wills, R.B.H., Francke, R.A., & Walker, B.P. (1982) *J. Agric. Food Chem.* **30**, 1242–1243

(21)   DeVries, J.W., Chang, H.L., Heroff, J.C., & Johnson, K.D. (1983) *J. Assoc. Off. Anal. Chem.* **66**, 197–198

(22)   Hurst, W.J., Martin, R.A. Jr., & Zopumas, B.L. (1979) *J. Food Sci.* **44**, 892–895

(23)   Vidal-Valverde, C., Martin-Billa, M.C., Herranz, J., & Rojas-Hidalgo (1981) *Z. Lebensm.-Unters. Forsch.* **172**, 93–95

(24)   Thean, J.E., & Funderburk, W.C. Jr. (1977) *J. Assoc. Off. Anal. Chem.* **60**, 838–841

(25)   Li, B.W., Schuhmann, P.J., & Wolf, W.R. (1983) *J. Agric. Food Chem.* **33**, 531–536

(26)   Black, L.T., & Glover, J.D. (1980) *J. Am. Oil Chem. Soc.* **57**, 143–144

(27)   Wilson, A.M., Work, T.M., Bushaway, A.A., & Bushway, R.J. (1981) *J. Food Sci.* **46**, 300–301

(28)   Martin-Villa, C., Vidal-Valverde, C., & Rojas-Hidalgo, E., (1982) *J. Food Sci.* **47**, 2086–2088

(29)   Smith, J.S., Villalobos, M.C., & Kottemann, C.M. (1986) *J. Food Sci.* **51**, 1373–1375

(30)   Verhaar, L.A., & Kuster, B.F.M. (1981) *J. Chromatog.* **210**, 279–290

(31)   Picha, D.H. (1985) *J. Food Sci.* **50**, 1189–90, 1210

(32)   Lee, Y.C. (1990) *Anal. Chem.* **189**, 151–162

(33)   Edwards, W.T., Pohl, C.A., & Rubin, R. (1987) *Tappi J.* **70**, 138–140

(34)   Rocklin, R.D., & Pohl, C.A. (1983) *J. Liq. Chromatogr.* **6**, 1577–1590

(35)   Joslyn, M.A. (1970) *Methods in Food Analysis, Physical, Chemical, and Instrumental Methods of Analysis*, 2nd Ed., Academic Press, New York, NY

(36)   Southgate, D.A.T. (1991) *Determination of Food Carbohydrates*, 2nd Ed., Applied Science Publishers, Ltd., London, UK

(37)   Anon. (1989) *Methods of Biochemical Analysis and Food Analysis*, Boehringer Mannheim GmbH Biochemica, Mannheim, Germany

(38)   Lee, S.C., & Prosky, L. (1992) *Cereal Foods World* **37**, 765–771

(39)   Prosky, L., Asp, N.-G., Furda, I., DeVries, J.W., Schweizer, T.F., & Harland, B. (1984) *J. Assoc. Off. Anal. Chem.* **67**, 1044–1052

(40)   Prosky, L., Asp, N-G., Schweizer, T.F., DeVries, J.W., & Furda, I. (1988) *J. Assoc. Off. Anal. Chem.* **71**, 1017–1023

(41)   Prosky, L., Asp, N.-G., Furda, I., DeVries, J.W., Schweizer, T.F., & Harland, B. (1992) *J. AOAC Int.* **75**, 360–367

(42)   Prosky, L., Asp, N.-G., Schweizer, T., DeVries, J.W., Furda, I., & Lee, S.C. (1993) *J. AOAC Int.* **76**, in press

(43)   Schweizer, T.F., Walter, E., & Venetz, P. (1988) *Mitt. Geb. Lebensmittelunters. Hyg.* **79**, 57–68

(44)   Lee, S.C., Prosky, L., DeVries, J.W. (1992) *J. AOAC Int.* **75**, 395–416

(45)   Kunita, N., Kojima, S., Kawamura, T., Kawai, S., Kamika, T., Tanaka, K., & Kawabata, N. (1988) *The 1988 Report of the Japan Association of Prefectural and Municipal Public Health Institutes*, General Office of the Osaka Public Health Institute, Osaka, Japan

(46)   Mongeau, R., & Brassard, R. (1990) *Cereal Foods World* **35**, 319–324

(47)   Prosky, L. (1992) *The Referee*, AOAC Internaional, Arlington, VA, **16**(11), p. 4

(48)   Li, B., & Cardozo, M.S. (1993) *J. AOAC Int.*, in press

(49)   Selvendran, R.R., Verne, A.V.F.V., & Faulks, R.M. (1989) "Plant Fibers," in *Modern Methods for Analysis of Dietary Fiber*, Vol. 10, H.F. Linskens & J.F. Jackson (Eds), Springer-Verlaj, Heildelberg, Germany, pp 234–259

(50)   Theander, O., & Westerlund, E.A. (1986) *J. Agric. Food Chem.* **34**, 330–336

(51)   Marlett, J.A., Chesters, J.G., Longaere, J.J., & Bodganski, J.J., (1989) *Am. J. Clin. Nutr.* **50**, 479–485

(52)   Southgate, D.A.T. (1969) *J. Sci. Food Agric.* **20**, 331–335

(53)   Englyst, H.N., & Hudson, G.J. (1987) *Food Chem.* **24**, 63–76

(54)   Englyst, H.N., Cummings, J.H., & Wood, R. (1990) Personal written communication; Novo-Nordisk Biolabs' Englyst Method Kit Manual

(55)   Marsden, W.L., Gray, P.P., Nippard, G.J., & Quinlan, M.R. (1982) *J. Chem. Technol. Biotechnol.* **32**, 1016–1022

(56)   Irick, T.J., West, K., Brownell, H., Schwald, W., & Saddler, J.N. (1988) *Appl. Biochem. Biotechnol.* **17**, 137–149

(57)   Breuil, C., & Saddler, T.N. (1985) *Enzyme Microb. Technol.* **7**, 327–332

(58)   Rivers, D.B., Gracheck, S.J., Woodford, L.C., & Emert, G.H. (1984) *Biotechnol. Bioeng.* **26**, 800–802

(59)   Forouhi, E., & Gunn, D. J. (1983) *Biotechnol. Bioeng.* **25**, 1905–1911

(60)   Leung, D.W., & Thorpe, T.A. (1984) *Phytochem.* **23**, 2949–2950

(61)   Englyst, H., Wiggins, H.S., & Cummings, J.H. (1982) *Analyst* **107**, 307–318

(62)   Englyst, H.N., & Cummings, J.H. (1984) *Analyst* **109**, 937–942

(63)   Englyst, H.N., Cummings, J., & Wood, R. (1987) *J. Assoc. Publ. Anal.* **25**, 59–71

(64)   Englyst, H.N., Cummings, J.H., & Wood, R. (1987) *J. Assoc. Publ. Anal.* **25**, 73–110

(65)   Mongeau, R., & Brassard, R. (1989) *J. Food Comp. Anal.* **2**, 189–199

(66)   Wolters, M.G.E., Verbeek, C., VanWesterop, J.M., Hermus, R.J.J., & Voragen, A.G.J. (1992) *J. AOAC Int.* **75**, 626–634

(67)   Hagglund, E., Lindberg, B., & McPherson, J. (1956) *Acta Chem. Scand.* **10**, 1160–1164

(68)   Gruppen, H., Hamer, R.J., & Voragen, A.G.J. (1991) *J. Cereal Sci.* **13**, 275

(69)   Woolard, G.R., Rathbone, E.B., & Novellie, L. (1977) *Phytochem.* **16**, 961–963

(70)   Garleb, K.A., Bourquin, L.D., & Fahey, G.C. (1989) *J. Agric. Food Chem.* **37**, 1287–1293

Chapter 5
Lipid Analysis

Donald E. Carpenter, Jerry Ngeh-Ngwainbi, and Sungsoo Lee

Introduction

The U.S. Food and Drug Administration (FDA) food labeling regulations, published in January 1993, defined fat for nutrition labeling purposes as the sum of fatty acids expressed as triglyceride equivalents. Saturated fat was defined as those fatty acids that do not contain a double bond. There are many official analytical methods for fat in various food matrixes and it is not always clear which method should be used. In addition, international definitions may differ from those adopted by the FDA, leading to different requirements for methodologies. This chapter presents the guidelines for selection of proper analytical methods of fat and other lipid components that are required to be or may be placed voluntarily on the nutrition panel. The issue relating to specific analyses are discussed, and guidance is provided for future methodologies.

Lipids

Lipids are a group of substances whose members are often unrelated physiologically or chemically but are classified together because of their solubility in nonpolar solvents. This group of naturally occurring compounds is not soluble in water but is soluble in organic solvents such as chloroform, benzene, ethers, and alcohol. The classical definition of total lipids refers to the sum of mono-, di-, and triglycerides, free fatty acids, phospholipids, glycolipids, terpenes, sterols, waxes, and other ether-soluble compounds (1). These are chemically distinct but have similar solubility characteristics. Over the years, many classification systems have been proposed based on chemical complexity or polarity characteristics. In 1920, Bloor (2) classified lipids into three groups: simple lipids (fats and waxes), compound lipids (phospholipids and glycolipids), and derived lipids (fatty acids, alcohols, and sterols). Other researchers classified lipids based on "acyl residue" or polarity characteristics. Three approaches generally accepted for lipid classification are presented in Table 1. The main (95%) component of dietary lipids are triglycerides, compounds composed of glycerol with three fatty acids esterified to glycerol. The remaining 5% of lipids in the diet consist of mono- and diglycerides, phospholipids, glycolipids, sterols, and others. The fatty acid moieties may be saturated or mono- or polyunsaturated (3). The triglycerides are classified by the nature of their esterified fatty acids. For example, a triglyceride containing polyunsaturated fatty acids is a polyunsaturated fat.

Table 1. Classification of Lipids:

Bloor Classification

I.   Simple lipids - esters of fatty acids with various alcohols.
    a.   Fats - esters of fatty acids with glycerol; commonly called triglycerides or neutral fats.
    b.   Waxes - esters of fatty acids with alcohols other than glycerol.

II.   Compound Lipids - esters of fatty acids containing groups in addition to an alcohol and fatty acid.
    a.   Phospholipids - substituted fats containing phosphoric acid and a nitrogen base.
        1.   Lecithin
        2.   Cephalin
        3.   Sphingomyelin

        b.   Glycolipids - compounds of fatty acids with a carbohydrate and containing a nitrogen base but, no phosphoric acid - cerebrosides.

        c.   Aminolipids, sulfolipids, etc. - groups of lipid compounds that, in many cases, are not well defined but contain amino acids, sulfur based compounds, etc.

III.   Derived lipids - substances derived from the above groups by hydrolysis.

        a.   Fatty acids of various series.

        b.   Sterols - mostly large molecular weight alcohols, found in nature combined with fatty acids; soluble in nonpolar solvents.

            1.   Cholesterol

            2.   Plant sterols

                (a)   Brassicasterol

                (b)   Sitosterol

                (c)   Campesterol

                (d)   Stigmasterol

Classification by Acyl Residue

I.   Simple lipids (not saponifiable)

Free fatty acids

Isoprenoid - lipids (sterols, carotenoid, monoterpenes)

II.   Acyl lipids constituents (saponifiable)

Triglyceride   three fatty acids plus glycerol

Diglyceride   two fatty acids plus glycerol

Monoglyceride   one fatty acid plus glycerol

Phospholipids   two fatty acids, phosphoric acid, a nitrogenous compound, and often glycerol.

Glycolipid   fatty acids, a nitrogen-containing alcohol, and a sugar

Sterol (free-form)   none

Sterol esters   one fatty acid and the free sterol

Waxes   long-chain fatty acids and monohydroxy alcohols of higher molecular weight

Classification by Polarity

I.   Neutral lipids   fatty acids (>C12) Mono-, di-, triacylglycerols, sterols, sterol esters, carotenoids, waxes, tocopherols.

II.   Polar lipids   glycerophospholipid, glyceroglycolipid, sphingophospholipid, sphingoglycolipid

III.   Tocopherols and quinone lipids are often considered as "redox lipids"

Fat

Fats are a subclass of lipids (4, 5), but 'fat' is often used interchangeably with 'lipid' (6, 7). Early descriptions were attempts to distinguish fat from other nutrients based on solubility in nonpolar solvents (4, 7). However, the debate continues as to which lipid compounds should be classified as fat. The National Academy of Science report on nutrition labeling (8) defines fats and oils as "complex organic molecules that are formed by combining three fatty acid molecules with one molecule of glycerol." The focus of nutritional concern has been the triglycerides, because they constitute most of the fat. For nutrition labeling purposes, fat has been variously defined as triglycerides, substances extracted with ether, or total lipids (8-10). On the other hand, the American Institute of Nutrition and the American Society of Clinical Nutrition define fat as "triglycerides and polar lipids" (11). This definition would include phospho- and glycolipids and is justified because they are also a source of fatty acids. The report of the Committee on Medical Aspects of Food Policy in the United Kingdom (12) included among its recommendations on dietary reference values (DRV) for fat the following. Total fat intake should be calculated from the sum of fatty acid intake and glycerol. Total fatty acid intake should, therefore, average 30%, and total fat intake including glycerol should average 33% of total dietary energy.

   All of the above mentioned reports clearly indicate that fatty acids, particularly from triglycerides, are a major nutrition concern in the diet. Triglycerides are a highly concentrated source of energy. The energy yield from complete oxidation of triglycerides is approximately 9 kcal/g, in contrast to about 4 kcal/g for carbohydrate and protein (1, 3, 13, 14). This large difference in caloric yield is due to the fatty acid moiety being in a higher state of reduction. Phospho-, di-, and monoglycerides containing only one or two fatty acid groups have lower caloric values than triglycerides containing three fatty acids (15). Thus, a more accurate assessment of caloric value is derived from total fatty acid content compared to total lipid. The declaration of "fat" as the sum of fatty acids expressed as triglycerides takes into account all the possible sources of fatty acids in a food.

Fatty Acids
Fatty acids are derived from glycerides, free fatty acids, phospho- and glycolipids, and sterol esters. Generally, they are straight chain, can be saturated, or contain double bonds. If unsaturated, the configuration at the double bond can be in the cis or trans form. The common names and International Union of Chemistry (IUC) names of fatty acids commonly present in food fats as well as their sources are presented in Table 2.

Table 2. Fatty Acids Commonly Found in Food

Common Name	IUC Name	Abbreviated Designation	Possible Sources
	Saturated Acids $C_nH_{2n+1}COOH$ Unbranched chain		
Butyric	butanoic	4:0	Butter
Caproic	hexanoic	6:0	Butter, coconut, and palm nut oils
Caprylic	octanoic	8:0	Butter, coconut, and palm nut oils
Capric	decanoic	10:0	Butter, coconut, and palm nut oils
Lauric	dodecanoic	12:0	Laurel oil, coconut oil, spermaceti
Myristic	tetradecanoic	14:0	Coconut oil, nutmeg oil, animal fats
Palmitic	hexadecanoic	16:0	Plant and animal fats
Stearic	octadecanoic	18:0	Plant and animal fats
Arachidic	eicosanoic	20:0	Peanut oil, rapeseed oil, butter, lard

Table 2. Fatty Acids Commonly Found in Food

Common Name	IUC Name	Abbreviated Designation	Possible Sources
Behenic	docosanoic	22:0	Oil of ben, peanut oil
Lignoceric	tetracosanoic	24:0	Peanut oil, glycolipids, phospholipids
Unsaturated Acids One double bond $C_nH_{2n-1}COOH$			
Myristoleic	*cis*-9-tetradecenoic	14:1(9)	Butter, sperm oil, fish liver oils
Palmitoleic	*cis*-9-hexadecenoic	16:1(9)	Butter, fish oils, animal fat
Oleic	*cis*-9-octadecenoic	18:1(9)	Plant and animal fats
Vaccenic	*cis*- and *trans*-11-octadecanoic	18:1 cort(11)	Butter
Gadoleic	*cis*-9-eicosenoic	20:1(9)	Brain phospholipids, fish liver oils
Erucic	*cis*-13-docosenoic	22:1(13)	Rapeseed oil, various seed oils
Two double bonds, C_nH_{2n-2}			
Linoleic	*cis*-9,*cis*-12-octadecadienoic	18:2(9,12)	Plant and animal fats
Three double bonds, $C_nH_{2n-5}COOH$			
Linolenic	Octadecatrienoic cis-9, cis-12, cis-15	18:3(9,12,15)	Linseed oil, mammal fats, fish liver oils
Eleostearic	9,11,13-octadecatrienoic	18:3(9,11,13)	Chinese wood oil, seed, fats
γ-Linolenic	6,9,12-octadecatrienoic	18:3(6,9,12)	Primrose seed oil
Four double bonds, $C_nH_{2n-7}COOH$			
Moroctic	4,8,12,15-octadecatetraenoic	18:4(4,8,12,15)	Fish oil
Arachidonic	5,8,11,14-eicosatetraenoic	20:4(5,8,11,14)	Animal phospholipids, fats
Five double bonds, C_nH_{2n-9}			
Timnodonic	4,8,12,15,18-eicosapentaenoic	20:5(4,8,12,15,18)	Sardine Oil
Clupanodonic	4,8,12,15,19-docosapentaenoic	22:5(4,8,12,15,19)	Brain and liver phospholipids

Table 2. Fatty Acids Commonly Found in Food

Common Name	IUC Name	Abbreviated Designation	Possible Sources
	Six double bonds, $C_nH_{2n-11}COOH$		
Nisinic	4,8,12,15,18,21-tetracosahexaenoic	20:6(4,8,12,15,18,21)	Sardine Oil

Fatty acids in higher plants and animals usually contain even numbers of carbon atoms, typically between 14 and 24, with 16- and 18- carbon fatty acids being most common. The hydrocarbon chain is almost invariably unbranched in fatty acids from higher plants and animals. The geometric configuration in the double bonds in most unsaturated fatty acids in nature is cis. The double bonds in polyunsaturated fatty acids are usually separated by at least one methylene group. Processed fats, especially hydrogenated fats, may contain a variety of geometric and position isomers. Tables 3A and 3B list fatty acid composition of common food fats. Table 4 also presents the major fatty acids that occur in food. Palmitic, oleic, and linoleic acids usually occur in high amounts, whereas the other acids are present in relatively small amounts. Unbranched, straight-chain molecules with an even number of carbon atoms, particularly palmitic, stearic and myristic acids, are predominant among the saturated fatty acids. The short-chain, low molecular weight fatty acids (<14:0) are commonly found only in fat and oil of dairy products, coconut and palmseed. In free form or esterified with low molecular weight alcohols, these aromatic substances occur only in small amounts in nature, particularly in fermented food products. Fatty acids with an odd number of carbon atoms, such as valeric (5:0) or enanthic (7:0) acids, are present in milk and a number of plant oils only in traces. Unsaturated fatty acids with an unusual structure are those with a trans double bond and/or conjugated double bonds. Such trans unsaturated acids are formed as artifacts in the industrial processing of oil or fat (heat treatment and oil hardening). However, there are natural trans unsaturated acids. For example, the trans analog of oleic acid is found in small amounts in mutton tallow. Conjugated fatty acids with diene, triene or tetraene systems occur frequently in several seed oils. Conjugated linoleic acid is reported to be anticarcinogenic (16).

Table 3A. Fatty Acid Composition of Common Food Fats, Animal Origin[a]

Trivial Name	Fatty Acid	Beef Tallow	Lard (Pork)	Butter
Butyric	4:0			2.6
Caproic	6:0			1.6
Caprylic	8:0			0.9
Capric	10:0		0.1	2.0
Lauric	12:0	0.9	0.2	2.3
Myristic	14:0	3.7	1.3	8.2
Palmitic	16:0	24.9	23.8	21.3
Stearic	18:0	18.9	13.5	9.8

Table 3A. Fatty Acid Composition of Common Food Fats, Animal Origin[a]

Trivial Name	Fatty Acid	Beef Tallow	Lard (Pork)	Butter
	16:1	4.2	2.7	1.8
Oleic	18:1	36.0	41.2	20.4
	20:1	0.3	1.0	
	22:1			
Linoleic	18:2	3.1	10.2	1.8
Linolenic	18:3	0.6	1.0	1.2

[a] (Amount in 100 gm, Edible Portion) Adapted from USDA Handbook No. 8.

Table 3B. Fatty Acid Composition of Common Food Fats, Plant Origin[a]

	Cocoa-Butter	Coconut Oil	Corn Oil	Cottonseed Oil	Olive Oil	Palm Oil	Peanut Oil	Soybean Oil
4:0								
6:0		0.6						
8:0		7.5						
10:0		6.0						
12:0		44.6				0.1		
14:0	0.1	16.8		0.8		1.0	0.1	0.1
16:0	25.4	8.2	10.9	22.7	11.0	43.5	9.5	10.3
18:0	33.2	2.8	1.8	2.3	2.2	4.3	2.2	3.8
16:1	0.2			0.8	0.8	0.3	0.1	0.2
18:1	32.6	5.8	24.2	17.0	72.5	36.6	44.8	22.8
20:1					0.3	0.1	1.3	0.2
22:1								
18:2	2.8	1.8	58.0	51.5	7.9	9.1	32.0	51.0
18:3	0.1		0.7	0.2	0.6	0.2		6.8

[a] (Amount in 100 gm, Edible Portion) Adapted from USDA Handbook No. 8.

Table 4. Structures and Distribution of Major Fatty Acids in Food[a]

Common Name	Abbreviated Designation	Structure[b]	Proportion (%)[c]
Myristic	14:0	$CH_3(CH_2)_{12}COOH$	2
Palmitic	16:0	$CH_3(CH_2)_{14}COOH$	11
Stearic	18:0	$CH_3(CH_2)_{16}COOH$	4
Oleic	18:1(9)	$CH_3(CH_2)_7\text{-}CH=CH\text{-}CH\text{-}(CH_2)_6\text{-}COOH$	34
Linoleic	18:2(9,12)	$CH_3(CH_2)_4\text{-}CH=CH\text{-}CH_2)_2\text{-}(CH_2)_6\text{-}COOH$	34
Linolenic	18:3(9,12,15)	$CH_3CH_2(CH=CH\text{-}CH_2)_3\text{-}(CH_2)_6\text{-}COOH$	5

[a] Adapted from Belitz, H.D. and Grosch, W. (1987) in *Food Chemistry*, Springer-Velag, Berlin, pp. 128–200.
[b] Numbering of carbon atoms starts with carboxyl group - C as number 1.
[c] A percentage estimate based on worldwide production of edible oils. These figures may not necessarily represent the percentage of fatty acids actually consumed.

Fat Substitutes

Recently, lipoid-like fat substitutes have been introduced. Two fundamental approaches have been used to design molecular fat substitutes that exhibit organoleptic properties that mimic triglycerides but have lower caloric content (17). The first approach was to design a molecule to which fatty acids were attached in a way that preserved their functional properties but hindered digestion. The second approach was to use the glycerol esterified with moieties that were not digested or fatty acids that contributed less than nine calories per gram. Conventional fat methods give an overestimate of the "true" fat content in products that contain ether extractable fat substitutes. To obtain the "true" value, an independent measurement of the fat substitute must be made and subtracted from the total value of the fat extract.

Low Fat Issues

FDA, through the Nutritional Labeling and Educational Act of 1990 (NLEA), has defined a number of descriptors to be used by food manufacturers. These include light, lite, free, low, reduced, and less (18). Fat-free according to these regulations can only be used for food with less than 0.5 g per serving. Low fat is applicable only for food with less than 3 g per serving and less than 1 g saturated fat per serving. Additionally, foods low in saturated fat cannot contribute more than 15% of the calories from saturated fat. Foods low in cholesterol cannot have more than 20 mg of cholesterol per serving.

In many other countries, the designation "fat-free" is reserved for foods with a fat level less than the U.S. limit of 0.5 g per serving. For example, in Canada, this level is 0.1% (19); in the United Kingdom, it is 0.15% (9), and for CODEX, the level is 0.15% (20). At these levels, the accuracy and precision of the method becomes very critical.

These descriptors and the levels defined demand that better analytical methods capable of accurately determining fat at these levels be developed. Current methods were developed and collaboratively studied at much higher levels. At very low fat levels, <0.5 g per serving, the methods are not accurate or precise.

Summary of NLEA Regulations

Final nutrition labeling regulations published in the *Federal Register* on January 6, 1993, defined total fat as the sum of all lipid fatty acids expressed as triglycerides, i.e., the fatty acids from mono-, di-, and triglycerides, fatty acids, phospholipids and sterol esters. Saturated fat is defined as the sum of all fatty acids containing no double bonds. Total fat and saturated fat are required on the label. Voluntary label declarations are as follows: polyunsaturated fat (*cis-, cis*-methylene interrupted polyunsaturated fatty acids) and monounsaturated fatty acids (*cis*-monounsaturated fatty acids). At this point in time, trans fatty acids are included with total fat and are declared as neither saturated nor unsaturated fatty acids. Total fat is declared as the sum of fatty acids expressed as triglycerides, and saturated fat and unsaturated fats are all expressed in grams per serving.

Introduction of Fat Methodology

A number of gravimetric methods are available for measuring fat and lipid. Fat along with moisture and protein is one of the proximate methods, and thus, it is dependent on the particular methodology. In addition to the methodology, product matrix factors affect the material that is extracted and called fat.

Method specific factors that influence fat extraction include the polarity of extraction solvents, sample pretreatment (whether or not samples are hydrolyzed or digested prior to extraction), and re-extraction or 'washing' procedures. Water insolubility (21–23) is generally the physical property used for the separation of lipids from proteins and carbohydrates. In practice, the wide range of polarity of lipids due to their various structures makes solvent selection quite difficult, and the choice of a solvent for fat and/or lipid extraction remains one of the most critical steps in the determination of fat in various matrixes. Complete extraction might occasionally require longer extraction times or a series or combination of solvents so that lipids can be solubilized from the matrix. Typical solvents include anhydrous diethyl ether, petroleum ether, chloroform–methanol, and tetrachloroethylene. All of these solvents extract triglycerides, whereas ether extracts simple glycerides such as mono-, di-, and triglycerides, sterols, and, usually, free fatty acids. The more polar solvents such as chloroform–methanol also extract the more polar lipids, including phospholipids, sterols, terpenes, waxes, hydrocarbons and other nonlipid materials (24, 25). Other solvents such as acetone, methylene chloride, and tetrachloromethane are used for more rapid fat analysis of meat products [*see Official Methods of Analysis* (1990) 15th ed., **948.16, 976.21, 985.15**].

Food matrixes are often treated prior to extraction to make the lipids more available to the solvent. These treatments include addition of alkali to solubilize protein or addition of acid to break emulsions or hydrolyze complex lipids and matrixes. The chloroform–methanol procedure for lipids (**983.23**) uses enzymes to hydrolyze protein, and polysaccharide matrixes making it easier to extract the lipids. Selectivity for fat can be improved by prewashing sugar-containing samples with water or drying the solvent and re-extracting with a solvent of different polarity, thus leaving behind the sugar by-products. Other factors might also affect the outcome of the fat value. Drying conditions must also be clearly specified and controlled to reduce loss of the more volatile lower chain fatty acids and to minimize air oxidation.

A number of matrix specific factors hinder the extraction of lipid or contribute to high fat values. Particle size, product moisture and formulation may all affect the extraction process. For example, the moisture content of a product and the extraction time may influence the amount of lipid removed from the product or sample (26). The type of processing or the addition of processing aids during the manufacture of a food product may encapsulate or hinder complete extraction of lipid. In addition, a number of studies indicate that the apparent fat content of many samples can be affected by particle size (24, 26). These studies report improved fat extraction in more finely ground samples regardless of the analytical method or solvent extraction system used. Apparently, the smaller particle size allows more intimate contact of the solvent with the lipid in the sample, thus improving extraction performance.

Because of the nonspecific nature of the fat extraction procedure, different components are probably extracted and called fat. For example, some polysaccharide or protein-containing matrixes may preclude complete removal of fat with ether and thus require more vigorous procedures, such as hydrolysis prior to extraction. However, acid hydrolysis of high carbohydrate-containing products prior to ether extraction may lead to high fat values due to extraction of sugar or sugar by-products (24). Re-extraction procedures to remove the unwanted by-products may give an accurate fat determination but will need verification. It has been recognized for some time that the ether extract is not necessarily pure fat (27). For example, oil-soluble flavor, vitamin, and color compounds may be extracted with nonpolar solvents and called fat. Recently, the AOAC INTERNATIONAL Task Force on Methods for Nutrient Labeling Analyses examined all Official Methods for fat and determined which of these methods are applicable (28, 29). They further recommended that AOAC work to validate methods that most accurately measure the food components defined as fat.

Chloroform–Methanol

There is general agreement that chloroform–methanol mixtures extract total lipid more exhaustively than other solvents currently in use and that the extract can be used for further lipid characterization. Cholesterol and other sterols are not destroyed in this process, and the probability of changing the structure of any particular class of lipid is very low. In addition, this method is widely used in the dairy industry as a extractant because of its effectiveness for very low carbon number fatty acids. The chloroform–methanol method (983.23) is an approved AOAC procedure for "composite foods and foods for which methods of analysis for fat or lipids are not specified. Method is for lipids, not fats (triglycerides and other ether-soluble materials)." This method uses Clarase (an enzyme mixture of the starch degrading α-amylase and a protease) prior to homogenization. The FDA Lipid Manual (10) uses a method that is similar to the AOAC procedure but omits the use of the enzyme pretreatment. In some baked products, this method does not extract all of the lipid material (30). Another similar procedure (969.24) uses the chloroform–methanol extraction without the enzyme pretreatment.

Although chloroform–methanol is an excellent solvent for lipids, it does have drawbacks. The ratio of chloroform–methanol–water is critical for quantitative extraction of fat (31); therefore, moisture must be determined before extraction. There are environmental concerns with the halogenated hydrocarbons, including the cost of disposal (32). Studies are underway to develop more environmentally friendly extraction procedures without sacrificing the efficiency of extraction. Tables 5A–5C list organic solvents that are toxic or carcinogenic to varying degrees.

Table 5A. Organic Solvents Used in Lipid Extraction Known to be Carcinogenic of Mutagenic[a]

Solvent	Mutagenic[b]	Carcinogenic[c]
1. Chloroform	X	X
2. Benzene	X	X
3. Toluene	X	X
4. Xylene	X	X
5. Carbon tetrachloride	X	
6. Most chlorinated hydrocarbons	X	Usually
7. Most aromatic hydrocarbons	X	Usually

Table 5B. Organic Solvents Used in Lipid Extraction Known to be Toxic[a]

Solvent	Toxicity
1. Chloroform	Medium
2. Benzene	High
3. Toluene	High
4. Xylene	Medium
5. Carbon tetrachloride	Low to medium
6. Methanol	High
7. Acetic acid	Concentrated, high; dilute, low
8. Diethyl ether	Medium
9. Ethyl alcohol	Low to medium

| 10. Chlorinated hydrocarbons | Medium to very high |
| 11. Aromatic hydrocarbons | Medium to very high |

Table 5C. Organic Solvents of Lower Environmental Hazard and Lower Toxicity[a]

Solvent	Comments
1. Saturated, streight-chain hydrocarbons (pentane, hexane, up to octane)	Chains > 8 carbons are poor lipid solvents; high boiling, lower chain are skin irritants
2. Isopropanol	May be toxic if consumed
3. Butanol, isobutanol	high boiling, inconvenient to remove from extract
4. Acetone	may be a skin irritant on contact, particularly the eyes
5. Isooctane	may be toxic if consumed
6. Methyl ethyl ketone	may be toxic if consumed, skin irritant
7. Cyclohexane	poor lipid solvent

[a]See references 16 and 17.
[b]Ames test.
[c]Animal studies.

Adapted from Sax, N.I. (1984) in *Dangerous Properties of Industrial Materials*, Van Reinhold, N.Y., pp. 1764-1765 and Torkelson, T.R. and V.K. Rowe (1978) in *Patty's Industrial Hygiene and Toxicology*, 3rd ed. Vol. IIB, G.D. Clayton and F.F. Clayton (Ed) John Wiley & Sons, N.Y., pp. 3462-3469.

Ether Extraction

The ether extraction methods are suitable for analysis of fat in animal feed (**920.39B,C**); raw cereal grains (**945.38F**) such as "wheat, rye, oats, corn, buckwheat, rice, barley, soybeans, and their products except cereal adjuncts, etc."; cereal adjuncts (**945.18A**); meats and meat products (**960.39**); confections (**963.15, 925.07, 920.177**); butter (**938.06**); nuts (**948.22**); and spices (**920.172**). These methods use diethyl or petroleum ether to remove the fat by continually refluxing ether (diethyl or petroleum) through the ground sample for 12–78 h. After extraction, the solvent is evaporated under a stream of nitrogen, and the residual fat is determined by gravimetric procedures. Modifications of the Soxhlet method use semi-automated equipment (Soxtec) to reduce the extraction time. These methods extract mono-, di-, and triglycerides, most sterols, and glycolipids. They may not quantitatively extract polar lipids such as phospholipids and free fatty acids, depending on the food matrix.

However, ether extraction methods may underestimate the amount of fat in some baked products (33). It was suggested that the ether solvent cannot penetrate the hard-baked glutinous particles formed during the baking process in order to extract all of the fat. In addition, the presence of water-soluble carbohydrates, certain sugars, glycerol, lactic acid, and similar materials is thought to interfere with the extraction of fat in the Soxhlet procedure (30). Samples known to contain any of these compounds should be washed to remove interfering substances and dried prior to determining the fat content. The extraction time, rinse time, sample particle size and the temperature of the condenser water may affect the results of the Soxtec method (26). At the present level of performance, all of the total fatty acids are not always extracted and may result in under-reporting of the fat content of some products. If samples are high in sugar, methods that use a water prewash such as **920.39C** and **945.38F** should be used. If samples are high in other nonfat ether extractable substances, Method **920.177**, which is for fat in confectionery products and uses a re-extraction procedure, should be used to remove the nonfat material.

Acid Hydrolysis

The acid hydrolysis Methods (**950.54, 925.32, 922.06, 925.12, 935.39D, 935.38, 948.15** and **945.44**) are used for fat determination in flour, baked, fruit-filled baked products, egg products including macaroni and salad dressings, process cheese, and a variety of other foods. Digestion with hydrochloric acid liberates fatty acids from glycerides, glyco- and phospholipids, and sterol esters. It also assists the extraction of fat by hydrolyzing protein and polysaccharide and disrupting cell walls. The released fat is usually extracted with a mixture of diethyl and petroleum ether. The solvents are evaporated, and the remaining residue is determined by gravimetric procedures.

Acid hydrolysis followed by ether extraction removes fat as neutral lipids. However, this procedure also extracts nonfat material such as glycerol, low molecular weight carbohydrates and their polymerization products (including sugars and their derivatives that are formed during acid digestion), amino acids, and urea salts. Results using these methods can be higher than true fat values. The contribution of extracted nonfat materials can become a serious issue in low fat products and can require accurate analyses for assignment of the proper descriptor. Separate clean-up steps capable of removing these artifacts include column chromatography, electrophoresis, dialysis and a second extraction with a solvent of different polarity. Modifications of these methods, including re-extraction with ether (**945.44**) to remove some of the nonlipid material yields acceptable results for many matrixes.

Alkaline Treatment (Roese-Gottlieb and Mojonnier)

Many of the dairy products, including cheese, use an alkali pretreatment, usually ammonium hydroxide, which breaks the fat emulsion, neutralizes any acid, and solubilizes the protein prior to extraction with ether. These methods are the Roese-Gottlieb (**905.02**) and Mojonnier (**989.05**) procedures, both of which use a mixed ether to extract an ethanolic ammonium solution. The Mojonnier flask/centrifugation aids in breaking the emulsion and subsequent removal of the ether layer. The Roese-Gottlieb procedure measures only the petroleum ether soluble fat, whereas the Mojonnier method measures the total fat extracted by a mixture of diethyl and petroleum ether.

Official Methods **933.05, 905.02, 989.05, 956.25, 920.111A, 952.06, 945.48G, 932.06, 920.125, 986.25** and **948.22** are all methods that involve alkali treatment prior to extraction. These methods are often used for the extraction of fat from dairy products such as milk, milk-based products, cheese, butter and milk-based infant formula.

Alkaline treatment is usually the first step in each of these methods, followed by an ether extraction of the lipids. Keister found that addition of ammonia makes fat removal more difficult and requires an extra extraction step that is included in the Official Method (34). Mono-, di-, and triglycerides and traces of other lipids are extracted quite efficiently from dairy products. The values obtained from these methods are crude fat values and should be adequate for normal fat containing products. These methods are recommended until new fatty acid methodology is available.

Volumetric Analysis for Fat (Babcock)

The Babcock procedures are used for many dairy products. They are fast and do not require extensive equipment or solvents. The principle of the procedures is to destabilize and release the fat from the emulsion with strong sulfuric acid. The less dense lipid material rises in the calibrated neck of the bottle and is measured volumetrically in a graduated and calibrated Babcock bottle (**920.111B, 989.04**). In addition, Method **964.12** is a Babcock procedure that measures fat in fish products. When the main sources of fat are glycerides, the fat values should be acceptable. However, the Babcock method for milk gives a slightly higher value for fat when compared to the modified Mojonnier method (35). For other products, validation is required to ensure that all of the fatty acids are being measured.

Spectroscopic-Based Fat Methods

Other methods for fat determination are based on physical phenomena such as turbidimetry and infrared (IR) spectroscopy. Examples of this type are Methods **969.16** and **972.16** for analysis of fat in milk. In both the turbidimetric and IR methods, the light scattering must be carefully controlled. The turbidimetric procedure eliminates the light scattering from casein micelles by addition of ethylenediaminetetraacetic acid and homogenization to make uniform-sized fat globules. These methods rely on a standard reference method and must be calibrated against methodology that is validated for the new NLEA definition of fat. Fat must be well-determined by the reference method, because this can be a significant source of error in the spectroscopic procedures.

Fatty Acids

The fatty acid methods are used to determine saturated, unsaturated, and polyunsaturated fatty acid content for several labeling purposes. In addition, because of NLEA and the new definition of fat, total fat methods are being developed based on the sum of fatty acids. The fatty acid methods start with an isolated oil or fat. Modification or adaptation may be required for some food matrixes. The classical procedure for obtaining fatty acids from fats and oils has been through saponification. This produces an alkali salt of the fatty acids and glycerol. The fatty acids are subsequently obtained by acidification of the mixture. These procedures are slow at room temperature and the double bonds tend to isomerize at elevated temperatures. Transmethylation procedures are more popular and methyl esters have lower boiling points than the corresponding acids. Sheppard gives a general extraction scheme (10) for foods, and care must be taken to achieve a representative profile of fatty acids in the extract. Method **969.33** deals with the preparation of the fatty acid methyl esters, and **963.22** deals with the chromatography of the methyl esters, using a packed column. The method is applicable for carbon numbers 8–24 and, thus, is not adequate under the new NLEA regulations for foods containing shorter chain fatty acids. The new NLEA definition for saturated fatty acids includes all fatty acids that do not contain a double bond. The preparation of the methyl esters is not suitable for conjugated polyunsaturated fatty acids due to partial destruction of these groups. The preferred sample size for chromatography on the packed column is about 350 mg. Low fat samples will require a large initial sample size.

A chromatographic procedure using a polar, carbowax 20 m bonded-phase capillary column has been developed and can measure fatty acids with carbon numbers 4–24. However, the method has not been subjected to the AOAC collaborative study process (36). The methyl esters of the short chain fatty acids are volatile and care must be exercised to ensure quantitative recovery. Because of their lower volatility, the butyl esters may be the preferred route of derivitization. There are several American Oil Chemists' Society (AOCS) procedures for fatty acid determination that may be applicable for some food products. These include the method for marine oils (AOCS Ce1b-89) applicable to carbon numbers 14–24; however, it may be applicable to less than 8 carbons if care is taken to retain the volatile fatty acid esters. AOCS method Ce1c-89 measures the cis,cis- and trans-isomers, and method Ce1d-91 is for the determination of n-3 and n-6 unsaturated fatty acids in vegetable oils. All of these are capillary gas chromatographic methods.

For fat analysis to be reliable, all the required steps from extraction, derivatization and final chromatographic analysis must be done accurately and reproducibly. A total lipid extract is still the most crucial step in the procedure, but subsequent conversion into the corresponding fatty acid methyl esters or fatty acids is equally critical for the success of the entire method. To meet the new fat definition, the fatty acid values on a whole product basis must be converted to triglycerides. The factors for converting the fatty acid methyl esters into the corresponding triglycerides are outlined in Table 6. In expressing fatty acids or fatty acid methyl esters as triglycerides, different factors have to be used. In the past, it was generally acceptable to use an average factor for all fatty acids. The error associated with the use of an average is quite small, but in doing such calculations, the nature and profile of the acids must first be determined quantitatively.

Table 6. Fatty acid (FA), fatty acid ester (ME), and triglyceride (TRIG) molecular weights and factors for conversion of fatty acids and fatty acid esters to their corresponding triglycerides[a]

ID[c]	Molecular Weight[b]			Conversion Factor	
	FA	ME	TRIG	FA→TRIG	ME→TRIG
Saturated Fatty Acid Series					
4:0	86.108	102.135	302.373	1.143948	0.986841
5:0	102.135	116.162	344.454	1.124179	0.988430
6:0	116.162	130.189	386.535	1.109184	0.989677
7:0	130.189	144.216	428.616	1.097420	0.990681
8:0	144.216	158.243	470.697	1.087944	0.991507
9:0	158.243	172.270	512.778	1.080149	0.992198
10:0	172.270	186.297	554.859	1.073623	0.992786
11:0	186.297	200.324	596.940	1.068079	0.993291
12:0	200.324	214.351	639.021	1.063312	0.993730
13:0	214.351	228.378	681.102	1.059169	0.994115
14:0	228.378	242.405	723.183	1.055535	0.994456
15:0	242.405	256.432	765.264	1.052322	0.994759
16:0	256.432	270.459	807.345	1.049460	0.995031
17:0	270.459	284.486	849.426	1.046894	0.995276
18:0	284.486	298.513	891.507	1.044582	0.995498
19:0	298.513	312.540	933.588	1.042487	0.995700
20:0	312.540	326.567	975.669	1.040580	0.995884
21:0	326.567	340.594	1017.750	1.038837	0.996054
22:0	340.594	354.621	1059.831	1.037238	0.996210
23:0	354.621	368.648	1101.912	1.035765	0.996354
24:0	368.648	382.675	1143.993	1.034404	0.996488
Monoenoic Fatty Acid Series					
4:1	86.108	100.135	296.373	1.147292	0.986578
5:1	100.135	114.162	338.454	1.126659	0.988227
6:1	114.162	128.189	380.535	1.111097	0.989515

Table 6. Fatty acid (FA), fatty acid ester (ME), and triglyceride (TRIG) molecular weights and factors for conversion of fatty acids and fatty acid esters to their corresponding triglycerides[a]

ID[c]	Molecular Weight[b]			Conversion Factor	
	FA	ME	TRIG	FA→TRIG	ME→TRIG
7:1	128.189	142.216	422.616	1.098940	0.990550
8:1	142.216	156.243	464.697	1.089181	0.991398
9:1	156.243	170.270	506.778	1.081175	0.992107
10:1	170.270	184.297	548.859	1.074488	0.992707
11:1	184.297	198.324	590.940	1.068818	0.993223
12:1	198.324	212.351	633.021	1.063951	0.993671
13:1	212.351	226.378	675.102	1.059727	0.994063
14:1	226.378	240.405	717.183	1.056026	0.994409
15:1	240.405	254.432	759.264	1.052757	0.994718
16:1	254.432	268.459	801.345	1.049848	0.994994
17:1	268.459	282.486	843.426	1.047244	0.995242
18:1	282.486	296.513	885.507	1.044898	0.995467
19:1	296.513	310.540	927.588	1.042774	0.995672
20:1	310.540	324.567	969.669	1.040842	0.995859
21:1	324.567	338.594	1011.750	1.039077	0.996031
22:1	338.594	352.621	1053.831	1.037458	0.996189
23:1	352.621	366.648	1095.912	1.035968	0.996334
24:1	366.648	380.675	1137.993	1.034952	0.996469
Dienoic Fatty Acid Series					
8:2	140.216	154.234	458.697	1.090453	0.991286
9:2	154.243	168.270	500.778	1.082227	0.992013
10:2	168.270	182.297	542.859	1.075373	0.992627
11:2	182.297	196.324	584.940	1.069573	0.993154
12:2	196.324	210.351	627.021	1.064602	0.993611
13:2	210.351	224.378	669.102	1.060294	0.994010
14:2	224.378	238.405	711.183	1.056525	0.994363

Table 6. Fatty acid (FA), fatty acid ester (ME), and triglyceride (TRIG) molecular weights and factors for conversion of fatty acids and fatty acid esters to their corresponding triglycerides[a]

ID[c]	Molecular Weight[b]			Conversion Factor	
	FA	ME	TRIG	FA→TRIG	ME→TRIG
15:2	238.405	252.432	753.264	1.053199	0.994676
16:2	252.432	266.459	795.345	1.050243	0.994956
17:2	266.459	280.486	837.426	1.047598	0.995208
18:2	280.486	294.513	879.507	1.045218	0.995437
19:2	294.513	308.540	921.588	1.043064	0.995644
20:2	308.540	322.567	963.669	1.041107	0.995833
21:2	322.567	336.594	1005.750	1.039319	0.996007
22:2	336.594	350.621	1047.831	1.037680	0.996167
23:2	350.621	364.648	1089.912	1.036173	0.996314
24:2	364.648	378.675	1131.993	1.034781	0.996451
Trienoic Fatty Acid Series					
8:3	138.216	152.243	452.697	1.091762	0.991172
9:3	152.243	166.270	494.778	1.083308	0.991917
10:3	166.270	180.297	536.859	1.076280	0.992546
11:3	180.297	194.324	578.940	1.070345	0.993084
12:3	194.324	208.351	621.021	1.065267	0.993549
13:3	208.351	222.378	663.102	1.060873	0.993956
14:3	222.378	236.405	705.183	1.057034	0.994315
15:3	236.405	250.432	747.264	1.053649	0.994633
16:3	250.432	264.459	789.345	1.050644	0.994918
17:3	264.459	278.486	831.426	1.047958	0.995174
18:3	278.486	292.513	873.507	1.045543	0.995405
19:3	292.513	306.540	915.588	1.043359	0.995616
20:3	306.540	320.567	957.669	1.041375	0.995807
21:3	320.567	334.594	999.750	1.039564	0.995983
22:3	334.594	348.621	1041.831	1.037906	0.996145

Table 6. Fatty acid (FA), fatty acid ester (ME), and triglyceride (TRIG) molecular weights and factors for conversion of fatty acids and fatty acid esters to their corresponding triglycerides[a]

	Molecular Weight[b]			Conversion Factor	
ID[c]	FA	ME	TRIG	FA→TRIG	ME→TRIG
23:3	348.621	362.648	1083.912	1.036380	0.996294
24:3	362.648	376.675	1125.993	1.034973	0.996432
Tetraenoic Fatty Acid Series					
11:4	178.297	192.324	572.940	1.071134	0.993012
12:4	192.324	206.351	615.021	1.065946	0.993487
13:4	206.351	220.378	657.102	1.061463	0.993901
14:4	220.378	234.405	699.183	1.057511	0.994266
15:4	234.405	248.432	741.264	1.054107	0.994590
16:4	248.432	262.459	783.345	1.051052	0.994879
17:4	262.459	276.486	825.426	1.048324	0.995139
18:4	276.486	290.513	867.507	1.045872	0.995374
19:4	290.513	304.540	909.588	1.043657	0.995587
20:4	304.540	318.567	951.669	1.041646	0.995781
21:4	318.567	332.594	993.750	1.039813	0.995959
22:4	332.594	346.621	1035.831	1.038134	0.996123
23:4	346.621	360.648	1077.912	1.036590	0.996273
24:4	360.648	374.675	1119.993	1.035167	0.996413
Pentaenoic Fatty Acid Series					
16:5	246.432	260.459	777.345	1.051467	0.994840
17:5	260.459	274.486	819.426	1.048695	0.995104
18:5	274.486	288.513	861.507	1.046207	0.995342
19:5	288.513	302.540	903.588	1.043960	0.995558
20:5	302.540	316.567	945.669	1.041922	0.995754
21:5	316.567	330.594	987.750	1.040064	0.995935
22:5	330.594	344.621	1029.831	1.038364	0.996100
23:5	344.621	358.648	1071.912	1.036803	0.996253

Table 6. Fatty acid (FA), fatty acid ester (ME), and triglyceride (TRIG) molecular weights and factors for conversion of fatty acids and fatty acid esters to their corresponding triglycerides[a]

ID[c]	Molecular Weight[b]			Conversion Factor	
	FA	ME	TRIG	FA→TRIG	ME→TRIG
24:5	358.648	372.675	1113.993	1.035363	0.996394
Hexaenoic Fatty Acid Series					
16:6	244.432	258.459	771.345	1.051888	0.994800
17:6	258.459	272.486	813.426	1.049072	0.995068
18:6	272.486	286.513	855.507	1.046546	0.995309
19:6	286.513	300.540	897.588	1.044267	0.995528
20:6	300.540	314.567	939.669	1.042201	0.995727
21:6	314.567	328.594	981.750	1.040319	0.995910
22:6	328.594	342.621	1023.831	1.038598	0.996077
23:6	342.621	356.648	1065.912	1.037018	0.996232
24:6	356.648	370.675	1107.993	1.035562	0.996374

Example: Calculation of a typical conversion factor for the calculation of triglyceride from fatty acid data
The conversion of palmitic to its equivalent triglyceride weight.

Molecular weight of palmitic acid: 256.432
Molecular weight of tripalmitin: 807.345

Three molecules of palmitic acid are required to form one molecule of tripalmitin. Therefore, the amount of palmitic acid required is 3(256.432) for a total of 769.296.
Calculation of the conversion factor:

$$\frac{Mol.\ weight\ of\ tripalmitin}{3(Mol.\ weight\ of\ palmitic\ acid)} = \frac{807.345}{3(256.432)} = 1.049460$$

Application of conversion factor:

100 grams of palmitic acid found in sample.
How many grams of tripalmitin is this 100 grams of palmitic acid equivalent to?
The solution is as follows:
100(1.049460) = 104.946 grams of tripalmitin

[a] Adapted from Sheppard (10).
[b] Molecular weights based on atomic weights of 1.008, 16.000, and 12.011, respectively, for hydrogen, oxygen, and carbon.
[c] Number of carbons in fatty acid chain:number of double bonds.

In the U.S. food labeling regulations (18), FDA has defined fat as the sum of fatty acids expressed as triglyceride equivalents for nutrition labeling purposes. This regulation has intensified the need for up-to-date information on the fatty acid contents of food and triglyceride equivalents.

In the U.S. Department of Agriculture Handbook No. 8, total lipids, their fatty acid composition and lipid conversion factors are listed for the majority of food matrixes.

Conjugated polyunsaturated fatty acids are analyzed by AOAC Official Methods **979.19** or **957.13**. The former procedure measures the *cis-,cis*-methylene interrupted polyunsaturated fatty acids. The *cis-,cis*-polyunsaturated fatty acids are oxidized by lipoxidase to the hydroperoxides and determined by spectrophotometry at 234 nm. As with the chromatographic procedures, the method starts with an isolated oil or fat and care must be exercised in extraction of the fat from the food matrix. The latter is a spectrophotometric method for fats and oils and detects conjugated polyunsaturated fatty acids by UV absorption. It is applicable to fats and oils containing cis isomers and is not applicable (or with caution) to fats and oils containing trans isomers.

Cholesterol

The AOAC Official Method for cholesterol, **976.26**, is applicable for all foods with a sensitivity of at least 10 mg of cholesterol per 100 g. This procedure is a mixed solvent extraction followed by saponification. The derivatized cholesterol is chromatographed on a packed column. Another method is currently under collaborative study. It involves direct saponification (which may help release tightly bound cholesterol) prior to extraction, derivatization and chromatography on a capillary column (37). Other methods that have not been through the AOAC collaborative study procedure but that may be more easily automated are by Tsui (38) and Oles et al. (39). These procedures involve direct saponification followed by solid-phase extraction prior to derivatization and separation by capillary chromatography.

Future Fat Methods

The current fat methodologies should at least be used until new validated procedures are in place to meet the NLEA definition of fat. Because of their speed and cost-effectiveness, the traditional solvent methods will continue to be used even after validated total fat methods based on fatty acids are in place. However, the solvent extraction methods may need to be modified to ensure accuracy for the measurement of total fatty acids. Extraction of fat from food is not always easy. A total lipid extract is crucial to accurate total fat analysis. The degree of difficulty in obtaining a total lipid extract will vary depending on the solvent system used and the nature of the sample. A complete extraction protocol needs to be established for each case. Depending on the matrix and the method of extraction, the extracts may contain varying amounts and kind of nonlipid material. The challenge for the analytical chemist is to separate out the nonlipid impurities from the extract and accurately determine the total fatty acid content. This may be accomplished via chromatography of the fatty acid derivatives or by washing or re-extraction procedures.

Supercritical fluid extraction is an emerging technology that shows promise as a fat extractant. This technique offers the luxury of a "solvent-less" extraction by using liquid carbon dioxide as an extractant. This is an active area of study, and more work needs to be done to demonstrate recovery and reliability for a wide range of food matrixes. Instrumentation is expensive but can be automated to reduce operating costs.

References

(1)   Linscheer, W.G., & Vergroesen, A.J. (1988) in *Lipids In Modern Nutrition in Health and Disease*, M.E. Shils and V.R. Young (Eds), Lea & Febriger, Philadelphia, PA, pp. 72–107

(2)   Bloor, W.R. (1920) *Proc. Soc. Exp. Biol. Med.* **17**, 138–140

(3)   Stryer, L. (1981) in *Biochemistry, 2nd Edition*, W.H. Freeman and Company, New York, NY, pp. 383–406

(4)   Aurand, L.W., Woods, A.E., & Wells, M.R. (1987) in *Food Composition and Analysis*, Van Nostrand Rienhold Co., New York, NY, pp. 178–231

(5)   National Academy of Sciences (1989) *Diet and Health, Implications for Reducing Chronic Disease Risk*, Report of the Committee on Diet and Health, National Research Council, National Academy Press, Washington, DC

(6)   Marini, D. (1992) in *Food Analysis by HPLC*, L.M.L. Nollet (Ed.), Marcel Dekker, Inc., New York, NY, pp. 169–240

(7)   DeMan, J.M. (1991) in *Encyclopedia of Food Science and Technology* 2, Y.H. Hui (Ed.), John Wiley & Sons, Inc., New York, NY, pp. 818–828

(8)   National Academy of Sciences (1990) *Nutritional Labeling: Issues and Directions for the 1990's*, Report of the Committee on the Nutrition Components of Food Labeling, Food and Nutrition Board, Institute of Medicine, National Research Council, National Academy Press, Washington, DC

(9)   Saccomandi, V. (1990) *Off. J. Eur. Comm.* **276**, 40–44

(10)   Sheppard, A.J. (1992) *Lipid Manual, Methodology Suitable for Fatty Acid - Cholesterol Analysis*, Wm. C. Brown Publishers, Dubuque, IA

(11)   American Institute of Nutrition and American Society for Clinical Nutrition (1990) *Position Statement on Nutrition Labeling*, Bethesda, MD

(12)   The United Kingdom Department of Health (1991) *Dietary Reference Values for Food Energy and Nutrients for the United Kingdom,* Report of the Panel on Dietary Reference Values of the Committee on Medical Aspects of Food Policy, HMSO, London, England

(13)   National Academy of Sciences (1989) *Recommended Dietary Allowances*, 10th Ed., The Report of the Subcommittee on the Tenth Edition of the RDAs, Food and Nutrition Board, Commission on Life Sciences National Research Council, National Academy Press, Washington, DC

(14)   Whitney, E.N., & Rolfes, S.R. (1993) *Understanding Nutrition*, 6th Ed., West Publishing Co., St. Paul, MN, pp. 1–26

(15)   Krisnamoorthy, R.V., Venkataramiah, A., Lakshmi, G.J., & Biesiot, P. (1979) *J. Agric. Food Chem.* **27**, 1125–1127

(16)   Ha, Y.L., Grimm, N.K., & Pariza, M.W. (1988) *Carcinogenesis* **8**, 1881–1887

(17)   Best, D. (1992) *Prepared Foods* **162**, 59–62

(18)   *Federal Register* (1993) U.S. Government Printing Office **58**, 2079

(19)   Anonymous (1988) *Nutritional Labeling Handbook*, Food Division, Consumer Products Branch, Consumer and Corporate Affairs, Canada, December

(20)   World Health Organization (1992) Codex Alimentarius Commission, Proposed Draft General Guidelines on Nutrition and Health Claims for Food Labeling, Food and Agriculture Organization of the United Nations, CX/NFSOU 92/7

(21)   Bender, A.E. (1982) *Dictionary of Nutrition and Food Technology*, Butterworths, London, England, 5th Ed., p. 97

(22)   Sonntag, N.O.V. (1979) in *Baily's Industrial Oil and Fat Products*, D. Swern (Ed.), Interscience Publishers, New York, NY, pp. 1–98

(23)   Lundberg, W.O. (1951) in *The Chemistry and Technology of Food and Food Products*, Jacobs, N.B. (Ed.), Vol. 1, Interscience Publishers, Inc., New York, NY, pp. 104–138

(24)   McGhee, J.E., Black, L.T., & Brekke, O.L. (1974) *Cereal Chem.* **51**, 472–477

(25)   Hubbard, W.D., Shepard, A.J., Newkirk, D.R., Prosser, A.R., & Osgood, T. (1977) *J. Amer. Oil Chem. Soc.* **54**, 81–83

(26)   Finney, K.F., Pomeranz, Y., & Hoseney, R.C. (1976) *Cereal Chem.* **53**, 383–338

(27)   Lepper, H.A., & Waterman, H.C. (1925) *J. Assoc. Off. Agric. Chem.* **8**, 705–710

(28)   *The Referee* (1992) AOAC INTERNATIONAL Task Force on Methods for Nutrient Labeling Analyses Final Report, AOAC INTERNATIONAL, Arlington, VA, **16**(7), pp. 1, 7–12

(29)   *The Referee* (1992) AOAC Official Methods and Determination of Fat, AOAC INTERNATIONAL, Arlington, VA, **16**(9), pp. 1, 5-9

(30)   Pomeranz, Y., & Meloan, C.E. (1987) in *Food Analysis Theory and Practice*, 2nd Ed. pp. 691-748

(31)   Daugherty, C.E., & Lento, H.G. (1983) *J. Assoc. Off. Anal. Chem.* **66**, 927-932

(32)   Perkins, E.G. (1991) in *Analysis of Fats, Oils and Lipopriteins*, E.G. Perkins (Ed.), American Oil Chemists Society, Champaign, IL, pp. 1-59

(33)   Hertwig, R. (1923) *J. Assoc. Off. Agric. Chem.* **6**, 508-510

(34)   Keister, J.T. (1922) *J. Assoc. Off. Agric. Chem.* **5**, 507-509

(35)   Barbano, D.M., Clark, J.L., & Dunham, C.E. (1988) *J. Assoc. Off. Anal. Chem.* **71**, 898-914

(36)   Keith Meyer, Personal Communication

(37)   Adams, M.L., Sullivan, D.M., Smith, R.L., & Richter, E.F. (1986) *J. Assoc. Off. Anal. Chem.* **69**, 844-846

(38)   Tsui, I.C. (1989) *J. Assoc. Off. Anal. Chem.* **72**, 421-424

(39)   Oles, P., Gates G., Kensinger, S., Patchell, J., Schumacher, D., Showers, T., & Silcox, A. (1990) *J. Assoc. Off. Anal. Chem.* **73**, 724-728

Chapter 6
Proximate and Mineral Analysis

Darryl M. Sullivan

Introduction

For the most part, the analysis of food products for their proximate composition is fairly well defined. There are a number of methods that can be used for the determination of protein, moisture, and ash. The determination of fat under the new Nutrition Labeling and Education Act (NLEA) regulations is very complicated and is discussed in detail in Chapter 5, *Lipid Analysis*. Analyses of soluble, insoluble, and total dietary fiber and specific carbohydrates such as sugars are discussed in Chapter 4, *Carbohydrate/Dietary Fiber Analysis*. A number of new options for calculating carbohydrates and calories will be presented.

AOAC has a wide variety of methods for the determination of essential cations and trace elements in food. A number of atomic absorption spectrophotometry (AAS) and inductively coupled argon plasma atomic emission spectrophotometry (ICP) procedures will be discussed in this chapter. Regardless of which technology an analyst uses to measure inorganic analytes, the sample oxidation procedures play a major role in the precision and accuracy of these assays. Depending on the type of food being analyzed, a number of chemical or thermal oxidation procedures will provide adequate sample preparation for inorganic analysis.

Protein

All types of protein, from both animal and plant sources, are made up of about 20 common amino acids. The relative compositions of these amino acids vary with each protein source. Amino nitrogen accounts for approximately 16% of the weight of these various proteins. Methods for the determination of protein measure the amount of nitrogen present in the food and use this ratio (N $\times$ 6.25) to calculate the quantity of protein. Specific food proteins have greater (cereals) or lesser (milk) percentages of nitrogen. Individual nitrogen factors can be used depending on the type of food being analyzed (1).

The most commonly used procedure for the determination of protein is the Kjeldahl method. In this procedure, the food sample is digested with sulfuric acid in the presence of a catalyst, and the liberated ammonia is distilled and measured titrimetrically or colorimetrically. Many of the AOAC Kjeldahl methods use a mercury catalyst (**981.10, 955.04, 977.02, 978.04, 920.152, 920.87, 945.18B, 950.36, 930.33, 930.29, 928.08, 977.14, 950.48,** and **935.39**). Because of recent disposal problems associated with mercury, several methods were approved that use a copper based catalyst (**991.20, 991.22,** and **991.23**). Studies are in progress to investigate the potential for use of copper based catalysts in many of the other AOAC Official Methods.

The most current protein methods use combustion procedures (**992.15** for meat products and **990.03** for animal feeds). Combustion methods determine nitrogen released at high temperature into pure oxygen and then measure the nitrogen by thermal conductivity. These procedures can be highly automated and do not have waste disposal problems. Other types of protein methods, which are acceptable for dairy products, include dye binding (**967.12** and **975.17**) and infrared spectrophotometry (**975.18** and **972.16**).

Corrected Protein

To list a percent daily value (DV) for protein on a nutrition label, a "corrected protein" must be determined. The total amount of protein in a food product is corrected using the "amino acid score" and the "protein digestibility." These two factors combine to derive the Protein Digestibility Corrected Amino Acid Score (PDCAAS).

The amino acid score is calculated from an amino acid profile. Method **982.30** is an acceptable procedure. An analyst must use the "limiting" amino acid to determine the amino acid score. (The essential amino acid in the least concentration.)

Protein digestibility factors for some common types of protein can be found in the NLEA regulations (2). The digestibility of all other types of protein must be determined using a rat bioassay (3). Method **991.29** is the AOAC rat bioassay procedure.

Moisture

The vast majority of methods for the determination of moisture are based on oven drying techniques. Even though the steps to these procedures vary widely, the procedures themselves are not truly measuring water. Instead, they are measuring "volatile" matter (4).

Oven moisture methods use convection, forced air, or vacuum ovens. Some of the methods provide parameters for several types of ovens. The temperatures used for drying are matrix specific and fall into three categories: 60°C for high sugar samples, 70°C for vegetable samples, and 100–135°C for all other food types. The time specified for drying depends on the type of oven used and the oven temperature.

Two types of methods do not rely on weight loss after drying but instead measure water directly. The first type of direct moisture procedure is the Karl Fischer method (**977.10** and **984.20**). These procedures titrate against water that is solubilized in methanol or a similar solvent. The second type of direct moisture determination is accomplished with toluene distillation (**925.04** and **986.21**). When using these methods, water is distilled away from the food after suspension in a toluene solution.

Other types of moisture determinations include conductivity (**972.20**), microwave oven drying (**985.14** and **985.26**), and an infrared spectroscopy (**972.16**).

Ash

The percent ash in food products is determined by weight loss after ignition at 525–550°C. Some types of food matrices call for slightly higher temperatures, and numerous sample preparation techniques are recommended for certain types of food products.

Fat

See Chapter 5, *Lipid Analysis*.

Dietary Fiber

See Chapter 4, *Carbohydrate/Dietary Fiber Analysis*.

Total and Other Carbohydrates

Total carbohydrate content is calculated by subtracting the sum of the crude protein, total fat, moisture, and ash from the total weight of the food. The term "other carbohydrate" is defined as the difference between total carbohydrate and the sum of dietary fiber, sugars, and sugar alcohol (if measured).

Calories

The calorie value for nutrition labeling can be determined by any one of four different ways: calculation using the general factors of protein × 4, carbohydrates × 4, and fat × 9; calculation subtracting the insoluble dietary fiber using protein × 4, (carbohydrates − IDF) × 4, and fat × 9; calculation using the specific food factors for particular foods or ingredients approved by the U.S. Food and Drug Administration (5); and using bomb calorimetry (6) and subtracting 1.25 calories per gram of protein to correct for incomplete digestibility.

Calcium

Dairy products contribute more than 55% of the calcium intake of a normal population (7). Other good sources of calcium include some leafy green vegetables (such as broccoli, kale, and collards), lime-processed tortillas, calcium precipitated tofu, and calcium fortified foods.

The determination of calcium in food products has been well validated. The analyst can choose between AAS, ICP, and titrimetric procedures. AAS methods include **968.08**, **975.03**, **965.09**, **991.25**, and **985.35**. These are fairly straight forward methods that prepare the food samples using both wet and dry ashing procedures.

The multielement techniques prepare the samples in the same manner as the AAS methods. They include ICP Methods **985.01** and **984.27** and emission spectrophotometric Methods **980.03** and **953.01**.

Calcium can also be determined using titration Methods **921.01**, **983.19**, **968.31**, **945.41**, or **944.03**.

Copper

Even though copper is an essential nutrient, severe copper deficiency is quite rare in humans (8). Organ meats, especially liver, are the richest sources of copper in the diet, followed by seafoods, nuts, and seeds.

Copper is often found in very low concentrations in some food, and care should be taken to avoid laboratory contamination, particularly when using wet ashing sample preparation. Copper can also be lost during dry ashing sample preparation if the furnace temperature exceeds 525°C.

Acceptable instrumental methods for the determination of copper include AAS Methods **985.35**, **968.08**, **985.40**, and **990.05**; ICP methods **984.27** and **985.01**, and emission spectrophotometric Methods **980.03** and **953.01**. Copper can also be measured colorimetrically with Methods **960.40** or **953.03**.

Iodine

Iodine, an integral part of the thyroid hormones thyroxine and triiodothyronine, is an essential micronutrient for all animal species, including humans (9). It is present in food and water predominantly as iodide and, to a lesser degree, organically bound to amino acids. Iodine deficiency can lead to a wide spectrum of diseases, ranging from severe cretinism with mental retardation to barely visible enlargement of the thyroid. Endemic goiter and the more severe forms of iodine deficiency disorders continue to be a worldwide problem.

The environmental levels of iodine and their contribution to human intake vary widely in different parts of the world. In coastal areas, seafoods, water, and ocean mist containing iodine are important sources. In most inland areas, the iodine content of plant and animal products is variable, depending on the geochemical environment. In areas where it is available, the most reliable source of iodine is from iodized table salt.

The analysis of iodine is probably the most difficult of the inorganic analyses. The only AOAC Official Method that is validated for food is in infant formula (**992.22**). This procedure does not have useful application to many other food products.

The most common method for iodine analysis in food uses a classical chemical procedure (10). This analysis is accomplished by colorimetrically measuring the extent of the reaction between arsenic (III) and cerium (IV) as catalyzed by the presence of iodide. This assay procedure is very technique oriented but has been used successfully in a wide variety of food products. It has not, however, been collaboratively studied.

Iron

Because iron is a constituent of hemoglobin, myoglobin, and a number of enzymes, it is an essential nutrient for humans (11). Iron deficiency occurs primarily during four periods of life: from about 6 months to 4 years of age, because the iron content of milk is low and the body is growing rapidly; during the rapid growth of early adolescence; during the female reproductive period because of menstrual iron losses; and during pregnancy, because of the expanding blood volume of the mother.

Iron is widely distributed in the world food supply; meat, eggs, vegetables, and cereals (especially fortified cereal products) are the principal dietary sources.

Methods for the determination of iron of food are very well documented. The only concern in using these methods in the food laboratory is caused by contamination from rusted metal fixtures or lab furniture. Instrumental techniques for measuring iron include AAS Methods **968.08**, **975.03**, **965.09**, **985.35**, and **990.05**; ICP Method **984.27**; and emission spectroscopic Methods **980.03** and **953.01**. Iron can also be determined using spectrophotometric Methods **945.40**, **950.39**, or **944.02B**.

Magnesium

Almost all unprocessed foods contain magnesium, and purely dietary magnesium deficiency has not been reported in people consuming natural diets. The highest concentrations of magnesium are found in whole seeds such as nuts, legumes, and unmilled grains. More than 80% of the magnesium is lost by removal of the germ and outer layers of cereal grains (12).

Magnesium can be effectively determined using AAS Methods **975.03**, **965.09**, **991.25**, and **985.35**; ICP Methods **985.01** and **984.27**; and emission spectrographic methods **980.03** and **953.01**.

Phosphorus

Phosphorus is an essential component of bone mineral. It also plays an important role in many different chemical reactions in the body. Phosphorus is present in soft tissues as soluble phosphate ion; in lipids, proteins, carbohydrates, and nucleic acid in an ester or anhydride linkage; and in enzymes as a modulator of their activities.

Phosphorus is present in nearly all foods. The amount available in the food supply from unprocessed commodities has been relatively constant during the past 75 years. Major contributors of phosphorus are protein-rich foods (milk, meat, poultry, and fish) and cereal grains.

The determination of phosphorus is generally accomplished by using ICP Methods **985.01** and **984.27** or any of a wide variety of colorimetric/spectrophotometric methods. Both approaches have produced acceptable results in almost all types of food.

Potassium

Potassium is the principal intracellular cation in all of the cells of the human body. It is widely distributed in foods, because is an essential constituent of all living cells. The richest dietary sources are unprocessed foods, especially fruits, many vegetables, and fresh meats.

Methods for the determination of potassium include AAS Methods **985.35** and **975.03**; ICP Methods **985.03** and **984.27**; emission spectrographic Methods **953.01**, **980.03**, and **990.23**; and flame photometric Methods **956.01**, **965.30**, and **969.23**.

Sodium

Sodium, the principal cation of extracellular fluid, is the primary regulator of extracellular fluid volume in the human body. Foods and beverages containing sodium chloride are the primary sources of sodium. The highest salt intakes are normally associated with a diet high in processed foods and the lowest intakes are normally associated with diets emphasizing fresh fruits, vegetables, and legumes.

All of the methods that were listed under *Potassium* work equally well for the determination of sodium. In addition to these, an ion-specific electrode Method (**976.025**) can be used on certain types of food.

The accurate determination of low levels of sodium can be critical for specialty foods or foods designed as "low" or "reduced" sodium. To avoid analytical variability, samples should be dry ashed in platinum crucibles or wet ashed with ultra-pure acid prior to sodium analysis.

Zinc

Zinc is a constituent of enzymes involved in most major human metabolic pathways. The bioavailability of zinc in different foods varies greatly. Meat, liver, eggs, and seafoods (especially oysters) are good sources of available zinc, whereas whole grain products contain the element in a less available form.

Zinc can be accurately measured in food by using AAS Methods **968.08**, **975.03**, **965.09**, **986.15**, **969.32**, and **985.35** or ICP Method **985.01**. Other Methods include emission spectrography (**980.03** and **953.01**) and colorimetry (**944.09**, **941.03**, and **953.04**).

References

(1)   *Agriculture Handbook Series 8* (1976-89) Agricultural Research Service, United States Department of Agriculture, Washington, DC

(2)   *Federal Register* (1993) U.S. Government Printing Office **58**, 2193–2195

(3)   *Protein Quality Evaluation, Report of a Joint FAO/WHO Expert Consultation* (1990) Food Agriculture Organization of the United Nations, Rome, Italy, and World Health Organization, Geneva, Switzerland

(4)   *The Referee* (1993) "AOAC Methods and Determination of Moisture," **17**(1), 5–9

(5)   *Federal Register* (1993) U.S. Government Printing Office **58**, 2175–2176

(6)   *USDA Handbook No. 74* (1973) Agriculture Research Service, U.S. Department of Agriculture, Washington, DC

(7)   Block, G., Dresser, C.M., Hartman, A.M., & Caroll, M.D. (1985) *Am. J. Epidemiol.* **122**, 13–26

(8)   Danks, D.M. (1988) *Annu. Rev. Nutr.* **8**, 235–257

(9)   Hetzel, B.S., & Maberly, G.F. (1986) "Iodine," in *Trace Elements in Human and Animal Nutrition*, 5th Ed., W. Mertz (ed.), Academic Press, New York, NY, pp 139–208

(10)   Binnerts, W.T. (1954) *Anal. Chim. Acta* **10**, 78

(11)   Bothwell, T.H., Charlton, R.W., Cook, J.D., & Finch, C.A. (1979) *Iron Metabolism in Man*, Blackwell, Oxford, UK

(12)   Marier, J.R. (1986) *Magnesium* **5**, 1–8

Chapter 7
Reference Materials

Wayne R. Wolf

Introduction

The role of reference materials in AOAC INTERNATIONAL activities results from AOAC's expanded mission statement "to promote quality measurements and method validation in the analytical sciences."

To ensure the accuracy of an analytical method for nutrition labeling, the method must be verified at three different points: (*1*) When the method is first developed and collaboratively validated; Can it generate the correct (accurate) number? (*2*) When the method is implemented in a different laboratory (after becoming an AOAC Official Method); Can it generate the correct (accurate) number under different use conditions or by a different analyst? (*3*) When the method is routinely used; Can it generate the correct (accurate) number each time it is used?

Determination of method accuracy during development and a collaborative study validation are the first steps to promoting quality measurements. Proof of accuracy is usually considered to be the responsibility of the method developer before the validation process begins. Such proof is often left to studies showing quantitative recovery of added analyte. Recovery studies are known to be unreliable in many cases, especially when the naturally occurring analyte is bound to the matrix but the added analyte is not bound in the same fashion.

The collaborative study process is predominately designed to assure reproducibility of analytical results among a number of laboratories. Again, the issue of accuracy is generally discussed through determination of recovery of spikes. But again, confidence in the accuracy of the data can only be obtained by the ability of the method to obtain known values on appropriate reference materials, as used in different hands. Reference materials can be incorporated in the validation study to give this information.

Verification of method accuracy with each new implementation is the second step. Historically, AOAC has validated analytical methods and incorporated them into the *Official Methods of Analysis* but has not been involved in the method's further implementation and use. However, when a method is applied by the user in a specific situation and laboratory, it must be revalidated for accuracy in that particular situation. If a suitable reference material is available, either having been independently validated or characterized in the collaborative study, this verification process is a simple one for the user laboratory.

Verification of method accuracy in each use of the method is the third step to promoting quality measurements. The growing trend toward laboratory accreditation incorporates the demonstration of validation of methods used. Quality measurements depend on establishment of quality control procedures within a quality assurance system. The periodic use of well defined reference materials to confirm accuracy is well understood. Confidence in the accuracy of data generated by use of a specific analytical method can only be assured by the ability to obtain known values of an appropriate reference material or by independent verification of analytical results on a reference sample using independent techniques.

Technical Division on Reference Materials

In order for reference material activities to be initiated and carried out, a Technical Division on Reference Materials was approved by the AOAC INTERNATIONAL Board of Directors on March 23, 1993. For further information about activities of membership in the Technical Division, contact AOAC headquarters.

Task Force Addresses Reference Materials

In addition to the activities directed toward evaluation of suitability of AOAC Official Methods for nutrient analyses, the AOAC Task Force on Methods for Nutrient Labeling Analyses also addressed several issues relating to reference materials. A survey of available Certified Reference Materials available from the National Institute of Standards and Technology (NIST) and from the European Community Bureau of Reference (BCR) was compiled and published in the August 1992 issue of *The Referee*. This survey is included below for reference.

Work was initiated by a subcommittee to define a food matrix system for collaborative studies. The system is very important in that it is a way of defining a reasonable number of matrixes that constitute foods reflecting behavior on a chemical basis rather than a commodity basis. Evaluation of need for reference materials and providing appropriate reference material matrixes will more logically flow from this system of definition. The final report of this subcommittee was published in the July 1993 issue of *The Referee* and is included here for reference.

Another NLEA Task Force subcommittee generated a set of guidelines for preparation of in-house quality control materials. These values are very useful for establishing an accuracy based quality control program. The report of this subcommittee was published in the May 1993 issue of *The Referee* and is included here for reference.

Future AOAC Activities on Reference Materials

As the AOAC Technical Division on Reference Materials becomes established, many activities are anticipated. As these unfold and information becomes available, it will be reported in *The Referee*, and in the *Journal of AOAC INTERNATIONAL* when appropriate. Updates of this manual are planned as new information becomes available. Appropriate updated information of reference materials is also planned for inclusion in future editions of *Official Methods of Analysis*.

[Excerpted and revised from Wolf, W.R. (1992) The Referee, AOAC International, 16(8), pp. 4,5]

Reference Materials for Nutrition Labeling

Analysis of appropriate reference standards using the AOAC Official Methods allows assessment and validation of the accuracy of these measurements. Tables 1–3 are a selected listing of some of the presently or soon to be available reference materials that cover a variety of the analyte/matrix combinations noted in the compiled list of AOAC Official Methods. Values in the tables are given mainly for the mandatory components of the U.S. Nutrition Labeling and Education Act.

Information and catalogs about these reference materials can be obtained from:

■ Standard Reference Materials Program, NIST, Gaithersburg, MD 20899, Sales Office, telephone 301/975-6776, fax 301/948-3730.

■ Community Bureau of Reference (BCR), Commission of the European Communities, Rue de la Loi, 200, B-1049, Brussels, Belgium, telephone 32-2-295-3115, fax 32-2-295-8072.

Analysts may also have success in obtaining a number of reference materials including BCR CRMs by contacting either of the organizations listed below, both of which have extensive catalogs and supply materials on a wide basis:

■ The Office of Reference Materials, Laboratory of the Government Chemist, Queens Road, Teddington, Middlesex TW11 OLY, UK, telephone 44-81-943-7565, fax 44-81-943-2767.

■ Promochem GMBH, Postfach 1246, D 4230 Wesel, Germany, telephone 49-281-530081, fax 49-281-89993.

A number of reference materials are available from other sources, particularly for elemental content, which may be of valuable use in these analyses.

Several additional matrixes with specific analytes for nutrition labeling also warrant special note. BCR has three materials with Fatty Acid Profiles, namely CRM 162 Soy-Maize Oil, CRM 163 Beef-Pig Fat, and CRM 164 Milk Fat. BCR also has CRM 422 Cod Muscle and CRM 278 Mussel Tissue as marine food matrixes with sodium, potassium, calcium, and iron certified values. A particularly interesting matrix is the Swedish Meat material, which is a canned fresh pork material certified for total fat, protein, sodium and ash. Information on obtaining this material is available from Kurt Kolar, Swedish Meat Research Institute, Analytical Services, PO Box 504, S-244, Kavlinge, Sweden, telephone 046-73-22-30, fax 046-73-61-37.

Further compilation and evaluation of a range of materials including the availability of pure analyte standards will be future activities of the task force and will be reported later.

-Wayne R. Wolf

Table 1. Standard reference materials for nutritional labeling[a]

Components related to nutritional labeling	SRM 1548 total diet	SRM 1549 nonfat dry milk	SRM 1563 cholesterol and fat soluble vitamins in coconut oil	SRM 1567a wheat flour	SRM 1568a rice flour	SRM 1577b bovine liver	SRM 1845 cholesterol in whole egg
Calories, kcal/g	5.22	—	—	—	—	—	—
Total fat weight, %	20.6	—	—	—	—	—	—
Saturated fat	—	—	—	—	—	—	—
Cholesterol, mg/kg	—	—	642	—	—	—	19000
Total carbohydrate weight, %	—	—	—	—	—	—	—
Sugars weight, %	—	(49) lactose	—	—	—	—	—
Dietary fiber weight, %	3.69	—	—	—	—	—	—
Kjeldahl N weight, %	3.44	—	—	—	—	—	—
Sodium, mg/kg	6250	4970	—	6.1	6.6	2420	—
Potassium weight, %	0.606	1.69	—	0.133	0.128	0.994	—
Calcium, mg/kg	1740	13000	—	19	12	116	—
Iron, mg/kg	32.6	1.78	—	14.1	7.4	184	—
Vitamin A, mg/kg	—	—	12.2 retinyl acetate	—	—	—	—
Vitamin C, mg/kg	—	(53)	—	—	—	—	—

[a] Distributed by NIST Gaithersburg, MD.

Table 2. U.S./Canada collaborative reference materials[a]

Components related to nutritional labeling	RM 8413 corn kernel	RM 8414 bovine muscle powder	RM 8415 whole egg powder	RM 8418 wheat gluten	RM 8433 corn bran	RM 8435 whole milk	RM 8436 durum wheat flour
Calories, kcal/g	—	—	—	—	—	—	—
Total fat weight, %[b]	—	(9.22)	(44.8)	(4.84)	(2.88)	(23.2)	(2.70)
Saturated fat	—	—	—	—	—	—	—
Cholesterol, mg/kg	—	—	—	—	—	—	—
Total carbohydrate weight, %[b]	—	0	(9.34)	(10.8)	(85.9)	(42.2)	(73.0)
Sugars weight, %	—	—	—	—	—	—	—
Dietary fiber weight, %	—	—	—	—	—	—	—
Protein weight, %[b]	(8.59)[c] Kjel. N × 6.25	(80.1)	(37.9)	(75.9)	(5.32)	(25.3)	(13.7)
Sodium weight, %[d]	—	(0.20)	(0.37)	(0.14)	(0.040)	(0.37)	(0.001)
Potassium weight, %[d]	(0.36)[c]	(1.40)	(0.32)	(0.050)	(0.060)	(1.30)	(0.33)
Calcium, mg/kg[d]	(42)[c]	(140)	(2400)	(0.037)	(0.042)	(8800)	(0.026)
Iron, mg/kg	(23)[c]	—	—	—	—	—	—
Vitamin A, mg/kg	—	—	—	—	—	—	—
Vitamin C, mg/kg	—	—	—	—	—	40.6	—

[a] Distributed by NIST, Gaithersburg, MD. Available in October 1993.
[b] Informative Values from Tanner, J.T., et al. (1988) *Fresenius Z. Anal. Chem.* **332**, 701–703.
[c] Information Values from M. Ihnat, Report of Analysis—RM 8413, NIST.
[d] Information Values from Ihnat, M., & Stoeppler, M. (1990) *Fresenius Z. Anal. Chem.* **338**, 455–460. See Individual Reports of Analysis for Best Estimate Values.

Table 3. Certified reference materials for nutritional labeling[a]

Components related to nutritional labeling	BCR CRM 380 whole milk powder	BCR CRM 381 rye flour	BCR CRM 382 wheat flour	BCR CRM 383 haricot beans	BCR CRM 384 lyoph pork muscle	BCR CRM 184 bovine muscle	BCR CRM 185 bovine liver
Calories, kcal/g	—	—	—	—	—	—	—
Total fat weight, %	26.9	1.06	1.26	—	10.8	4.4	10.3
Saturated fat	—	—	—	—	—	—	—
Cholesterol, mg/kg	—	—	—	—	—	—	—

Table 3. Certified reference materials for nutritional labeling[a]

Components related to nutritional labeling	BCR CRM 380 whole milk powder	BCR CRM 381 rye flour	BCR CRM 382 wheat flour	BCR CRM 383 haricot beans	BCR CRM 384 lyoph pork muscle	BCR CRM 184 bovine muscle	BCR CRM 185 bovine liver
Total carbohydrate weight, %	—	(90) Avail. CHO	(89) Avail. CHO	(79) Avail. CHO	—	—	—
Sugars weight, %	36.3 lactose	—	—	—	—	—	—
Dietary fiber weight, %	—	8.22	3.25	11.91	—	—	—
Kjeldahl N weight, %	4.50	1.25	2.12	1.05	13.69	86.6[b]	63.1[b]
Sodium, mg/kg	(3920)	19	—	5	2820	(2000)	(2100)
Potassium, mg/kg	(12450)	2850	(1750)	7750	15530	(16600)	(11200)
Calcium, mg/kg	(9450)	220	(1510)	2850	230	(150)	(131)
Iron, mg/kg	—	—	—	—	—	79	214
Vitamin A, mg/kg	—	—	—	—	—	—	—
Vitamin C, mg/kg	—	—	—	—	—	—	—

[a] Distributed by the Community Bureau of Reference (BCR), Brussels, Belgium
[b] Total protein.

[From Ikins, W., DeVries, J., Wolf, W.R., Oles, P., Carpenter, D., Fraley, N., Ngeh-Ngwainbi, J. (1993) The Referee, AOAC International, 17(7), pp. 1,6,7]

A Food Matrix Organizational System Applied to Collaborative Studies

Purpose

Currently, no systematic procedure exists for validating analytical methods as applicable to all foods. Clearly, such a systematic procedure is needed. AOAC Associate Referees must assure the methods they validate and recommend are, or are not, applicable to all foods, and AOAC Official Method Committees must judge the applicability range of the methods. Further, such a system should be designed to minimize the effort required for collaborative studies while maximizing the value of the resulting data to AOAC Official Method users.

The Subcommittee on Food Definition of the AOAC Task Force on Methods for Nutrient Labeling Analyses investigated systematic approaches to validate analytical methods as applicable to all foods and food products. This Subcommittee report describes a system that better reflects how foods vary on a chemical basis rather than on a commodity basis, thereby reducing the number of samples that would represent all foods to a manageable number. The Subcommittee recommended this system for studies applicable to all food.

Discussion

The prospect of coordinating a collaborative study involving 40 or more different foods may discourage many researchers from fully exploring the scope of applicability of their method. As a result, researchers may limit the scope of the study to a few food groups to reduce the analytical burden on the participating laboratories.

Many of the 40 or more foods selected to represent all foods for a collaborative study may be very similar to one another on a dry basis, and may behave chemically, and thus analytically, in a very similar way. In any analytical procedure, water can be added or subtracted to suit the requirements of the method. Ash, in general, does not have a great impact on the performance of analytical methods for organic material in foods. Thus, the behavior of a given food in an analytical method is primarily determined by the relative proportions of protein, fat, and carbohydrate.

Figure 1 depicts a scheme by which all foods can be organized according to their relative levels of these three major classes of food components. The points of the triangle represent 100% of either protein, fat, and carbohydrate (moisture and ash are excluded for the reasons cited above). The triangle is divided into nine sectors that serve to group foods according to their basic chemical makeup. Table 1 contains a listing of some of the foods found in the U.S. Department of Agriculture Handbook No. 8 that might be useful for a collaborative study. The foods have been categorized into each of the nine sectors of the triangle. Careful selection of two foods or food products from each sector will cover the entire range of carbohydrate, protein, and fat, as well as other food attributes.

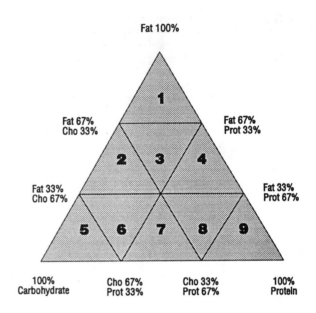

Figure 1. Schematic layout of food matrixes suggested for a collaborative study based on protein, fat, and carbohydrate content, excluding moisture and ash.

If a diagram such as Figure 1 were to be used to select samples for a collaborative study, two samples from a sector could be selected to account for variation in the type of protein, fat, or carbohydrate that may have an impact on the performance of the method. Examples of these variations within carbohydrates are high fiber foods vs high sugar foods. Other variations include fats containing significant amounts of short chain fatty acids vs those containing predominantly long chain fatty acids, or foods containing more hydrophilic proteins as opposed to those containing predominantly hydrophobic proteins. In addition, two foods may be selected within a sector that vary according to the extent of processing each has undergone.

Example

Figure 2 illustrates how this system can be used with the Youden concept for statistical evaluation of an analyte of interest. For the purposes of this example, the U.S. Department of Agriculture Handbook No. 8 was used to select representative foods that fell within each of the nine sectors. Samples containing similar levels of the analyte of interest will be ultimately paired for statistical purposes. The actual percent of protein, fat, and carbohydrate used to construct Figure 2 are shown in Table 2.

When conducting a collaborative study to validate a method to be used on all foods or a particular subset of matrixes, a system such as that depicted in Figure 1 can be used to select foods for the validation study. In doing so, samples that are truly chemically different from one another can be used to test the limitations of a method. If a method fails for food matrixes located within certain sectors, those factors that cause the method to be ineffective can be more clearly understood and delineated.

Recommendation

The AOAC Task Force on Methods for Nutrient Labeling Analyses recommends the four AOAC food committees and the Official Methods Board adopt this systematic approach for validating methods for all foods. Adoption of this approach will minimize the efforts required for collaborative studies while maximizing the value of the resulting method to its users.

Comments from AOAC members, volunteers, and method users are cordially invited. Please contact Nancy Palmer, AOAC Technical Director, at the AOAC offices.

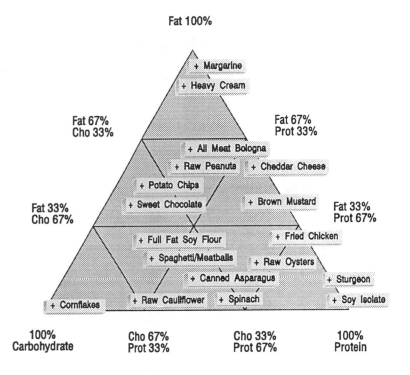

Figure 2. Schematic layout of food matrixes to be used in a collaborative study based on protein, fat, and carbohydrate content, excluding moisture and ash.

Table 1. Selected example foods from U.S. Department of Agriculture Handbook No. 8 and their corresponding sectors in the triangle[a]

Sector	ITEM	PROT%	FAT%	CHO'S%
1		0-33%	67-100%	0-33%
	Cooking oil	0	100	0
	Margarine	1	99	0
	Cream/heavy whipping	5	88	7
	Avocados/California	9	67	24
	Bacon	11	88	1
2		0-33%	33-67%	33-67%
	Potato chips	6	42	53
	Chocolate/sweet	5	36	59

117

Table 1. Selected example foods from U.S. Department of Agriculture Handbook No. 8 and their corresponding sectors in the triangle[a]

Sector	ITEM	PROT%	FAT%	CHO'S%
3		0-33%	33-67%	0-33%
	Dried almonds	20	59	21
	Raw peanuts	28	52	20
	All-meat bologna	33	57	9
4		33-67%	33-67%	0-33%
	Brown mustard	34	36	30
	Blue cheese	40	56	4
	Cheddar cheese	42	54	4
	Hamburger	46	54	0
	Raw eggs	51	45	4
	Caviar	60	33	7
	Canned turkey	63	37	0
5		0-33%	0-33%	67-100%
	Bananas	5	1	94
	Rice bran	6	1	92
	Cornflakes	8	0	91
	Noodles	14	5	81
	Canned lima beans	23	1	76
	Frozen biscuit dough	9	18	74
	Raw cauliflower	33	2	64
6		0-33%	0-33%	33-67%
	Plain cocoa	19	27	54
	Spaghetti with meatballs	24	20	56
	Whole milk yogurt	27	30	43
	Wheat germ	33	13	54
	Baby food-chicken/vegetables	39	24	38
	Canned asparagus	39	6	55

Table 1. Selected example foods from U.S. Department of Agriculture Handbook No. 8 and their corresponding sectors in the triangle[a]

Sector	ITEM	PROT%	FAT%	CHO'S%
7		33-67%	0-33%	33-67%
	Skim milk	41	1	58
	Spinach	41	4	55
	Full-fat soy flour	42	23	35
	Defatted peanut flour	54	10	36
8		33-67%	0-33%	0-33%
	Fried chicken (dark meat)	64	29	7
	Raw oysters	62	13	25
9		67-100%	0-33%	0-33%
	Raw beef liver	69	13	18
	Soy protein isolate	83	0	17
	Cottage cheese	66	20	14
	Dried chipped beef	84	16	0
	Raw catfish	85	15	0
	Sturgeon	91	10	0
	Canned tuna in water	97	3	0
	Gelatin	100	0	0

[a]Percent of protein, fat, and carbohydrate, excluding moisture and ash, are normalized to 100%.

Table 2. Selected example foods from the USDA Handbook No. 8 and their corresponding sectors in the triangle[a]

ITEM	SECTOR	PROT%	FAT%	CHO's %
Margarine	1	1	99	0
Cream/heavy whipping	1	5	88	7
Potato chips	2	6	42	53
Chocolate/sweet	2	5	36	59
Raw peanuts	3	28	52	20
All-meat bologna	3	33	57	9
Brown mustard	4	34	36	30

Table 2. Selected example foods from the USDA Handbook No. 8 and their corresponding sectors in the triangle[a]

ITEM	SECTOR	PROT%	FAT%	CHO's %
Cheddar cheese	4	42	54	4
Cornflakes	5	8	0	91
Raw cauliflower	5	33	2	64
Spaghetti with meatballs	6	24	20	56
Canned asparagus	6	39	6	55
Spinach	7	41	4	55
Full-fat soy flour	7	42	23	35
Fried chicken (dark meat)	8	64	29	7
Raw oysters	8	62	13	25
Soy protein isolate	9	83	0	17
Sturgeon	9	91	10	0

[a]Percent of protein, fat, and carbohydrate, excluding moisture and ash, are normalized to 100%.

[Excerpted and revised from Craft, N., & Boyer, K. (1993) The Referee, AOAC International, 17(5), pp. 6–8]

Preparation of In-House Quality Assurance Control Materials for Food Analysis

A. Purpose

To provide guidelines for the preparation and use of affordable, well-characterized, stable foods or food-like materials for use as quality assurance control materials (CM) in nutritional analyses of foods.

B. Desirable Properties

Matrix.—A CM matrix should mimic real samples, with respect to both macro- and micronutrient content. Macro- and/or micronutrients may be added if no source can be found to mimic major food classes or matrix types, but spiking should be avoided where natural sources are available. The addition of nutrients does not necessarily mimic the form and compartmentalization of a real food matrix. Lyophilized materials may be used to improve storage and stability only if comparability to the original matrix has been demonstrated.

Stability.—Candidate CMs should be stable at normal laboratory room temperatures, or well-defined instructions should be determined for keeping the material stable over time with respect to macro- and micro-nutrient content. It is always better to err on the side of conservatism when packaging and storing CMs (i.e., if the influence of exposure to light on an analyte is unknown, then protect the CM from light).

C. Sources and Selection of Matrixes for Characterization

Major data bases.—Major data bases such as the U.S. Department of Agriculture Handbook 8, can be searched for foods that provide the best combination of nutrients and macro components (fat, carbohydrate, protein, and moisture) to represent broad classes of foods. This information may be used to locate food items within the "Food Triangle" which is being considered by AOAC INTERNATIONAL as a means of identifying a small number of foods that are representative of all food matrixes. Each vertex of the triangle represents 100% of fat, carbohydrate, or protein. The triangle is divided into 9 subsections that serve to group foods according to their basic chemical make-up. One must bear in mind that such data bases may lack information or contain less reliable information for micro-nutrients.

Starting materials.—Starting materials should be selected that represent major food groups (or "Food Triangle" subtriangles) and are already very homogeneous, or can easily be made homogeneous. Examples of foods already homogeneous that can represent major food groups include: (*1*) *Baby foods.*—Beef and chicken can be used to represent cooked meats and poultry; (*2*) *Flour.*—Fortified cereal grains, such as Cheerios or Corn Flakes, can represent grain products, and fortified components in a cereal grain matrix; (*3*) *Sugars.*—Mixed and blended pure powdered sugars (dextrose, fructose, sucrose, lactose, etc.) may be analyzed directly, or dissolved in deionized water to give the desired concentration of sugars for analysis as a laboratory CM; (*4*) *Fats.*—Lard, vegetable oils, and saturated fats can be melted together to provide uniform mixtures containing tocopherols and saturated/unsaturated fatty acids after hydrolysis; and (*5*) *Formulas.*—These can be used as CMs for infant formula, enteral feedings, or semipurified diets. They may also be blended with other major food materials to simulate supplemented dietary components.

D. Matrix Preparation and Homogenization

If a matrix exists that is appropriately prepared, homogenized, and packaged, it may be used without further manipulation.

If a matrix is a liquid or fine suspension, it should be mixed thoroughly prior to and during dispensing (preferably under inert environment) to ensure uniformity. It can then be dispensed into individual use containers appropriate for the storage requirements of the CM.

Nonuniform materials can be made uniform by using grinding, milling, homogenizing, and sieving techniques that minimize degradation of labile compounds due to heat buildup or oxidation by air. The material should be mixed/agitated prior to and during dispensing to minimize settling. It can then be dispensed into single use containers appropriate for storage requirements of the CM.

Batch size should be determined on the basis of analyte stability and the rate at which the CM would be used in a given laboratory. For samples that are not limited by analyte stability, at least a 12 month supply should be prepared due to the effort necessary to prepare and characterize CMs. Samples susceptible to instability must be prepared or revalidated more frequently.

Homogeneity criteria must be established for each food matrix prepared for use as a laboratory CM. Analysis of representative samples can be performed on homogeneity-indicating nutrients, such as calcium, fat, moisture, etc., to assess if further homogenization is needed. It is not necessary to measure all analytes during homogeneity assessment. To test homogeneity, analytes should be selected that are representative of one or more classes of compounds and for which highly precise methods exist. Good method precision will permit the detection of sample inhomogeneity that might go undetected if analytes of poor analytical precision were selected.

All materials are inhomogeneous below a given sample size. Minimum sample size should be determined and specified such that the sample portion of a CM used for the measurement of a given analyte is large enough to be representative of the entire batch of CM or equal to that specified in AOAC Official Methods.

Final product homogeneity should be determined by analyzing stratified random samples throughout the dispensing process.

E. Characterization

Priority for full characterization of each material is as follows: (*1*) Major components — fat, protein, carbohydrate, and moisture — This "classifies" the matrix; (*2*) All remaining **mandatory nutritional labeling parameters,** plus any voluntary parameters, such as soluble and insoluble dietary fiber, that can be obtained most conveniently with the mandatory parameters; (3) All remaining voluntary nutritional labeling parameters; and (4) Any other components that are of food composition interest, but not required by nutritional labeling, such as preservatives, other sterols, and other carotenoids.

It is recommended that a preliminary mean and standard deviation for each analyte be established using duplicate analyses on randomly selected samples over at least 10 independent analysis sample sets or runs using a calibrated method. Where possible, normal quality assurance steps, including running blanks, spikes, and other control samples, should be included. If a Standard Reference Material is available, it should be included to validate the method and assist in value-assigning the CM.

F. Packaging and Storage

CMs should be packaged and stored to minimize degradation, e.g., stored sealed under inert environment, in containers that exclude light, and, where applicable, in freezers to slow degradation due to heat and/or in desiccators to maintain constant humidity.

CMs should be packaged in clearly labeled single use containers or in quantities small enough that the sample is consumed in a relatively short time (e.g., during one week's analytical runs). Appropriate containers might include: glass ampoules, bottles with Teflon-lined screw top caps, or baby-food jars. Some analytes may not require exclusion of air and light or containers composed of glass and Teflon, but, if in doubt, these precautions are recommended.

G. Documentation

Proper documentation is an essential part of preparing and using CMs. Each step of producing a new batch of a CM should be carefully documented for problem solving or later reference. It is suggested that producers of CMs record the following, at a minimum, for each batch of CM that is prepared: (1) Source, date, physical description, and condition of starting material as received; (2) Details of homogenization and preparation procedures used; (3) Details of packaging procedures and containers used; (4) Details of storage conditions and history; (5) and References for analytical methods used during the initial determination of analyte concentrations; and (6) A "Record of Analysis" (including mean, standard deviation, 95% confidence interval, and date analyzed) of all analytes for which the CM will be used, on the basis of at least 10 independent analyses of the CM. Also a statement of intended use, estimated expiration date, storage and handling conditions required, and any other special instructions for use of the CM should be included with the Record of Analysis.

Users should maintain a running control chart of analytical results for each analyte to judge when a CM is changing or when an analysis is out of control.

Detailed specific information about the preparation and use of CMs may be shared with other AOAC members (through *The Referee*, the Reference Materials Technical Division, or directly) as a benefit to all parties interested in nutritional analysis of foods. Because AOAC Official Methods are specified in the U.S. nutritional labeling regulations, AOAC INTERNATIONAL is the best vehicle for exchange of information about the use of CMs with AOAC Official Methods.

H. Additional Comments

At a minimum, CMs should be used with each batch of samples run to verify that the method is in control (prior to measuring actual samples, when possible). In addition, it may be useful to include CMs at the end of, and possibly interspersed within, a batch of samples, depending on the risk of a particular method drifting out of control and on the size of the analytical batch of samples.

A new CM should be prepared far enough in advance and characterized while using a current CM to establish a new control chart *before* the current CM lot is depleted.

Chapter 8
Fat-Soluble Vitamins

Edward H. Waysek

Introduction

The accurate determination of fat-soluble vitamins in foods poses a difficult challenge to the analytical chemist. Sampling, extraction, separation from interferences, and potential complications from isomerization and degradation are all concerns that must constantly be kept in mind. The fat-soluble vitamins have common properties that contribute to these concerns. They generally are not stable in their pure states and are sensitive to air, light, acids, and trace metals. To overcome handling, processing, and stability concerns, fat-soluble vitamins are usually added to foods as stabilized product forms. This stabilization is accomplished through chemical means such as the formation of stable esters and/or product formulations that protect the vitamin by coating, encapsulation, or providing antioxidant systems. These product forms for fat-soluble vitamins include beadlets, microcapsules, adsorbates, oils, emulsions, and spray-dried products. Often for the analyst, the same techniques used to stabilize fat-soluble vitamins for food fortification applications are the main factors that make their analysis more difficult. Specific problems will be discussed under the individual vitamins.

The presence of structurally related forms or vitamers of fat-soluble vitamins can also be a source of confusion and analytical error. For example, vitamers of vitamin E not only include the most active form, α-tocopherol, but also other tocopherols and tocotrienols. Similarly, the vitamin A vitamers include retinol, retinaldehyde, 3-dehydroretinol, and their cis/trans isomers. Lastly, the vitamers of vitamin D include ergocalciferol, cholecalciferol, and their previtamin isomers. Because the various vitamers and forms of the fat-soluble vitamins do not have equivalent biological activities, care must be taken with how analytical results are expressed and what units are used. The commonly reported unit for vitamins E and D is International Units (IU), and for vitamin A it is retinol equivalents (RE). Their definitions and conversion factors will be discussed under the individual vitamins. For additional background information regarding fat-soluble vitamins, the analyst is referred to reviews by Ball (1) for analysis, Gaby et al. (2) for human health and nutrition information, and the *Encyclopedia of Food Science and Technology* (3) for general information.

The information presented in this section deals with the analytical determination of the fat-soluble vitamins and the findings of the AOAC INTERNATIONAL Task Force on Methods for Nutrient Labeling Analyses regarding the applicability of the vitamin methods described in *AOAC Official Methods of Analysis* for compliance with the Nutrition Labeling & Education Act of 1990 (NLEA). The fat-soluble vitamins A, D, E, and β-carotene, their applicable AOAC methods, and some insights into the application of these methods are discussed.

Vitamin A

Vitamin A is essential for normal growth, reproduction, vision, and the development and proper functioning of the skin and mucous membranes.

The determination of the total vitamin A content of a food involves the determination of naturally occurring vitamin A compounds and added or supplemental vitamin A. Although the provitamin A carotenoids, especially β-carotene, may contribute significantly to the total vitamin A activity, they usually are determined separately. Unless there is a need for the determination of a specific vitamin A ester, most procedures use a saponification step and determine preformed vitamin A as retinol. If the procedure does not involve a saponification step and the food contains supplemental vitamin A, care must be taken to be sure that the product form that has been used is properly dispersed before extraction, because many vitamin A products are encapsulated to protect the vitamin. Regardless of the procedure used, the analyst should always keep in mind the sensitivity of vitamin A to oxidation and UV light and take proper precautions.

The latest edition and supplements of *Official Methods of Analysis*, 15th Ed., list the following methods for the determination of vitamin A (4): **960.45**, Vitamin A in Margarine (Spectrophotometric Method); **974.29**, Vitamin A in Mixed Feeds, Premixes, and Foods (Colorimetric Method); **992.04**, Vitamin A (Retinol Isomers) in Milk and Milk-Based Infant Formula (LC Method); and **992.06**, Vitamin A (Retinol) in Milk-Based Infant Formula (LC Method).

Method **960.45**, Vitamin A in Margarine, is listed as "Surplus 1980." A "surplus" method is considered not currently in use. Surplus methods, however, have gone through the collaborative study process and still retain official status. A full description of this method is reported in *Official Methods of Analysis*, 14th Ed. (5). Basically, the method consists of saponification, extraction, and column chromatographic separation of vitamin A from carotenoids and other interferences, followed by spectrophotometric determination of vitamin A. "Carotenes" may also be determined spectrophotometrically. Although not as specific, sensitive, or widely applicable as **974.29** (colorimetric), the method is less technique dependent and does not require the use of antimony trichloride.

The AOAC Task Force on Methods for Nutrient Labeling Analyses found **974.29** generally adequate for the determination of vitamin A in a variety of matrixes, including baby foods (meats), cheese, dairy products, fish, infant formula/medical diet, meat (beef/pork/fowl), mixed dinners (TV dinners), and shellfish. Method **992.04** was found adequate for dairy products and infant formula/medical diet. Method **992.06** was found adequate for dairy products. The need for an official liquid chromatographic (LC) method for the determination of vitamin A in all matrixes was identified.

Method **974.29**, the colorimetric (commonly known as "Carr-Price") method for vitamin A in mixed feeds, premixes, and foods is a time-tested, reliable procedure for vitamin A providing the method is properly applied and performed. The procedure is based on the formation of an intense blue reaction product between vitamin A and antimony trichloride; the product's absorbance at 620 nm is a function of vitamin A concentration. The colorimetric method has a number of disadvantages and shortcomings that the analyst should be aware. The procedure is not to be used when the sample contains carotenes as the main source of vitamin A activity or for high potency vitamin A concentrates. *cis*-Retinol isomers have the same response as all-*trans*-retinol. Because cis isomers of vitamin A have less biological activity than the trans form, products containing significant amounts of cis isomers will have their vitamin A activity overestimated. Carotenoids, retinaldehyde, dehydroretinol, and related compounds present will cause positive interferences. Sterols and tocopherols may inhibit color development. The method is also very technique dependent and requires a high level of manipulative analytical skill. The Carr-Price reagent must be carefully handled and added rapidly to the sample solution using the dispenser specified. Absorbance or transmittance measurements must be performed using the instrumentation specified and the techniques described. The blue color produced fades rapidly. The antimony trichloride reagent is extremely sensitive to trace amounts of water, which results in the formation of insoluble antimony hypochlorite and causes turbidity and an opaque coating on the colorimeter tube.

The majority of procedures for the determination of vitamin A currently being reported or under development involve the use of LC. Both reversed-phase and normal-phase LC procedures have been developed for the determination of vitamin A in foods. The source of vitamin A (naturally present vs supplemental), the matrix, and the information required should be taken into account before a method is chosen. Most reversed-phase procedures will not separate the various vitamin A isomers, although nonaqueous reversed-phase methods may do so depending on the particular column and mobile phase used (6). Many reversed-phase methods are generally more rugged than normal-phase procedures, especially when a laboratory cannot dedicate an instrument to normal-phase and must switch between aqueous and nonaqueous procedures. If isomers are separated, extreme care must be taken with standards or response factors.

Vitamin A potency or content has traditionally been expressed in IU. One IU of vitamin A is defined as the activity of the following: 0.300 μg of all-*trans*-retinol, 0.344 μg of all-*trans*-retinyl acetate, 0.55 μg of all-*trans*-retinyl palmitate, or 0.6 μg of all-*trans*-β-carotene.

The vitamin A content of foods can now be expressed in terms of retinol equivalents (RE). One RE of vitamin A is defined as the following: 1 μg of all-*trans*-retinol (3.33 IU vitamin A activity) or 6 μg of all-*trans*-β-carotene (10 IU vitamin A activity from all-*trans*-β-carotene).

The cis isomers of vitamin A possess less biological activity than the all-trans form. The relative biopotencies of vitamin A acetate isomers (%), as determined by rat growth and rat liver bioassays, are the following (7): All-*trans*-, 100; 13-*cis*- (neo), 75; 9-*cis*-, 21; 9,13-di-*cis*-, 24; 11-*cis*-, 24; and 11,13-di-*cis*-, 15.

β-Carotene

Because of β-carotene's important role in human health and nutrition, it is the most important member of a class of naturally occurring compounds referred to as carotenoids. In addition to its role as a commonly used, stable food color, β-carotene also provides a safe source of vitamin A. Because the body converts β-carotene to vitamin A in a regulated way, the risk of hypervitaminosis A is eliminated. B-Carotene is also a very effective antioxidant that not only quenches singlet oxygen but also reacts directly with free radicals. It is an effective treatment for a particular genetic light-sensitive skin disorder and may play an important role in the reduction of certain chronic disease risks such as cancer. (8)

β-Carotene must be properly extracted from the food matrix without change or destruction. Accordingly, care must be taken to avoid exposure of β-carotene solutions to air, light, acids, free halogens, and excessive heat. B-Carotene is also sensitive to isomerization. Significant amounts of β-carotene isomers are known to be formed during normal cooking procedures and consequently their occurrence should be accounted for in an analytical procedure.

The following methods for the determination of carotenes are described in *Official Methods of Analysis*, 15th Ed.: **941.15**, Carotenes in Fresh Plant Materials and Silages (Spectrophotometric Method); **970.64**, Carotenes and Xanthophylls in Dried Plant Materials and Mixed Feeds (Spectrophotometric Method); **958.05**, Color of Egg Yolks; **925.13**, Coloring Matter in Macaroni Products; and **938.04**, Carotenoids in Macaroni Products (Colorimetric Method).

The AOAC Task Force on Methods for Nutrient Labeling Analyses found Method **941.15**, "Carotene in Fresh Plant Materials and Silages, Spectrophotometric Method," adequate for the determination of naturally occurring carotenoids in the following matrixes: baby foods (fruits), baby foods (vegetables), fruits, potatoes and products, and vegetables. Its usefulness, however, may be limited to a degree, because the commercial availability of the activated magnesia adsorbent specified is a problem. The method is not applicable to the determination of supplemental β-carotene in foods, especially when it is added as a stabilized product form such as a beadlet. To determine β-carotene accurately when it is added as a beadlet product, the beadlets first must be "opened" or dispersed completely. This step can be accomplished by enzyme treatment or mild alkaline hydrolysis. Care, however, must be taken to insure complete dispersion of the beadlets without degrading or isomerizing the β-carotene present. Because an official AOAC method for supplemental β-carotene does not exist, it is recommended that recovery studies be conducted when determining supplemental β-carotene.

Carotenoids have been the subject of chromatographic investigations since the advent of these techniques. Alumina (9), calcium hydroxide (10), and nonaqueous reversed-phase methods (11, 12) were applied to the determination of carotenoids. Epler et al. (13) performed an extensive study of reversed-phase LC columns for the separation and recovery of carotenoids. LC procedures were developed for the separation of the various carotenes, xanthophylls, and their positional isomers such as alpha- and β-carotene. Rizzolo and Polesello (14) and Furr et al. (15) provided overall reviews of LC application to the analysis of carotenoids. However, to date no LC procedures have been collaboratively studied by AOAC.

The most difficult problem in carotenoid analysis is the accurate determination of the geometrical (cis/trans) isomers. An accurate, reliable, and practical LC procedure suitable for the determination of *cis-β*-carotene isomers in a variety of food matrixes has not yet been developed. Problems encountered include lack of column-to-column reproducibility, inadequate resolution and separation of individual isomers, unclear identification of individual isomers, and the lack of satisfactory reference materials. O'Neil and Schwartz (16) completed a thorough review on the current status of the chromatographic analysis of cis/trans carotenoid isomers and concluded that additional method development work is needed in this area.

Food processing that involves heat will result in the formation of cis isomers. Of the *β*-carotene isomers, cis forms are reported to have less vitamin A activity that the all-trans form (17). Weiser and Kormann used epithelial protection tests with vitamin A deficient rats to comparatively evaluate the provitamin A activity of various carotenoids and *β*-carotene isomers (18). For *cis-β*-carotene isomers, the following relative provitamin A biological activities (%), as compared to all-*trans-β*-carotene, were obtained: all-*trans*-, 100; 13-*cis*-, 42; 15-*cis*-, 36; 13,15-di-*cis*-, 31; 9-*cis*-, 26; 9,15-di-*cis*-, 15; and 9,9-di-*cis*-, 10. Sufficient data are not yet available to allow extrapolation of a direct relationship to their biological activity in humans. Further study is necessary to determine how to use the data as correction factors in reporting *β*-carotene analyses. For additional information regarding carotenoids and their biological activity, the analyst is referred to Bauernfeind (19).

Vitamin D

Vitamin D is essential for proper calcium and phosphorus homeostasis and absorption, which results in proper bone formation and health. Poor vitamin D status in children results in a disease known as rickets. An equivalent disease in adults, osteomalacia, can result from vitamin D deficiency.

The term vitamin D generally refers to two compounds, ergocalciferol (vitamin D_2) and cholecalciferol (vitamin D_3). The variation in chemical structure between the two molecules occurs in the C-17 side chain, in which vitamin D_2 has a double bond with an additional methyl group in the C-28 position. A major distinguishing factor between the two compounds is that vitamin D_2 is not biologically active in birds. However, both vitamin D_2 and vitamin D_3 exhibit equal biological activity in humans. The biologically active form of vitamin D that occurs in nature is the 5,6-*cis*- form. The trans form of vitamin D does not have significant antirachitic activity. The IU of vitamin D is defined as the activity of 0.025 µg of crystalline cholecalciferol (vitamin D_3). Vitamin D_2 crystals have a potency of 40 IU per µg.

In solution, Vitamin D is susceptible to reversible thermal transformation resulting in the formation of previtamin D. Previtamin D is biologically active and must be included in the calculation to determine total vitamin D potency properly. The transformation of vitamin D to previtamin D is a function of time and temperature. The ratio of vitamin D/previtamin D in the resulting equilibrium mixture was found to be dependent on temperature (20). At 20°C, the equilibrium ratio of previtamin D to vitamin D is 7:93; whereas at 60°C, the ratio is 16:84. The times required to reach equilibrium are 30 days at 20°C and 12 h at 60°C. The conversion of vitamin D to previtamin D during the saponification step of an analytical procedure must be taken into account, and the proper correction factor must be used in the calculation of vitamin D potency. AOAC methods **981.17**, Vitamin D in Fortified Milk and Milk Powder, and **982.29**, Vitamin D in Mixed Feeds, Premixes, and Pet Foods, use a correction factor of 1.25 for previtamin D formed during refluxing for saponification. Method **980.26**, an LC procedure for vitamin D in multivitamin preparations, determines a response factor for previtamin D by comparing the peak heights of previtamin D_3 and vitamin D_3 obtained from a heated vitamin D_3 standard solution to the peak height of vitamin D_3 obtained from the same, unheated standard solution. Butylated hydroxytoluene is added to the standard solution before it is heated, and the solution is kept under a nitrogen atmosphere during the entire heating period to minimize degradation. Because vitamin D is sensitive to oxygen, light, acidity, and water, exposure of vitamin D solutions to actinic light should be avoided throughout the entire determination.

The following methods for the determination of vitamin D are described in *Official Methods of Analysis*, 15th Ed.: **982.29**, Vitamin D in Mixed Feeds, Premixes, and Pet Foods (Liquid Chromatographic Method); **981.17**, Vitamin D in Fortified Milk and Milk Powder (Liquid Chromatographic Method); **936.14**, Vitamin D in Milk, Vitamin Preparations, and Food Concentrates (Rat Bioassay); **980.26**, Vitamin D in Multivitamin Preparations (Liquid Chromatographic Method); **985.27**, Vitamin D in Vitamin AD Concentrates (Liquid Chromatographic Method); **979.24**, Vitamin D in Vitamin Preparations (Liquid Chromatographic Method); **975.42**, Vitamin D in Vitamin Preparations (Colorimetric Method); **932.16**, Vitamin D_3 in Poultry Feed Supplements (Chick Bioassay).

The AOAC Task Force on Methods for Nutrient Labeling Analyses found Method **982.29**, Vitamin D in Mixed Feeds, Premixes and Pet Foods, LC Method, adequate for the determination of vitamin D in all fortified food matrixes considered; however, some concern has been expressed by the laboratories surveyed that this method may need revision for certain foods, especially low level unfortified products. Because the quality of the chromatogram is very column dependent, the system suitability test must be performed with care. Method **936.14**, Rat Bioassay, is likewise generally regarded as satisfactory for all food matrixes. Method **981.17**, Vitamin D in Fortified Milk and Milkpowder, LC Method, is regarded as satisfactory for the determination of vitamin D in cheese, dairy products, and infant formula/medical diet.

Vitamin E

Vitamin E is essential for a number of physiological functions (21). It serves as an antioxidant that can inhibit free radical chain reactions in tissue membranes, inhibit the formation of mutagens, and protect membranes from oxidative damage. It also plays an important role in the prevention of neuromuscular deficits, in maintaining proper red blood cell lifetime, and in the prevention of abnormal platelet activity. Recent studies also indicated a relationship between vitamin E and reduced risk of certain forms of cancer and heart disease. The role vitamin E plays in immunity, infection, and in reducing cataract formation is also under investigation.

The term vitamin E refers to all tocol and tocotrienol derivatives qualitatively exhibiting the biological activity of α-tocopherol. New nomenclature rules for vitamin E replaced the traditional ones and include the following: The term "tocopherol" is not synonymous with the term "vitamin E," *d*-α-tocopherol should be designated *RRR*-α-tocopherol, and *dl*-α-tocopherol should be designated *all-rac*-α-tocopherol. The analyst is referred to **972.31** in *Official Methods of Analysis*, 15th Ed., for a more thorough explanation of nomenclature rules for vitamin E (22).

The determination of the total vitamin E content of a food requires the determination of both naturally occurring and supplemental vitamin E vitamers. There are eight vitamers of vitamin E: four tocopherols (α-, β-, γ-, and δ-) and four corresponding tocotrienols. Because of their varying biological activities, the vitamers cannot be added together to arrive at a "total" vitamin E value. Quantitation of the eight individual isomers is complicated by the unavailability of satisfactory reference standards. Because α-tocopherol and its esters (acetate and succinate) are the most significant sources of vitamin E activity, the customary practice in the vast majority of cases is to quantify α-tocopherol only. Because tocopherols are sensitive to oxidation induced by light, heat, alkaline pH, and metal ions such as iron (Fe^{3+}) and copper (Cu^{2+}), the following standard precautions should be followed: Complete all steps of the analytical procedure as rapidly as possible. If the entire analysis cannot be completed within one day, all solutions must be stored in the dark at $-20\,^\circ$C. Evaporate tocopherol solutions with nitrogen or under vacuum, **not** with air. Because tocopherol in a thin film is quite sensitive to oxidation, do not allow the residue that remains after tocopherol solutions are evaporated to dryness to stand more than 2–3 s. Perform thin-layer chromatography (TLC) in darkness or very subdued light.

Because the basic chemical structure of α-tocopherol contains three asymmetric carbon atoms, there are eight possible diastereoisomers. The forms of most interest and significance to the analyst are *all-rac*-α-tocopheryl acetate (dl), *all-rac*-α-tocopherol (dl), *RRR*-α-tocopheryl acetate (d), and *RRR*-α-tocopherol (d). Analytical results for vitamin E assays are often expressed in IU. One IU of vitamin E is defined as 1 mg of *all-rac*-α-tocopheryl acetate. The relative biological activities (IU/mg) of the above forms are as follows (23): *all-rac*-α-tocopheryl acetate (dl), 1.00; *all-rac*-α-tocopherol (dl), 1.10; *RRR*-α-tocopheryl acetate (d), 1.36; and *RRR*-α-tocopherol (d), 1.49. Proper care must be taken when expressing the vitamin E content of supplemented foods and feeds in IU. The stereo isomeric form of the supplement must be known before the potency can be calculated.

The first colorimetric procedure for the determination of vitamin E was reported by Emmerie and Engel in 1938 (24). The procedure is based upon the reduction by tocopherols and tocotrienols of ferric ions to ferrous ions, which form a red complex with 2,2'-bipyridyl that is measured at 520 nm. Although widely used for the determination of vitamin E, especially in food products, the procedure has a number of shortcomings, such as interferences, the stability of the complex, and the possibility of photo-reduction of excess ferric ions. The latter two shortcomings were greatly improved by Tsen (25). Tsen used bathophenanthrolone, in place of 2,2'-bipyridyl, to provide a more stable and sensitive complex and orthophosphoric acid to stabilize excess ferric ions. However, interferences such as vitamin A, carotenoids, and sterols are still a problem. Tocopherol dimers and trimers that are biologically inactive will also interfere (26). Hence, Method **971.30**, a colorimetric method for α-tocopherol and α-tocopheryl acetate in foods and feeds, incorporates a TLC step to separate α-tocopherol from other unsaponifiable matter present, including the above potential interferences.

The following methods for the determination of vitamin E are described in *Official Methods of Analysis*, 15th Ed.: **971.30**, α-Tocopherol and α-Tocopheryl Acetate in Foods and Feeds (Colorimetric Method); **975.43**, Identification of *RRR*- or *all-rac*-α Tocopherol in Drugs and Food or Feed Supplements (Polarimetric Method); **948.26**, α-Tocopheryl Acetate (Supplemental) in Foods and Feeds (Colorimetric   Method); **988.14**, Tocopherol Isomers in Mixed Tocopherols Concentrate (Gas Chromatographic Method); **989.09**, α-Tocopheryl Acetate in Supplemental Vitamin E Concentrates (Gas Chromatographic Method); **969.40**, Vitamin E in Drugs (Gas Chromatographic Method); and **992.03**, Vitamin E Activity in Milk-Based Infant Formula (LC Method).

The AOAC Task Force on Methods for Nutrient Labeling Analyses found Method **971.30**, A-Tocopherol and A-Tocopheryl Acetate in Foods and Feeds, Colorimetric Method, satisfactory for the determination of vitamin E in all food matrixes considered. However, the method is technique dependent and reported to be difficult and tedious. Method **992.03**, Vitamin E Activity in Milk-Based Infant Formula, LC Method, is adequate for the determination of vitamin E in infant formula/medical diet. A normal-phase LC assay was developed by Cort et al. (27) for the determination of vitamin E in feedstuffs. The method uses fluorescence detection and can individually separate the four tocopherols and four tocotrienols. The procedure was applied to food products (28, 29), but a collaborative study is required.

Vitamin K

There are currently no AOAC validated methods deemed adequate for vitamin K.

Acknowledgements

The author acknowledges the contributions of the AOAC Task Force on Methods for Nutrient Labeling Analyses and thanks William J. Mergens for many fruitful discussions and reviews.

References

(1)   Ball, G.F.M. (1988) *Fat-Soluble Vitamin Assays in Food Analysis - A Comprehensive Review*, Elsevier Applied Science

(2)   Gaby, S.K., Bendich, A., Singh, V.N., & Machlin, L.J. (1991) *Vitamin Intake and Health - A Scientific Review*, Marcel Dekker, Inc., New York, NY

(3)   *Encyclopedia of Food Science and Technology, Vitamins* (1991) John Wily & Sons, Inc., Parts 1–8, Vol. 4, p. 2687

(4)   *Official Methods of Analysis* (1990) 15th Ed., AOAC, Arlington, VA, p. 1045

(5)   *Official Methods of Analysis* (1984) 14th Ed., AOAC, Arlington, VA, p. 830

(6)   DeVries, J.W., Egberg, D.C., & Heroff, J.C. (1979) "Concurrent Analysis of Vitamin A and Vitamin E by Reversed-Phase High Performance Liquid Chromatography" in *Liquid Chromatographic Analysis of Food and Beverages: Volume 2*, G. Charalambous (ed.), Academic Press, p. 477

(7)   Ames, S.R. (1966) *J. Assoc. Off. Anal. Chem.* **49**, 1071–1078

(8)   *Encyclopedia of Food Science and Technology, Vitamins* (1991) John Wily & Sons, Inc., Chapter 3, p. 2920

(9)   Vecchi, M., Englert, G., Maurer, R., & Meduna, V. (1981) *Helv. Chim. Acta* **64**, 2746–2758

(10)   Tsukida, K., & Kayoko, S. (1982) *J. Chromatogr.* **245**, 359–364

(11)   Quackenbush, F.W. (1987) *J. Liq. Chromatogr.* **10**, 643–653

(12)   Craft, N.E., Wise, S.A., & Soares, J.A. Jr. (1992) *J. Chromatogr.* **589**, 171–76

(13)   Epler, K.S., Sander, L.C., Ziegler, R.G., Wise, S.A., & Craft, N.E. (1992) *J. Chromatogr.* **595**, 89

(14)   Rizzolo, A., & Polesello, S. (1992) *J. Chromatogr.* **624**, 103–152

(15)   Furr, H.C., Barva, A.B., & Olson, J.A. (1992) *Retinoids and Carotenoids in Modern Chromatographic Analysis of Vitamins*, 2nd Ed., A.P. DeLeenheer, W.E. Lambert, & H.J. Nelis (eds), Marcel Dekker, Inc., New York, NY, pp. 1–71

(16)   O'Neil, J.P., & Schwartz, S.J. (1992) *J. Chromatogr.* **624**, 235–252

(17)   Sweeney, J.P., & Marsh, A.C. (1973) *J. Nutr.* **103**, 20–25

(18)   Weiser, H., & Kormann, A.W. (1993) *Provitamin A Activities of Carotenoids in Animal Models,* 10th International Symposium on Carotenoids, Trondheim, Norway, June 20–25, 1993

(19)   Bauernfeind, J.C. (1981) *Carotenoids as Colorants and Vitamin A Precursors, Technological and Nutritional Applications*, Academic Press, New York, NY

(20)   Mulder, F.J., deVries, E.J., & Borsje, B. (1971) *J. Assoc. Off. Anal. Chem.* **54**, 1168–1174

(21)   Gaby, S.K., Bendich, A., Singh, V.N., & Machlin, L.J. (1991) *Vitamin Intake and Health - A Scientific Review*, Marcel Dekker, Inc., New York, NY, p. 71

(22)   *Official Methods of Analysis* (1990) 15th Ed., AOAC, Arlington, VA, pp. 1070–1071

(23)   Bieri, J.G., & McKenna, M.C. (1981) *Am. J. Clin. Nutr.* **34**, 289–295

(24)   Emmerie, A., & Engel, C. (1938) *Rec. Trav. Chim.* **57**, 1351

(25)   Tsen, C.C. (1961) *Anal. Chem.*, **33**, 849

(26)   Ball, G.F.M. (1988) *Fat-Soluble Vitamin Assays in Food Analysis - A Comprehensive Review*, Elsevier Applied Science, p. 114

(27)   Cort, W.M., Vicente, T.S., Waysek, E.H., & Williams, B.D. (1983) *J. Agric. Food Chem.* **31**, 1330–1333

(28)   Waysek, E.H., Keating, J.P., & Gerenz, C.N. (1987) *Liquid Chromatographic Determination of Supplemental Vitamin E in Foods*, 101st AOAC Annual International Meeting, Sept. 14–17, San Francisco, CA

(29)   Kirkegaard, P.D., & Jabusch, J.A. (1987) *HPLC/Fluorescence Determination of α-Tocopherol in Selected Food Products*, 101st AOAC Annual International Meeting, Sept. 14–17, San Francisco, CA

Chapter 9
Water-Soluble Vitamins

Jonathan W. DeVries

Introduction

Unlike analyses that characterize the levels of fat, protein, moisture, carbohydrate, and ash (the macronutrients) in foods, analysis of the water-soluble vitamins presents challenges to the food analyst because these vitamins are often present in trace quantities. The quantities to be measured in a given food portion can range from the 100% (or greater) daily value level of 60 mg for vitamin C, to the 2% (the minimum considered nutritionally significant) daily value level of 0.12 mcg for vitamin B_{12}. This certainly presents a wide range of analyte levels. Of course, accurate and precise quantitation becomes difficult to achieve at the parts per billion level (2% daily value of B_{12} in a 100 g portion of food) so the utmost of care must be exercised by the analyst to produce quality results. Adding to the difficulties of quantitating low levels is the fact that vitamins, by nature, are very functional chemically, are often very labile molecules, and often serve as antioxidants and/or reaction intermediates in the body. Therefore, numerous precautions must be taken when handling samples and sample extracts containing water-soluble vitamins. This handling will assure that minimal vitamin degradation results from exposure to heat, light, oxygen, or other factors. In the case of some of the water-soluble vitamins, certain isomers of the vitamins, (i.e. isoascorbic acid) will have little or no vitamin activity or a different level of vitamin activity than other isomers. These isomers will show up as interferents to the analytical method or will require special treatments or methods to assure the that true vitamin activity is being measured. Carefully following the validated procedures and good laboratory techniques will overcome these difficulties and produce satisfactory results.

Vitamin C

Vitamin C is essential to a wide variety of human body functions. When deficiency of vitamin C occurs, the resulting symptoms are collectively defined as the malady scurvy. Individuals suffering from the deficiency disease exhibit weakness, fatigue, listlessness, shortness of breath, and aching in the bones, joints, and muscles. Hemorrhagic skin conditions appear along with gingival lesions in the mouth, often accompanied by loss of teeth. Hippocrates described the symptoms of vitamin C deficiency, but the deficiency became a major health problem with the development of ocean-going ships that allowed long sea voyages and the subsequent lack of access to fresh fruits and vegetables. Although the relationship of the disease state to vitamin C was not known, the British Navy realized the deficiency relationship to the lack of intake of fruits and vegetables and provided their seaman with rations of lemon (called limes) juice to ward off the malady, hence the nickname for British sailors of "limies." The deficiency disease shows up most frequently in individuals dining alone during those months when fresh fruits and vegetables are not available (late winter and early spring). Resumption of adequate intake begins a rapid reversal of the symptoms.

In addition to its role in prevention of scurvy, vitamin C is a powerful antioxidant, being itself easily oxidized. As such it often serves a sacrificial role in foods, preventing the oxidation of other nutrients present. This ease of oxidation presents the most significant problem to the analyst during the analysis of vitamin C. Oxidation of ascorbic acid is observed almost immediately upon extraction, and the rate depends on the relative concentration of the analyte in solution, the presence of metal ions that might act as catalysts, and the quantity of oxygen dissolved in the extraction media. Agents such as *m*-phosphoric acid added to chelate metal ions and the proper adjustment of pH help reduce, but do not eliminate, oxidation; therefore, proper handling of the samples, extracts, and timing of analytical steps is of the essence for quality results.

Vitamin C has two active forms: ascorbic acid and its first oxidation product, dehydroascorbic acid. Both are considered to have equal vitamin C activity. Further oxidation yields inactive products. Isoascorbic acid (erythrobic acid), often used as an antioxidant in foods, exhibits only 5% of the vitamin C activity of ascorbic acid.

AOAC INTERNATIONAL Official Methods **967.21** and **985.33** are based on the ease of oxidation of ascorbic acid. The acid is titrated with the mild, colored, oxidizing agent 1,2-dichloroindophenol. Only ascorbic acid is measured using these procedures. The vitamin C level of foods containing dehydroascorbic acid will be underestimated. Highly colored products such as colored fruit juices cannot be analyzed because of the difficulty of determining the endpoint. The presence of other easily oxidized substances such as Maillard browning intermediates and products (often called reductones) present in the sample will give artificially high results because they consume the indophenol titrant.

Methods **984.26** and **967.22** both measure the total vitamin C content of the sample. Ascorbic acid is oxidized to dehydroascorbic acid. The total dehydroascorbic acid is then reacted with phenylene diamine to produce the measurable fluorescent adduct. If the analyst desires to measure only dehydroascorbic acid, the oxidation step can merely be omitted. Therefore, ascorbic acid can be analyzed by measuring the total vitamin C and the dehydroascorbic acid and then calculating the difference.

Isoascorbic acid, if present, is analyzed as vitamin C by all four methods mentioned above, thereby rendering the methods of little value if isoascorbic acid has been added to the food product. Numerous analysts have turned to high performance liquid chromatography (HPLC) as a potential means of handling this problem, but methods development has been difficult because of the handling difficulties with this vitamin (1, 2).

Niacin

Pellagra, one of the health states resulting from deficient intake of niacin, is a dermatological condition of cracking, pigmentation changes, and sometimes lesions that occur where skin is exposed to sunlight. In addition to pellagra, deficient individuals experience malfunctions of the gastrointestinal tract and the nervous system. Anemia, anxiety, depression, and fatigue are often symptoms found. Niacin is an essential component of the enzyme systems for the metabolism of carbohydrates, fatty acids, and amino acids.

Tryptophan also serves as a source (by conversion in the body) of niacin in the diet and is considered a part of the overall niacin nutrient content of the food.

Method **960.46** combined with **944.13** and Method **985.34** are microbiological assay methods suitable for the determination of niacin in all food types. Microbiological methods are preferred over colorimetric methods for foods containing high levels of Maillard browning products (for example, cocoa containing products), which give high blanks with the colorimetric procedure. The AOAC INTERNATIONAL Task Force on Methods for Nutrient Labeling Analyses, in its deliberations on the microbiological methods for niacin, recommended a collaborative study on the use of *L. planarum* for all matrices with the **960.46/985.24** combination.

Aside from samples with high levels of browning products, Methods **961.14**, **981.16**, and **975.41**, which use colorimetry for the determinative step, give comparable results to the microbiological method, as evidenced by collaborative study results. Although the microbiological methods may provide higher levels of sensitivity for niacin in some samples, the daily dietary requirements for the vitamin are sufficiently high that both methods will measure nutritionally significant levels.

HPLC methods for niacin have been considered and evaluated. Despite the difficulty with achieving retention times that assure chromatographic separation of the analyte, there is an ongoing interest in developing this technique and validating Official Methods that use HPLC (3).

Tryptophan can be determined microbiologically using Method **960.46**. A collaborative study is recommended on the use of **960.46** combined with a digestion using *L. plantarum* to measure both the free and bound forms of tryptophan in foods.

Method **988.15**, an ion-exchange method, is adequate for all foods for nutrition labeling. Method **982.30** can also be used for quantitation of tryptophan. Analyst time may be saved when amino acids are being run on the sample for protein labeling purposes, and tryptophan data is also used to calculate the niacin equivalents represented by the tryptophan.

Pantothenate

Because of the widespread availability of pantothenic acid in normal food sources, deficiency effects resulting from insufficient intake of this nutrient are rarely observed. Only in cases of severe malnourishment does insufficiency occur. The primary symptom of insufficiency is a burning sensation on the soles of the feet. Pantothenic acid has been found in measurable quantities in all commodity food groups.

The microbiological methods (Method **960.46** combined with **945.74**) are validated as suitable for the free forms of pantothenic acid only. Attention must be paid to the steps for discarding outliers and qualifying data outlined in **960.46H** to assure proper method performance. For total pantothenic acid content, and enzymatic digestion of the sample with *L. plantarum* and *A. suboxydaus* is recommended. The enzymatic digestion procedure has not been validated through collaborative study. Care must be taken to avoid spoilage in the food sample before analysis, because pantothenic acid levels have been shown to increase with spoilage.

Vitamin B$_6$ (Pyridoxine)

Although vitamin B$_6$ has been proven, through a substantial body of animal studies, to be involved in multiple and numerous aspects of metabolic processes, no particular deficiency related to B$_6$ has been identified in humans, apparently because of the vitamin's presence in a wide variety of foods at significant levels. The vitamin occurs in three vitamer forms, pyridoxine (free alcohol), pyridoxal, and pyridoxamine, as well as their respective phosphates. Analysis of each of the different forms are carried out microbiologically based on the selective differential response of different microorganisms or by chromatographic separation of the vitamers followed by growth response measurements using a single microbe strain. The latter method may be advantageous in assuring against the presence of factors that promote growth in a microorganism but not in humans.

Method **960.46** combined with **961.15** and Method **985.32** rely on microbiological growths rates as the means of quantitating vitamin B$_6$. Satisfactory results can be obtained for the quantitation of all three vitamer forms of vitamin B$_6$.

Vitamin B$_2$ (Riboflavin)

Deficiency diseases associated with lack of sufficient intake of riboflavin have been recognized for some time, and treatment for the symptoms is the consumption of yeast products. The deficiency disease manifests itself in facial lesions (particularly in folds of the skin around the mouth and nose), soreness of the tongue, scrotal and vulval dermatitis and lesions, and conjunctivitis, lacrimation, and itching of the eyes. All symptoms of the deficiency disease respond rapidly to adequate dietary intake of riboflavin. Riboflavin occurs in the free form as well as in the form of riboflavin phosphate in food samples. Analytical schemes must include a phosphate ester hydrolysis step to assure the total riboflavin present in the sample is measured by whatever quantitation technique is chosen for the determination.

Methods **970.65**, **981.15**, and **985.31** all depend on the natural fluorescence of the riboflavin molecule for their determinative step. The key to successful analysis using these procedures is the removal of interfering fluorescence resulting from other compounds present. Elimination of interfering fluorescence is accomplished by two means. First, the extract of the sample is treated with potassium permanganate to oxidize interferences susceptible to such oxidation (riboflavin is not). Excess potassium permanganate is then destroyed, and the fluorescence of the solution is measured (*Caution*: Gas bubbles may form during the permanganate destruction step and must be removed from cuvettes before taking fluorescence readings to prevent light scattering and erroneous readings). The solution is treated with dithionate solution to destroy the riboflavin present. Any fluorescence remaining in the solution is measured and subtracted as a blank from the initial readings. The automated method provides a convenient means of handling a substantial number of samples in a short time frame.

The microbiological assay procedure for riboflavin, a combination of Methods **960.46** and **960.33**, gives identical results to the fluorimetric method on the basis of a collaborative study comparing the two methods. For adequate method performance, close attention must be paid to the steps for discarding outlier results and qualifying the data.

Although a substantial number of reports have appeared on the use of HPLC for the separation and quantitation of riboflavin from foods or food extracts, none of the methods has been collaboratively studied to date.

Vitamin B$_1$ (Thiamine)

Thiamine occurs in nature in a wide variety of foodstuffs at widely varying levels. Meat and fish, whole cereal grains, nuts and legumes, brewer's yeast, eggs, and fruits and vegetables all contain measurable levels of this nutrient. Deficiencies of the vitamin are rare, with the exception of individuals in cultures whose diet consists almost solely of polished rice. The deficiency disease, called beriberi, usually manifests itself as edema (swelling).

All of the Official Methods for thiamine (**942.23**, **957.17**, **953.17**, and **986.27**) depend on fluorimetry of thiochrome (oxidation product of thiamine) as the final determinative step of the analysis. Method **942.23** is considered adequate for nutrition labeling analysis for all foods, Method **986.27** for infant formula and medical diets, and Methods **957.17** and **953.17** for cereals, sweet mixes, and cereal products.

Folacin

A shortage of folate intake results in anemia, retarded growth, weakness, depression, dermatological lesions, and (if deficiency occurs during pregnancy) birth defects in offspring. Folate is found in a wide variety of foods of both animal and plant origin, with especially high levels present in liver, brewer's yeast, and vegetables. Insufficient supplies of zinc in the diet reduce the functional effectiveness of the folate present in the body.

Method **960.46**, when combined with method **944.12**, will provide satisfactory results for free folate on a routine basis. Close attention must be paid to the steps for discarding outliers and qualifying data, as outlined in **960.46H**. For total folacin content, an enzymatic digestion of the sample with *K. apriculata* is recommended, although this digestion step has not been collaboratively studied. Such a collaborative study is recommended. Folate is sensitive to freeze/thaw/freeze cycles and also degrades rapidly after extraction. Analysts need to provide proper samples storage (avoid self defrosting freezers that allow samples to thaw) and to analyze sample extracts in as short a time frame as possible.

An additional microbiological method (**992.05**) for free folate has been given official status.

Biotin

Deficiency of intake of biotin in humans results in dermatitis, mild depression, and muscle aches. This is followed by slight anemia and increases in serum cholesterol. Insufficient biotin intake is not the only cause of biotin deficiency. If the intake of anti-biotin (Avidin protein that binds biotin, such as that found in egg whites) exceeds the intake of biotin, deficiency can also result.

Currently, no Official Methods are considered adequate for the analysis of biotin in foods. Most analysts working with this nutrient use modifications (*L. plantarum* is recommended) of Method **960.46**. A collaborative study of appropriate methodology for this nutrient has been recommended by the AOAC Task Force on Methods for Nutrient Labeling Analyses.

Vitamin B$_{12}$ (Cyancobalamine)

Insufficient body stores of vitamin B$_{12}$ manifest themselves in the form of the vitamin deficiency disease called pernicious anemia, a disease state affecting not only the red blood cells but also the nervous system and the stomach. The vitamin is widely found in animal based food sources; therefore, deficiency usually is experienced only by those on vegetarian diets. In addition to pernicious anemia, animal studies show that vitamin B$_{12}$ is an important growth factor; however, because of the much slower growth rate of humans, it is difficult to ascertain whether deficient levels of the vitamin are responsible for the subnormal growth rates.

Microbiological assay is the only officially validated methodology for the analysis of vitamin B$_{12}$. Method **960.46** combined with **952.20** and **986.23** will provide satisfactory results for vitamin B$_{12}$ on a routine basis. Particular attention must be paid to the steps involved with discarding outliers and qualifying all data, as described in **960.46H**, to assure proper method performance. Vitamin B$_{12}$ is formed by bacteria; therefore, improper storage and/or sample spoilage may increase the apparent level of the vitamin in the food sample being analyzed.

References

(1)   Vanderslice, J.T., & Higgs, D.J. (1993) *J. Nutr. Biochem* **4**, 184–190

(2)   Pelletier, O. (1985) "Vitamin C (L-Ascorbic and L-Dehydroascorbic Acids," in *Methods of Vitamin Assay*, 4th Ed., Augustin, J., Klein, B.P., Becker, D.A., & Vanugopal, P.B. (eds), John Wiley and Sons, New York, NY, p. 318

(3)   DeVries, J.W. (1985) "Chromatographic Assay of Vitamins," in *Methods of Vitamin Assay*, 4th Ed., Augustin, J., Klein, B.P., Becker, D.A., & Vanugopal, P.B. (eds), John Wiley and Sons, New York, NY, p. 87

*Official Methods
of Analysis*

Chapter 10
Ash

10.1   **940.26A—Ash of Fruits and Fruit Products**
Final Action

A. Ash

Proceed as in **900.02A** or **B**, ashing at ≤525°, using 25 g juices, fresh fruits, or canned fruits, and 10 g jellies, sirups, preserves, jams, marmalades, or dried fruits.

If ash of H_2O-soluble portion only is desired, evaporate 100 mL prepared solution, **920.149(b)** or (**c**), to dryness on steam bath. Proceed as in **900.02A** or **B**.

NOTE: The Task Force on Methods for Nutrient Labeling Analyses has recommended that all references to 900.02A and 900.02B be replaced by 923.03 (see 10.20).

I. **900.02A** [Ash of Sugars and Sirups; from *Official Methods of Analysis* (1984) 14th ed., **31.012**]
Heat sample of appropriate weight for product being examined (usually 5–10 g) in 50–100 mL Pt dish at 100° until H_2O is expelled; add few drops pure olive oil and heat *slowly* over flame or under IR lamp until swelling stops. Place dish in furnace at ca 525° and leave until white ash is obtained. Moisten ash with H_2O, dry on steam bath and then on hot plate, and re-ash at 525° to constant weight.

II. **900.02B** [Ash of Sugars and Sirups; from *Official Methods of Analysis* (1984) 14th ed., **31.013**]
Carbonize sample of appropriate weight for product being examined (usually 5–10 g) in 50–100 mL Pt dish at ca 525° and treat charred mass with hot H_2O to dissolve soluble salts. (In case of low-purity products, addition of few drops of pure olive oil, as in **31.012**, may be desirable.) Filter through ashless paper, ignite paper and residue to white ash, add filtrate of soluble salts, evaporate to dryness, and ignite at ca 525° to constant weight.

III. **920.149(b)** and (**c**)
(**b**) *Jellies and sirups.*—Mix thoroughly to ensure uniform sample. Prepare solution by weighing 300 g thoroughly mixed sample into 2 L flask and dissolve in H_2O, heating on steam bath if necessary. Apply as little heat as possible to minimize inversion of sucrose. Cool, dilute to volume, mix thoroughly by shaking, and use aliquots for the various determinations. If insoluble material is present, mix thoroughly and filter first.
(**c**) *Fresh fruits, dried fruits, preserves, jams, and marmalades.*—Pulp by passing through food chopper, or by use of soil dispersion mixer, Hobart mixer, or other suitable mechanical mixing apparatus, or by grinding in large mortar, and mixing thoroughly, completing operation as quickly as possible to avoid loss of moisture. With dried fruits, pass sample through food chopper 3 times, mixing thoroughly after each grinding. Set burrs or blades of food chopper as close as possible

without crushing seeds. Grind entire contents of No. 10 or smaller container. Mix contents of larger containers thoroughly by stirring and remove portion for grinding. With stone fruits, remove pits and determine their proportion in weighed sample.

Prepare solution by weighing into 1.5–2 L beaker 300 g fresh fruit, or equivalent of dried fruit, preserves, jams, and marmalades, well-pulped and mixed in blender or other suitable type of mechanical grinder; add ca 800 mL H_2O; and boil 1 hr, replacing at intervals H_2O lost by evaporation. Transfer to 2 L volumetric flask, cool, dilute to volume, and filter. With unsweetened fruit, ashing is facilitated by addition of sugar before boiling; therefore, weigh 150 g fruit, add 150 g sugar and 800 mL H_2O, and proceed as above.

Reference: JAOAC **23,** 314(1940).

10.2 920.153—Ash of Meat
Final Action

Proceed as in **900.02A** or **B** (*see* 10.1).

10.3 925.51A—Ash of Canned Vegetables

Proceed as in **900.02A** or **B** (*see* 10.1).

10.4 950.14A—Ash of Nonalcoholic Beverages
Final Action

Proceed as in **900.02A** or **B** (*see* 10.1).

10.5 920.100A,B—Ash in Tea
Final Action

A. Ash

Proceed as in **900.02A** or **B** (*see* 10.1).

B. Soluble and Insoluble Ash

Proceed as in **900.02D**, using the ash obtained in **920.100A**.

900.02D [Ash of Sugars and Sirups; from *Official Methods of Analysis* (1984) 14th ed., **31.015**]

Ash sample as in **900.02A** or **B**. Add 10 mL H_2O to ash in the Pt dish, heat nearly to boiling, filter through ashless paper, and wash with hot H_2O until combined filtrate and washings measure ca 60 mL. Return paper and contents to Pt dish, ignite carefully, cool, and weigh. Calculate % H_2O-soluble and H_2O-insoluble ash.

10.6   925.49A,C,D—Confectionary
Final Action

A. Preparation of Sample

If composition of entire sample is desired, grind and mix thoroughly. If sample is composed of layers or of distinctly different portions and it is desired to examine these individually, separate with knife or other mechanical means as completely as possible, and grind and mix each portion thoroughly.

C. Ash

Proceed as in **900.02A** or **B** (*see* 10.1).

D. Soluble and Insoluble Ash

Proceed as in **900.02D** (*see* 10.5).

10.7   972.15—Ash of Cacao Products
First Action 1972
Final Action 1974
*AOAC-Office International du Cacao
et du Chocolat Method*

A. Determination

Accurately weigh 2–5 g prepared sample, **970.20**, into 25–50 mL Pt, quartz, or Vycor dish previously heated to 600°, covered with watch glass, cooled in desiccator, and weighed. Carbonize by either (*1*) slowly bringing temperature of furnace to 600° in hood with exhaust vent open or door not completely closed; or (*2*) heating under IR lamps until smoking ceases and then transferring to 600° furnace. Heat 2 h. Moisten cooled ash with alcohol, dry under IR lamps or on steam bath, and re-ash at 1 h intervals until change in weight is <1 mg, or overnight. Cover with watch glass, cool in desiccator, and weigh as soon as room temperature is attained.

970.20 (Preparation of Sample, Procedure)

(a) *Powdered products.*—Mix thoroughly and preserve in tightly stoppered bottles.

(b) *Chocolate products.*—(*1*) Chill ca 200 g sweet or bitter chocolate until hard, and grate or shave to fine granular condition. Mix thoroughly and preserve in tightly stoppered bottle in cool place. Alternatively—(*2*) Melt ca 200 g bitter, sweet, or milk chocolate by placing in suitable container and partly immersing container in bath at ca 50°. Stir frequently until sample melts and reaches temperature of 45–50°. Remove from bath, stir thoroughly, and while still liquid, remove portion for analysis, using glass or metal tube, 4–10 mm diameter, provided with close-fitting plunger to expel sample from tube, or disposable plastic syringe.

Reference: JAOAC **53,** 388(1970).

B. Soluble and Insoluble Ash

Proceed as in **900.02D** (*see* 10.5), using ash from **972.15A**.

Reference: JAOAC **55,** 1027(1972).

10.8 945.18C—Cereal Adjuncts
Final Action

C. Ash

Proceed as in **923.03** (*see* 10.20).

10.9 930.22—Ash of Bread
Final Action

Use 3–5 g prepared sample, **926.04,** and proceed as in **923.03** (*see* 10.20) or **936.07B.**

I. **926.04** (Preparation of Sample)

(a) *All types of bread not containing fruit.*—Cut loaf, or ½ loaf, of bread into slices 2–3 mm thick. Spread slices on paper and let dry in warm room until sufficiently crisp and brittle to grind well in mill. Grind entire sample to pass No. 20 sieve, mix well, and keep in air-tight container. References: JAOAC **9,** 42(1926); **15,** 72(1932); **17,** 65(1934).

(b) *Raisin bread.*—Proceed as in (a), except comminute by passing twice through food chopper instead of grinder.

II. **936.07** (Ash of Flour, Magnesium Acetate Method)

A. Reagent

Magnesium acetate solution.—Dissolve 4.054 g $Mg(OAc)_2 \cdot 4H_2O$ in 50 mL H_2O and dilute to 1 L with alcohol.

B. Determination

From buret add 5 mL of the reagent to 3–5 g flour, bread, etc., or 10 mL to 1 g bran, wheat germ, etc. Let stand 1–2 min, evaporate excess alcohol, and place in furnace at 700°, closing door after flaming ceases. When incineration is complete, place dish in desiccator until cool; then weigh. Determine blank on solution and deduct blank from weight ash. Evaporate blank cautiously.

References: JAOAC **19,** 85(1936); **20,** 69(1937); **22,** 522(1939).

Reference: JAOAC **9,** 42(1926).

10.10   935.42—Ash of Cheese
Gravimetric Method
Final Action

Weigh 3–5 g prepared sample, **955.30**, into Pt dish, place on steam bath, and dry ca 1 h. (If cheese is high in fat, place small amount of absorbent cotton in dish.) Ignite cautiously to avoid spattering and remove burner while fat is burning. When flame ceases, complete ignition in furnace at ≤550°, cool, and weigh.

955.30 (Preparation of Samples, Procedure)

Cut wedge sample into strips and pass 3 times through food chopper. Grind plugs in food chopper (preferable method), or cut or shred very finely and mix thoroughly.

With creamed cottage and similar cheeses, place 300–600 g sample at <15° in 1 L (1 qt) cup of high-speed blender and blend for minimum time (2–5 min) required to obtain homogeneous mixture. Final temperature should be ≤25°. This may require stopping blender frequently after channeling and spooning cheese back into blades until blending action starts. (Use of variable transformer in line to permit slow speed at first minimizes channeling when speed is increased later.)

References: JAOAC **18,** 401(1935); **20,** 339(1937).

10.11   945.46—Ash of Milk
Gravimetric Method
Final Action

Into suitable Pt dish weigh ca 5 g prepared sample, **925.21**, and evaporate to dryness on steam bath. Ignite in furnace at ≤550° until ash is C-free. Cool in desiccator, weigh, and calculate % ash.

925.21 (Preparation of Milk Sample, Procedure)

Bring sample to ca 20°, mix until homogeneous by pouring into clean receptacle and back repeatedly, and promptly weigh or measure test portion. If lumps of cream do not disperse, warm sample in H_2O bath to ca 38° and keep mixing until homogeneous, using policeman, if necessary, to reincorporate any cream adhering to container or stopper. Where practical and fat remains dispersed, cool warmed samples to ca 20° before transferring test portion.

When Babcock method, **989.04C** (*see* Chapter 18.12), is used, adjust both fresh and composite samples to ca 38°, mix until homogeneous as above, and immediately pipet portions into test bottles.

References: JAOAC **23**, 453(1940); **28**, 211(1945); **34**, 239(1951).

10.12 920.117—Casein, Ash, and Salt in Butter
Final Action

Cover crucible containing residue from fat determination by indirect method, **938.06A** (*see* Chapter 18.10); heat, gently at first, and gradually raise temperature to ≤500°. Remove cover and continue heating until residue is white. Loss in weight represents casein; residue in crucible represents mineral matter. Dissolve residue in H_2O slightly acidified with HNO_3 and determine Cl, either gravimetrically as in **928.04B** [*see Official Methods of Analysis* (1990) 15th Ed.], or volumetrically as in **915.01B** [*see Official Methods of Analysis* (1990) 15th Ed.], and calculate % NaCl.

CAS-9000-71-9 (casein)
CAS-7647-14-5 (sodium chloride)

10.13 930.30—Ash of Dried Milk
Final Action

Ignite 1 g sample at ≤550° until C-free. If suitable dish was used for moisture determination, **927.05**, ash may be determined on same portion. Cool in desiccator and weigh.

927.05 (Moisture in Dried Milk, Final Action)

Weigh 1–1.5 g sample into round, flat-bottom metal dish (≥5 cm diameter and provided with tight-fitting slip-in cover). Loosen cover and place dish on metal shelf (dish resting directly on shelf) in vacuum oven at 100°. Dry to constant weight (ca 5 h) under pressure ≤100 mm (4″) of Hg. During drying, admit slow current of air into oven (ca 2 bubbles/sec), dried by passing through H_2SO_4. Stop vacuum pump and carefully admit dried air into oven. Press cover tightly into dish, remove from oven, cool, and weigh. Calculate % loss in weight as moisture.

References: JAOAC **10**, 308(1927); **11**, 289(1928).

10.14   **920.108—Ash of Cream**
                          Final Action

Proceed as in **945.46** (*see* 10.11).

10.15   **945.48B,D,E—Evaporated Milk (Unsweetened)**
                          Final Action

B. Preparation of Sample—Procedure, IDF-ISO-AOAC Method
   (**a**) Temper unopened can in H_2O bath at ca 60°. Remove and vigorously shake can every 15 min. After 2 h, remove can and let cool to room temperature. Remove entire lid and thoroughly mix by stirring contents in can with spoon or spatula. (If fat separates, sample is not properly prepared.)
   (**b**) Dilute 40 g prepared mixture (**a**) with 60 g H_2O and mix thoroughly.
   References: JAOAC **28**, 207(1945); **52**, 239(1969).

D. Total Solids, IDF-ISO-AOAC Method
   Proceed as in **925.23A**, using 4–5 g diluted sample, **945.48B(b)**. Correct result for dilution.
   References: JAOAC **23**, 453(1940); **28**, 211(1945); **34**, 239(1951).

   925.23A [Solids (Total) in Milk, IDF-ISO-AOAC Method]
        A. Method I—Final Action
        Weigh 2.5–3 g prepared sample, **925.21** (*see* 10.11), into weighed flat-bottom dish ≥5 cm diameter; use ca 5 g and Pt dish if ash is to be determined on same portion. Heat on steam bath 10–15 min, exposing maximum surface of dish bottom to live steam; then heat 3 h in air oven at 98–100°. Cool in desiccator, weigh quickly, and report % residue as total solids.

E. Ash
   Ignite residue from total solids determination, **945.48D**, at temperature ≤550° until ash is C-free. Correct result for dilution.

References: JAOAC **23**, 453(1940); **28**, 211(1945); **34**, 239(1951).

10.16   **920.115E—Sweetened Condensed Milk**
                          Final Action

E. Ash
   Evaporate 10 mL prepared solution, **920.115B(b)**, to dryness on H_2O bath and ignite residue as in **900.02A** or **B** (*see* 10.1). Correct result for dilution.

920.115B

B. Preparation of Sample—Procedure

(a) Temper unopened can in H_2O bath at 30–35° until warm. Open, scrape out all milk adhering to interior of can, transfer to dish large enough to permit stirring thoroughly, and mix until whole mass is homogeneous.

(b) Weigh 100 g thoroughly mixed sample into 500 mL volumetric flask, dilute to volume with H_2O, and mix thoroughly. If sample will not emulsify uniformly, weigh out separate portion of (a) for each determination.

10.17   938.08—Ash of Seafood
Final Action

Dry sample containing ca 2 g dry material and proceed as in **900.02A** or **B** (*see* 10.1), using temperature ≤550°. If material contains large amount of fat, make preliminary ashing at low enough temperature to allow smoking off of fat without burning.

References: JAOAC **21,** 85(1938); **23,** 589(1940).

10.18   986.25A—Proximate Analysis of Milk-Based Infant Formula
First Action 1986
Final Action 1988

A. Ash

Proceed as in **945.46** (*see* 10.11).

10.19   950.49—Ash of Nuts and Nut Products
Gravimetric Method
First Action

Proceed as in **900.02A,** or **B** (*see* 10.1) if added chlorides are present.

References: JAOAC **33,** 753(1950); **34,** 357(1951).

10.20

923.03—Ash of Flour
Direct Method
Final Action

Weigh 3–5 g well-mixed sample into shallow, relatively broad ashing dish that has been ignited, cooled in desiccator, and weighed soon after reaching room temperature. Ignite in furnace at ca 550° (dull red) until light gray ash results, or to constant weight. Cool in desiccator and weigh soon after reaching room temperature. Reignited CaO is satisfactory drying agent for desiccator.

Reference: JAOAC **7**, 132(1923).

10.21

935.39B—Baked Products
Final Action

(Other than bread; not containing fruit)

B. Ash

Proceed as in **923.03** (*see* 10.20).

References: JAOAC **16**, 518(1933); **17**, 404(1934); **23**, 537(1940); **35**, 687(1952).

10.22

941.12—Ash of Spices
Gravimetric Methods
Final Action

A. Determination

(**a**) *Most spices.*—Accurately weigh ca 2 g sample in flat-bottom dish, preferably Pt. Place dish in entrance of open furnace so that sample fumes off without catching fire. Then ash in furnace 30 min at 550°, break up ash with several drops H_2O, evaporate carefully to dryness, and heat in furnace 30 min. If previous wetting showed ash to be C-free, remove dish to desiccator containing fresh, efficient desiccant (H_2SO_4 or anhydrous $Mg(ClO_4)_2$ is satisfactory), let cool to room temperature, and weigh soon. If first wetting showed C, repeat wetting and heating until no specks of C are visible; then heat 30 min after disappearance of C. If C persists, leach ash with hot H_2O, filter through quantitative paper, wash paper thoroughly, transfer paper and contents to ashing dish, dry, and ignite at 550° until ash is white. Cool dish, add filtrate, evaporate to dryness on steam bath, and heat in furnace 30 min. Cool, and weigh as previously.

(**b**) *Nutmeg, mace, ginger, and cloves.*—Proceed as in (**a**), but heat at 600°.

(**c**) *Ground mustard or mustard flour.*—Ignite as in (**a**) and heat 30 min at 550°. Leach ash with hot H_2O, filter, and wash thoroughly. Transfer paper and contents to ashing dish, dry, and heat in furnace 30 min. Remove dish, let cool, add 5–10 drops HNO_3, evaporate to dryness, and heat in furnace 30 min. Repeat

HNO_3 and heating treatment until residue is white. Add filtrate, evaporate to dryness, and heat in furnace 30 min. Cool, and weigh as in (**a**).

Reference: JAOAC **24,** 667(1941).

B. Soluble and Insoluble Ash

Proceed as in **900.02D** (*see* 10.5), using ash obtained in **941.12A.**

C. Ash Insoluble in Acid

Boil H_2O-insoluble residue, **941.12B**, or total ash, **941.12A**, with 25 mL HCl (2 + 5) 5 min, covering dish with watch glass to prevent spattering; collect insoluble matter on gooch or ashless filter, wash with hot H_2O until washings are acid-free, ignite until C-free, cool, and weigh.

Chapter 11
β-Carotene

11.1   **941.15—Carotenes in Fresh Plant Materials and Silages**
Spectrophotometric Method
Final Action

(*Caution: See Appendix* for safety notes on blenders, distillation, flammable solvents, acetone, and hexane.)

A. Reagents

(**a**) *Acetone.*—Dry, alcohol-free. To dry, treat with anhydrous Na_2SO_4 and distil over granular ca "10 mesh" Zn.
(**b**) *Commercial hexane.*—Bp 60–70°; distilled over KOH.
(**c**) *Adsorbent.*—Activated magnesia (Sea Sorb 43; Fisher Scientific Co., No. S-120).
(**d**) *Diatomaceous earth.*—Hyflo Super-Cel.

B. Extraction

Finely cut material with scissors or knife, or grind in food chopper to assure representative sample. If analysis cannot be performed immediately, blanch in boiling H_2O 5–10 min and store in frozen condition. Place 2–5 g weighed sample in high-speed blender; add 40 mL acetone, 60 mL hexane, and 0.1 g $MgCO_3$, and blend 5 min. Filter with suction or let residue settle and decant into separator. Wash residue with two 25 mL portions acetone, then with 25 mL hexane, and combine extracts. Wash acetone from extract with five 100 mL portions H_2O, transfer upper layer to 100 mL volumetric flask containing 9 mL acetone, and dilute to volume with hexane. If desired, alcohol may be used instead of acetone for extraction. Use 80 mL alcohol and 60 mL hexane in blender; other volumes same as for acetone.

C. Separation of Pigments

Pack activated magnesia-diatomaceous earth mixture (1 + 1) in chromatographic tube 22 mm od × 175 mm sealed to 10 mm od tube at bottom. To prepare column, place small glass wool or cotton plug inside tube, add loose adsorbent to 15 cm depth, attach tube to suction flask, and apply full vacuum of H_2O pump. Use flat instrument (such as inverted cork mounted on rod or tamping rod) to gently press adsorbent and flatten surface (packed column should be ca 10 cm deep). Place 1 cm layer anhydrous Na_2SO_4 above adsorbent.

With vacuum continuously applied to flask, pour extract into column. Use 50 mL acetone–hexane (1 + 9), or slightly more, if necessary, to develop chromatogram and wash visible carotenes through adsorbent. Keep top of column covered with layer of solvent during entire operation (conveniently done by clamping inverted volumetric flask full of solvent above column with neck 1–2 cm above surface of adsorbent).

Collect entire eluate. (Carotenes pass rapidly through column; bands of xanthophylls, carotene oxidation products, and chlorophylls should be present in column when operation is complete.) Transfer eluate, which has been reduced in volume by loss of vapor through H_2O pump, to 100 mL volumetric flask, dilute to volume with acetonehexane $(1 + 9)$, and determine carotene content photometrically.

D. Determination

Determine A of solution as soon as possible with spectrophotometer at 436 nm or with instrument having suitable filter system, such as Klett photo-meter with No. 44 filter, or Evelyn photoelectric colorimeter with 440 nm filter. Calibrate these instruments first with solutions of high purity β-carotene as shown by characteristic absorption curve (J. Biol. Chem. **144,** 21(1942)). Prepare calibration chart and convert A of solution to be determined to carotene concentration from chart.

When determinations are made with properly calibrated spectrophotometer at 436 nm,

$$C = (A \times 454)/(196 \times L \times W)$$

where C = concentration carotene (mg/lb) in original sample, L = cell length in cm, and W = g sample/mL final dilution. Report results as mg β-carotene/lb. Multiply by 2.2 to give ppm or by 1667 to give International Units/lb.

References: Ind. Eng. Chem. Anal. Ed. **13,** 600(1941); **15,** 18(1943); **16,** 513(1944); **19,** 170(1947). J. Biol. Chem. **164,** 2(1946). JAOAC **25,** 573, 886(1942); **26,** 77(1943); **27,** 542(1944); **28,** 563(1945); **29,** 18(1946); **30,** 412(1947); **31,** 459, 621, 623, 633, 776(1948); **32,** 480, 766, 775, 804(1949); **33,** 647(1950); **34,** 387, 460(1951); **35,** 736, 826(1952); **36,** 857(1953); **37,** 753, 756, 880, 887, 894(1954); **38,** 694(1955); **39,** 139(1956); **40,** 865(1957); **41,** 600(1958); **42,** 528(1959); **45,** 219(1962); **48,** 168(1965); **53,** 181, 186(1970).
CAS-36-88-4 (carotene)

Chapter 12
Calcium

12.1
968.08—Minerals in Animal Feed
Atomic Absorption Spectrophotometric Method
First Action 1968
Final Action 1969

(*Caution: See Appendix* for safety notes on AAS.)

A. Apparatus

Atomic absorption spectrophotometer.—See **965.09A** (*see* 12.3).

B. Operating Parameters

See Table **965.09**, except use fuel-rich air-C_2H_2 flame for Ca and Mg, and ranges of operation for μg element/mL solution are: Ca 5–20, Cu 2–20, Fe 5–20, Mg 0.5–2.5, Mn 5–20, and Zn 1–5.

C. Reagents

(*See* introduction to **965.09B**. Commercial prepared standard solutions may be used.)

(**a**) *Calcium standard solutions.*—Prepare as in **965.09B(a)**.

(**b**) *Copper, iron, magnesium, manganese, and zinc standard solutions.*—Prepare stock solutions as in **965.09B(b)**, (**c**), (**e**), (**f**), and (**g**), and dilute aliquots with 0.1–0.5N HCl to make $\geq$4 standard solutions of each element within range of determination.

D. Preparation of Sample Solution

(**a**) *Dry ashing* (*not applicable to mineral-mix feeds*).—Ash 2–10 g sample in well-glazed porcelain dish. Start in cold furnace, bring to 550°, and hold 4 h. Cool, add 10 mL 3N HCl, cover with watch glass, and boil gently 10 min. Cool, filter into 100 mL volumetric flask, and dilute to volume with H_2O. Subsequent dilutions with 0.1–0.5N HCl may be necessary to bring sample solutions into analytical range, except for Ca. Final Ca dilution must contain enough La solution, **965.09B(d)**, to provide 1% La concentration after dilution to volume with H_2O.

(**b**) *Wet digestion.*—Proceed as in **935.13A(a)**, adding 25 mL HNO_3 for each 2.5 g sample and diluting to 100 mL with H_2O. Digestion can be made at low heat on hot plate, using 600 mL beaker covered with watch glass. Subsequent dilutions with 0.1–0.5N HCl may be necessary to bring sample solutions into analytical range, as in (**a**).

> **935.13A(a)**
>
> *A. Preparation of Solution*
>
> (*Caution: See Appendix* for safety notes on nitric acid and perchloric acid.)

(a) Weigh 2.5 g sample into 500 or 800 mL Kjeldahl flask. Add 20–30 mL HNO_3 and boil gently 30–45 min to oxidize all easily oxidizable matter. Cool solution somewhat and add 10 mL 70–72% $HClO_4$. Boil very gently, adjusting flame as necessary, until solution is colorless or nearly so and dense white fumes appear. Use particular care not to boil to dryness (Danger!) at any time. Cool slightly, add 50 mL H_2O, and boil to drive out any remaining NO_2 fumes. Cool, dilute, filter into 250 mL volumetric flask, dilute to volume, and mix thoroughly.

E. Determination and Calculation
See **965.09D–E**.

References: JAOAC **51**, 776(1968); **54**, 666(1971); **59**, 937(1976); **60**, 465(1977).
CAS-7440-70-2 (calcium)
CAS-7440-50-8 (copper)
CAS-7439-89-6 (iron)
CAS-7439-96-5 (manganese)
CAS-7440-66-6 (zinc)

12.2   975.03—Metals in Plants
Atomic Absorption Spectrophotometric Method
First Action 1975
Final Action 1988

(Applicable to calcium, copper, iron, magnesium, manganese, potassium, and zinc)

A. Apparatus and Reagents
Deionized H_2O may be used. See **965.09A** and **B** (see **12.3**), and following:

(a) *Potassium stock solution.*—1000 μg K/mL. Dissolve 1.9068 g dried (2 h at 105°) KCl in H_2O and dilute to 1 L. Use following parameters for Table **965.09**: 7665 A, air-C_2H_2 flame, and 0.04–2 μg/mL range.

(b) *Calcium stock solutions.*—Prepare Ca stock solution and working standards as in **965.09B**.

(c) *Cu, Fe, Mg, Mn, and Zn stock solutions.*—Prepare as in **965.09B(b)**, (c), (e), (f), and (g).

(d) *Working standard solutions.*—Dilute aliquots of solutions (c) with 10% HCl to make ≥4 standard solutions of each element within range of determination.

B. Preparation of Sample
(a) *Dry ashing.*—Accurately weigh 1 g sample, dried and ground as in **922.02(a)**, into glazed, high-form porcelain crucible. Ash 2 h at 500°, and let cool. Wet ash with 10 drops H_2O, and carefully add 3–4 mL HNO_3 (1 + 1). Evaporate excess HNO_3 on hot plate set at 100–120°. Return crucible to furnace and ash additional 1 h at 500°. Cool crucible, dissolve ash in 10 mL HCl (1 + 1), and transfer quantitatively to 50 mL volumetric flask.

922.02(a) (Preparation of Sample)

(a) *For mineral constituents.*—Thoroughly remove all foreign matter from material, especially adhering soil or sand, but to prevent leaching, avoid excessive washing. Air- or oven-dry as rapidly as possible to prevent decomposition or weight loss by respiration, grind, and store in tightly stoppered bottles. If results are to be expressed on fresh weight basis, record sample weights before and after drying. When Cu, Mn, Zn, Fe, Al, etc. are to be determined, avoid contaminating sample by dust during drying and from grinding and sieving machinery.

(b) *Wet ashing.*—Accurately weigh 1 g sample, dried and ground as in **922.02(a)**, into 150 mL Pyrex beaker. Add 10 mL HNO_3 and let soak thoroughly. Add 3 mL 60% $HClO_4$ and heat on hot plate, slowly at first, until frothing ceases. (*Caution: See Appendix* for safety notes on wet oxidation.) Heat until HNO_3 is almost evaporated. If charring occurs, cool, add 10 mL HNO_3, and continue heating. Heat to white fumes of $HClO_4$. Cool, add 10 mL HCl (1 + 1), and transfer quantitatively to 50 mL volumetric flask.

C. Determination

To solution in 50 mL volumetric flask, add 10 mL 5% La solution, and dilute to volume. Let silica settle, decant supernate, and proceed as in **965.09D**.

Make necessary dilutions with 10% HCl to obtain solutions within range of instrument.

D. Calculations

$$\text{ppm Element} = (\mu g/mL) \times F/g \text{ sample}$$
$$\% \text{ Element} = \text{ppm} \times 10^{-4}$$

where F = (mL original dilution × mL final dilution)/mL aliquot if original 50 mL is diluted.

Reference: JAOAC **58,** 436(1975).

12.3   980.03—Metals in Plants
Direct Reading Spectrographic Method
Final Action 1988

A. Apparatus

(a) *Spark excitation source.*

(b) *Spectrograph.*—1.5 m grating spectrograph with spark stand and disk attachment rotating at 30 rpm.

(c) *Electrode sharpener.*

(d) *Disk electrode.*—High purity graphite disk 0.492″ diameter and 0.200″ thick.

(e) *Upper (pin) electrode.*—Point appropriate lengths of standard grade spectrographic C rods, 0.180″ diameter, in pencil sharpener equipped with pin stop to produce 1/16″ diameter flat tip.

(f) *Porcelain boat.*—60 mm long, 10 mm wide, and 8 mm high (Coors No. 2, or equivalent).

B. Reagents

(a) *Buffer.*—Dissolve 50 g Li_2CO_3 in 200 mL HNO_3, and dilute to 1 L with H_2O. (*Caution: See Appendix* for safety notes on nitric acid.)

(**b**) *Element stock standard solutions.*—On basis of expected sample concentration range, prepare stock solutions from individual pure nitrates, chlorides, or carbonate salts, or metal of respective elements, as indicated in Table **980.03A**.

Table 980.03A Preparation of Stock Standard Solutions

Element	Salt	Element, g/L	Salt, g/L	Solvent
K	KCl	125	238.36	H_2O
Ca	$CaCO_3$	40	99.89	1 N HNO_3
Mg	MgO	20	33.16	1 N HNO_3
P	H_3PO_4	10	31.64	H_2O
Na	NaCl	10	25.42	H_2O
Fe	Fe metal	1	1.00	1 N HNO_3
Mn	MnO	1	1.29	1 N HNO_3
Al	Al metal	1	1.00	1 N HNO_3
Zn	Zn metal	1	1.00	1 N HNO_3
Cu	Cu metal	1	1.00	1 N HNO_3
Ba	$BaCl_2$	1	1.52	H_2O
Sr	$SrCO_3$	1	1.68	1 N HNO_3
B	H_3BO_3	1	5.72	H_2O
Mo	$(NH_4)_6Mo_7O_{24} \cdot H_2O$	0.1	1.29	H_2O

(**c**) *Mixed element standard solutions.*—Prepare 5 standard solutions containing % or ppm element indicated in Table **980.03B** as follows: Dissolve 50 g Li_2CO_3 in 200 mL HNO_3, pipet in indicated aliquots, and dilute to 1 L with H_2O. Prepare fresh every 6 months.

Table 980.03B Preparation of Mixed Element Standard Solutions

Element	Element, g/L	Standard Solution Number				
		1	2	3	4	5
		mL to give (%)[a]				
K (CAS-7440-09-7)	125	2(0.5)	4(1.0)	8(2.0)	12(3.0)	20(5.0)
Ca (CAS-7440-70-2)	40	100(2.0)	50(1.0)	30(0.6)	10(0.2)	15(0.3)
Mg (CAS-7439-95-4)	20	100(1.0)	70(0.7)	50(0.5)	20(0.2)	10(0.1)
P (CAS-7723-14-0)	10	2(0.1)	4(0.2)	6(0.3)	10(0.5)	14(0.7)
		mL to give (ppm)[a]				
Na (CAS-7440-23-5)	10	1(50)	2(100)	10(500)	20(1000)	40(2000)
Fe (CAS-7439-89-6)	10	10(500)	4(200)	2(100)	1(50)	6(300)
Mn (CAS-7439-96-5)	10	0.4(20)	1(50)	2(100)	4(200)	10(500)
Al (CAS-7429-90-5)	10	0.6(30)	1(50)	2(100)	4(200)	10(500)
Zn (CAS-7440-66-6)	1	2(10)	4(20)	6(30)	10(50)	20(100)
Cu (CAS-7440-50-8)	1	1(5)	2(10)	4(20)	10(50)	14(70)
Ba (CAS-7440-39-3)	1	20(100)	10(50)	4(20)	2(10)	1(5)
Sr (CAS-7440-24-6)	1	40(200)	20(100)	10(50)	6(30)	3(15)
B (CAS-7440-42-8)	1	1(5)	2(10)	4(20)	10(50)	14(70)
Mo (CAS-7439-98-7)	0.1	2(1)	4(2)	8(4)	12(6)	20(10)

[a] Concentration based on 1 g sample taken up in 5 mL buffer.

C. Preparation of Sample

Dry plant material 24 h at 80° and grind in Wiley mill with No. 20 stainless steel sieve. Store in air-tight containers or in coin envelopes in dry atmosphere.

Weigh 1.0 g prepared sample into 30 mL high form crucible (porcelain is satisfactory). Ash ≥4 h at 500° with crucible resting on asbestos plate rather than on floor of furnace. Cool, add 5.0 mL buffer solution, (a), stir, and let stand 30 min.

D. Determination

(a) *Excitation.*—Align and space electrodes 4 mm apart in holders; position pin electrode over disk electrode. Set source parameters to give uniform breakdown voltage at tandem air gap with operating parameters at 4 breaks/cycle and 4 amp (parameters may vary with source for best operating efficiency).

Place aliquot of prepared solution in porcelain boat, set boat on arc stand, and raise to immerse 1/16″ of disc in solution. Spark 10 sec to condition electrodes and photomultiplier tubes and then spark additional 30 sec for integration.

(b) *Calibration.*—Calibration technique varies with instrument. Use mixed element standard solutions and known plant tissue standards to calibrate spectrograph by same technique as for samples. Prepare standard curves to cover desired concentration range, using ratio to internal standard and background correction for best results.

12.4   965.09—Nutrients (Minor) in Fertilizers
Atomic Absorption Spectrophotometric Method
First Action 1965
Final Action 1969

(*Caution: See Appendix* for safety notes on atomic absorption spectrophotometer.)

A. Apparatus and Reagent

(a) *Atomic absorption spectrophotometer.*—Several commercial models are available. Since each design is somewhat different, with varying requirements of light source, burner flow rate, and detector sensitivity, only general outline of operating parameters is given in Table **965.09**. Operators must become familiar with settings and procedures adapted to their own apparatus and use table only as guide to concentration ranges and flame conditions.

(b) *Disodium EDTA solution.*—2.5%. Dissolve 25 g Na_2H_2EDTA in 1 L H_2O and adjust to pH 7.0 with $5N$ NaOH, using pH meter.

Table 965.09 Operating Parameters

Element	Wavelength, Å	Flame	Range, μg/mL	Remarks
Ca	4227	Rich Air-C_2H_2	2-20	1% La, 1% HCl
	4227	Rich N_2O-C_2H_2	2-20	Requires special burner
Cu	3247	Air-C_2H_2	2-20	

Table 965.09 Operating Parameters

Element	Wavelength, Å	Flame	Range, μg/mL	Remarks
Fe	2483	Rich Air-C_2H_2	2-20	
Mg	2852	Rich Air-C_2H_2	0.2-2	May need La
Mn	2795	Air-C_2H_2	2-20	
Zn	2138	Air-C_2H_2	0.5-5	

B. Standard Solutions

(Do not use <2 mL pipets or <25 mL volumetric flasks. Automatic dilution apparatus may be used. Prepare standard solutions in 0–20 μg range fresh daily.)

(a) *Calcium solutions.—(1) Stock solution.*—25 μg Ca/mL. Dissolve 1.249 g $CaCO_3$ in minimum amount 3N HCl. Dilute to 1 L. Dilute 50 mL to 1 L. (2) *Working standard solutions*—0, 5, 10, 15, and 20 μg Ca/mL containing 1% La. To 25 mL volumetric flasks add 0, 5, 10, 15, and 20 mL Ca stock solution. Add 5 mL La stock solution and dilute to 25 mL.

(b) *Copper stock solution.*—1000 μg Cu/mL. Dissolve 1.000 g pure Cu metal in minimum amount HNO_3 and add 5 mL HCl. Evaporate almost to dryness and dilute to 1 L with 0.1N HCl.

(c) *Iron stock solution.*—1000 μg Fe/mL. Dissolve 1.000 g pure Fe wire in ca 30 mL 6N HCl with boiling. Dilute to 1 L.

(d) *Lanthanum stock solution.*—50 g La/L. Dissolve 58.65 g La_2O_3 in 250 mL HCl, adding acid slowly. Dilute to 1 L.

(e) *Magnesium stock solution.*—1000 μg Mg/mL. Place 1.000 g pure Mg metal in 50 mL H_2O and slowly add 10 mL HCl. Dilute to 1 L.

(f) *Manganese stock solution.*—1000 μg Mn/mL. Dissolve 1.582 g MnO_2 in ca 30 mL 6N HCl. Boil to remove Cl and dilute to 1 L.

(g) *Zinc stock solution.*—1000 μg Zn/mL. Dissolve 1.000 g pure Zn metal in ca 10 mL 6N HCl. Dilute to 1 L.

(h) *Other standard solutions.*—Dilute aliquots of solutions (b), (c), (e), (f), and (g) with 0.5N HCl to make ≥4 standard solutions of each element within range of determination.

C. Preparation of Sample Solutions

(*Caution: See Appendix* for safety notes on wet oxidation, hydrofluoric acid, and perchloric acid.)

(a) *Inorganic materials and mixed fertilizers.*—Dissolve 1.00 g well ground sample in 10 mL HCl in 150 mL beaker. Boil and evaporate solution nearly to dryness on hot plate. *Do not bake residue.* Redissolve residue in 20 mL 2N HCl, boiling gently if necessary. Filter through fast paper into 100 mL volumetric flask, washing paper and residue thoroughly with H_2O. Measure absorption of solution directly, or dilute with 0.5N HCl to obtain solutions within ranges of instrument. If Ca is to be determined, add enough La stock solution to make final dilution 1% La (i.e., 5 mL La to 25 mL flask, 20 mL to 100 mL flask, etc.).

(b) *Fertilizers containing organic matter (tankage, corncobs, cottonseed hulls, etc.).*—Place 1.00 g sample in 150 mL beaker (Pyrex, or equivalent). Char on hot plate and ignite 1 h at 500° with muffle door propped open to allow free access of air. Break up cake with stirring rod and dissolve in 10 mL HCl as in (a).

(c) *Fertilizers containing fritted trace elements.*— Dissolve ≤1.00 g well ground sample in 5 mL $HClO_4$ and 5 mL HF. Boil and evaporate to dense $HClO_4$ fumes. Dilute carefully with H_2O, filter, and proceed as in (a). Alternatively, dissolve sample in 10 mL HCl, 5 mL HF, and 10 mL methyl alcohol. Evaporate to dryness. Add 5 mL HCl and evaporate. Repeat HCl addition and evaporation. Dissolve residue as in (**a**). (Normally Pt ware should be used; Pyrex or other glassware may be used if Na, K, Ca, and Fe are not to be determined.)

(**d**) *For manganese.—(1) Acid-soluble, for both Mn²⁺ and Mn⁴⁺.—See* (**a**), (**b**), and (**c**), and **972.02(b)**. *(2) Acid-soluble, for Mn²⁺ only.—See* **972.02(a)**, **940.02**, and **941.02**. *(3) Water-soluble, for Mn²⁺ only.—See* **972.03**.

I. **972.02** (Manganese [Acid-Soluble] in Fertilizers, AAS Method)

(**a**) *Applicable to Mn²⁺ only.*—Prepare sample solution as in **940.02**, omitting the 50 mL H_3PO_4 (1 + 9). Proceed as in **965.09D**, using standard solutions prepared as in **965.09B(f)** and (**h**), substituting $0.5N$ H_2SO_4 for $0.5N$ HCl in **965.09B(h)**.

(**b**) *Applicable to total Mn²⁺ and Mn⁴⁺.*—Prepare sample solution as in **965.09C**. Proceed as in **965.09D**, using standard solutionss prepared as in **965.09(f)** and (**h**).

Reference: JAOAC **55,** 695(1972).

II. **940.02** (Manganese [Acid-Soluble] in Fertilizers, Colorimetric Method)

(Applicable to samples containing Mn²⁺ only and with ≤5% Mn)

A. *Reagent*

Potassium permanganate standard solution.—500 ppm Mn. Prepare and standardize as in **940.35**, except use 1.4383 g $KMnO_4$ and 0.12 g sodium oxalate. Transfer aliquot containing 20 mg Mn to beaker. Add 100 mL H_2O, 15 mL H_3PO_4, and 0.3 g KIO_4, and heat to bp. Cool, and dilute to 1 L. Protect from light. Dilute this solution containing 20 ppm Mn with H_2O (previously boiled with 0.3 g KIO_4/L) to make convenient working standards in range of concentrations to be compared.

940.35 (Standard Solution of Potassium Permanganate)

A. *Preparation of Standard Solution*

Dissolve slightly more than desired equivalent weight (3.2 g for $0.1N$) of $KMnO_4$ in 1 L H_2O. Boil solution 1 h. Protect from dust and let stand overnight. Thoroughly clean 15 cm glass funnel, perforated porcelain plate from Caldwell crucible, and glass-stoppered bottle (preferably of brown glass) with warm chromic acid cleaning solution. Digest asbestos for use in gooches on steam bath 1 h with ca $0.1N$ $KMnO_4$ that has been acidified with few drops H_2SO_4 (1 + 3). Let settle, decant, and replace with H_2O. To prepare glass funnel, place porcelain plate in apex, make pad of asbestos ca 3 mm thick on plate, and wash acid-free. (Pad should not be too tightly packed and only moderate suction should be applied.) Insert stem of funnel into neck of bottle and filter $KMnO_4$ solution directly into bottle without aid of suction.

B. *Standardization*

For $0.1N$ solution, transfer 0.3 g dried (1 h at 105°) Na oxalate (NIST SRM 40) to 600 mL beaker. Add 250 mL

H_2SO_4 (5 + 95), previously boiled 10–15 min and then cooled to 27 $\pm$ 3°.

Stir until $Na_2C_2O_4$ dissolves. Add 39–40 mL $KMnO_4$ solution at rate of 25–35 mL/min, stirring slowly. Let stand until pink disappears (ca 45 s). If pink persists because $KMnO_4$ solution is too concentrated, discard and begin again, adding few mL less of $KMnO_4$ solution. Heat to 55–60°, and complete titration by adding $KMnO_4$ solution until faint pink persists 30 s. Add last 0.5–1 mL dropwise, letting each drop decolorize before adding next.

Determine excess of $KMnO_4$ solution required to turn solution pink by matching with color obtained by adding $KMnO_4$ solution to same volume of boiled and cooled diluted H_2SO_4 at 55–60°. This correction is usually 0.03–0.05 mL. From net volume $KMnO_4$, calculate normality:

$$\text{Normality} = g\ Na_2C_2O_4 \times 1000/mL\ KMnO_4 \times 66.999$$

Refs.: JAOAC **23**, 543(1940); **31**, 568(1948). J. Research NBS **15**, 493(1935), Research Paper No. 843.

B. Determination

Place 1 g sample in 200 mL wide-neck volumetric flask or 250 mL beaker. Add 10 mL H_2SO_4 and 30 mL HNO_3. Heat gently until brown fumes diminish; then boil 30 min. If organic matter is not destroyed, cool, add 5 mL HNO_3, and boil. Repeat process until no organic matter remains, and boil until white fumes appear. Cool slightly, and add 50 mL H_3PO_4 (1 + 9). Boil few min. Cool, dilute to 200 mL in volumetric flask, mix, and let stand to allow precipitation of $CaSO_4$.

Pipet 50 mL clear solution into beaker. Heat nearly to bp. With stirring or swirling, add 0.3 g *KIO*₄ for each 15 mg Mn present, and hold 30–60 min at 90–100°, or until color development is complete. Cool, and dilute to measured volume that will provide satisfactory concentration for colorimetric measurement by instrument chosen (usually <20 ppm Mn). Compare in colorimeter against standard $KMnO_4$ solution, or in spectrophotometer at 530 nm. Calculate to Mn.

Reference: JAOAC **23**, 249(1940).

CAS-7439-96-5 (manganese)

III. **941.02** (Manganese [Acid-Soluble] in Fertilizers, Bismuthate Method)
Surplus 1970
(Applicable to Mn^{2+} only)

See **2.127–2.128** [*Official Methods of Analysis* (1970) 11th Ed.]

IV. **972.03** (Manganese [Water-Soluble] in Fertilizers, AAS Method)
(Applicable to Mn^{2+} only)

Place 1 g sample in 50 mL beaker, wet with alcohol, add 20 mL H_2O, and let stand 15 min, stirring occasionally. Transfer to 9 cm Whatman No. 5 paper, and wash with small portions H_2O until filtrate measures ca 230 mL. Let each portion pass through paper before adding more. Add 3–4 mL H_2SO_4 to filtrate. Proceed as in **965.09D**, using standard solutions prepared as in **965.09B(f)** and (**h**), substituting $0.5N$ H_2SO_4 for $0.5N$ HCl in **965.09B(h)**.
Reference: JAOAC **55**, 695(1972).

(**e**) *For iron and zinc.*—(*1*) *Aqueous extraction.*—Place 1.00 g sample in 250 mL beaker, add 75 mL H_2O, and boil 30 min. Filter into 100 mL volumetric flask, washing paper with H_2O. Dilute to volume and redilute if necessary. (*2*) *Chelation extraction.*—Place 1.00 g sample in 250 mL beaker, and add 5 cm (2″) magnetic stirrer bar and 100 mL 2.5% EDTA solution. Stir exactly 5 min, and filter through Whatman No. 41 paper, or equivalent. If filtrate is cloudy, refilter immediately through fine paper (Whatman No. 5, or equivalent). Redilute, if necessary, with $0.5N$ HCl.

D. Determination

(P interferes in Ca and may interfere in Mg determination with air-C_2H_2 burners. Eliminate interference by adding La stock solution to standard and sample solutions so that final dilutions contain 1% La. P does not interfere with Ca determination when N_2O-C_2H_2 flame is used.)

Set up instrument as in Table **965.09**, or previously established optimum settings for apparatus to be used. Less sensitive secondary lines (Gatehouse, and Willis, *Spectrochim. Acta* **17**, 710(1961)) may be used to reduce necessary dilution, if desired. Read ≥ 4 standard solutions within analysis range before and after each group of 6–12 samples. Flush burner with H_2O between samples, and re-establish 0 absorption point each time. Prepare calibration curve from average of each standard before and after sample group. Read concentration of samples from plot of absorption against $\mu g/mL$.

E. Calculations

% Element $= (\mu g/mL) \times (F/\text{sample wt}) \times 10^{-4}$

F = mL original dilution $\times$ mL final dilution/mL aliquot, if original 100 mL volume is diluted.

References: JAOAC **48**, 406, 1100(1965); **50**, 401(1967); **51**, 847(1968); **58**, 928(1975).
CAS-7440-70-2 (calcium)
CAS-7440-50-8 (copper)
CAS-7439-89-6 (iron)
CAS-7439-95-4 (magnesium)
CAS-7439-96-5 (manganese)
CAS-7440-66-6 (zinc)

12.5   953.01—Metals in Plants
General Recommendations for Emission Spectrographic Methods
Final Action 1988

(Applicable to aluminum, barium, boron, calcium, copper, iron, magnesium, manganese, molybdenum, phosphorus, potassium, sodium, strontium, and zinc)

(a) *Instrumental technique*—If, because of equipment limitations, described methods cannot be followed in detail, or if determination of other elements is desired, following protocol is recommended: Determine experimentally, with available facilities, potentials of various sample preparations and excitation conditions with relation to element detectability and general concentration requirements. Select analysis lines on basis of desirable intensity and freedom from spectral interference by other elements, as determined by preparing spectrum of each component element at average concentration at which it occurs in samples to be analyzed. Line and phototube characteristics are usually determined by instrument manufacturer.

(b) *Precision.*—Standardize all conditions of technique and determine reproducibility of results by making ca 20 successive exposures on sample of representative composition. For each element, calculate standard deviation of single exposure and divide by square root of number of individual exposures that will be averaged in practice to constitute 1 determination. From this estimate of standard deviation of single determination, calculate coefficient of variation for each element. Following upper limits for precision error of spectrographic determinations in analysis of plant material are satisfactory in relation to other routine methods or to practical requirements: Coefficients of variation (%)—Ca, Mg, Mn, and Mo, 3–7; B, Ba, Cu, K, P, and Zn, 7–15; and Al, Fe, and Na, >15. Coefficients of variation vary from instrument to instrument for each element; above values were obtained from standard plant tissue by 11 different instruments.

(c) *Accuracy.*—Precise technique is essential but not only factor involved in accuracy. Reliability and appropriateness of standards and judgment used in reference method are of utmost importance. Failure in any of these respects can result in serious calibration error for otherwise satisfactory method.

Carefully prepare synthetic standards from highest grade H_2O-free analyzed chemicals, collectively blanked for minor and trace elements. Preferably confirm values assigned to natural standards by results of >1 laboratory.

Matrix similarity between standards and samples, or closely controlled correction system for matrix differences, is essential. Check correction scales frequently against standards which closely match particular types of plant materials being analyzed.

Precision error of technique applies to reference exposures as well as to samples. For this reason, base fiducial adjustments on as many reference exposures as may be feasibly included in each series of samples.

References: JAOAC **36,** 411(1953); **37,** 721(1954); **58,** 764(1975).

12.6   985.01—Metals and Other Elements in Plants
Inductively Coupled Plasma Spectroscopic Method
First Action 1985
Final Action 1988

(Applicable to B, Ca, Cu, K Mg, Mn, P, Zn)

A. Principle

Sample is dry-ashed, treated with HNO_3, and dissolved in HCl; elements are determined by ICP emission spectroscopy.

B. Reagents and Apparatus

(a) *Stock solutions.*—1000 $\mu g/mL$. Weigh designated reagent into separate 1 L volumetric flasks, dissolve in minimum amount of dissolving reagent, and dilute to volume with H_2O.

Element	Reagent	g	Dissolving reagent
B	H_3BO_3	5.7192	H_2O
Ca	$CaCO_3$	2.4973	6N HCl
Cu	Pure metal	1.0000	HNO_3
K	KCl	1.9067	H_2O
Mg	$MgSO_4 \cdot 7H_2O$	10.1382	H_2O
Mn	MnO_2	1.5825	6N HCl
P	$NH_4H_2PO_4$	3.7138	H_2O
Zn	Pure metal	1.0000	6N HCl

(b) *Standard solutions.*—Pipet following volumes of stock solution into 1 L volumetric flasks. Add 100 mL HCl and dilute to volume with H_2O.

Element	Std soln 1 Stock soln, mL	Std soln 1 Final concn, $\mu g/mL$	Std soln 2 Stock soln, mL	Std soln 2 Final concn, $\mu g/mL$
B	0	0	10	10
Ca	5	5	60	60
Cu	0	0	1	1
K	5	5	60	60
Mg	1	1	20	20
Mn	0	0	10	10
P	5	5	60	60
Zn	0	0	10	10

Make any needed subsequent dilutions with 10% HCl (1 + 9).

161

(c) *ICP emission spectrometer.*—Suggested operating parameters: forward power, 1.1 kilowatts; reflected power, <10 watts; aspiration rate, 0.85—3.5 mL/min; flush between samples, 15—45 s; integration time, 1—10 s.

Element	Wavelength, Å
B (CAS-7440-42-8)	2496
Ca (CAS-7440-70-2)	3179
Cu (CAS-7440-50-8)	3247
K (CAS-7440-09-7)	7665
Mg (CAS-7439-95-4)	2795
Mn (CAS-7439-96-5)	2576
P (CAS-7723-14-0)	2149
Zn (CAS-7440-66-6)	2138

C. Dry Ashing

Accurately weigh 1 g sample, dried and ground as in **922.02(a)**, into glazed, high-form porcelain crucible. Ash 2 h at 500°. Wet ash with 10 drops of H_2O, and carefully add 3-4 mL HNO_3 (1 + 1). Evaporate excess HNO_3 on hot plate set at 100-120°. Return crucible to furnace and ash additional 1 h at 500°. Cool crucible, dissolve ash in 10 mL HCl (1 + 1), and transfer quantitatively to 50 mL volumetric flask. Dilute to volume with H_2O.

922.02(a) (*Preparation of Sample*)

(a) *For mineral constituents.*—Thoroughly remove all foreign matter from material, especially adhering soil or sand, but to prevent leaching, avoid excessive washing. Air- or oven-dry as rapidly as possible to prevent decomposition or weight loss by respiration, grind, and store in tightly stoppered bottles. If results are to be expressed on fresh weight basis, record sample weights before and after drying. When Cu, Mn, Zn, Fe, Al, etc., are to be determined, avoid contaminating sample by dust during drying and from grinding and sieving machinery.

References: Botan. Gaz. **73**, 44(1922). Proc. Am. Soc. Hort. Sci. 1927, p. 191. JAOAC **13**, 224(1930); **16**, 71(1933); **19**, 70(1936).

D. Determination

Elemental determination is accomplished by inductively coupled plasma emission spectroscopy. Calibration of instrument is done through use of known calibration standards. After calibration is complete, samples can be analyzed. Check calibration after every 10 samples. If instrument has drifted out of calibration (>3% of original values), recalibrate.

Calculate concentration for each element of each diluted sample as μg/mL.

Reference: JAOAC **68**, 499(1985).

12.7   921.01—Calcium in Plants
Titrimetric Micro Method
Final Action

Weigh 2 g sample into small crucible and ignite in furnace at 500–550°. Dissolve ash in HCl (1 + 4) and transfer to 100 mL beaker. Add 5 mL HCl and evaporate to dryness on steam bath to dehydrate SiO_2. Moisten residue with 5 mL HCl, add ca 50 mL H_2O, heat few min on steam bath, transfer to 100 mL volumetric flask, cool quickly to room temperature, dilute to volume, shake, and filter, discarding first portion of filtrate.

Pipet 15 mL aliquot into conical-tip centrifuge tube containing 2 mL saturated $(NH_4)_2C_2O_4$ solution and 2 drops methyl red, (dissolve 1 g methyl red in 200 mL alcohol). Add 2 mL CH_3COOH (1 + 4), rotating tube to mix contents thoroughly. Add NH_4OH (1 + 4), while intermittently rotating tube, until solution is faintly alkaline; then add few drops of the CH_3COOH until color is faint pink (pH 5.0). (It is important at this point to rotate tube so that last bit of liquid in conical tip has required color.) Let stand ≥4 h; then centrifuge 15 min. (Precipitate should be in firm lump in tip of tube.) Remove supernate, using suction device, Fig. **921.01**, taking care not to disturb precipitate. Wash precipitate by adding 2 mL NH_4OH (1 + 49), rotating tube to break up precipitate. (It may be necessary to jar tube sharply.) Centrifuge 10 min, again remove supernate, and wash with reagent as before. Repeat washing of precipitate 3 times.

After removing last supernate, add 2 mL H_2SO_4 (1 + 4) to tube, break up precipitate as before, heat on steam bath to 80–90°, and titrate in tube with 0.02N $KMnO_4$, rotating liquid during titration to attain proper end point. If tube cools to <60° during

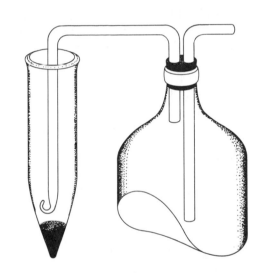

Figure 921.01—Suction device used in micro method for determining calcium.

titration, as indicated by slow reduction of $KMnO_4$, reheat in steam bath few min and complete titration. Perform blank on identical volume H_2SO_4 in similar tube heated to same temperature to determine volume $KMnO_4$ solution necessary to give end point color. Subtract this value from buret reading. 1 mL 0.02N $KMnO_4$ = 0.000400 g Ca. Report as % Ca.

References: J. Biol. Chem. **47**, 475(1921); **50**, 527, 537(1922). JAOAC **14**, 216(1931); **16**, 71(1933); **19**, 71(1936). CAS-7440-70-2 (calcium)

12.8   983.19—Calcium in Mechanically Separated Poultry and Beef
Titrimetric Method
First Action 1983
Final Action 1985

A. Reagents

(a) *Ethylenedinitrilotetraacetic acid dihydrate (EDTA).*—0.02M. Dissolve 7.44 g EDTA (99+% purity) in H_2O in 1 L volumetric flask and dilute to volume. Standardize with ACS $CaCO_3$ primary standard as in **967.30A(d)** (3 significant figures) [*see* **968.31A** (12.9)].

(b) *Hydroxy naphthol blue indicator.*—Mallinckrodt Chemical Works.

(c) *KOH–KCN solution.*—Dissolve 280 g KOH in 500 mL H_2O. Cool, add 66 g KCN, dissolve, and dilute to 1 L in H_2O. *Caution:* Use care in handling of KCN. HCN is evolved on contact with acid or moisture. Flush titrated solution down drain in fume hood with ample *cold* H_2O.

(d) *Calcium carbonate.*—0.02M. Weigh 2.000 g ACS primary standard $CaCO_3$ (dried 2 h at 100°) and transfer to 1 L volumetric flask. Add 500 mL H_2O and 10–12 mL HCl (1 + 1). Heat just to boiling to dissolve $CaCO_3$. Cool and dilute to volume with H_2O. Pipet 25 mL aliquot of EDTA (a) into 400 mL beaker and determine ratio of EDTA to $CaCO_3$ by titration as under *Determination* beginning ". . . add ca 50 mL H_2O, place on magnetic stirrer . . ." Use average of 3 determinations.

B. Determination

Weigh 10 g sample, transfer to 300 mL tall form beaker, add 30 mL HCl (1 + 1), several glass beads, cover with watch glass, and place on hot plate in fume hood. Bring to boil slowly, digest 20 min, cool, and filter (Whatman No. 4 paper) into 200 mL volumetric flask. Wash filter paper with H_2O until 190 mL is obtained. Dilute to volume and mix. Pipet 20 mL aliquot into 400 mL beaker, add ca 50 mL H_2O, place on magnetic stirrer, and add 200–300 mg hydroxy naphthol blue indicator, stir, and adjust pH to 12.5 ± 0.2 with KOH–KCN solution. (Do not exceed pH 12.7, to prevent precipitation. If precipitation occurs, discard and repeat.) Add 10–25 mL 0.02M EDTA accurately measured to provide back-titration of minimum of 3 mL. Mix on magnetic stirrer and titrate sample with 0.02M $CaCO_3$ to permanent purple end point. If back-titration is <3 mL, repeat with larger aliquot of EDTA solution.

$$\% \text{ Calcium (Ca)} = (A - B \times R) \times M \times 4$$
$$\% \text{ Bone (for poultry)} = (\%\text{Ca} - 0.015)F$$

where A = mL EDTA added; B = mL $CaCO_3$ of back titration; R = EDTA:$CaCO_3$ ratio; M = molarity of EDTA solution; 4 = meq. weight Ca (0.040 g) × 100(%); 0.015 = correction for natural Ca in poultry tissue; F = Ca-to-bone conversion factor (6.25 for young chickens and 4.55 for turkeys and mature chickens).

Reference: JAOAC **66,** 989(1983).

12.9   **968.31—Calcium in Canned Vegetables**
                              Titrimetric Method
                              First Action 1968
                              Final Action 1969

(Applicable to canned lima beans, potatoes, and tomatoes)

A. Reagents and Apparatus
Proceed as in **967.30A,B**.

967.30A,B (Calcium and Magnesium in Drugs, Titrimetric Method)
(Applicable to pharmaceuticals and vitamin-mineral preparations)
A. Reagents
Use H_2O redistilled from glass (preferable) or deionized H_2O.
(a) *Calcium carbonate.*—Primary standard grade, dried 2 h at 285°.
(b) *Hydroxy naphthol blue.*—Ca indicator (Mallinckrodt Chemical Works No. 5630 in dispenser bottle ready for use, or equivalent). Store in dark and replace after 1 year.
(c) *Calmagite.*—Ca + Mg indicator (Mallinckrodt No. 4283 in dispenser bottle ready for use, or equivalent). Store in dark and replace after 1 year.
(d) *Disodium dihydrogen ethylenediamine tetraacetate (EDTA) standard solution.*—0.01M. Dissolve 3.72 g $Na_2H_2EDTA\cdot 2H_2O$ (99+% purity) in H_2O in 1 L volumetric flask, dilute to volume, and mix. Accurately weigh enough $CaCO_3$ (ca 40 mg) to give ca 40 mL titration with 0.01M EDTA and transfer to 400 mL beaker. Add 50 mL H_2O and enough HCl (1 + 3) to dissolve the $CaCO_3$. Dilute to ca 150 mL with H_2O and add 15 mL 1N NaOH, disregarding any precipitate or turbidity. Add ca 200 mg hydroxy naphthol blue indicator and titrate from pink to deep blue end point, using magnetic stirrer. Add last few mL EDTA solution dropwise. Molarity EDTA solution = mg $CaCO_3$/(mL EDTA × 100.09).
(e) *Buffer solution.*—pH 10. Dissolve 67.5 g NH_4Cl in 200 mL H_2O, add 570 mL NH_4OH, and dilute to 1 L.
(f) *Potassium hydroxide–potassium cyanide solution.*—Dissolve 280 g KOH and 66 g KCN in 1 L H_2O.
(g) *Potassium cyanide solution.*—2%. Dissolve 2 g KCN in 100 mL H_2O.

B. Apparatus
(a) *Titration standard.*—Fluorescent illuminated.
(b) *Ion exchange column.*—Approximately 20 × 600 mm, fitted with coarse porosity fritted glass disk and Teflon stopcock. Place 30–40 g moist Amberlite IR-4B resin (anion exchange resin with high phosphate capacity) from fresh bottle in 600 mL beaker and exhaust with three 250 mL portions 5% Na_2CO_3 or NaOH. Wash with H_2O until excess base is removed. Treat resin with three 250 mL portions 5% HCl (3 + 22), mixing thoroughly after each treatment. Rinse with H_2O until color is removed, and transfer with H_2O to column. Column is ready for use after draining H_2O to top of resin column. (Exchange capacity for phosphate is ca 1500 mg; therefore, number of aliquots can be passed through column before regeneration is necessary. Rinse column with ca 250 mL H_2O before each use until eluate is colorless.)

B. Preparation of Sample

Thoroughly comminute entire contents of can (representative portion if larger than No. 303 size can) in high-speed blender. Weigh 50 g sample (100 g in absence of declaration of added Ca) into Pt or porcelain dish. Evaporate to dryness, using forced-draft oven, IR radiation, or other convenient means. Ash and treat as in **967.30C**.

967.30C

C. Preparation of Sample

Transfer 2 g well-mixed sample to 100 mL Pt or porcelain dish. Ash at $\leq 525°$ until apparently C-free (gray to brown). Cool, add 20 mL H_2O, stir with stirring rod, and add 10 mL HCl cautiously under watch glass. Rinse off watch glass into dish and evaporate to dryness on steam bath. Add 50 mL HCl $(1 + 9)$, heat on steam bath 15 min, and filter through quantitative paper into 200 mL volumetric flask. Wash paper and dish thoroughly with hot H_2O. Cool filtrate, dilute to volume, and mix.

C. Determination

Transfer 100 mL aliquot prepared sample solution to 250 mL beaker and adjust to pH 3.5 with 10% KOH solution added dropwise, using pH meter and magnetic stirrer. Pass sample solution through resin column (column is in chloride form), collecting effluent in 400 mL beaker at flow rate of 2–3 mL/min. Wash column with two 50 mL portions H_2O, passing first portion through at same rate as sample solution and second at 6–7 mL/min. Finally pass enough H_2O freely through column to make 250–300 mL final volume. Adjust to pH 12.5–13.0, using pH meter and magnetic stirrer, with KOH–KCN solution (dissolve 280 g KOH and 66 g KCN in 1 L H_2O). Add 0.100 g ascorbic acid and 200–300 mg hydroxynaphthol blue indicator. Titrate immediately with 0.01M EDTA solution through pink to deep blue end point, using magnetic stirrer.

$$\% \text{ Ca} = \text{mL EDTA} \times (\text{molarity EDTA solution}/0.01)$$
$$\times 0.4008 \times 2 \times 100/\text{mg sample}$$

References: JAOAC **49**, 287(1966); **50**, 787(1967); **51**, 796(1968); **53**, 720(1970). CAS-7440-70-2 (calcium)

12.10   945.41—Calcium in Bread
Final Action

Proceed as in **944.02C**.

944.02 (Iron in Flour, Spectrophotometric Method)

(Applicable to enriched, enriched self-rising, and phosphated flours. Rinse all flasks, beakers, funnels, etc., with H_2O before use, and filter all reagents to remove suspended matter.)

A. Reagents

(a) *Orthophenanthroline solution.*—Dissolve 0.1 g *o*-phenanthroline in ca 80 mL H_2O at 80°, cool, and dilute to 100 mL.

(b) *Alpha,alpha-dipyridyl solution.*—Dissolve 0.1 g α,α-dipyridyl in H_2O and dilute to 100 mL.

(Reagents (**a**) and (**b**) kept in cool, dark place will remain stable several weeks.)

(**c**) *Iron standard solution.*—0.01 mg Fe/mL. (*1*) Dissolve 0.1 g anhydrous grade Fe wire in 20 mL HCl and 50 mL H_2O, and dilute to 1 L. Dilute 100 mL of this solution to 1 L. Or—(*2*) Dissolve 3.512 g $Fe(NH_4)_2(SO_4)_2 \cdot 6H_2O$ in H_2O, add 2 drops HCl, and dilute to 500 mL. Dilute 10 mL of this solution to 1 L.

(**d**) *Hydroxylamine hydrochloride solution.*—Dissolve 10 g $H_2NOH \cdot HCl$ in H_2O and dilute to 100 mL.

(**e**) *Magnesium nitrate solution.*—Dissolve 50 g $Mg(NO_3)_2 \cdot 6H_2O$ in H_2O and dilute to 100 mL.

(**f**) *Acetate buffer solution.*—Dissolve 8.3 g anhydrous NaOAc (previously dried at 100°) in H_2O, add 12 mL CH_3COOH, and dilute to 100 mL. (It may be necessary to redistil the CH_3COOH and recrystallize the NaOAc from H_2O, depending on amount of Fe present.)

(**g**) *Sodium acetate solution.*—2*M*. Dissolve 272 g $NaOAc \cdot 3H_2O$ in H_2O and dilute to 1 L.

(**h**) *Buffer solution, pH 3.5.*—Dilute 6.4 mL 2*M* NaOAc solution, (**g**), and 93.6 mL 2*M* CH_3COOH (120 g/L) to 1 L with H_2O.

B. Preparation of Standard Curve

Prepare 11 solutions containing 0.0, 2.0, 5.0, 10.0, 15.0, 20.0, 25.0, 30.0, 35.0, 40.0, and 45.0 mL, respectively, of the final diluted Fe standard solution, plus 2.0 mL HCl, in 100 mL. Using 10 mL of each of these solutions, proceed as in **944.02C**, beginning ". . . add 1 mL $H_2NOH \cdot HCl$. . . ." Plot concentration against scale reading.

C. Determination

(**a**) *By dry ashing.*—Ash 10.0 g flour in Pt, SiO_2, or porcelain dish (ca 60 mm diameter, 35 mL capacity) as in **923.03**. (Porcelain evaporating dishes of ca 25 mL capacity are satisfactory. Do not use flat-bottom dishes of diameter >60 mm.) Cool, and weigh if % ash is desired. Continue ashing until practically C-free. To diminish ashing time, or for samples that do not burn practically C-free, use one of following ash aids:

Moisten ash with 0.5–1.0 mL $Mg(NO_3)_2$ solution or with redistilled HNO_3. Dry and carefully ignite in furnace, avoiding spattering. (White ash with no C results in most cases.) Do not add these ash aids to self-rising flour (products containing NaCl) in Pt dish because of vigorous action on dish. Cool, add 5 mL HCl, letting acid rinse upper portion of dish, and evaporate to dryness on steam bath. Dissolve residue by adding 2.0 mL HCl, accurately measured, and heat 5 min on steam bath with watch glass on dish. Rinse watch glass with H_2O, filter into 100 mL volumetric flask, cool, and dilute to volume.

Pipet 10 mL aliquot into 25 mL volumetric flask, and add 1 mL $H_2NOH \cdot HCl$ solution; in few min add 5 mL buffer solution, (**f**), and 1 mL *o*-phenanthroline or 2 mL dipyridyl solution, and dilute to volume. Determine *A* in spectrophotometer or photometer at ca 510 nm. From reading, determine Fe concentration from equation of line representing standard points or by reference to standard curve for known Fe concentration. Determine blank on reagents and make correction. Calculate Fe in flour as mg/lb.

923.03 (Ash of Flour, Direct Method)

Weigh 3–5 g well mixed sample into shallow, relatively broad ashing dish that has been ignited, cooled in desiccator, and weighed soon after reaching room temperature. Ignite in furnace at ca 550° (dull red) until light gray ash results, or to constant weight. Cool in desiccator and weigh soon after reaching room temperature. Reignited CaO is satisfactory drying agent for desiccator. Reference: JAOAC 7, 132(1923).

(b) *By wet digestion.*—(*Caution: See Appendix* for safety notes on distillation, wet oxidation, nitric acid, and sulfuric acid.) Transfer 10.00 g flour to 800 mL Kjeldahl flask, previously rinsed with dilute acid, then with H_2O; add 20 mL H_2O and mix; pipet 5 mL H_2SO_4 into flask and mix; add 25 mL HNO_3 and mix well. After few min, heat flask very gently at brief intervals (to avoid foaming out of flask) until heavy evolution of NO_2 fumes ceases. Continue to heat gently until material begins to char; then add few mL HNO_3 cautiously at intervals until SO_3 fumes evolve and colorless or very pale yellow liquid is obtained (60–65 mL HNO_3 total in ca 2 h). Cool, add 50 mL H_2O and 1 Pyrex glass bead, and heat to SO_3 fumes; cool, add 25 mL H_2O, and filter quantitatively through 11 cm paper into 100 mL volumetric flask; cool, and dilute to volume.

Pipet 10 mL into 25 mL volumetric flask, add 1 mL $H_2NOH \cdot HCl$ solution, rotate flask, and let stand few min. Add 9.5 mL 2M NaOAc solution, (g), and 1 mL *o*-phenanthroline solution, dilute to volume, and mix. Let stand $\geq$5 min and determine A in spectrophotometer or photometer at ca 510 nm.

With self-rising flour, the 9.5 mL 2M NaOAc solution, (g), may be reduced to 8.0 mL. To determine exact amount of buffer solution, (g), needed to adjust each digest to most desirable pH range, mix 10 mL aliquot of sample with measured amount of buffer solution, (g), dilute with H_2O to 25 mL, and determine pH either potentiometrically or colorimetrically.

For colorimetric determination, add 5 drops bromophenol blue indicator, (grind 0.1 g powder with 1.5 mL 0.1N NaOH and dilute to 25 mL) to solution and compare color with that of equal volume of pH 3.5 buffer solution, (h), also treated with 5 drops indicator. Although color develops from pH 2–9, avoid pH <3.0 and preferably work at pH 3.5–4.5. With cereal products, 9.5 mL buffer solution, (g), is satisfactory. With samples high in Fe, aliquot of 5 mL instead of 10 mL may be used with 4.8 mL buffer solution, (g).

Conduct digestion so as to avoid contamination with Fe, and determine blank. After correction for blank, calculate as mg Fe/lb.

References: JAOAC **27,** 86, 396(1944); **28,** 77(1945).
CAS-7439-89-6 (iron)

12.11

944.03—Calcium in Flour
Titrimetric Method
Final Action

(Applicable to enriched, enriched self-rising, and phosphated flours)

Ash 10 g flour or air-dried bread as in **923.03**, and proceed as in **944.02C(a)** (*see* 12.10), through "Rinse watch glass with H_2O . . ." then filter into 400 mL beaker; or transfer 50 mL solution from Fe determination to 400 mL beaker. Dilute to ca 150 mL.

923.03 (Ash of Flour, Direct Method)

Weigh 3–5 g well-mixed sample into shallow, relatively broad ashing dish that has been ignited, cooled in desiccator, and weighed soon after reaching room temperature. Ignite in furnace at ca 550° (dull red) until light gray ash results, or to constant weight. Cool in desiccator and weigh soon after reaching room temperature. Reignited CaO is satisfactory drying agent for desiccator. Reference: JAOAC 7, 132(1923).

Add 8–10 drops bromocresol green indicator, **941.17A**, and enough *20% NaOAc solution* to change pH to 4.8–5.0 (blue). Cover with watch glass and heat to bp. Precipitate Ca slowly by adding *3% oxalic acid solution,* 1 drop every 3–5 s, until pH is 4.4–4.6 (optimum for Ca oxalate precipitation) as indicated by distinct green shade. (Avoid excess of oxalic acid indicated by yellow tints, showing undesirable displacement of pH.) Boil 1–2 min and let mixture settle until clear or overnight. Filter supernate through quantitative paper, gooch, or fine fritted glass filter, and wash beaker and precipitate with ca 50 mL NH_4OH (1 + 50) in small portions, using wash bottle delivering very small stream. Break point of filter and wash filter or crucible with mixture of 125 mL H_2O and 5 mL H_2SO_4 at 80–90°. Titrate at 70–90° with $0.05N$ $KMnO_4$ until slight pink is obtained, add filter paper, and continue titration if necessary. Correct for blank and calculate Ca as mg/lb. 1 mL $0.05N$ $KMnO_4$ = 1 mg Ca.

941.17A (Standard Buffers and Indicators for Colorimetric pH Comparisons

A. Preparation of Sulfonphthalein Indicators

	X	pH
Bromocresol green	14.3	3.8–5.4
Chlorophenol red	23.6	4.8–6.4
Bromothymol blue	16.0	6.0–7.6
Phenol red	28.2	6.8–8.4

X = mL 0.01N NaOH/0.1 g indicator required to form mono-Na salt. Dilute to 250 mL for 0.04% reagent.

References: JAOAC **27**, 402(1944); **28**, 77(1945).
CAS-7440-70-2 (calcium)

12.12   991.25—Calcium, Magnesium, and Phosphorus in Cheese
Atomic Absorption Spectrophotometric and Colorimetric Methods
First Action 1991

(*Caution*: *See Appendix* for safety note on magnesium.)

(Applicable to determination of calcium, magnesium, and phosphorus in processed American, mozzarella, cheddar, Romano, and Parmesan cheeses at levels studied.)

Method Performance:

   Calcium, 608–1107 mg/100 g

   s_r = 9.9–17.8; s_R = 15.1–32.6; av. RSD_r = 1.5%; av. RSD_R = 2.6%

   Magnesium, 23.9–25.1 mg/100 g

   s_r = 0.91–1.06; s_R = 1.08–1.27; av. RSD_r = 4.0%; av. RSD_R = 4.8%

   Magnesium, 40.0–50.6 mg/100 g

   s_r = 0.29–0.56; s_R = 1.01–1.17; av. RSD_r = 0.9%; av. RSD_R = 2.4%

   Phosphorus, 444–695 mg/100 g

   s_r = 5.9–7.6; s_R = 7.6–9.6; av. RSD_r = 1.2%; av. RSD_R = 1.6%

A. Principle

Sample is dried and ashed. Residue is dissolved and diluted in acidified aqueous solution. Portions are diluted for colorimetric (P) and AAS (Ca and Mg) determinations.

B. Apparatus

Note: Before use, rinse all glassware (volumetric flasks, stoppers, and pipets) and crucibles with HCl (1 + 1) and then with water.

(a) *Atomic absorption spectrophotometer.*—Capable of determining absorbance response to 3 decimal places and of integrating response for 9 s. Determine Ca at 422.7 nm and Mg at 285.2 nm using an air–acetylene flame. Allow 5 min warm-up with flame and source lamp lit.

   Several commercial models are available, which have varying requirements of light source, burner flow rate, and detector sensitivity. Operators must become familiar with settings and procedures for their apparatus. Linear range and detector response must be comparable with manufacturer's specifications.

(b) *Spectrophotometer.*—With 1 cm glass cuvets. Capable of measuring absorbance response to 3 decimal places. Determine P at 400 nm. Allow 5 min warm-up with source lit.

C. Reagents

Note: Reagents for Ca, P, and Mg standards must be ultra-pure (99.95%). Opened reagents should be resealed and stored in desiccator in inert atmosphere.

(a) *Calcium carbonate.*—$CaCO_3$, 99.95% pure. Dry overnight at 200°.

(b) *Ammonium dihydrogen phosphate.*—$(NH_4)H_2PO_4$, 99.99% pure. Dry overnight at 110°.

(c) *Magnesium metal.*—99.95% pure.

(d) *Magnesium stock solution.*—1000 mg Mg/L. Place 1.0000 g pure Mg metal, (c), in 50 mL H_2O and slowly add 10 mL HCl. Dilute solution to 1 L.

(e) *Concentrated stock solution.*—500 mg Ca/L, 300 mg P/L, and 25 mg Mg/L. To 1 L volumetric flask, add 1.249 g $CaCO_3$, (a), 1.114 g $(NH_4)H_2PO_4$, (b), and 25 mL Mg stock solution, (d). Add 30 mL HCl (1 + 3), mix until dissolved, and dilute to volume. Store solution in clean Nalgene or poly(ethylene) bottle.

(f) *Dilute stock solution.*—20 mg Ca/L, 12 mg P/L, and 1 mg Mg/L. Dilute 20 mL concentrated stock solution, (e), to 500 mL with water.

(g) *Molybdovanadate reagent.*—Dissolve 60 g ammonium molybdate tetrahydrate in 900 mL hot H_2O, cool to 20°, and dilute to 1 L. Dissolve 1.5 g ammonium metavanadate in 690 mL hot H_2O, add 300 mL HNO_3, cool to 20°, and dilute to 1 L. While stirring, gradually add molybdate solution to vanadate solution. Store at room temperature in poly(ethylene) or glass-stopper Pyrex bottle. (*Note:* Reagent is stable indefinitely in poly(ethylene) bottle; in Pyrex bottle, precipitate gradually forms after several months. Discard reagent if precipitate forms.)

(**h**) *Lanthanum stock solution.*—1% La. Dissolve 11.73 g La_2O_3 in 25 mL HNO_3, adding acid slowly. Dilute solution to 1 L.

D. Sample Preparation

Thoroughly mix cheese as in **955.30**. Weigh ca 1 g cheese to nearest mg in 100 mL Vycor® dish or Pt crucible and dry 1 h in 100° forced air oven. Char dried cheese on hot plate. Ash in furnace overnight (16 h) at 525°, and cool in desiccator.

Dissolve ash in 1 mL HNO_3. Transfer to 250 mL volumetric flask and dilute to volume (Solution A).

955.30 (Preparation of Samples, Procedure)

Cut wedge sample into strips and pass 3 times through food chopper. Grind plugs in food chopper (preferable method), or cut or shred very finely and mix thoroughly.

With creamed cottage and similar cheeses, place 300–600 g sample at <15° in 1 L (1 qt) cup of high-speed blender and blend for minimum time (2–5 min) required to obtain homogeneous mixture. Final temperature should be ≤25°. This may require stopping blender frequently after channeling and spooning cheese back into blades until blending action starts. (Use of variable transformer in line to permit slow speed at first minimizes channeling when speed is increased later.)

E. Determination of Phosphorus

(**a**) *Standard curve.*—Pipet 0, 5, 10, 15, 20, 25, 30, and 35 mL portions of dilute stock solution, **C(f)**, into series of 50 mL volumetric flasks. Add 10 mL molybdovanadate reagent, **C(g)**, to each flask. Mix each solution and dilute each to volume to obtain 0, 1.2, 2.4,...8.4 ppm P standards. Read absorbance of each solution within 1 h. Set spectrophotometer at 400 nm and adjust instrument to 0 A with 0 ppm standard. Plot A vs ppm P.

Linear regression analysis of this curve should yield coefficient of variation of ≥0.99980, with intercept 0 ± 0.004 AU.

(**b**) *Samples.*—Pipet 10 mL Solution A into 50 mL volumetric flask. Develop color and read absorbance as for standard curve. Determine ppm P from standard curve. (*Note:* Although standards and molybdovanadate reagent are stable for several months, periodically check reproducibility of curve by concurrently running 4.8 ppm standard with assay. Prepare new curve if absorbance of this standard differs from curve by ±1%.)

Calculate mg P/100 g cheese as follows:

$$\text{Phosphorus, mg/100 g} = (Y \times 125)/W$$

where Y = ppm P in assay solution as extrapolated from standard curve and W = weight of cheese taken, g. Report results to nearest mg.

F. Determination of Calcium and Magnesium

(**a**) *Standard curve.*—Pipet 0, 5, 10, 15, 20, 25, and 30 mL portions of dilute stock solution, **C(f)**, into series of 100 mL volumetric flasks. To each flask, add 10 mL La stock solution, **C(h)**, and dilute to volume to obtain 0–6 ppm Ca and 0–0.3 ppm Mg in 0.1% La. Use 4 or 5 standards in range that approximates anticipated assay level. Adjust instrument to 0 A with 0 ppm standard and run samples along with standards under conditions in **B(a)**. Plot A vs ppm Ca and ppm Mg.

Linear regression analysis of these curves should yield correlation coefficient of ≥ 0.99960 with intercept 0 ± 0.002 AU.

(b) *Samples*.—Pipet 10 mL Solution A into 100 mL volumetric flask. Add 10 mL La stock solution and dilute to volume. With AAS system set for optimum response, determine ppm Ca and Mg in Solution A vs 4 or 5 standards of respective material. Periodically check absorbance of 4.0 ppm Ca (0.2 ppm Mg) standard. Response should not differ by more than 1%. If absorbance of sample is beyond range of curve [above 6.0 ppm Ca (0.3 ppm Mg)], use smaller portion of Solution A for assay.

Calculate mg Ca/100 g and mg Mg/100 g cheese as follows:

$$\text{Calcium or magnesium, mg/100 g} = (Z \times 2500)/(W/V)$$

where Z = ppm Ca or Mg in assay solution as extrapolated from standard curve; W = weight of cheese taken, g; and V = volume of Solution A taken for assay, mL. Report Ca results to nearest mg and Mg results to nearest 0.1 mg.

Ref.: JAOAC **74**, 27(1991).
CAS-7440-70-2 (calcium)
CAS-7439-95-4 (magnesium)
CAS-7723-14-0 (phosphorus)

12.13 984.27—Calcium, Copper, Iron, Magnesium, Manganese, Phosphorus, Potassium, Sodium, and Zinc in Infant Formula
Inductively Coupled Plasma Emission Spectroscopic Method
First Action 1984
Final Action 1986

(*Caution: See Appendix* for safety notes on wet oxidation, nitric acid, and perchloric acid.)

A. Principle

Sample is digested in $HNO_3/HClO_4$ and elements are determined by ICP emission spectroscopy.

B. Reagents

(a) *Water*.—Distilled, deionized. Use throughout.

(b) *Perchloric acid*.—Double-distilled (G. Frederick Smith Chemical Co., or equivalent). Dilute 10 mL to 50 mL with H_2O.

(c) *Standards*.—(All preparations yield 1000 μg/mL).

    (*1*) *Calcium*.—Place 2.4973 g $CaCO_3$ in 1 L volumetric flask with 300 mL H_2O, add 10 mL HCl, and after CO_2 has been released, dilute to 1 L.

    (*2*) *Copper*.—Dissolve 1.000 g Cu in 10 mL HCl plus 5 mL H_2O to which HNO_3 is added dropwise until dissolution is complete. Boil to expel fumes, cool, and dilute to 1 L with H_2O.

    (*3*) *Iron*.—Dissolve 1.000 g Fe wire in 20 mL 5M HCl; dilute to 1 L with H_2O.

    (*4*) *Potassium*.—Dissolve 1.9067 g KCl in H_2O and dilute to 1 L with H_2O.

    (*5*) *Magnesium*.—Dissolve 1.000 g Mg in 50 mL 1M HCl and dilute to 1 L with H_2O.

(*6*) *Manganese.*—Dissolve 1.000 g Mn in 10 mL HCl plus 1 mL HNO_3 and dilute to 1 L with H_2O.

(*7*) *Sodium.*—Dissolve 2.5421 g NaCl in H_2O and dilute to 1 L with H_2O.

(*8*) *Phosphorus.*—Dissolve 4.263 g $(NH_4)_2HPO_4$ in H_2O and dilute to 1 L with H_2O.

(*9*) *Zinc.*—Dissolve 1.000 g Zn in 10 mL HCl and dilute to 1 L with H_2O.

Commercially available certified standards may be substituted for any of the above elements.

(**d**) *Calibration standards.*—Prepare to concentration indicated in Table **984.27**, using standards above. All calibration standards should be prepared to contain 20% $HClO_4$ to approximate $HClO_4$ concentration in diluted, digested samples.

Table 984.27 Suggested Operating Parameters for ICP Emission Spectroscopy

| Element | Wavelength, nm | Background Correction[a] | Stds, μg/mL | |
			Low	High
Ca	317.9	N	0	200
Cu	324.7	H	0	5
Fe	259.9	N	0	10
K	766.5	N	0	200
Mg	383.2	N	0	5
Mn	257.6	N	0	5
Na	589.0	N	0	200
P	214.9	N	0	100
Zn	213.8	H	0	5

[a] H = high side; N = no correction.

C. Apparatus

(**a**) *ICP emission spectrometer.*—Model 975 Plasma Atom Comp (Jarrell-Ash Co., 8E Forge Pkwy, PO Box 9101, Franklin, MA 02038-9101), or equivalent, capable of simultaneous or sequential determination of Ca, Cu, Fe, K, Mg, Mn, Na, P, and Zn. Minipuls 2 peristaltic pump (Gilson Medical Electronics, PO Box 27, 3000 W Beltline Highway, Middleton, WI 53562), or equivalent, used to feed glass crossflow nebulizer. Suggested operating parameters: warmup time (plasma on), 30 min; exposure time, 5 s; integration cycles, 1 cycle (2 on line exposures, 1 off line exposure); forward power, 1.1 KW; reflected power, <5 watts; sample uptake rate (w/pump), 0.8 mL/min; observation height: 16 mm above load coil (optimized for Mn).

(**b**) *Controllable heating mantle and acid scrubber.*—Labconco 60301, (Labconco, 8811 Prospect, Kansas City, MO 64132), or equivalent.

(**c**) *Glassware.*—Soak overnight in 10% HNO_3 and thoroughly rinse with H_2O.

D. Procedure

Vigorously shake container of infant formula to ensure complete mixing. Measure 15.0 mL of ready to feed (10.0 mL if concentrated, 1.5 g if powdered) infant formula into 100 mL Kjeldahl flask. Add 30 mL HNO_3–$HClO_4$ (2 + 1) to flask along with 3 or 4 glass boiling beads. Let samples sit overnight in acid. Carry 2 reagent blanks through entire procedure along with samples.

Before starting digestion, have ice bath available for cooling Kjeldahl flasks. HNO_3 should also be readily available. To start digestion, place each Kjeldahl flask on heating mantle set at low temperature. Once boiling is initiated, red-orange fumes of NO_2 will be driven off. Continue gentle heating until HNO_3 and H_2O have been driven off, and sample is contained in $HClO_4$. At this point effervescent reaction occurs between sample and $HClO_4$. Place flask on cool heating mantle and let digestion proceed with occasional heating from mantle. It is important that reaction between sample and $HClO_4$ not go too fast, because charring will occur. If sample chars, immediately place flask in ice bath to stop digestion. Add 1 mL HNO_3 and resume gentle heating.

After reaction of sample with $HClO_4$ is complete (identified by cessation of effervescent reaction between sample and $HClO_4$) apply high heat to sample for ca 2 min. Avoid heating sample to dryness because this can cause explosion. Remove flask from heating mantle and let cool.

Transfer each digested sample to 50 mL volumetric flask and dilute to volume with H_2O. Some precipitation is likely to occur (especially with high salt content samples) after dilution. Precipitate will dissolve if shaken and allowed to sit overnight. Final acid content of samples is ca 20% $HClO_4$.

Elemental determination is accomplished by inductively coupled plasma (ICP) emission spectroscopy (see Table **984.27** for parameters). Calibration of instrument is done through use of known calibration standards. Calibration standards may be used as single standards (i.e., one element per standard) or as mixed standard containing 2 or more elements. Whether single or mixed standards should be used for calibration will depend on computer software requirements of particular ICP system in use.

After calibration is complete, samples can be analyzed. Calibration of instrument should be checked after every 10 samples by analyzing calibration standards. If reanalysis of calibration standards indicates that instrument has drifted out of calibration (>3% of original values), instrument should be recalibrated.

Computer will calculate concentration for each element of each diluted sample as μg/mL. Use following equation to convert this value to μg/mL if original sample was ready-to-feed or concentrated formula or μg/g if sample was powder.

$$C = A \times (50 \text{ mL}/B)$$

where A = concentration (μg/mL) of element as determined by ICP; B = volume or weight of sample as mL or g; C = elemental concentration in sample, μg/mL or μg/g, depending on value of B.

Reference: JAOAC **67,** 985(1984).

12.14   985.35—Minerals in Ready-to-Feed Milk-Based Infant Formula
Atomic Absorption Spectrophotometric Method
First Action 1985
Final Action 1988

(Applicable to Ca, Mg, Fe, Zn, Cu, Mn, Na, and K)

A. Apparatus

(a) *Glassware.*—Thoroughly clean all glassware by soaking overnight in 20% HNO_3. Rinse all glassware 3 times with distilled-deionized or 18 MΩ resistance H_2O.

(**b**) *Evaporating dish.*—100 mL unetched Vycor (or Pt), flat-bottom, with pour spout, which withstands temperatures to 600°.

(**c**) *Atomic absorption spectrophotometer.*—Perkin-Elmer 503, or equivalent.

(**d**) *Furnace.*—With pyrometer to control temperature range of 250–600° ± 10°.

B. Reagents

(**a**) *Water.*—Distilled, deionized, or 18 MΩ resistance (DD), for preparation of standard or sample solutions.

(**b**) *Standard stock solutions.*—Commercially prepared, certified AA standards, or prepared in laboratory by one of the following methods: Na, **969.23A(c)**; K, from Spex Industries, Inc., 3880 Park Ave, Edison, NJ 08820; Mn, **965.09(f)**; Zn, **965.09B(g)**.

> **969.23A(c)** (Sodium and Potassium in Seafood, Flame Photometric Method)
>
> *A. Apparatus and Reagents*
>
> (**c**) *Sodium standard solutions.*—(*1*) *Stock solution.*—1 mg Na/mL. Dry reagent grade NaCl 2 h at 110°; cool in desiccator. Weigh 2.5421 g into 1 L volumetric flask and dilute to volume with H_2O. (*2*) *Working solutions for flame emission.*—0.01, 0.03, and 0.05 mg Na/mL. Pipet 1, 3, and 5 mL Na stock solution into separate 100 mL volumetric flasks; add 7 mL K stock solution and 2 mL HNO_3 to each flask; dilute to volume with H_2O. (*3*) *Working solutions for flame absorption.*—0.00003, 0.0001, 0.0003, and 0.0005 mg Na/mL. Pipet 1 mL Na stock solution into 100 mL volumetric flask and dilute to volume with H_2O. Pipet 0.3, 1.0, 3.0, and 5.0 mL diluted stock solution into separate 100 mL volumetric flasks and dilute to volume with H_2O.

(**c**) *Nitric acid.*—Unless specified otherwise, use redistilled or ultrapure.

(**d**) *Lanthanum oxide.*—La_2O_3, 99.99%; AAS quality (Alfa Products, Morton-Thiokol, Inc., 152 Andover St, Danvers, MA 01923, Stock No. 87808).

(**e**) *Lanthanum chloride solution.*—$LaCl_3$, 1% weight/volume. Weigh 11.7 g (±100 mg) La_2O_3 and transfer to 1 L volumetric flask. Add sufficient DD H_2O to wet powder and then slowly add 50 mL concentrated HCl (Caution: Exothermic reaction.). Let powder dissolve and then dilute to volume with DD H_2O and mix. Make fresh every six months or purchase from Spex Industries, Inc.

(**f**) *Cesium chloride solution.*—CsCl 10% weight/volume. Weigh 12.7 g (±100 mg) CsCl (Spex Industries Cat. No. Cs-35) and transfer to 100 mL volumetric flask. Dilute to volume with DD H_2O and mix. Make fresh every 6 months.

(**g**) *Filter pulp.*—Analytically ash-free (Scientific Products Inc., Div. Baxter Healthcare Corp., 1430 Waukegan Rd, McGaw Park, IL 60085, or equivalent).

C. Ashing Procedure

Place composite aliquot in previously cleaned Vycor evaporating dish (which may contain 5 g filter pulp for ease of handling). Exact amount of composite required will depend on concentration of minerals present. In general, 25 mL will be adequate. If some minerals, in particular Fe, Cu, or Mn, are at very low levels, larger sample size (up to 50 mL) may be necessary.

    Dry aliquot in 100° oven overnight or in microwave oven (programmed over ca 30 min). After sample is dry, heat on hot plate until smoking ceases. Place sample in 525° furnace (carefully avoiding ignition) for minimum time necessary to obtain ash that is white and free from C, normally 3–5 h, but <8 h. Remove sample from furnace and let cool. Ash should be white and free from C. If ash contains C particles (i.e., it is gray), wet with DD H_2O and add 0.5–3 mL HNO_3. Dry on hot plate or steam bath and return sample to 525° furnace 1–2 h. Repeat until ash is white. (This step should be avoided if possible because K may be lost.)

Dissolve in 5 mL 1N HNO_3, warming on steam bath or hot plate 2–3 min to aid in solution. Add solution to 50 mL volumetric flask and repeat with 2 additional portions of 1N HNO_3. Dilute to 50 mL with 1N HNO_3.

D. Determination

Add $LaCl_3$ solution to each standard and sample final dilution to make 0.1% weight/volume La for determination of Ca and Mg only. Add CsCl solution to each standard and sample final dilution to make 0.5% weight/volume Cs (0.04M) for determination of Na and K only.

Prepare blanks representing all reagents and glassware, and carry through entire procedure.

Prepare calibration curve (concentration vs A) for each mineral to be determined. using wavelength and flame specified in Table **985.35**. Optimize flame parameters in accordance with instrument manufacturer's instructions. Prepare solutions for calibration of instrument to cover linear range of calibration curve. See instrument instruction manual.

Table 985.35. Wavelength and Flame Parameters for AAS Determination of Minerals in Infant Formula

Element	Wavelength, nm (instrument setting UV/vis range)	Flame
Ca (CAS-7440-70-2)	422.7 (211-vis)	reducing air-C_2H_2
Cu (CAS-7440-50-8)	324.7 (325-UV)	oxidizing air-C_2H_2
Fe (CAS-7439-89-6)	248.3 (248-vis)	oxidizing air-C_2H_2
K (CAS-7440-09-7)	766.5 or 769.9 (383-vis)	oxidizing air-C_2H_2
Na (CAS-7440-23-5)	589.0 (295-vis)	oxidizing air-C_2H_2
Mg (CAS-7439-95-4)	285.2 (285-UV)	oxidizing air-C_2H_2
Mn (CAS-7439-96-5)	279.5 (279-UV)	oxidizing air-C_2H_2
Zn (CAS-7440-66-6)	213.9 (214-UV)	oxidizing air-C_2H_2

Assay samples in similar manner. Determine concentration of each mineral from its calibration curve, and calculate concentration in sample, taking into account sample size and dilutions.

Reference: JAOAC **68**, 514(1985).

Chapter 13
Cholesterol

13.1   **976.26—Cholesterol in Multicomponent Foods**

Gas Chromatographic Method
First Action 1976
Final Action 1977

A. Principle

Lipid is extracted from sample by mixed solvent and saponified. Unsaponifiable fraction containing cholesterol and other sterols is extracted with benzene. Sterols are derivatized to form trimethylsilyl (TMS) ethers which are determined quantitatively by GC, using 5α-cholestane as internal standard.

B. Apparatus

(a) *Centrifuge tubes.*—Pyrex No. 13, 15 mL. Silanize tubes as follows: Rinse clean tubes with anhydrous methyl alcohol and dry 30 min at 110°. Transfer tubes to desiccator. Fill tubes with 10% solution of dimethyldichlorosilane (DMCS) in toluene, stopper tubes, and let stand 1 h. Drain tubes and rinse thoroughly with anhydrous methyl alcohol. Dry in 110° oven before use. After use, clean tubes with methyl alcohol, H_2O, and methyl alcohol, in that order. Dry tubes in 100° oven before use. Tubes can be re-used without silylation as long as strong alkali wash is avoided.

(b) *Gas chromatograph.*—With H flame ionization detector, on-column injection system, and 2.4 m (8′) × 3 mm id U-shaped glass column packed with 0.5% Apiezon L (No. 08304, Applied Science Laboratories, Inc.) on 80–100 mesh Gas-Chrom Q (No. 02002, Applied Science). Alternative column: 1.8 m (6′) × 4 mm id U-shaped glass column packed with 1% SE-30 on 100–120 mesh Gas-Chrom Q (No. 12409, Applied Science). Operating conditions: temperatures (°)—flash heater 275, detector 275, column 230; flow rates (mL/min)—N (ultra high purity grade) ca 50, to elute cholesterol in 9–11 min, H ca 35, air 350; electrometer sensitivity 1×10^{-9} amp full-scale deflection with 1 mV recorder.

(c) *Homogenizer.*—Sorvall Omnimixer (DuPont Instrument Co., Sorvall Operations, Peck's Ln, Newton, CT 06470), or equivalent, for use with 12 oz (350 mL) wide-mouth screw-cap jars.

(d) *Magnetic stirrer-hot plate.*—With variable speed and heat controls.

(e) *Rotary evaporator.*—With glass condenser flask between concentration flask and metal shaft.

(f) *Test tube mixer.*—Vortex-Genie mixer (No. 12-812, Fisher Scientific Co.), or equivalent.

C. Reagents

(*Caution:* Silanes are toxic. Avoid contact with skin and eyes. Use effective fume removal device.)

(a) *Cholesterol standard solutions.*—Standard cholesterol available as No. 21502, Applied Science. (*1*) *Stock solution.*—1.0 mg/mL DMF. (*2*) *Working solutions.*—Dilute stock solution with DMF to obtain concentration range from 0.05 to 0.5 mg/mL.

(b) *5α-Cholestane internal standard solutions.*—Standard 5α-cholestane available as No. 19505, Applied Science. (*1*) *Stock solution.*—1.0 mg/mL *n*-heptane. (*2*) *Working solution.*—0.2 mg/mL. Dilute stock solution with *n*-heptane to obtain concentration of 0.2 mg/mL.

(c) *Dimethyldichlorosilane.*—No. 18008, Applied Science, or equivalent.

(d) *Dimethylformamide.*—Distilled in glass (Burdick & Jackson Laboratories, Inc.; Anspec Co., Inc., PO Box 7730, Ann Arbor, MI 48107; or equivalent).

(e) *Glass wool.*—Silane-treated (No. 14502, Applied Science, or equivalent).

(f) *n-Heptane.*—Distilled in glass (Burdick & Jackson, Eastman Kodak Co., No. 2215, or equivalent).

(g) *Hexamethyldisilazane (HMDS).*—No. 18006, Applied Science, Pierce Chemical Co., or equivalent.

(h) *Concentrated potassium hydroxide solution.*—Dissolve 60 g KOH in 40 mL H_2O.

(i) *Reagent alcohols.*—ethyl alcohol-methyl alcohol-isopropanol (90 + 5 + 5). Following reagent alcohols are satisfactory: EM Diagnostics, A Div. of EM Industries, Inc., 480 Democrat Rd, Gibbstown, NJ 08027; Wilkens-Anderson Co., 4525 W Division St, Chicago IL 60651; No. 7019 or No. 7006, Mallinckrodt Chemical Works.

(j) *Toluene.*—Nanograde, distilled in glass (Mallinckrodt Chemical Works, or equivalent).

(k) *Trimethylchlorosilane (TMCS).*—No. 18010, Applied Science, or equivalent.

(l) *Trimethylsilyl (TMS) reagent.*—HMDS-TMCS-pyridine (9 + 6 + 10).

(m) *Adsorbent.*—Celite 545, acid-washed (Johns-Manville Products Corp.), or equivalent, is usually suitable for column chromatography. When interfering materials are present, purify as follows: place pad of glass wool in base of chromatographic tube ≥100 mm diameter and add siliceous earth to height ca 5 times diameter. Add volume HCl equal to ca ⅓ volume of earth, and let percolate. Wash with methyl alcohol, using small volumes at first to rinse walls of tube, and then until washings are neutral to moistened indicator paper. Extrude into shallow dishes, heat on steam bath to remove methyl alcohol, and dry at 105° until material is powdery and methyl alcohol free. Store in tightly closed containers.

D. Preparation and Packing of Gas Chromatographic Column

(*Caution: See Appendix* for safety notes on hydrofluoric acid and isooctane.)

Attach empty column to aspirator and draw through 5% HF solution. Stop vacuum with pinch clamp, quickly cap both ends of column with rubber stoppers, and let column stand filled with 5% HF solution 10 min.

Attach column to aspirator again, draw off 5% HF solution, and rinse with ca 150 mL H_2O followed by 150 mL anhydrous methyl alcohol. Finally, rinse column with 150 mL isooctane. Draw air through column until dry. Fill column with TMS reagent, (**l**), by pulling it through slowly with aspirator. Plug both ends of column and let stand 30 min. Draw TMS reagent through and rinse immediately with 100 mL anhydrous methyl alcohol, followed by 200 mL isooctane. Let column dry under vacuum.

Use commercially prepared column packing of 0.5% Apiezon L on 80–100 mesh Gas-Chrom Q (Applied Science), or prepare as follows: Weigh 0.5 g Apiezon L into 100 mL beaker, add 80 mL toluene, stir magnetically until it dissolves completely, and transfer to 500 mL Erlenmeyer, rinsing beaker with four 5 mL portions toluene. Weigh 10 g 80–100 mesh Gas-Chrom Q and add to Apiezon L solution. Stopper flask and shake to make slurry. Immediately pour slurry through Buchner-type fritted glass Pyrex filter (medium porosity) under vacuum, stirring continuously until all liquid is drawn off. Measure filtrate in graduate and determine amount Apiezon L adsorbed. Let stand under vacuum, stirring occasionally until almost dry. Transfer packing to porcelain evaporation dish and dry completely in 110–120° oven. Store in glass bottle until ready to use.

Heat packing 15 min in 100° oven. Plug detector end of silanized column with 6 mm silanized glass wool and attach to aspirator. Add warm packing through funnel attached to column and gently tap column. Finally, plug injection port end with silanized glass wool. Condition column 24 h at 235° with N flow.

E. Moisture Determination

Accurately weigh ca 5.0 g sample into tared Al dish, place in circulating-type 100° air oven, and dry overnight or 3 h at 110°. Cover, and let cool in desiccator. Weigh accurately and determine moisture content to adjust for H_2O to be added in **976.26F**.

F. Extraction of Lipid

(*Caution: See Appendix* for safety notes on distillation, diethyl ether, chloroform, methanol, and pentane.)

(**a**) *For foods other than dried whole egg solids, mayonnaise, and nonfat dry milk.*—Accurately weigh known amount sample containing ca 0.5–1 g fat and transfer quantitatively to homogenizer cup with 100.0 mL anhydrous methyl alcohol. On basis of moisture determination, add enough H_2O to bring total H_2O content in extraction to 40 mL. Add 50 mL $CHCl_3$ and blend 3 min at high speed. (Ratio of $CHCl_3$-methyl alcohol-H_2O must be 50–100–40 in this single-phase extraction.) Add additional 50 mL $CHCl_3$ and blend 0.5 min at medium speed. Then add 50 mL H_2O and again blend 0.5 min at medium speed. Filter homogenate under vacuum into 1 L suction flask through buchner fitted with Whatman No. 1 paper containing 2 g diatomaceous earth. Pour filtrate into 500 mL graduate. Re-extract filter cake and paper with ca 90 mL $CHCl_3$ and filter extract without diatomaceous earth. Rinse cup and filter cake with two 15 mL portions $CHCl_3$. Add these rinses to original filtrate and let layers separate. (If emulsion develops, centrifuge filtrate 5 min at 2500 rpm.) Record volume of $CHCl_3$ (lower) layer and aspirate aqueous alcohol layer. (Total volume of $CHCl_3$ layer should be ca 200 mL.) Proceed as in **976.26G**.

(**b**) *For dried whole egg solids.*—Use acid hydrolysis, **925.32A(b)**, and proceed as in **976.26G**, par. 2.

> I. **925.32A(b)** (Fat in Eggs, Acid Hydrolysis Method)
>
> *A. Preparation of Solution*
>
> (**a**) *Liquid eggs.*—From well mixed sample, **925.29(a)** or (**b**), accurately weigh, by difference, into Mojonnier fat-extraction tube ca 2 g yolks, 3 g whole eggs, or 5 g whites. Slowly, with vigorous shaking, add 10 mL HCl, set tube in H_2O bath heated to 70°, bring to boiling, and continue heating at bp 30 min, shaking tube carefully every 5 min. Remove tube, add H_2O to nearly fill lower bulb of tube, and cool to room temperature.
>
> (**b**) *Dried eggs.*—Transfer 1 g well mixed sample to fat-extraction tube, slowly add 10 mL HCl (4 + 1), washing down any egg particles adhering to sides of tube, and proceed as in (**a**).

> II. **925.29** (Sampling of Eggs, Collection and Preparation of Sample)
>
> No simple rules can be made for collection of sample representative of average of any particular lot of egg material, as conditions may differ widely. Experienced judgment must be used in each instance. For large lots, preferably draw several samples for separate analyses rather than attempt to get one composite representative sample. Sampling for microbiological examination, if required, should be performed first; *see* **939.14A–B** [*Official Methods of Analysis* (1990) 15th Ed.].
>
> (**a**) *Liquid eggs.*—Obtain representative container or containers. Mix contents of container thoroughly and draw ca 300 g. (Long-handle dipper or ladle serves well.) Keep sample in hermetically sealed jar in freezer or with solid CO_2. Report odor and appearance.

(b) *Frozen eggs.*—Obtain representative container or containers. Examine contents as to odor and appearance. (Condition of contents can be determined best by drilling to center of container with auger and noting odor as auger is withdrawn. If impossible to secure individual containers, samples may consist of composite of borings from contents of each container.) Take borings diagonally across can from ≥ 3 widely separated parts, starting 2–5 cm in from edge and extending to opposite side as near to bottom as possible. Pack shavings tightly into sample jar and fill it completely to prevent partial dehydration of sample. Seal jar tightly and store in freezer or with solid CO_2. Before analyzing, warm sample in bath held at $<50°$, and mix well.

(c) *For mayonnaise.*—Accurately weigh ca 1.2–1.5 g sample and transfer quantitatively to homogenizer cup with 100.0 mL anhydrous methyl alcohol. Add 40 mL H_2O and 50 mL $CHCl_3$ and blend 3 min at medium speed. Add additional 50 mL $CHCl_3$ and blend 0.5 min at medium speed. Then add 50 mL H_2O and again blend 0.5 min at medium speed. Transfer homogenate to 500 mL separator. Rinse cup with three 20 mL portions $CHCl_3$ and add these rinses to separator. Mix by gently rotating separator end to end. Let layers separate. Drain $CHCl_3$ (lower) layer into graduate. Rinse aqueous methyl alcohol layer with 40 mL $CHCl_3$, add rinse to graduate, and mix. Record volume of $CHCl_3$ layer. Proceed as in **976.26G**, using 150 mL aliquot $CHCl_3$-lipid extract and 250 mL beaker.

(d) *For nonfat dry milk.*—Accurately weigh ca 25 g sample and transfer quantitatively to 300 mL Erlenmeyer containing 100 mL H_2O. Stir to mix thoroughly, and refrigerate overnight. Pour reconstituted milk into 1 L separator, add 100 mL reagent alcohol, (**i**), and shake 1 min. Add 100 mL ether and shake 1 min. Add 100 mL pentane and shake 1 min. Let layers separate. Drain aqueous (lower) layer into second separator. Repeat extraction with 100 mL ether and 100 mL pentane, shaking 1 min after each addition. If layers do not separate, add 40 mL reagent alcohol, gently rotate end over end 10 times, and let stand 5 min. Discard aqueous layer. Filter combined ether extracts through column of anhydrous Na_2SO_4 into 600 mL beaker. Evaporate to ca 10 mL under gentle N stream on 70° H_2O bath. Transfer extract to 300 mL glass-stoppered erlenmeyer, rinsing beaker with pentane. Evaporate to dryness under gentle N stream on steam bath, and proceed as in **976.26G**, paragraph 2.

G. Saponification and Extraction of Unsaponifiable Fraction

(*Caution: See Appendix* for safety notes on distillation, pipets, benzene, and petroleum ether.)

Filter 100 mL aliquot $CHCl_3$-lipid extract through glass funnel containing small pledget of glass wool and ca 25 g anhydrous Na_2SO_4 into 150 mL beaker. Rinse Na_2SO_4 with 15 mL $CHCl_3$ and evaporate extract to dryness under gentle N stream on 90° H_2O bath or steam bath. Dissolve residue in ca 70 mL petroleum ether and filter through Whatman No. 1 paper containing ca 20 g anhydrous Na_2SO_4 into 300 mL glass-stoppered erlenmeyer. Rinse beaker and Na_2SO_4 with several 10 mL portions petroleum ether. Evaporate to dryness under gentle N stream on steam bath.

Introduce magnetic stirring bar into erlenmeyer and place on magnetic stirrer-hot plate. With gentle stirring, slowly add 8 mL concentrated KOH solution, (**h**), and 40 mL reagent alcohol, (**i**). Attach condenser, turn on magnetic stirrer-hot plate, and reflux solution 1 h. Turn off heat and add 60 mL reagent alcohol through condenser into saponified solution while stirring and cooling. When sample ceases to reflux, remove condenser, and pipet 100 mL benzene into sample while slowly stirring. Remove stirring bar, stopper flask, and shake vigorously 30 s.

Pour into 500 mL separator without rinsing. Add 200 mL 1N KOH and shake vigorously 10 s. Let layers separate and discard aqueous (lower) layer (will be turbid). Wash benzene layer with 40 mL 0.5N KOH, rotate gently end to end 10 s, and discard aqueous (lower) layer. Pour benzene layer into 250 mL separator. Back-wash benzene layer with 40 mL H_2O by gently rotating separator end to end 10 times. Repeat H_2O wash 3 more times. pH of last H_2O wash should be ca 7. Pour benzene extract from top of separator, filtering through Whatman No. 4 paper containing ca 15 g anhydrous Na_2SO_4 into 125 mL glass-stoppered erlenmeyer. Add ca 20 g anhydrous Na_2SO_4; stopper and shake flask vigorously. Let stand 15 min.

Pipet 50 mL aliquot into 100 mL round-bottom glass-stoppered flask and evaporate to dryness on rotary evaporator at 40°. Add 3 mL acetone and again evaporate to dryness. Dissolve residue in 3 mL DMF.

H. Derivatization of Cholesterol Standards and Gas Chromatographic Calibration

Transfer 1.0 mL of each cholesterol working standard solution, **976.26C(a)(2)**, to 15 mL silanized centrifuge tube. (Keep DMCS-silanized centrifuge tubes clean and dry.) Add 0.2 mL HMDS and 0.1 mL TMCS. Stopper tube and shake vigorously on test tube mixer, **976.26B(f)**, or by hand for 30 s. Let solution stand undisturbed 15 min. Add 1.0 mL 5α-cholestane internal standard working solution, **976.26C(b)(2)**, and 10 mL H_2O to tube. Shake vigorously 1 min and centrifuge 2 min.

Inject duplicate 3 μL or other appropriate volumes (use same volume throughout for all standards and samples) heptane layer into gas chromatograph. Adjust GC parameters to give retention times of ca 5 min for 5α-cholestane and 10 min for cholesterol. Determine area of each peak by using height-width measurement or digital integrator. Divide cholesterol peak area by internal standard peak area to obtain standard response ratio. Average results for duplicate determinations. Plot average response ratio (y-axis) against cholesterol concentration (mg/mL) (x-axis). Standard response ratio plot should bracket sample response ratio.

I. Derivatization and Analysis of Samples

Transfer 1.0 mL sample solution, **976.26G**, to 15 mL silanized centrifuge tube and proceed as in **976.26H**, beginning "Add 0.2 mL HMDS. . . ." If GC response is beyond scope of standard calibration, dilute sample solution and derivatize again.

mg Cholesterol/100 g sample = (mg/mL cholesterol in sample from standard curve
× 100)/(g/mL sample used for derivatization)

References: JAOAC **58,** 804(1975); **59,** 46(1976).
CAS-57-88-5 (cholesterol)

Chapter 14
Copper

14.1   985.35—Minerals in Ready-to-Feed Milk-Based Infant Formula
Atomic Absorption Spectrophotometric Method
First Action 1985
Final Action 1988

See Chapter 12.14.

14.2   984.27—Calcium, Copper, Iron, Magnesium, Manganese, Phosphorus, Potassium, Sodium, and Zinc in Infant Formula
Inductively Coupled Plasma Emission Spectroscopic Method
First Action 1984
Final Action 1986

See Chapter 12.13.

14.3   960.40—Copper in Food
Colorimetric Method
First Action 1960
Final Action 1965
International Union of Pure and Applied Chemistry—AOAC Method

A. Principle

Sample is digested with HNO_3 and H_2SO_4. Cu is isolated and determined colorimetrically at pH 8.5 as diethyldithiocarbamate in presence of chelating agent, EDTA. Bi and Te also give colored carbamates at pH 8.5 but are decomposed to colorless compounds with $1N$ NaOH. Cu complex is stable. Range of color development is 0–50 μg. Blank is ca 1 μg Cu.

B. Precautions

Clean glassware with hot HNO₃. Use white petrolatum to lubricate stopcocks of separators, and do not use brass chains. Purify H_2O and HNO_3 by distillation in Pyrex.

C. Reagents

(**a**) *Sodium diethyldithiocarbamate* (*carbamate solution*).—Dissolve 1 g of the salt in H_2O, dilute to 100 mL, and filter. Store in refrigerator and prepare weekly.

(**b**) *Citrate-EDTA solution.*—Dissolve 20 g dibasic ammonium citrate and 5 g Na_2EDTA (Eastman Kodak Co.) in H_2O and dilute to 100 mL. Remove traces of Cu by adding 0.1 mL carbamate solution and extracting with 10 mL CCl_4. Repeat extraction until CCl_4 extract is colorless.

(**c**) *Copper standard solutions.*—(*1*) *Stock solution.*—1 mg/mL. Place 0.2000 g Cu wire or foil into 125 mL Erlenmeyer. Add 15 mL HNO_3 (1 + 4), cover flask with watch glass, and let Cu dissolve, warming to complete solution. Boil to expel fumes, cool, and dilute to 200 mL. (*2*) *Intermediate solution.*—100 μg/mL. Dilute 20 mL stock solution to 200 mL. (*3*) *Working solution.*—2 μg/mL. Prepare daily by diluting 5 mL intermediate standard solution to 250 mL with $2.0N\ H_2SO_4$.

(**d**) *Ammonium hydroxide.*—6N. Purify as in (**b**).

(**e**) *Thymol blue indicator.*—0.1%. Dissolve 0.1 g thymol blue in H_2O, add enough 0.1N NaOH to change color to blue, and dilute to 100 mL.

D. Preparation of Sample

(*Caution: See Appendix* for safety notes on nitric acid and sulfuric acid.)

Weigh sample containing ≤20 g solids, depending upon expected Cu content. If sample contains <75% H_2O, add H_2O to obtain this dilution. Add initial volume HNO_3 to equal ca 2 times dry sample weight and 5 mL H_2SO_4, or as many mL H_2SO_4 as g dry sample, but ≥5 mL. Digest as in **963.21C**.

963.21C (Arsenic in Food, Kjeldahl Flask Digestion)

C. Preparation of Sample

(*Caution: See Appendix* for safety notes on wet oxidation, nitric acid, and sulfuric acid.) (For details of convenient churn-type washer that will remove arsenical spray residues from firm fruits or vegetables with an aqueous NH_4NO_3-HNO_3 solution, *see* JAOAC **26**, 150(1943). Digest aliquot of "strip" solution and proceed as in (**a**).

All digestions can be greatly facilitated by following optional method, JAOAC **47**, 629(1964): Proceed as in (**a**) until mixture no longer turns brown or darkens. Cool, add 0.5 mL 70% $HClO_4$ (*Caution: See Appendix* for safety notes on perchloric acid), and heat until fuming occurs and digest is clear. Cool, and add 2 additional 0.5 mL portions $HClO_4$, heating each time as above. Finish digestion with H_2O and saturated ammonium oxalate as in (**a**). Conduct ≥1 blank determination with samples. Blanks should not show >1 μg As.)

(**a**) *For fresh fruits* (*apples, pears, or similar products*).—Weigh and peel representative sample (1–5 lb; 0.5–2 kg). At blossom and stem ends cut out all flesh thought to be contaminated with As compounds and include with peelings, if desired. Place peelings in 1 or more 800 mL Kjeldahl flasks. (As-free Pyrex glassware and "wet ashing" apparatus of Duriron are available.) Add 25–50 mL HNO_3; then cautiously add 40 mL H_2SO_4 (20 mL if Gutzeit method is used). Place each flask on asbestos mat with 5 cm hole. Warm slightly and discontinue heating if foaming becomes excessive.

When reaction has quieted, heat flask cautiously and rotate occasionally to prevent caking of sample upon glass exposed to flame. Maintain oxidizing conditions in flask at all times during digestion by cautiously adding small amounts of HNO_3 whenever mixture turns brown or darkens. Continue digestion until organic matter is destroyed and SO_3 fumes are copiously evolved. (Final solution should be colorless, or at most light straw color.) Cool slightly, and add 75 mL H_2O and 25 mL saturated ammonium oxalate solution to assist in expelling oxides of N from solution. Evaporate again to point where fumes of SO_3 appear in neck of flask. Cool, and dilute with H_2O to 500 or 1000 mL in volumetric flask.

(**b**) *For dried fruit products.*—Prepare sample by alternately grinding and mixing 4–5 times in food chopper. Place 35–70 g portions in 800 mL Kjeldahl flasks, and add 10–25 mL H_2O, 25–50 mL HNO_3, and 20 mL H_2SO_4. Continue digestion as in (**a**). Dilute digested solution to 250 mL.

(**c**) *For small fruits, vegetables, etc.*—Use 70–140 g sample and digest as in (**a**) or (**b**).

(**d**) *For materials other than* (**a**), (**b**), *or* (**c**).—Digest 5–50 g, according to moisture content and amount of As expected, as in (**a**) or (**b**). Dilute to definite volume determined by As concentration expected.

(**e**) *For products containing stable organic As compounds, products liable to yield incompletely oxidized organic derivatives that inhibit arsine evolution, or products that are difficult to digest.*—Shrimp, tobacco, oils, and some other products require special treatment to complete oxidation of organic As to inorganic As_2O_5, or to destroy organic interferences previous to As determination. For details consult: Ind. Eng. Chem., Anal. Ed. **5**, 58(1933); **6**, 280, 327 (1934); JAOAC **20**, 171(1937); **47**, 629(1964).

Dilute As solutions obtained by these special methods of preparation to definite volume.

(**f**) *For ultra-micro quantities of As, very labile forms of As, and vacuum-accelerated Gutzeit reduction system for mercuric bromide spot filtration.*— Consult Ind. Eng. Chem., Anal. Ed. **16**, 400(1944).

When sample contains large amount of fat, make partial digestion with HNO_3 until only fat is undissolved. Cool, filter free of solid fat, wash residue with H_2O, add H_2SO_4 to filtrate, and complete digestion as above. After digestion, cool, add 25 mL H_2O, and remove nitrosylsulfuric acid by heating to fumes. Repeat addition of 25 mL H_2O and fuming. If after cooling and diluting, insoluble matter is present, filter through acid-washed paper, rinse paper with H_2O, and dilute to 100 mL.

Prepare reagent blank similarly.

E. Isolation and Determination of Copper

Pipet 25 mL sample solution into 100 or 250 mL short-stem separator and add 10 mL citrate-EDTA reagent. Add 2 drops thymol blue indicator, **C**(**e**), and 6N NH_4OH dropwise until solution turns green or blue-green. Cool, and add 1 mL carbamate solution and 15 mL CCl_4. Shake vigorously 2 min. Let layers separate and drain CCl_4 through cotton pledget into glass-stoppered tube or flask. Determine A or T in suitable instrument at ca 400 nm.

If >50 μg Cu is present in 25 mL aliquot, use smaller aliquot and dilute to 25 mL with 2.0N H_2SO_4. Highest accuracy is obtained at ca 25 μg Cu level (A ca 0.3 in 1 cm cell).

To test for Bi and Te, return CCl_4 solution to separator, add 10 mL 5% KCN solution, and shake 1 min. If CCl_4 layer becomes colorless, Bi and Te are absent.

If test is positive, develop color in another 25 mL aliquot as above (without KCN). Drain CCl_4 layer into second separator, add 10 mL $1N$ NaOH, and shake 1 min. Let layers separate and drain CCl_4 into third separator. Again wash CCl_4 extract with 10 mL $1N$ NaOH. Determine A or T of CCl_4 layer and convert to μg Cu.

F. Preparation of Standards and Calibration Curves

Transfer 0, 1, 2.5, 5, 10, 15, 20, and 25 mL of Cu standard solution (2 μg/mL) to separators and add $2.0N$ H_2SO_4 to make total volume of 25 mL.

Add 10 mL citrate-EDTA reagent and proceed as in **960.40E**, beginning "Add 2 drops thymol blue indicator . . . ."

Plot A against μg Cu on ordinary graph paper. If readings are in % T, use semilog paper, and plot T on log scale. Since there is usually some deviation from linearity, read sample values from smoothed curve.

Reference: JAOAC **43,** 695(1960).
CAS-7440-50-8 (copper)

14.4

968.08—Minerals in Animal Feed
Atomic Absorption Spectrophotometric Method
First Action 1968
Final Action 1969

See Chapter 12.1.

14.5

975.03—Metals in Plants
Atomic Absorption Spectrophotometric Method
First Action 1975
Final Action 1988

See Chapter 12.2.

14.6

980.03—Metals in Plants
Direct Reading Spectrographic Method
Final Action 1988

See Chapter 12.3.

14.7 953.01—Metals in Plants
General Recommendations for Emission Spectrographic Methods
First Action 1988

See Chapter 12.5.

14.8 985.01—Metals and Other Elements in Plants
Inductively Coupled Plasma Spectroscopic Method
First Action 1985
Final Action 1988

See Chapter 12.6.

14.9 953.03—Copper in Plants
Colorimetric Method
Final Action 1965

A. Reagents

Those listed in **951.01A** and following:

(a) *Sodium diethyldithiocarbamate solution.*—0.1%. Freshly prepared in redistilled H_2O, **951.01A(a)**.

(b) *Copper standard solution.*—1 µg/mL. Dissolve 0.3929 g $CuSO_4 \cdot 5H_2O$ in redistilled H_2O, **951.01A(a)**, add 5 mL H_2SO_4, dilute to 1 L, and mix. Take 10 mL aliquot, add 5 mL H_2SO_4, dilute to 1 L, and mix.

951.01A (Cobalt in Plants, Nitrosocresol Method)

(*Caution: See Appendix* for safety notes on distillation, toxic solvents, carbon tetrachloride, and nitroaromatics.)

A. Reagents

(Make all distillations in Pyrex stills with ᛏ joints. Store reagents in glass-stoppered Pyrex bottles.)

(a) *Redistilled water.*—Distil twice, or pass through column of ion exchange resin (IR-100A, H-form, or equivalent) to remove heavy metals.

(b) *Hydrofluoric acid.*—48%. Procurement in vinyl plastic bottles is advantageous.

(c) *Perchloric acid.*—60%. No further purification necessary.

(d) *Hydrochloric acid.*—(1 + 1). Add equal volume HCl to distilled H_2O and distil.

(e) *Ammonium hydroxide.*—(1 + 1). Distil concentrated NH_4OH into equal volume redistilled H_2O.

(f) *Ammonium hydroxide.*—0.02N. Add 7 mL of the NH_4OH (1 + 1) to 2.5 L redistilled H_2O.

(g) *Carbon tetrachloride.*—Distil over CaO, passing distillate through dry, acid-washed filter paper. Used CCl_4 may be recovered as in **941.03A(a)**.

> **941.03A(a)** (Zinc in Plants, Mixed Color Method)
>
> *A. Reagents*
>
> (Redistil all H_2O from Pyrex. Treat all glassware with HNO_3 (1 + 1) or fresh chromic acid cleaning solution. Rinse repeatedly with ordinary distilled H_2O and finally with Zn-free H_2O.)
>
> (**a**) *Carbon tetrachloride.*—Use ACS grade without purification. If technical grade is used, dry with anhydrous $CaCl_2$ and redistil in presence of small amount CaO. (Used CCl_4 may be reclaimed by distillation in presence of NaOH (1 + 100) containing small amounts of $Na_2S_2O_3$, followed by drying with anhydrous $CaCl_2$ and fractional distillation in presence of small amounts of CaO.) (*Caution: See Appendix* for safety notes on distillation and carbon tetrachloride.)

(**h**) *Dithizone.*—Dissolve 0.5 g dithizone in 600–700 mL CCl_4 (technical grade is satisfactory). Filter into 5 L separator containing 2.5–3.0 L 0.02N NH_4OH, shake well, and discard CCl_4 layer. Shake with 50 mL portions redistilled CCl_4 until CCl_4 phase as it separates is pure green. Add 1 L redistilled CCl_4 and acidify slightly with the HCl (1 + 1). Shake the dithizone into CCl_4 layer and discard aqueous layer. Store in cool, dark place, preferably in refrigerator.

(**i**) *Ammonium citrate solution.*—40%. Dissolve 800 g citric acid in 600 mL distilled H_2O, and, while stirring, slowly add 900 mL NH_4OH. Reaction is exothermic; take care to prevent spattering. Adjust pH to 8.5, if necessary. Dilute to 2 L and extract with 25 mL portions dithizone solution until aqueous phase stays orange and CCl_4 remains predominantly green. Then extract solution with CCl_4 until all orange is removed.

(**j**) *Hydrochloric acid.*—0.1N. Dilute 16.6 mL of the HCl (1 + 1) to 1 L with redistilled H_2O.

(**k**) *Hydrochloric acid.*—0.01N. Dilute 100 mL of the 0.1N HCl to 1 L with redistilled H_2O.

(**l**) *Sodium hydroxide solution.*—1N. Dissolve 40 g NaOH in 1 L redistilled H_2O.

(**m**) *Borate buffer.*—pH 7.8. Dissolve 20 g H_3BO_3 in 1 L redistilled H_2O. Add 50 mL 1N NaOH and adjust pH, if necessary. Equal volumes borate buffer and 0.01N HCl should give solution of pH 7.9.

(**n**) *Borate buffer.*—pH 9.1. To 1 L borate buffer, pH 7.8, add 120 mL 1N NaOH and adjust pH, if necessary.

(**o**) *Skellysolve B.*—Essentially *n*-hexane. Purify by adding 20–30 g silica gel/L, let stand several days, and distil.

(**p**) *Cupric acetate solution.*—Dissolve 10 g $Cu(CH_3COO)_2 \cdot H_2O$ in 1 L redistilled H_2O.

(**q**) *o-Nitrosocresol solution.*—Dissolve 8.4 g anhydrous $CuCl_2$ and 8.4 g $NH_2OH \cdot HCl$ in 900 mL H_2O. Add 8 mL *m*-cresol (practical grade) and stir vigorously while slowly adding 24 mL 30% H_2O_2. Stir mechanically 2 h at room temperature. (Standing for longer periods results in excessive decomposition.) Add 25 mL HCl and extract *o*-nitrosocresol with four 150 mL portions Skellysolve B, (**o**), in large separator. Then add additional 25 mL HCl and again extract with four 150 mL portions Skellysolve B. Wash combined Skellysolve B extracts twice with 50–100 mL portions 0.1N HCl and twice with 50–100 mL portions redistilled H_2O. Shake o-nitrosocresol solution with successive 50–100 mL portions 1% $Cu(CH_3COO)_2$ solution until aqueous phase is no longer deep blood-red. When light purple is evident, extraction is complete. Discard Skellysolve B phase, acidify aqueous solution of Cu salt with 25 mL HCl, and extract reagent with two 500 mL portions Skellysolve B; wash twice with 150–200 mL portions 0.1N HCl and several times with 150–200 mL portions redistilled H_2O. Store o-nitrosocresol solution in refrigerator at ca 4°. Reagent is stable ≥6 months.

(**r**) *Sodium o-nitrosocresol solution.*—Extract 100 mL o-nitrosocresol by shaking with two 50 mL portions borate buffer, pH 9.1, in separator. (If this is carried out as 2 extractions, resulting reagent is more concentrated. It is important that total volume o-nitrosocresol solution equal total volume buffer.)

(**s**) *Cobalt standard solutions.*—(*1*) *Stock solution.*—Heat $CoSO_4 \cdot 7H_2O$ in oven at 250–300° to constant weight (6–8 h). Weigh exactly 0.263 g of the $CoSO_4$ and dissolve in 50 mL redistilled H_2O and 1 mL H_2SO_4. Dilute to 1 L. (*2*) *Working solution.*—0.5 μg/mL. Transfer 5 mL stock solution to 1 L volumetric flask and dilute to volume with redistilled H_2O.

(**t**) *Hydroxylamine acetate buffer.*—pH 5.1±0.1. Dissolve 10 g $NH_2OH \cdot HCl$ and 9.5 g anhydrous $NaCH_3COO$ in 500 mL redistilled H_2O.

B. Determination

Transfer aliquot (0.5–1 g dry material) from solution obtained from **951.01F** or **953.02C** to 125 mL separator. Add 2 mL ammonium citrate solution, 1 drop phenolphthalein, 5 mL sodium diethyldithiocarbamate solution, and NH_4OH (1 + 1), **951.01(e)**, until pink. Add 10 mL CCl_4 and shake 5 min. Drain CCl_4, centrifuge 5 min, transfer to absorption cell, and read at maximum A, ca 430 nm.

I. 951.01F (Dithizone Extraction)

(Caution: *See Appendix* for safety notes on distillation, perchloric acid, and carbon tetrachloride.)

Transfer suitable aliquot (2–3 g dry material) to 120 mL separator (use petroleum jelly as stopcock lubricant). Add 5 mL ammonium citrate solution and 1 drop phenolphthalein; adjust to pH 8.5 with NH_4OH (1 + 1). If precipitate forms, add additional ammonium citrate. Add 10 mL dithizone in CCl_4 and shake 5 min. Drain CCl_4 phase into 100 mL beaker. Repeat as many times as necessary, using 5 mL dithizone solution and shaking 5 min each time. Extraction is complete when aqueous phase remains orange and CCl_4 phase remains predominantly green. Then add 10 mL CCl_4, shake 5 min, and combine with CCl_4 extract. Final 10 mL CCl_4 should be pure green. If not, extraction was incomplete and must be repeated.

Add 2 mL $HClO_4$ to combined CCl_4 extracts, cover beaker with Pyrex watch glass, and digest on hot plate until colorless. Remove cover glass and evaporate slowly to dryness. (If sample is heated any length of time at high temperature when dry, losses of Co may occur. Heat only enough to evaporate completely to dryness. If free acid remains, it interferes with next step where pH control is important.)

Add 5 mL 0.01N HCl to residue. Heat slightly to assure solution. If Cu is to be determined, transfer with redistilled H_2O to 25 mL volumetric flask, and dilute to volume. Transfer 20 mL aliquot to 50 mL glass-stoppered centrifuge tube or 60 mL separator and reserve remainder for Cu determination, **953.03B**. If Cu is not to be determined, transfer entire acid solution with redistilled H_2O to centrifuge tube or separator.

II. **953.02C** (Cobalt in Plants, Nitroso-R-Salt Method)

C. Dithizone Extraction

Transfer entire solution to 120 mL separator, and proceed as in **951.01F**, through "If free acid remains . . . pH control is important." Dissolve in 1 mL citric acid solution, (**d**), transfer to 25 mL volumetric flask, and dilute to volume with redistilled H_2O, **951.01A(a)**.

> *Note:* **953.02A(d)** is *Citric acid solution.*—0.2N. Use special reagent grade Pb-free citric acid.

Prepare standard curve with 0, 1, 5, 10, 15, and 20 μg Cu treated as above.

Reference: JAOAC **36,** 405(1953).
CAS-7440-50-8 (copper)

14.10

985.40—Copper in Liver
Atomic Absorption Spectrophotometric Method
First Action 1985
Final Action 1987

A. Principle

One g liver tissue is digested overnight at 60° in 5 mL HNO_3, then diluted to 25 mL with H_2O and analyzed by AAS.

B. Apparatus and Reagents

(**a**) *Atomic absorption spectrophotometer (AAS).*—Equipped with nebulizer and 10 cm, air-C_2H_2 burner head. Monitor performance by assuring that 4.0 mg Cu/L standard produces ≥ 0.200 absorbance unit.

(**b**) *External control.*—Standard Reference Material (SRM 1577) Bovine Liver (193 $\pm$ 10 mg Cu/kg; NIST, Washington, DC 20243), or equivalent.

(**c**) *Nitric acid.*—Concentrated and diluted (1 + 4).

(**d**) *Teflon screw-cap bottles.*—30 mL wide mouth (Cole-Parmer, K-6103-30), or equivalent.

(**e**) *Copper standard solutions.*—(*1*) *Stock standard solution.*—1000 mg Cu/L. Dissolve 1.000 g Cu metal in 10 mL HNO_3-H_2O (1 + 1). Dilute to 1000 mL with 1% HNO_3. (*2*) *Intermediate standard solution.*—100 mg Cu/L. Dilute 10 mL stock standard solution to 100 mL with H_2O. *(3) Working standard solutions.*—Dilute 0.0, 0.25, 0.5, 1.0, 2.0, and 4.0 mL intermediate standard solution to 100 mL with HNO_3-H_2O (1 + 4) to give Cu standards containing 0.0, 0.25, 0.5, 1.0, 2.0, and 4.0 mg Cu/L, respectively.

C. Sample Preparation

Rinse all glassware with 2N HCl. Mix samples thoroughly before weighing. Into separate Teflon screw-cap bottles, accurately weigh 1.0 g liver tissue and 0.25 g external control for each 10 samples or fraction thereof. (*Note:* Complete digestion will not occur for >0.5 g dry weight of samples or controls.) Add 5 mL concentrated HNO_3 to each bottle, tighten cap, and place bottles overnight in 60°, ventilated oven.

Remove bottles from oven and cool to room temperature. Using H_2O to rinse bottles, transfer sample digests to 25 mL volumetric flasks, allowing any fat to remain adhering to digestion bottles. Dilute flasks to volume with H_2O.

D. Determination

Analyze by AAS using following conditions: wavelength 324.7 nm; slit 0.7 nm; flame air-C_2H_2 (lean-blue). Aspirate series of working standard solutions, external control solutions, and sample dilutions. Prepare standard curve of concentration (mg Cu/L) vs *A* and determine sample solution concentrations. Dilute with HNO_3 (1 + 4) any samples above range of working standards. Repeat analysis if external control Cu value is not within accepted range. Calculate mg Cu/kg tissue *(X)*:

$$X = (C \times 25 \times D)/W$$

where *C* = sample solution concentration (mg Cu/L); *D* = additional sample dilution, if necessary; and *W* = tissue weight (g).

Reference: JAOAC **68,** 44(1985)
CAS-7440-50-8 (copper)

14.11   990.05—Copper, Iron, and Nickel in Edible Oils and Fats
Direct Graphite Furnace
Atomic Absorption Spectrophotometric Method
First Action 1990
IUPAC-AOAC Method

(Applicable to Cu, Fe, and Ni in oils and Cu and Fe in fats
at ≥5 μg/kg for Cu and ≥10 μg/kg for Fe and Ni)

Method Performance:

Copper in oils, 40–140 μg/kg
s_r = 5.4–10.7; s_R = 7.6–21.4; av. RSD_r = 10.6%; av. RSD_R = 17.4%
Iron in oils, 150–750 μg/kg
s_r = 30.7–46.5; s_R = 39.7–147.1; av. RSD_r = 12.1%; av. RSD_R = 21.8%
Nickel in oils, 140–800 μg/kg
s_r = 25.8–49.3; s_R = 33.7–129.9; av. RSD_r – 11.0%; av. RSD_R = 18.8%
Copper in fat, 40–150 μg/kg
s_r = 4.5–9.7; s_R = 7.9–27.0; av. RSD_r = 7.7%; av. RSD_R = 18.7%
Iron in fat, 150–850 μg/kg
s_r = 17.9–66.9; s_R = 36.3–183.4; av. RSD_r = 9.8%; av. RSD_R = 22.7%

A. Principle

Test portion is vaporized in graphite furnace connected to AAS previously calibrated using standard solutions of organocompounds of Cu, Fe, and Ni. Metal content is determined from measured absorbances at selected wavelengths. Elements are determined sequentially.

B. Apparatus

(a) *Atomic absorption spectrophotometer.*—Equipped with either peak height mode and printer or continuous mode and pen recorder (full scale response in 0.2 s) together with appropriate hollow cathode lamps and deuterium background corrector. Spectrophotometer should be located in dust-free atmosphere.

(b) *Graphite furnace atomizer and graphite tubes.*—Use uncoated tubes for Cu and Ni determinations. For Fe, coat tubes with Nb as follows: Use micropipettor to inject 100 μL Nb solution, **C(g)**, into furnace. Start temperature program to dry at 100° for 60 s and then atomize at 2700° for 5 s. Repeat this procedure until 300 μL Nb solution has been injected. Atomize at 2700° to constant absorbance (to remove any Fe contamination).

(c) *Chromatographic columns.*—Diameter:height ratio 1:10.

(d) *Electric oven.*—Regulated at 60 $\pm$ 2°, and suitable for heating at 150°.

(e) *Poly(ethylene) or poly(propylene) bottles.*—20 and 50 mL, with caps. Make bottles metal free as follows: Thoroughly clean bottles with warm HNO_3, **C(f)**, rinse with water, and dry in oven at ca 80°.

(f) *Micropipettors.*—20 and 50 μL, with pipettor tips.

C. Reagents

(a) *n-Heptane.*—Analytical grade.

(b) *Light petroleum.*—Analytical grade, bp 40–60°.

(c) *Aluminum oxide.*—Chromatographic grade (Merck No. 1077 is suitable). Activate by heating 14 h in 150° oven.

(d) *Argon.*—Purity $\geq$99.9%. If argon is not available, nitrogen may be used as purge gas. (*Caution:* At temperatures above 2300°, nitrogen forms toxic cyanogen gas. Provide continuous ventilation in furnace area.)

(e) *Sunflower oil.*—Refined, or similar, stable liquid oil with low metal content. Prepare as follows: Dissolve 1 part oil in 3 parts light petroleum (w/v). Prepare aluminum oxide column, **B(c)**, using twice weight of activated aluminum oxide, **(c)**, as weight of oil to be purified. Add oil solution to column and elute with 5 parts (v) of light petroleum. Evaporate light petroleum of eluate on heated water bath under gentle stream of nitrogen (2–5 L/min), **(d)**. Remove final traces of light petroleum under vacuum.

(f) *Nitric acid.*—2M. Free from traces of Fe, Ni, and Cu.

(g) *Niobium solution.*—Nb AAS standard in aqueous matrix, 1000 mg Nb/L. (Solution is available from Alfa Division, 152 Andover St, Danvers, MA 01923 [Code 88083].)

(h) *Standard solutions.*—*(1) Stock solutions.*—10 mg Fe/kg, 10 mg Ni/kg, and 2 mg Cu/kg. Prepare by appropriate dilution of organometallic standards with sunflower oil, **(e)**. (Suitable standards are available from, e.g., Continental Oil Co., Ponca City, OK [Conostan, 5000 mg/kg] or Merck, D-6100 Darmstadt, West Germany [metal in standard oil, 1000 mg/kg].) Stock solutions are stable for 1 month.

(2) Working solutions.—Prepare daily by diluting stock solutions with sunflower oil: Cu, 0.05, 0.1, and 0.2 mg/kg; Fe, 0.25, 0.5, and 1.0 mg/kg; Ni, 0.25, 0.5, and 1.0 mg/kg.

D. *Determination*

(a) *AAS start-up.*—Switch on spectrophotometer and D_2 corrector. Follow manufacturer's instructions to adjust lamp current, slit, wavelength, and amplification. Required wavelengths are (nm): Cu, 324.7; Fe, 302.1; Ni, 232.0.

Optimize position of graphite furnace atomizer in spectrophotometer and set required program for furnace as follows:

Element	Step	Temp., °	Ramp time, s	Hold time, s	Int. gas flow, mL/min
Cu	1	900	50	30	300
	2	2700	1	5	50
Fe, Ni	1	1200	50	30	300
	2	2700	1	5	50

If it is not possible to program the furnace exactly as shown, use comparable program suitable for equipment. *Note:* If in this case, background correction fails, dilute blank, standards, and test portions with organic fat solvent, e.g., heptane, **C(a)**, to maximum of 1:2 (w/w) and work at ambient temperature.

Use uncoated graphite tube for copper and nickel. Graphite tube for determination of iron must be coated with niobium as in **B(b)** to ensure that total amount of iron is determined. With uncoated tube, result will vary according to type of iron compound present in oil.

(b) *Samples and standard solutions.*—Place all samples and working standard solutions in 60° oven during period of determination. Shake samples vigorously before analysis.

If metal content of oil is known to be outside range specified for working standard solutions, **C(h)(2)**, dilute sample with sunflower oil, **C(e)**, to bring metal content within that range.

Use micropipettor and pipettor tip to make all injections. Pretreat pipettor tip by pipetting and then discarding 20 µL heptane. Film of heptane remaining on wall of tip facilitates reproducible transfer of oil sample. Tip must be pretreated before each injection of oil sample.

(c) *Procedure.*—Record absorbance, if any, of graphite tube and autozero this absorbance.

Table 990.05. Repeatability (r) and Reproducibility (R)

Element	Substrate	r	R
Cu	Oil	0.0102 + 0.140m[a]	0.0085 + 0.358m
	Fat	0.007 + 0.109m	0.0028 + 0.492m
Fe	Oil	0.077 + 0.081m	0.040 + 0.480m
	Fat	0.026 + 0.196n	0.031 + 0.543m
Ni	Oil	0.056 + 0.127m	0.027 + 0.442m

[a] m = corresponding mean concentration value.

Inject 20 µL low-metal oil, **C(e)**, into graphite furnace. Start temperature program and record absorbance.

Inject 20 µL portions of the 3 working standard solutions of metal being determined into graphite furnace. Record absorbance.

(1) *Oil samples.*—Inject 20 µL oil sample into graphite furnace. Initiate temperature program and record absorbance.

(2) Fat samples (mp >40°).—Introduce extra temperature programming step; hold time 20 s; temperature 60°; internal gas flow 0 mL/min. Initiate temperature program. Within first program step, introduce 20 μL melted fat into graphite furnace, let tip remain in injection opening to liquefy fat, and then inject. Record absorbance. *Note:* Normal, minimum limit of detection can be improved by either greater scale expansion or by repeated injections of sample at end of ashing step, then allowing program to proceed to completion. If metal content is too high (i.e., exceeds calibration curve), measure absorbance after further dilution of sample with sunflower oil.

Carry out 2 determinations in rapid succession.

E. Calculations

Measure peak height on recorder chart or read from display or printer. Draw calibration curve by plotting absorbance of the 3 working standard solutions, corrected for the blank, against their respective metal contents. (Some systems may have provision for autocalibration.)

Read metal content of sample from relevant calibration curve.

Report as final result, mean of results of 2 determinations, provided requirements for repeatability, **F**, are met. Report result in mg/kg oil or fat corrected for any required dilutions. If requirements are not met, discard results and carry out another 2 determinations on test portion.

F. Repeatability and Reproducibility

Repeatability.—Differences between values obtained for 2 single determinations, carried out in rapid succession by same operator, using same apparatus for analysis of same test sample, should not be greater than repeatability value (r) calculated as in Table **990.05**, which expresses precision in relation to determined mean value.

Reproducibility.—Difference between values for final results, obtained by 2 (or more) laboratories for analysis by this method of same laboratory sample, should not be greater than reproducibility value (R) calculated from formulas in Table **990.05**, which expresses precision in relation to determined mean value.

Refs.: Pure Appl. Chem. **60**, 893(1988). JAOAC **73**, 320(1990).

Chapter 15
Cyanocobalamine

15.1

960.46—Vitamin Assays
Microbiological Methods
Final Action

(Throughout all stages, except where otherwise directed, protect solutions from undue exposure to light.)

A. Stock Solutions for Basal Media

(Store all solutions in dark at ca 10°. Store all solutions except those containing alcohol under toluene. Proportionate amounts may be prepared.)

(a) *Acid-hydrolyzed casein solution.*—(*Caution: See Appendix* for safety notes on distillation and vacuum.) Mix 400 g vitamin-free casein with 2 L constantly boiling HCl (ca 5N) and either reflux 8–12 h or autoclave 8–12 h at 121–123°. Remove HCl from mixture by distillation under reduced pressure until thick paste remains. Redissolve paste in H_2O, adjust solution to pH 3.5 ± 0.1 with ca 10% NaOH solution, and dilute with H_2O to 4 L. Add 80 g activated charcoal, stir 1 h and filter. Repeat treatment with activated charcoal. Filter solution if precipitate forms upon storage. (Some commercial sources of vitamin-free acid-hydrolyzed casein have been found satisfactory.)

(b) *Adenine-guanine-uracil solution.*—Dissolve 1.0 g each of adenine sulfate, guanine·HCl, and uracil in 50 mL warm HCl (1 + 1), cool, and dilute with H_2O to 1 L.

(c) *Asparagine solution.*—Dissolve 10 g L-asparagine·H_2O in H_2O and dilute to 1 L.

(d) *Cystine solution.*—Suspend 2 g L-cystine in ca 750 mL H_2O, heat to 70–80°, and add HCl (1 + 1), dropwise, with stirring, until solid dissolves. Cool, and dilute with H_2O to 1 L.

(e) *Cystine-tryptophan solution.*—Suspend 8 g L-cystine and 2 g L-tryptophan (or 4 g D,L-tryptophan) in ca 1.5 L H_2O, heat to 70–80°, and add HCl (1 + 1), dropwise, with stirring, until solids dissolve. Cool, and dilute with H_2O to 2 L.

(f) *Manganese sulfate solution.*—Dissolve 2 g $MnSO_4$·H_2O in H_2O and dilute to 200 mL.

(g) *Photolyzed peptone solution.*—Dissolve 100 g peptone in 625 mL H_2O, add solution of 50 g NaOH in 625 mL H_2O, and mix in vessel (such as crystallizing dish) of such size that depth of solution is 1–2 cm. Place 100–500 watt bulb, fitted with reflector, ca 30–50 cm from solution, and expose solution, with occasional stirring, to light from bulb until riboflavin is destroyed (4–10 h may be enough). Maintain solution at ≤25° during this treatment. Adjust solution to pH 6.0–6.5 with CH_3COOH, add 18 g anhydrous NaOAc, stir until solid dissolves, dilute with H_2O to 2 L, and filter if solution is not clear.

(h) *Polysorbate 80 solution.*—Dissolve 25 g polysorbate 80 (polyoxyethylene sorbitan monooleate) in alcohol to make 250 mL.

(i) *Salt solution A.*—Dissolve 50 g anhydrous KH_2PO_4 and 50 g anhydrous K_2HPO_4 in H_2O, dilute to 1 L, and add 10 drops HCl.

(j) *Salt solution B.*—Dissolve 20 g $MgSO_4$·$7H_2O$, 1 g NaCl, 1 g $FeSO_4$·$7H_2O$, and 1 g $MnSO_4$·H_2O in H_2O, dilute to 1 L, and add 10 drops HCl.

(**k**) *Tryptophan solution.*—Suspend 2.0 g L-tryptophan (or 4.0 g D,L-tryptophan) in 700–800 mL H_2O, heat to 70–80°, and add HCl (1 + 1), dropwise, with stirring, until solid dissolves. Cool, and dilute with H_2O to 1 L.

(**l**) *Vitamin solution I.*—Dissolve 25 mg riboflavin, 25 mg thiamine·HCl, 0.25 mg biotin, and 50 mg niacin in 0.02N CH_3COOH to make 1 L.

(**m**) *Vitamin solution II.*—Dissolve 50 mg *p*-aminobenzoic acid, 25 mg Ca pantothenate, 100 mg pyridoxine·HCl, 100 mg pyridoxal·HCl, 20 mg pyridoxamine·2HCl, and 5 mg folic acid in 25% alcohol to make 1 L.

(**n**) *Vitamin solution III.*—Dissolve 10 mg *p*-aminobenzoic acid, 40 mg pyridoxine·HCl, 4 mg thiamine·HCl, 8 mg Ca pantothenate, 8 mg niacin, and 0.2 mg biotin in ca 300 mL H_2O. Add 10 mg riboflavin dissolved in ca 200 mL 0.02N CH_3COOH. Then add solution containing 1.9 g anhydrous NaOAc and 1.6 mL CH_3COOH in ca 40 mL H_2O, and dilute with H_2O to 2 L.

(**o**) *Vitamin solution IV.*—Dissolve 20 mg riboflavin, 10 mg thiamine·HCl, and 0.04 mg biotin in 0.02N CH_3COOH to make 1 L.

(**p**) *Vitamin solution V.*—Dissolve 10 mg *p*-aminobenzoic acid, 20 mg Ca pantothenate, and 40 mg pyridoxine·HCl in 25% alcohol to make 1 L.

(**q**) *Vitamin solution VI.*—Dissolve 10 mg *p*-aminobenzoic acid, 50 mg niacin, and 40 mg pyridoxine·HCl in 25% alcohol to make 1 L.

(**r**) *Xanthine solution.*—Suspend 1.0 g xanthine in 150–200 mL H_2O, heat to ca 70°, add 30 mL NH_4OH (2 + 3), and stir until solid dissolves. Cool, and dilute with H_2O to 1 L.

(**s**) *Yeast supplement solution.*—Dissolve 20 g H_2O-soluble yeast extract in 100 mL H_2O, add solution of 30 g Pb subacetate in 100 mL H_2O (solution is turbid), and mix. Filter, and adjust filtrate to pH 10 with NH_4OH (1 + 2). Filter, and adjust filtrate to pH 6.5 with CH_3COOH. Precipitate excess Pb with H_2S, filter, and dilute filtrate with H_2O to 200 mL.

B. Culture and Suspension Media

(**a**) *Liquid culture medium.*—Dissolve 15 g peptonized milk, 5 g H_2O-soluble yeast extract, 10 g anhydrous glucose, and 2 g anhydrous KH_2PO_4 in ca 600 mL H_2O. Add 100 mL filtered tomato juice, and adjust to pH 6.5–6.8 with NaOH solution. Add, with mixing, 10 mL polysorbate 80 solution, **A** (**h**), and dilute with H_2O to 1 L. Add 10 mL portions solution to test tubes, cover to prevent contamination, sterilize 15 min in autoclave at 121–123°, and cool tubes as rapidly as practicable to keep color formation at minimum. Store in dark at ca 10°. (Difco Lactobacilli Broth AOAC, Difco Laboratories, has been found satisfactory.)

(**b**) *Agar culture medium.*—To 500 mL liquid culture medium, (a), add 5.0–7.5 g agar, and heat with stirring on steam bath until agar dissolves. Add ca 10 mL portions hot solution to test tubes, cover to prevent contamination, sterilize 15 min in autoclave at 121–123°, and cool tubes in upright position as rapidly as practicable to keep color formation at minimum. Store in dark at ca 10°. (Difco agar culture medium for AOAC microbiological assays [Lactobacilli Agar AOAC] has been found satisfactory.)

(**c**) *Suspension medium.*—Dilute measured volume appropriate basal medium stock solution, Table **960.46**, with equal volume H_2O. Add 10 mL portions diluted medium to test tubes, cover to prevent contamination, sterilize 15 min in autoclave at 121–123°, and cool tubes as rapidly as practicable to keep color formation at minimum. Store in dark at ca 10°.

Table 960.46. Basal Media Stock Solutions for 250 mL (Proportionate Amounts May be Prepared)[a]

Ingredients (Stock Solutions, 960.46A)	(a) Cobalamin (Vitamin B_{12} Activity)	(b) Folic Acid (Pteroylglutamic Acid)	(c) Niacin and Niacinamide	(d) Pantothenic Acid	(e) Riboflavin (Vitamin B_2)
	mL	mL	mL	mL	mL
(a) Acid-hydrolyzed casein soln	25	25	25	25	
(b) Adenine-guanine-uracil soln	5	2.5	5	5	
(c) Asparagine soln	5	15			
(d) Cystine soln					25
(e) Cystine-tryptophan soln			25	25	
(f) Manganese sulfate soln		5			
(g) Photolyzed peptone soln					50
(h) Polysorbate 80 soln	5	0.25		0.25	
(i) Salt soln A	5		5	5	5
(j) Salt soln B	5	5	5	5	5
(k) Tryptophan soln		25			
(l) Vitamin soln I	10				
(m) Vitamin soln II	10				
(n) Vitamin soln III		50			
(o) Vitamin soln IV			5	5	
(p) Vitamin soln V			5		
(q) Vitamin soln VI				5	
(r) Xanthine soln	5	5			
(s) Yeast supplement soln					5
Solids	grams	grams	grams	grams	grams
Ascorbic acid	1				
L-Cysteine·HCl·H$_2$O		0.19			
L-Cystine	0.1				
Glucose, anhyd.	10	10	10	10	15
Glutathione		0.0013			
K$_2$HPO$_4$, anhyd.		1.6			
NaOAc·3H$_2$O	8.3		8.3	8.3	
Na citrate·2H$_2$O		13			
D,L-Tryptophan	0.1				

[a] Some commercial sources of basal media have been found satisfactory.

C. Stock Cultures of Test Organisms

For appropriate test organism, designated below, prepare stab culture in ≥1 tubes of *agar culture medium,* **960.46B(b)**. Incubate 6–24 h at any selected temperature between 30 and 40° held constant to within ± 0.5°, and finally store in dark at ca 10°. Before using new culture in assay, make several successive transfers of culture in 1–2 week period.

Prepare fresh stab culture ≥1 time weekly and do not use for preparing inoculum if >1 week old.

Activity of slow-growing culture may be increased by daily or twice-daily transfer of stab culture, and is considered satisfactory when definite turbidity in liquid inoculum can be observed 2–4 h after inoculation. Slow-growing culture seldom gives suitable response curve and may cause erratic results.

(**a**) *Lactobacillus leichmannii.*—ATCC No. 7830. For use in assay of cobalamin.

(**b**) *Streptococcus faecalis (faecium).*—ATCC No. 8043. For use in assay of folic acid.

(**c**) *Lactobacillus plantarum.*—ATCC No. 8014. For use in assay of niacin and pantothenic acid.

(**d**) *Lactobacillus casei* subsp. *rhamnosus.*—ATCC No. 7469. For use in assay of riboflavin.

D. Assay Tubes

Meticulously cleanse by suitable means (Na lauryl sulfate USP has been found satisfactory as detergent), hard-glass test tubes, ca 20 × 150 mm, and other necessary glassware. (Test organisms are highly sensitive to minute amounts of growth factors and to many cleansing agents. Therefore, it may be preferred to follow cleansing by heating 1–2 h at ca 250°. This is of particular importance in cobalamin assay.)

Prepare tubes containing appropriate standard solution as follows: To test tubes add, in duplicate (or replicate), 0.0 (for uninoculated blanks), 0.0 (for inoculated blanks), 1.0, 2.0, 3.0, 4.0, and 5.0 mL, respectively, of standard solution.

Prepare tubes containing appropriate assay solution as follows: To similar test tubes add, in duplicate (or replicate), 1.0, 2.0, 3.0, and 4.0 mL, respectively, of assay solution.

To each tube of standard solution and assay solution add H_2O to make 5.0 mL. Then add 5.0 mL appropriate basal medium stock solution, Table **960.46**, and mix. Cover tubes suitably to prevent bacterial contamination, and sterilize (10 min for titrimetric method, **960.46E**; or 5 min for turbidimetric method, **960.46G**) in autoclave at 121–123°, reaching this temperature in ≤10 min. Cool as rapidly as practicable to keep color formation at minimum. Take precautions to keep sterilizing and cooling conditions uniform throughout assay. Too close packing of tubes in autoclave, or overloading of it, may cause variation in heating rate.

Aseptically inoculate each tube, except 1 set of duplicate (or replicate) tubes containing 0.0 mL standard solution (uninoculated blanks), with 1 drop appropriate inoculum. Incubate for time period designated in titrimetric method, **960.46E**, or turbidimetric method, **960.46G**, at any selected temperature between 30 and 40° held constant to within ±0.5°. Contamination of assay tubes with any foreign organism invalidates assay.

Titrimetric Method

E. Determination

Incubate tubes 72 h and then titrate contents of each tube with 0.1N NaOH, using bromothymol blue indicator, or to pH 6.8 measured potentiometrically.

Disregard results of assay if response at inoculated blank level is equivalent to titration of >1.5 mL greater than that at uninoculated blank level. Response at 5.0 mL level of standard solution should be equivalent to titration of ca 8–12 mL.

Prepare standard concentration-response curve by plotting titration values, expressed in mL 0.1N NaOH for each level of standard solution used, against amount of reference standard contained in respective tubes.

Determine amount of vitamin for each level of assay solution by interpolation from standard curve. Discard any observed titration values equivalent to <0.5 mL or >4.5 mL, respectively, of standard solution. Proceed as in **960.46H**.

Turbidimetric Method

(Not applicable in presence of extraneous turbidity or color in amount that interferes with turbidimetric measurements)

F. Calibration of Photometer

Using inoculum and standard stock solution as prescribed for appropriate vitamin in following table, and using suspension medium **960.46B(c)**, proceed as directed below.

Vitamin	Inoculum	Std Stock Soln
Cobalamin	**952.20C**[a]	**952.20B**(a)
Folic acid	**944.12C**	**944.12B**(b)
Niacin	**944.13G**	**944.13B**(a)
Pantothenic acid	**945.74G**	**945.74B**(a)
Riboflavin	**940.33G**	**940.33B**(a)

[a] Proceed as in **952.20C**, except replace fifth sentence with the following: "Dil 0.2–1.0 mL aliquot of this suspension with 10 mL sterile suspension medium."

Aseptically add 1 mL inoculum to ca 300 mL sterile suspension medium containing 1.0 mL standard stock solution, and incubate mixture for same period and at same temperature to be employed in determination, **960.46G**. After incubating, centrifuge and wash cells 3 times with ca 50 mL portions 0.9% NaCl solution; then resuspend cells in the NaCl solution to make 25 mL.

Evaporate 10 mL aliquot of cell suspension on steam bath, and dry to constant weight at 110° in vacuum oven. Correcting for weight of NaCl, calculate dry weight of cells in mg/mL of suspension.

Dilute second measured aliquot of cell suspension with 0.9% NaCl solution so that each mL is equivalent to 0.5 mg dry cells. To test tubes add, in triplicate, 0.0 (for blanks), 0.5, 1.0, 1.5, 2.0, 2.5, 3.0, 4.0, and 5.0 mL, respectively, of this diluted cell suspension. To each tube add 0.9% NaCl solution to make 5.0 mL. Then add 5.0 mL appropriate basal medium stock solution, Table **960.46**, mix (1 drop of suitable *antifoam agent* may be added; 1–2% solution of Dow Corning Antifoam AF Emulsion or Antifoam B has been found satisfactory), and transfer to optical cell. With blanks set at 100% T, measure % T of each tube under same conditions to be used in respective assay. Prepare curve by plotting % T readings for each level of diluted cell suspension used against cell content (mg dry weight) of respective tubes.

Repeat appropriate calibration step at least twice more for photometer to be used in respective assay. Draw composite curve, best representing 3 or more individual curves, relating % T to mg dried cell weight for photometer under conditions of respective assay. Once appropriate curve for particular instrument is established, all subsequent relationships between % T and cell weight are determined directly from this curve. Respective assay limits expressed as mg dried cell weight/tube are so determined.

G. Determination

Incubate tubes 16–24 h until maximum turbidity is obtained, as demonstrated by lack of significant change during 2 h additional incubation period in tubes containing highest level of standard solution.

Determine T of tubes as follows: Thoroughly mix contents of each tube (1 drop of suitable antifoam agent solution may be added; 1–2% solution of Dow Corning Antifoam AF Emulsion or Antifoam B has been found satisfactory), and transfer to optical cell. Agitate contents, place cell in photometer set at any specific wavelength between 540 and 660 nm, and read % T when steady state is reached.

Steady state is observed a few seconds after agitation when galvanometer reading remains constant ≥ 30 s. Allow ca same time interval for reading on each tube.

With T set at 100% for uninoculated blank level, read % T of inoculated blank level. If this reading corresponds to dried cell weight >0.6 mg/tube, disregard results of assay. Then with T reset at 100% for inoculated blank level, read % T for each of remaining tubes. Disregard results of assay if % T observed at 5.0 mL level of standard solution (against inoculated blank) is equivalent to that for dried cell weight of <1.25 mg/tube.

Prepare standard concentration-response curve by plotting % T readings for each level of standard solution used against amount of reference standard contained in respective tubes.

Determine amount of vitamin for each level of assay solution by interpolation from standard curve. Discard any observed T values equivalent to <0.5 mL or >4.5 mL, respectively, of standard solution. Proceed as in **960.46H**.

H. Calculation for Both Titrimetric and Turbidimetric Methods

For each level of assay solution used, calculate vitamin content/mL of assay solution. Calculate average of values obtained from tubes that do not vary by $> \pm 10\%$ from this average. If number of acceptable values remaining is $< \frac{2}{3}$ of original number of tubes used in the 4 levels of assay solution, data are insufficient for calculating potency of sample. If number of acceptable values remaining is $\geq \frac{2}{3}$ of original number of tubes, calculate potency of sample from average of them.

CAS-68-19-9 (cobalamin; vitamin B_{12})
CAS-59-30-3 (folic acid)
CAS-59-67-6 (niacin)
CAS-79-83-4 (pantothenic acid)
CAS-83-88-5 (riboflavin)

15.2   952.20—Cobalamin (Vitamin B$_{12}$ Activity) in Vitamin Preparations
Microbiological Methods
Final Action 1960

(Applicable to materials containing ca ≥ 0.1 μg of vitamin B$_{12}$ activity/g or mL)

A. Basal Medium Stock Solution

Using ingredients in amounts prescribed for cobalamin, Table **960.46(a)** (*see* 15.1), proceed as directed below.

Dissolve L-cystine and D,L-tryptophan in 10 mL 1N HCl. Using solutions prepared as in **960.46A**, add, with mixing, and in following order: adenine-guanine-uracil solution, (**b**); xanthine solution, (**r**); vitamin solution I, (**l**); vitamin solution II, (**m**); salt solution A, (**i**); salt solution B, (**j**); asparagine solution, (**c**); and acid-hydrolyzed casein solution, (**a**). Add ca 100 mL H$_2$O and add, with mixing, anhydrous glucose, NaOAc·3H$_2$O, and ascorbic acid. When solution is complete, adjust to pH 6.0 with NaOH solution, add, with mixing, polysorbate 80 solution, (**h**), and dilute with H$_2$O to 250 mL.

Titrimetric Method

B. Cyanocobalamin Standard Solutions

(**a**) *Stock solution.*—100 ng/mL. Accurately weigh, in closed system, USP Cyanocobalamin Reference Standard equivalent to 50–60 μg cyanocobalamin, that has been dried to constant weight and stored in dark over P$_2$O$_5$ in desiccator. Dissolve in 25% alcohol, and dilute with additional 25% alcohol to make cyanocobalamin concentration exactly 100 ng/mL. Store in dark at ca 10°.

(**b**) *Intermediate solution.*—1 ng/mL. Dilute 10 mL stock solution, (**a**), with 25% alcohol to 1 L. Store in dark at ca 10°.

(**c**) *Working solution.*—Dilute suitable volume intermediate solution, (**b**), with H$_2$O to measured volume such that after incubation as in **960.46D** and **960.46E**, response at 5.0 mL level of this solution is equivalent to titration (as described in **960.46E**) of ca 8–12 mL. Designate this as standard solution. (This concentration is usually 0.01–0.04 ng cyanocobalamin/mL standard solution.) Prepare fresh standard solution for each assay.

C. Inoculum

Make transfer of cells from stock culture of *Lactobacillus leichmannii,* **960.46C(a)**, to sterile tube containing 10 mL liquid culture medium, **960.46B(a)**. Incubate 6–24 h at any selected temperature between 30 and 40° held constant to within ±0.5°. Under aseptic conditions, centrifuge culture and decant supernate. Wash cells with 3 ca 10 mL portions sterile 0.9% NaCl solution or sterile suspension medium, **960.46B(c)**. Resuspend cells in 10 mL sterile 0.9% NaCl solution or sterile suspension medium. Dilute aliquot with sterile 0.9% NaCl solution or sterile suspension medium to give T equivalent to that for dried cell weight (as described in **960.46F**) of 0.50–0.75 mg/tube when read against suspension medium set at 100% T. Cell suspension so obtained is inoculum.

D. Assay Solution

Prepare aqueous extracting solution just before use containing, in each 100 mL, 1.3 g anhydrous Na$_2$HPO$_4$, 1.2 g citric acid·H$_2$O, and 1.0 g *anhydrous Na metabisulfite,* Na$_2$S$_2$O$_5$. Place measured amount of sample in flask containing ≥ 25 mL extracting solution for each g or mL sample taken. If sample is not readily soluble, comminute to disperse it evenly in liquid; then agitate vigorously and wash down sides of flask with H_2O.

Autoclave mixture 10 min at 121–123° and cool. If lumping occurs, agitate mixture until particles are evenly dispersed. Dilute mixture to measured volume with H_2O, and let any undissolved particles settle, or filter or centrifuge if necessary. Take aliquot of clear solution, add H_2O, adjust to pH 6.0, and dilute with additional H_2O to measured volume containing, per mL, cobalamin activity ca equivalent to that of standard solution, **952.20B(c)**. Designate this as assay solution. Excess of bisulfite may affect test organism. Therefore, assay solution must contain ≤ 0.03 mg $Na_2S_2O_5$/mL.

E. Assay

Using standard solution, **952.20B(c)**, assay solution, **952.20D**, basal medium stock solution, **952.20A**, and inoculum, **952.20C**, proceed as in **960.46D**, **E**, and **H**.

Turbidimetric Method

F. Cyanocobalamin Standard Solution

Dilute suitable volume cyanocobalamin intermediate standard solution, **952.20B(b)**, with H_2O to measured volume such that after incubation as in **960.46D** and **960.46G**, with inoculated blank set at 100% T, % T at 5.0 mL level of this solution is equivalent to that for dried cell weight (as described in **960.46F**) of ≥ 1.25 mg. Designate this as standard solution. (This concentration is usually 0.01–0.04 ng cyanocobalamin/mL standard solution.) Prepare fresh standard solution for each assay.

G. Assay Solution

Proceed as in **952.20D**, except that where reference is made to concentration of cyanocobalamin activity ca equivalent to that of standard solution, **952.20B(c)**, replace by concentration of cyanocobalamin activity ca equivalent to that of standard solution, **952.20F**. Designate solution so obtained as assay solution.

H. Assay

Using standard solution, **952.20F**, assay solution, **952.20G**, basal medium stock solution, **952.20A**, and inoculum, **952.20C**, proceed as in **960.46D**, **G**, and **H**.

References: JAOAC **35**, 161, 169, 726(1952); **36**, 846(1953); **37**, 781(1954); **38**, 711(1955); **39**, 167, 172(1956); **40**, 856(1957); **41**, 61, 587(1958); **42**, 529(1959).
CAS-68-19-9 (cobalamin; cyanocobalamin; vitamin B_{12})

| 15.3 | 986.23—Cobalamin (Vitamin B₁₂ Activity) |

15.3   986.23—Cobalamin (Vitamin B_{12} Activity) in Milk-Based Infant Formula

Turbidimetric Method
First Action 1986
Final Action 1988

(Throughout all stages, except where otherwise noted, protect solutions from undue exposure to light.)

A. Stock Solutions for Basal Media

(a) *Adenine-guanine-uracil solution.*—Dissolve 1.0 g each of adenine sulfate, guanine·HCl, and uracil in 50 mL warm HCl (1 + 1), cool, and dilute with H_2O to 1 L.

(b) *Asparagine solution.*—Dissolve 10 g L-asparagine·H_2O in H_2O and dilute to 1 L.

(c) *Polysorbate 80 solution.*—Dissove 25 g polysorbate 80 (polyoxyethylene sorbitan monooleate) in alcohol to make 250 mL.

(d) *Salt solution A.*—Dissolve 50 g anhydrous KH_2PO_4 and 50 g anhydrous K_2HPO_4 in H_2O, dilute to 1 L, and add 10 drops of HCl.

(e) *Salt solution B.*—Dissolve 20 g $MgSO_4·7H_2O$, 1 g NaCl, 1 g $FeSO_4·7H_2O$, and 1 g $MnSO_4·H_2O$ in H_2O, dilute to 1 L, and add 10 drops of HCl.

(f) *Vitamin solution I.*—Dissolve 25 mg riboflavin, 25 mg thiamine·HCl, 0.25 mg biotin, and 50 mg niacin in 0.02N CH_3COOH to make 1 L.

(g) *Vitamin solution II.*—Dissolve 50 mg *p*-aminobezoic acid, 25 mg Ca pantothenate, 100 mg pyridoxine·HCl, 100 mg pyridoxal·HCl, 20 mg pyridoxamine·2HCl, and 5 mg folic acid in 25% alcohol to make 1 L.

(h) *Xanthine solution.*—Suspend 1.0 g xanthine in 150–200 mL H_2O, heat to ca 70°, add 30 mL NH_4OH (2 + 3), and stir until solid dissolves. Cool, and dilute to 1 L with H_2O.

(i) *Acid-hydrolyzed casein.*—Available as HY CASE AMINO from Humko Sheffield Chemical Div., PO Box 398, Memphis, TN 38101. Other commercial sources of vitamin-free, acid-hydrolyzed casein have been found satisfactory.

B. Culture and Suspension Media

(a) *Liquid culture medium.*—Dissolve 15 g peptonized milk, 5 g H_2O-soluble yeast extract, 10 g anhydrous glucose, and 2 g anhydrous KH_2PO_4 in ca 600 mL H_2O. Add 100 mL filtered tomato juice, and adjust to pH 6.5–6.8 with NaOH solution. Add, with mixing, 10 mL polysorbate 80 solution and dilute with H_2O to 1 L. (Difco Lactobacilli Broth AOAC, Difco Laboratories, has been found satisfactory.) Dilute measured amount with equal volume of H_2O containing 1 ng vitamin B_{12}/mL. Add 10 mL portions to 20 × 150 mm screw-cap test tubes, sterilize 15 min in autoclave at 121–123°, cool rapidly, and store in refrigerator.

(b) *Agar culture medium.*—To 500 mL liquid culture medium, (a), add 5.0–7.5 g agar, and heat with stirring on steam bath until agar dissolves. Add ca 10 mL portions of hot solution to test tubes, cover to prevent contamination, sterilize 15 min in autoclave at 121–123°, and cool tubes in upright position as rapidly as practicable to keep color formation at minimum. Store in dark at ca 10°. (Difco agar culture medium for AOAC microbiological assays [Lactobacilli Agar AOAC] has been found satisfactory.)

(c) *Suspension medium.*—Dilute measured volume appropriate basal medium stock solution, Table **960.46** (*see* 15.1), with equal volume H_2O. Add 10 mL portions diluted medium to test tubes, cover to prevent contamination, sterilize 15 min in autoclave at 121–123°, and cool tubes as rapidly as practicable to keep color formation at minimum. Store in dark at ca 10°.

C. Stock Culture of Test Organism

For *Lactobacillus leichmannii*, ATCC No. 7830, prepare stab culture in 1 or more tubes of agar culture medium, **986.23B(b)**. Incubate 6–24 h at 37° held constant to within 0.5°, and finally store in dark at ca 10°. Before using new culture in assay, make several successive transfers of culture in 1–2 week period. Prepare fresh stab culture at least once a week and do not use for preparing inoculum if >1 week old.

Activity of slow-growing culture may be increased by daily or twice-daily transfer of stab culture, and is considered satisfactory when definite turbidity in liquid inoculum can be observed 2–4 h after inoculation. Slow-growing culture seldom gives suitable response curve and may cause erratic results.

D. Assay Tubes

Meticulously cleanse by suitable means (Na lauryl sulfate USP has been found satisfactory as detergent), hard-glass test tubes, ca 20 × 150 mm, and other necessary glassware. (The test organism is highly sensitive to minute amounts of growth factors and to many cleansing agents. Therefore, it may be preferred to follow cleansing by heating 1–2 h at ca 250°.)

Prepare tubes containing standard solution as follows: To test tubes add, in duplicate (or replicate), 0.0 (for uninoculated blanks), 0.0 (for inoculated blanks), 1.0, 2.0, 3.0, 4.0, and 5.0 mL, respectively, of standard solution. Prepare tubes containing assay solution as follows: To similar test tubes add, in duplicate (or replicate), 1.0, 2.0, 3.0, and 4.0 mL, respectively, of assay solution.

To each tube of standard solution and assay solution, add H_2O to make 5.0 mL. Then add 5.0 mL basal medium stock solution and mix. Cover tubes suitably to prevent bacterial contamination, and sterilize 10 min in autoclave at 121–123°, reaching this temperature in not >10 min. Cool as rapidly as practicable to keep color formation at minimum. Take precautions to keep sterilizing and cooling conditions uniform throughout assay. Too close packing of tubes in autoclave, or overloading of it, may cause variation in heating rate.

Aseptically inoculate each tube, except 1 set of duplicate (or replicate) tubes containing 0.0 mL standard solution (uninoculated blanks), with 1 drop of inoculum. Incubate for 16–24 h at 37° held constant to within 0.5°. Contamination of assay tubes with any foreign organism invalidates assay.

E. Calibration of Photometer

Using inoculum, **986.23J**, and stock standard solution, **986.23I(a)**, proceed as directed below. Aseptically add 1 mL inoculum to ca 300 mL sterile suspension medium containing 1.0 mL standard stock solution, and incubate mixture for same period and at same temperature to be employed in determination, **986.23F**. After incubating, centrifuge and wash cells 3 times with ca 50 mL portions of 0.9% NaCl solution; then resuspend cells in the NaCl solution to make 25 mL.

Evaporate 10 mL aliquot cell suspension on steam bath, and dry to constant weight at 110° in vacuum oven. Correcting for weight of NaCl, calculate dry weight of cells in mg/mL of suspension.

Dilute second measured aliquot of cell suspension with 0.9% NaCl solution so that each mL is equivalent to 0.5 mg dry cells. To test tubes add, in triplicate, 0.0 (for blanks), 0.5, 1.0, 1.5, 2.0, 2.5, 3.0, 4.0, and 5.0 mL, respectively, of this diluted cell suspension. To each tube add 0.9% NaCl solution to make 5.0 mL. Then add 5.0 mL basal medium stock solution, mix (1 drop of suitable antifoam agent may be added; 1–2% solution of Dow Corning Antifoam AF Emulsion or Antifoam B has been found satisfactory), and transfer to optical cell. With blanks set at 100% T, measure % T of each tube under same conditions to be used in assay. Prepare curve by plotting % T readings for each level of diluted cell suspension used against cell content (mg dry weight) of respective tubes.

Repeat calibration step at least twice more for photometer under conditions of assay. Draw composite curve, best representing 3 or more individual curves, relating % T to mg dried cell weight for photometer under conditions of assay. Once curve for particular instrument is established, all subsequent relationships between $\%T$ and cell weight are determined directly from this curve. Assay limits expressed as mg dried cell weight/tube are so determined.

F. Determination

Incubate tubes 16–24 h until maximum turbidity is obtained, as demonstrated by lack of significant change during 2 h additional incubation period in tubes containing highest level of standard solution. Determine T of tubes as follows: Thoroughly mix contents of each tube (1 drop of suitable antifoam agent solution may be added; 1–2% solution of Dow Corning Antifoam AF emulsion or Antifoam B has been found satisfactory), and transfer to optical cell. Agitate contents, place cell in photometer set at any specific wavelength between 540 and 660 nm, and read $\%T$ when steady state is reached. Steady state is observed 3–4 s after agitation when galvanometer reading remains constant for >30 s. Allow ca same time interval for reading each tube.

With T set at 100% for uninoculated blank level, read $\%T$ of inoculated blank level. If this reading corresponds to dried cell weight >0.6 mg/tube, disregard results of assay. Then with T reset at 100% for inoculated blank level, read $\%T$ for each of remaining tubes. Disregard results of assay if $\%T$ observed at 5.0 mL level of standard solution (against inoculated blank) is equivalent to that for dried cell weight <1.25 mg/tube.

Prepare standard concentration-response curve by plotting $\%T$ readings for each level of standard solution used against amount of reference standard contained in respective tubes.

Determine amount of vitamin for each level of assay solution by interpolating from standard curve. Discard any observed T values equivalent to <0.5 mL or >4.5 mL, respectively, of standard solution. Proceed as in *Calculation*.

G. Calculation

For each level of assay solution used, calculate vitamin content/mL of assay solution. Calculate average of values obtained from tubes that do not vary by $>10\%$ from this average. If number of acceptable values remaining is $<\frac{2}{3}$ of original number of tubes used in 4 levels of assay solution, data are insufficient for calculating potency of sample. If number of acceptable values remaining is $\geq\frac{2}{3}$ of original number of tubes, calculate potency of sample from average of them.

H. Basal Medium Stock Solution

For each liter of vitamin B_{12}-free, double-strength basal medium to be prepared, add the following in order listed: 20 mL adenine–guanine–uracil solution, 20 mL asparagine solution, 20 mL salt solution A, 20 mL salt solution B, 40 mL vitamin solution I, 40 mL vitamin solution II, 20 mL xanthine solution, and 20 mL polysorbate 80 solution. Add H_2O to total volume ca 800 mL and mix well to prevent the following solids from precipitating when added. Then add the following in order listed: 10 g acid-hydrolyzed casein, 0.4 g L-cystine and 0.4 g D-L-tryptopahn dissolved together in minimum volume of dilute HCl (235 mL concentrated HCl/L), 40 g dextrose, 33.2 g Na acetate trihydrate, and 4 g ascorbic acid. Do not agitate solution vigorously after adding ascorbic acid. Swirl gently until all solids are dissolved. Adjust pH to 6.0 with either HCl or NaOH, using pH meter. Dilute to volume. Add polysorbate solution after pH adjustment when indicator is used because indicator is absorbed by polysorbate. Some commercial media have been found satisfactory.

I. Cyanocobalamin Standard Solutions

(a) *Stock solution.*—100 ng/mL. Accurately weigh, in closed system, USP Cyanocobalamin Reference Standard equivalent to 50–60 μg cyanocobalamin, which has been dried to constant weight, and store in dark over P_2O_5 in desiccator. Dissolve in 25% alcohol to make cyanocobalamin concentration exactly 100 ng/mL. Store in dark at ca 10°.

(c) *Working solutions.*—Dilute an aliquot of intermediate solution with H_2O to 500 mL. This primary standard solution is equivalent to 0.01–0.04 ng/mL and is ca equal to assay concentration of sample preparation. Similarly, prepare 2 additional secondary standards, one higher and one lower (e.g., 0.010 and 0.020 ng/mL) to provide wider working range for vitamin B_{12} concentrations in samples.

J. Inoculum

Make transfer of cells from stock culture of *Lactobacillus leichmannii*, **986.23C**, to 2 sterile tubes containing 10 mL liquid culture medium, **986.23B(a)**. Keep all transfers as sterile as possible. Incubate 6–24 h at 37° held constant to 0.5°. Under aseptic conditions, centrifuge culture and decant supernate. Wash cells with 3 ca 10 mL portions of sterile 0.9% NaCl solution or sterile suspension medium, **986.23B(c)**. Resuspend cells in 10 mL sterile 0.9% NaCl solution or sterile suspension medium. Dilute aliquot with sterile 0.9% NaCl solution or sterile suspension medium to give T equivalent to that for dried cell weight (as described in **986.23E**) of 0.50–0.75 mg/tube when read against suspension medium set at 100%T. Cell suspension so obtained is inoculum.

K. Assay Solution

Prepare aqueous extracting solution just before use containing, in each 100 mL, 1.3 g anhydrous Na_2HPO_4, 1.2 g citric acid·H_2O, and 1.0 g anhydrous Na metabisulfite, $Na_2S_2O_5$. Take amount of sample containing 50–100 ng vitamin B_{12} and transfer to beaker containing amount of extraction solution to contain not >0.03 mg $Na_2S_2O_5$/mL at final assay concentration between 0.01 and 0.04 ng vitamin B_{12}/mL.

Disperse sample solution evenly in liquid. Wash down sides of beaker with H_2O and cover with watch glass. Autoclave mixture 10 min at 121–123° and cool. If lumping occurs, agitate mixture until particles are evenly dispersed. Adjust mixture to pH 4.5 with vigorous agitation. Dilute mixture with H_2O to measured volume to obtain approximate vitamin B_{12} concentration of 0.2 ng/mL and filter.

Take aliquot of filtrate and check for dissolved protein by adding dropwise, first dilute HCl, and if no further precipitate forms, then with vigorous stirring, NaOH solution. Proceed as follows with aliquot:

(a) If no further precipitation occurs. add with vigorous stirring, NaOH solution to pH 6.0, dilute with H_2O to final measured volume containing vitamin B_{12} activity equivalent to ca 0.014 ng/mL.

(b) If further precipitation occurs, adjust mixture to point of maximum precipitation (ca pH 4.5), dilute with H_2O to measured volume, and filter. Take aliquot of clear filtrate and proceed as under (a).

L. Assay

Using standard solution, **986.23I(c)**, assay solution, **986.23K**, basal medium stock solution, **986.23H**, and inoculum, **986.23J**, proceed as in **986.23D**, **F**, and **G**.

Reference: JAOAC **69**, 777(1986).
CAS-68-19-9 (cobalamin; cyanocobalamin; vitamin B_{12})

Chapter 16
Dietary Fiber

16.1

985.29—Total Dietary Fiber in Foods
Enzymatic-Gravimetric Method
First Action 1985
Final Action 1986

A. Principle

Duplicate samples of dried foods, fat-extracted if containing >10% fat, are gelatinized with Termamyl (heat-stable α-amylase), and then enzymatically digested with protease and amyloglucosidase to remove protein and starch. (When analyzing mixed diets, always extract fat prior to determining total dietary fiber.) Four volumes of ethyl alcohol are added to precipitate soluble dietary fiber. Total residue is filtered, washed with 78% ethyl alcohol, 95% ethyl alcohol, and acetone. After drying, residue is weighed. One duplicate is analyzed for protein, and other is incinerated at 525° and ash is determined. Total dietary fiber = weight residue - weight (protein + ash).

B. Apparatus

(a) *Fritted crucible.*—Porosity No. 2 (Pyrex No. 32940, coarse, ASTM 40-60 μm; or Corning No. 36060 Buchner, fritted disk, Pyrex, 60 mL, ASTM 40-60 μm). Clean thoroughly, heat 1 h at 525°, and soak and then rinse in H_2O. Add ca 0.5 g Celite to air-dried crucibles and dry at 130° to constant weight ($\geq$ 1 h). Cool and store in desiccator until used.

(b) *Vacuum source.*—Vacuum pump or aspirator equipped with in-line double vacuum flask to prevent contamination in case of H_2O backup.

(c) *Vacuum oven.*—70°. Alternatively, 105° air oven can be used.

(d) *Desiccator.*

(e) *Muffle furnace.*

(f) *Water baths.*—(1) Boiling. (2) Constant temperature.—Adjustable to 60°, with either multistation shaker or multistation magnetic stirrer to provide constant agitation of digestion flasks during enzymatic hydrolysis.

(g) *Beakers.*—Tall-form, 400 or 600 mL.

(h) *Balance.*—Analytical, capable of weighing to 0.1 mg.

(i) *pH meter.*—Standardized with pH 7 and pH 4 buffers.

C. Reagents

(a) *98% Ethanol.*—Volume/volume, technical grade.

(b) *78% Ethanol.*—Place 207 mL H_2O into 1 L volumetric flask. Dilute to volume with 95% ethyl alcohol. Mix and dilute to volume again with 95% ethyl alcohol if necessary. Mix. One volume H_2O mixed with 4 volumes 95% ethyl alcohol will also give 78% ethyl alcohol final concentration.

(c) *Acetone.*—Reagent grade.

(**d**) *Phosphate buffer.*—0.08M, pH 6.0. Dissolve 1.400 g Na phosphate dibasic, anhydrous (Na_2HPO_4) (or 1.753 g dihydrate) and 9.68 Na phosphate monobasic monohydrate (NaH_2PO_4) (or 10.94 g dihydrate) in ca 700 mL H_2O. Dilute to 1 L with H_2O. Check pH with pH meter.

(**e**) *Termamyl (heat-stable α-amylase) solution.*—No. 120 L, Novo Laboratories, Inc., Wilton, CT 06897. Store in refrigerator.

(**f**) *Protease.*—No. P-3910, Sigma Chemical Co. Keep refrigerated.

(**g**) *Amyloglucosidase.*—No. A-9913, Sigma Chemical Co. Keep refrigerated. Alternatively, a kit containing all 3 enzymes (pretested) is available from Sigma Chemical Co., Kit No. TDF-100.

(**h**) *Sodium hydroxide solution.*—0.275N. Dissolve 11.00 g NaOH ACS in ca 700 mL H_2O in 1 L volumetric flask. Dilute to volume with H_2O.

(**i**) *Hydrochloric acid solution.*—0.325M. Dilute stock solution of known titer, e.g., 325 mL 1 M HCl, to 1 L with H_2O.

(**j**) *Celite C-211.*—Acid-washed, Fisher Scientific Co.

D. Enzyme Purity

To ensure absence of undesirable enzymatic activity in enzymes used in this procedure, run materials listed in table through entire procedure each time lot of enzymes is changed, or at maximum interval of 6 months to ensure that enzymes have not degraded.

Test Sample	Activity tested	Sample wt, g	Expected rec., %
Citrus pectin	pectinase	0.1	95–100
Stractan (larch gum)	hemicellulase	0.1	95–100
Wheat starch	amylase	1.0	0–1
Corn starch	amylase	1.0	0–2
Casein	protease	0.3	0–2
ß-Glucan (barley gum)[a]	ß-glucanase	0.1	95–100

[a] (Sigma Chemical Co.)

E. Sample Preparation

Determine total dietary fiber on dried sample. Homogenize sample and dry overnight in 70° vacuum oven, cool in desiccator, and dry-mill portion of sample to 0.3–0.5 mm mesh. If sample cannot be heated, freeze-dry before milling. If high fat content (>10%) prevents proper milling, defat with petroleum ether (3 times with 25 mL portions/g sample) before milling. Record loss of weight due to fat removal and make appropriate correction to final % dietary fiber found in determination. Store dry-milled sample in capped jar in desiccator until analysis is carried out.

F. Determination

Run blank through entire procedure along with samples to measure any contribution from reagents to residue.

Weigh duplicate 1 g samples, accurate to 0.1 mg, into 400 mL tall-form beakers. Sample weights should not differ >20 mg. Add 50 mL pH 6.0 phosphate buffer to each beaker. Check pH and adjust to pH 6.0 $\pm$ 0.2 if necessary. Add 0.1 mL Termamyl solution. Cover beaker with Al foil and place in boiling H_2O bath 15 min. Shake gently at 5 min intervals. Increase incubation time when number of beakers in boiling H_2O bath makes it difficult for beaker contents to reach internal temperature of 95–100°. Use thermometer to indicate that 15 min at 95–100° is attained. Total of 30 min in H_2O bath should be sufficient.

Cool solutions to room temperature. Adjust to pH 7.5 $\pm$ 0.2 by adding 10 mL 0.275N NaOH solution.

Add 5 mg protease. (Protease sticks to spatula, so it may be preferable to prepare enzyme solution (50 mg in 1 mL phophate buffer) and pipet 0.1 mL to each sample just before use.

Cover beaker with Al foil. Incubate 30 min at 60° with continuous agitation. Cool. Add 10 mL 0.325M HCl solution. Measure pH and dropwise add acid if necessary. Final pH should be 4.0–4.6. Add 0.3 mL amyloglucosidase, cover with Al foil, and incubate 30 min at 60° with continuous agitation. Add 280 mL 95% ethyl alcohol preheated to 60° (measure volume before heating). Let precipitate form at room temperature for 60 min.

Weigh crucible containing Celite to nearest 0.1 mg, then wet and redistribute bed of Celite in crucible by using stream of 78% ethyl alcohol from wash bottle. Apply suction to draw Celite onto fritted glass as even mat. Maintain suction and quantitatively transfer precipitate from enzyme digest to crucible.

Wash residue successively with three 20 mL portions of 78% ethyl alcohol, two 10 mL portions of 95% ethyl alcohol, and two 10 mL portions of acetone. Gum may form with some samples, trapping liquid. If so, break surface film with spatula to improve filtration. Time for filtration and washing will vary from 0.1 to 6 h, averaging ½ h per sample. Long filtration times can be avoided by careful intermittent suction throughout filtration.

Dry crucible containing residue overnight in 70° vacuum oven or 105° air oven. Cool in desiccator and weigh to nearest 0.1 mg. Subtract crucible and Celite weight to determine weight of residue.

Analyze residue from 1 sample of set of duplicates for protein by **960.52** (*see* 16.4), using N × 6.25 as conversion factor, except in cases where N content in protein is known.

Incinerate second residue sample of duplicate 5 h at 525°. Cool in desiccator and weigh to nearest 0.1 mg. Subtract crucible and Celite weight to determine ash.

G. Calculations

Determination of blank:

$$B = \text{blank, mg} = \text{weight residue} - P_B - A_B$$

where weight residue = average of residue weights (mg) for duplicate blank determinations; and P_B and A_B = weights (mg) of protein and ash, respectively, determined in first and second blank residues.

Calculate TDF as follows:

$$\text{TDF, \%} = [(\text{weight residue} - P - A - B)/\text{weight sample}] \times 100$$

where weight residue = average of weights (mg) for duplicate blank determinations; and P and A = weights (mg) of protein and ash, respectively, in first and second sample residues; and weight sample = average of 2 sample weights (mg) taken.

References: JAOAC **68,** 677(1985); **69,** 259(1986).

16.2   991.43—Total, Soluble, and Insoluble Dietary Fiber in Foods
Enzymatic-Gravimetric Method, MES-TRIS Buffer
First Action 1991

(Applicable to processed foods, grain and cereal products, fruits, and vegetables)

Method Performance
> *See* Table **991.43A** for method performance data.

A. Principle

Duplicate samples of dried foods, fat-extracted if containing >10% fat, undergo sequential enzymatic digestion by heat stable $\propto$-amylase, protease, and amyloglucosidase to remove starch and protein. For total dietary fiber (TDF), enzyme digestate is treated with alcohol to precipitate soluble dietary fiber before filtering, and TDF residue is washed with alcohol and acetone, dried, and weighed. For insoluble and soluble dietary fiber (IDF and SDF), enzyme digestate is filtered, and residue (IDF) is washed with warm water, dried and weighed. For SDF, combined filtrate and washes are precipitated with alcohol, filtered, dried, and weighed. TDF, IDF, and SDF residue values are corrected for protein, ash, and blank.

B. Apparatus

(a) *Beakers.*—400 or 600 mL tall form.

(b) *Filtering crucible.*—With fritted disk, coarse, ASTM 40–60 μm pore size, Pyrex 60 mL (Corning No. 36060 Buchner, Corning, Inc., Science Products, Corning, NY 14831, USA, or equivalent). Prepare as follows. Ash overnight at 525° in muffle furnace. Let furnace temperature fall below 130° before removing crucibles. Soak crucibles 1 h in 2% cleaning solution at room temperature. Rinse crucibles with H_2O and then deionized H_2O; for final rinse, use 15 mL acetone and then air-dry. Add ca 1.0 g Celite to dry crucibles, and dry at 130° to constant weight. Cool crucible ca 1 h in desiccator, and record weight, to nearest 0.1 mg, of crucible plus Celite.

(c) *Vacuum system.*—Vacuum pump or aspirator with regulating device. Heavy walled filtering flask, 1 L, with side arm. Rubber ring adaptors, for use with filtering flasks.

(d) *Shaking water baths.*—(*1*) Capable of maintaining 98 $\pm$ 2°, with automatic on-and-off timer. (*2*) Constant temperature, adjustable to 60°.

(e) *Balance.*—Analytical, sensitivity $\pm$ 0.1 mg.

(f) *Muffle furnace.*—Capable of maintaining 525 $\pm$ 5°.

(g) *Oven.*—Capable of maintaining 105 and 130 $\pm$ 3°.

(h) *Desiccator.*—With SiO_2 or equivalent desiccant. Biweekly, dry desiccant overnight at 130°.

(i) *pH meter.*—Temperature compensated, standardized with pH 4.0, 7.0, and 10.0 buffer solutions.

(j) *Pipetters.*—With disposable tips, 100–300 μL and 5 mL capacity.

(k) *Dispensers.*—Capable of dispensing 15 $\pm$ 0.5 mL for 78% EtOH, 95% EtOH, and acetone; 40 $\pm$ 0.5 mL for buffer.

(l) *Magnetic stirrers and stir bars.*

C. Reagents

Use deionized water throughout.

(a) *Ethanol solutions.*—(*1*) 85%. Place 895 mL 95% ethanol into 1 L volumetric flask, dilute to volume with H_2O. (2) 78%. Place 821 mL 95% ethanol into 1 L volumetric flask, dilute to volume with H_2O.

(b) *Heat-stable ∝-amylase solution.*—Cat. No. A 3306, Sigma Chemical Co., St. Louis, MO 63178, USA, or Termamyl 300L, Cat. No. 361-6282, Novo-Nordisk, Bagsvaerd, Denmark, or equivalent.

(c) *Protease.*—Cat. No. P 3910, Sigma Chemical Co, or equivalent. Prepare 50 mg/mL enzyme solution in MES/TRIS buffer fresh daily.

(d) *Amyloglucosidase solution.*—Cat. No. AMG A9913, Sigma Chemical Co., or equivalent. Store at 0–5°.

(e) *Diatomaceous earth.*—Acid washed (Celite 545 AW, No. C8656, Sigma Chemical Co., or equivalent).

(f) *Cleaning solution.*—Liquid surfactant-type laboratory cleaner, designed for critical cleaning (Micro®, International Products Corp., Trenton, NJ 08601, USA, or equivalent). Prepare 2% solution in H_2O.

(g) *MES.*—2-(*N*-Morpholino)ethanesulfonic acid (No. M-8250, Sigma Chemical Co., or equivalent.)

(h) *TRIS.*—Tris(hydroxymethyl)aminomethane (No. T-1503, Sigma Chemical Co., or equivalent).

(i) *MES/TRIS buffer solution.*—0.05M MES, 0.05M TRIS, pH 8.2 at 24°. Dissolve 19.52 g MES and 12.2 g TRIS in 1.7 L H_2O. Adjust pH to 8.2 with 6N NaOH, and dilute to 2 L with H_2O. (*Note:* It is important to adjust pH to 8.2 at 24°. However, if buffer temperature is 20°, adjust pH to 8.3; if temperature is 28°, adjust pH to 8.1. For deviations between 20 and 28°, adjust by interpolation.)

(j) *Hydrochloric acid solution.*—0.561N. Add 93.5 mL 6N HCl to ca 700 mL H_2O in 1 L volumetric flask. Dilute to 1 L with H_2O.

D. Enzyme Purity

To ensure absence of undesirable enzymatic activities and presence of desirable enzymatic activities, run standards listed in Table **991.43B** each time enzyme lot changes or at maximum interval of 6 months.

E. Sample Preparation and Digestion

Prepare samples as in **985.29E** (*see* 16.1) (if fat content of sample is unknown, defat before determining dietary fiber). For high sugar samples, desugar before determining dietary fiber by extracting 2–3 times with 85% EtOH, 10 mL/g, decanting, and then drying overnight at 40°.

Run 2 blanks/assay with samples to measure any contribution from reagents to residue.

Weigh duplicate 1.000 ± 0.005 g samples (M_1 and M_2), accurate to 0.1 mg, into 400 mL (or 600 mL) tall-form beakers. Add 40 mL MES/TRIS buffer solution, pH 8.2, to each. Stir on magnetic stirrer until sample is completely dispersed (to prevent lump formation, which would make test material inaccessible to enzymes).

Add 50 µL heat-stable ∝-amylase solution, stirring at low speed. Cover beakers with Al foil, and incubate in 95–100° H_2O bath 15 min with continuous agitation. Start timing once bath temperature reaches 95° (total of 35 min is normally sufficient).

Remove all beakers from bath, and cool to 60°. Remove foil. Scrape any ring from inside of beaker and disperse any gels in bottom of beaker with spatula. Rinse beaker walls and spatula with 10 mL H_2O.

Add 100 µL protease solution to each beaker. Cover with Al foil, and incubate 30 min at 60 ± 1° with continuous agitation. Start timing when bath temperature reaches 60°.

Remove foil. Dispense 5 mL 0.561N HCl into beakers while stirring. Adjust pH to 4.0–4.7 at 60°, by adding 1N NaOH solution or 1N HCl solution. (*Note:* It is important to check and adjust pH while solutions are 60° because pH will increase at lower temperatures.) (Most cereal, grain, and vegetable products do not require pH adjustment. Once verified for each laboratory, pH checking procedure can be omitted. As a precaution, check pH of blank routinely; if outside desirable range, check samples also.)

Add 300 µL amyloglucosidase solution while stirring. Cover with Al foil, and incubate 30 min at 60° ± 1° with constant agitation. Start timing once bath reaches 60°.

F. Determination of Total Dietary Fiber

To each digested sample, add 225 mL (measured after heating) 95% EtOH at 60°. Ratio of EtOH to sample volume should be 4:1. Remove from bath, and cover beakers with large sheets of Al foil. Let precipitate form 1 h at room temperature.

Wet and redistribute Celite bed in previously tared crucible **B(b)**, using 15 mL 78% EtOH from wash bottle. Apply suction to crucible to draw Celite onto fritted glass as even mat.

Filter alcohol-treated enzyme digestate through crucible. Using wash bottle with 78% EtOH and rubber spatula, quantitatively transfer all remaining particles to crucible. (*Note*: If some samples form a gum, trapping the liquid, break film with spatula.)

Using vacuum, wash residue 2 times each with 15 mL portions of 78% EtOH, 95% EtOH, and acetone. Dry crucible containing residue overnight in 105° oven. Cool crucible in desiccator ca 1 h. Weigh crucible, containing dietary fiber residue and Celite, to nearest 0.1 mg, and calculate residue weight by subtracting weight of dry crucible with Celite, **B(b)**.

Use one duplicate from each sample to determine protein, by method **960.52** (*see* 16.4) using N × 6.25 as conversion factor. For ash analysis, incinerate second duplicate 5 h at 525°. Cool in desiccator, and weigh to nearest 0.1 mg. Subtract weight of crucible and Celite, **B(b)**, to determine ash weight.

G. Determination of Insoluble Dietary Fiber

Wet and redistribute Celite bed in previously tared crucible, **B(b)**, using ca 3 mL H_2O. Apply suction to crucible to draw Celite into even mat.

Filter enzyme digestate, from **E**, through crucible into filtration flask. Rinse beaker, and then wash residue 2 times with 10 mL 70° H_2O. Combine filtrate and water washings, transfer to pretared 600 mL tall form beaker, and reserve for determination of soluble dietary fiber, **H**.

Using vacuum, wash residue 2 times each with 15 mL portions of 78% EtOH, 95% EtOH, and acetone. (*Note*: Delay in washing IDF residues with 78% EtOH, 95% EtOH, and acetone may cause inflated IDF values.)

Use duplicates to determine protein and ash as in **F**.

H. Determination of Soluble Dietary Fiber

Proceed as for insoluble dietary fiber determination through instruction to combine the filtrate and water washings in pretared 600 mL tall-form beakers. Weigh beakers with combined solution of filtrate and water washings, and estimate volumes.

Add 4 volumes of 95% EtOH preheated to 60°. Use portion of 60° EtOH to rinse filtering flask from IDF determination. Alternatively, adjust weight of combined solution of filtrate and water washings to 80 g by addition of H_2O, and add 320 mL 60° 95% EtOH. Let precipitate form at room temperature 1 h.

Follow TDF determination, **F**, from "Wet and redistribute Celite bed...."

I. Calculations

Blank (B, mg) determination:
$$B = [(BR_1 + BR_2)/2] - P_B - A_B$$
where BR_1 and BR_2 = residue weights (mg) for duplicate blank determinations; and P_B and A_B = weights (mg) of protein and ash, respectively, determined on first and second blank residues.

Dietary fiber (DF, g/100 g) determination:
$$DF = \{[(R_1 + R_2)/2] - P - A - B\}/[(M_1 + M_2)/2] \times 100$$

where R_1 and R_2 = residue weights (mg) for duplicate samples; P and A = weights (mg) of protein and ash, respectively, determined on first and second residues; B = blank weight (mg); and M_1 and M_2 = weights (mg) for samples.

Total dietary fiber determination: Determine either by independent analysis, as in **F**, or by summing IDF and SDF, as in **G** and **H**.

Ref.: J.AOAC Int. **75**, May/June issue(1992).

Table 991.43A. Method Performance for Total, Soluble, and Insoluble Dietary Fiber in Foods (Fresh Wt Basis), Enzymatic-Gravimetric Method, MES-TRIS Buffer

Food	Mean, g/100 g	s_r	s_R	RSD_r, %	RSD_R, %
Total dietary fiber (TDF)					
Barley	12.25	0.36	0.85	2.88	6.89
High fiber cereal	33.73	0.70	0.94	2.08	2.79
Oat bran	16.92	1.06	2.06	6.26	12.17
Soy bran	67.14	1.01	1.06	1.50	1.58
Apricots	1.12	0.01	0.01	0.89	0.89
Prunes	9.29	0.13	0.40	1.40	4.31
Raisins	3.13	0.09	0.15	2.88	4.79
Carrots	3.93	0.13	0.13	3.31	3.31
Green beans	2.89	0.07	0.07	2.42	2.42
Parsley	2.66	0.07	0.14	2.63	5.26
Soluble dietary fiber (SDF)					
Barley	5.02	0.40	0.62	8.01	12.29
High fiber cereal	2.78	0.44	0.56	15.83	20.14
Oat bran	7.17	0.72	1.14	10.04	15.90
Soy bran	6.90	0.30	0.60	4.35	8.70
Apricots	0.53	0.02	0.02	3.77	3.77
Prunes	5.07	0.11	0.31	2.17	6.11
Raisins	0.73	0.05	0.16	6.85	21.92
Carrots	1.10	0.07	0.18	6.36	16.36
Green beans	1.02	0.08	0.11	7.84	10.78
Parsley	0.64	0.03	0.10	4.69	15.63
Insoluble dietary fiber (IDF)					
Barley	7.05	0.61	0.61	8.62	8.62
High fiber cereal	30.52	0.44	0.71	1.44	2.33
Oat bran	9.73	0.85	1.17	8.74	12.02
Soy bran	60.53	0.70	0.70	1.16	1.16
Apricots	0.59	0.02	0.02	3.39	3.39
Prunes	4.17	0.07	0.09	1.68	2.16
Raisins	2.37	0.04	0.07	1.69	2.95
Carrots	2.81	0.09	0.16	3.20	5.69
Green beans	2.01	0.08	0.08	3.98	3.98
Parsley	2.37	0.12	0.24	5.06	10.13

Table 991.43A. Method Performance for Total, Soluble, and Insoluble Dietary Fiber in Foods (Fresh Wt Basis), Enzymatic-Gravimetric Method, MES-TRIS Buffer

Food	Mean, g/100 g	s_r	s_R	RSD$_r$, %	RSD$_R$, %
Total dietary fiber (SDF + IDF)					
Barley	12.14	0.39	0.70	3.21	5.77
High fiber cereal	33.30	0.63	0.90	1.89	2.70
Oat bran	16.90	0.99	1.49	5.86	8.82
Soy bran	67.56	0.56	0.94	0.83	1.39
Apricots	1.12	0.02	0.02	1.79	1.79
Prunes	9.37	0.12	0.30	1.28	3.20
Raisins	3.10	0.05	0.18	1.61	5.81
Carrots	3.92	0.11	0.13	2.81	3.32
Green beans	3.03	0.09	0.12	2.97	3.96
Parsley	3.01	0.12	0.23	3.99	7.64

Table 991.43B. Standards for Testing Enzyme Activity

Standard	Activity Tested	Wt of Std, g	Expected Rec. (%)
Citrus pectin	Pectinase	0.1–0.2	95–100
Arabinogalactan	Hemicellulase	0.1–0.2	95–100
β-Glucan	β-Glucanase	0.1–0.2	95–100
Wheat starch	α-Amylase + AMG	1.0	0–1
Corn starch	α-Amylase + AMG	1.0	0–1
Casein	Protease	0.3	0–1

16.3   991.42—Insoluble Dietary Fiber in Food and Food Products
Enzymatic–Gravimetric Method, Phosphate Buffer
First Action 1991

(Applicable to determination of insoluble dietary fiber in vegetables, fruit, and cereal grains)

Method Performance
    See Table **991.42** for method performance data.

A. Principle
    Duplicate test portions of dried foods, fat-extracted if they contain >10% fat, are gelatinized with Termamyl (heat-stable alpha-amylase) and then enzymatically digested with protease and amyloglucosidase to remove protein and starch. Soluble dietary fiber is removed by filtering and washing residue with water. Remaining residue, insoluble dietary fiber (IDF), is washed with 95% ethanol and acetone, dried, and weighed. One duplicate is analyzed for protein, and the other is incinerated at 525° to determine ash. IDF is weight of residue less weight of protein and ash.

B. Apparatus

See **985.29B** (*see* 16.1).

C. Reagents

See **985.29C** (*see* 16.1). (*Note:* Reagent (**e**), Termamyl solution, is available from Novo Nordisk Biolabs, 33 Turner Rd, Danbury, CT 06810, USA.)

(**a**) *85% Methanol.*—Place 105 mL H$_2$O into 1 L volumetric flask, dilute to volume with 95% ethanol.

D. Enzyme Purity

See **985.29D** (*see* 16.1).

E. Sample Preparation

Analyze dry samples without pretreatment whenever possible. Mill dry samples to 0.3–0.5 mm mesh. Homogenize and freeze-dry wet foods before milling. If high fat content (>10%) prevents proper milling, defat with petroleum ether (3 times with 25 mL portions/g sample) before milling. Determine residual moisture in milled samples by drying overnight in 70° vacuum oven, or 5 h in 105° air oven. Record weight loss due to fat and/or water, and make appropriate correction to final % total dietary fiber. (*Note:* For samples high in sugars that cannot be dried by lyophilization, extract 3 times each with 10 volumes of 85% methanol to remove sugars, which may interfere in determination.)

F. Determination

Run blank with samples to measure any contribution from reagents to residue. Weigh duplicate 1 g samples, accurate to 0.1 mg, into 400 mL tall-form beakers. Duplicate sample weights should not differ >20 mg. Add 50 mL phosphate buffer to each beaker. Check pH and adjust to pH 6.0 ± 0.2, by adding 0.275N NaOH or 0.325N HCl. Add 0.1 mL Termamyl solution to each beaker. Cover beakers with Al foil and place in boiling water bath. Shake beakers gently at 5 min intervals throughout incubation. When thermometer indicates beaker contents have reached 100°, continue incubation 15 min. Total of 30 min in bath is usually sufficient. Cool solutions to room temperature. Adjust to pH 7.5 ± 0.1 by adding ca 10 mL NaOH solution.

Add 5 mg protease to each solution. Protease sticks to spatula, so it may be preferable to prepare enzyme solution (50 mg in 1 mL phosphate buffer) just before use, and pipet 0.1 mL to each sample.

Cover beakers with Al foil. Incubate 30 min at 60° with continuous agitation. Cool. Check pH and adjust to pH 4.0–4.6 with ca 10 mL HCl solution. Add 0.3 mL amyloglucosidase, cover with Al foil, and incubate 30 min at 60° with continuous agitation.

Weigh crucible containing Celite to nearest 0.1 mg, then wet and redistribute bed of Celite in crucible using stream of water from wash bottle. Apply suction to draw Celite onto fritted glass as even mat. Apply enzyme mixture from beaker to crucible, filtering into suction flask. Wash residue 2 times with 10 mL water (removing soluble dietary fiber), 2 times with 10 mL 95% EtOH, and 2 times with 10 mL acetone. Break surface film that develops after addition of sample to Celite with spatula, to improve filtration. Careful intermittent suction throughout filtration and back-bubbling with air, if available, will speed up filtrations. Normal suction can be applied at washing.

Dry crucible containing residue overnight in 70° vacuum oven or 5 h in 105° air oven. Cool in desiccator and weigh to nearest 0.1 mg. Subtract crucible and Celite weights to determine residue weight.

Using 1 of duplicates, scrape sample, Celite, and fiber mat onto filter paper which can be folded shut, and analyze for protein by **960.52** (*see* 16.4). Use N × 6.25 as conversion factor.

Incinerate second of duplicates 5 h at 525°. Cool in desiccator and weigh to nearest 0.1 mg. Subtract crucible and Celite weights to determine ash.

G. Calculations

See **985.29G** (see 16.1), calculating IDF as described for TDF.

Table 991.42. Method Performance for Insoluble Dietary Fiber in Food and Food Products, Enzymatic-Gravimetric Method, Phosphate Buffer

Food/Food Product	No. Labs	IDF, av. %	s_r	s_R	RSD$_r$, %	RSD$_R$, %
Beans, butter	10	17.36	0.41	1.96	2.34	11.31
Beans, French	10	25.64	0.83	1.51	3.23	5.87
Beans, kidney	13	16.33	0.74	1.04	4.53	6.39
Brussels sprouts	15	30.23	0.69	2.39	2.27	7.89
Cabbage	9	21.60	0.86	1.68	4.00	7.79
Carrots	12	32.29	1.74	3.68	5.38	11.39
Chick peas	12	16.69	1.73	2.80	10.38	16.80
Okra	14	24.15	1.55	3.28	6.43	13.57
Onions	12	13.32	0.87	1.57	6.51	11.79
Parsley	12	34.39	1.22	4.69	3.56	13.64
Turnips	12	21.38	1.41	3.55	6.60	16.61
Apples	4	55.57	0.51	2.53	0.92	4.55
Apricots	5	44.92	0.39	3.69	0.86	8.22
Figs, Calimyrna	5	43.07	2.41	7.92	5.59	18.40
Figs, Mission	6	33.61	0.93	4.06	2.76	12.09
Peaches	6	39.53	0.86	2.44	2.17	6.16
Prunes	6	46.18	2.82	8.98	6.11	19.44
Raisins	8	49.18	2.71	9.49	5.51	19.30
Barley	12	4.30	0.43	0.62	9.92	14.33
Rye flour	15	11.81	0.58	1.02	4.87	8.62
Soy bran	13	65.24	0.91	2.40	1.40	3.68
Wheat germ	9	15.67	0.71	0.96	4.54	6.13

Ref.: J. AOAC Int. **75**, March/April issue(1992).

16.4   960.52—Microchemical Determination of Nitrogen
Micro-Kjeldahl Method
First Action 1960
Final Action 1961

(Not applicable to material containing N–N or N–O linkages)

A. Reagents

(a) *Sulfuric acid.*—Specific gravity 1.84, N-free.

(b) *Mercuric oxide.*—N-free.

(c) *Potassium sulfate.*—N-free.

(d) *Sodium hydroxide-sodium thiosulfate solution.*—Dissolve 60 g NaOH and 5 g $Na_2S_2O_3 \cdot 5H_2O$ in H_2O and dilute to 100 mL or add 25 mL 25% $Na_2S_2O_3 \cdot 5H_2O$ to 100 mL 50% NaOH solution.

(e) *Boric acid solution.*—Saturated solution.

(f) *Indicator solution.*—(*1*) *Methyl red-methylene blue.*—Mix 2 parts 0.2% alcoholic methyl red solution with 1 part 0.2% alcoholic methylene blue solution; or (*2*) *Methyl red-bromocresol green solution.*—Mix 1 part 0.2% alcoholic methyl red solution with 5 parts 0.2% alcoholic bromocresol green solution.

(g) *Hydrochloric acid.*—0.02*N*. Prepare as in **936.15A** and standardize as in **936.15E-G**.

936.15A, E–G (Standard Solution of Hydrochloric Acid)
A. Preparation of Standard Solutions

Following table gives approximate volumes of 36.5–38% HCl required to make 10 L standard solutions:

Approx. normality	mL HCl to be diluted to 10 L
0.01	8.6
0.02	17.2
0.10	86.0
0.50	430.1
1.0	860.1

E. Standardization

Accurately weigh enough standard $Na_2B_4O_7 \cdot 10H_2O$ to titrate ca 40 mL and transfer to 300 mL flask. Add 40 mL CO_2-free H_2O, **936.16B(a)**, and stopper flask. Swirl gently until sample dissolves. Add 4 drops methyl red and titrate with solution that is being standardized to equivalence point as indicated by reference solution.

Normality = g $Na_2B_4O_7 \cdot 10H_2O \times 1000$/mL acid $\times$ 190.69

936.16B (Standard Solution of Sodium Hydroxide)
B. Reagents

(a) *Carbon dioxide-free water.*—Prepare by one of following methods: (*1*) Boil H_2O 20 min and cool with soda-lime protection; (*2*) bubble air, freed from CO_2 by passing through tower of soda-lime, through H_2O 12 h.

Ref.: JAOAC **22**, 102, 563(1939).

Standard Sodium Carbonate Method

F. Reagents

(**a**) *Methyl orange indicator.*—0.1% in H_2O.

(**b**) *Reference solution.*—80 mL CO_2-free H_2O containing 3 or 4 drops methyl orange.

(**c**) *Anhydrous sodium carbonate.*—Heat 250 mL H_2O to 80° and add $NaHCO_3$ (ACS), stirring until no more dissolves. Filter solution through folded paper (use of hot H_2O funnel is desirable) into erlenmeyer. Cool filtrate to ca 10°, swirling constantly during crystallization. Fine crystals of trona that separate out have approximate composition: $Na_2CO_3 \cdot NaHCO_3 \cdot 2H_2O$. Decant supernate, drain crystals by suction, and wash once with cold H_2O.

Transfer precipitate, being careful not to include any paper fibers, to large flat-bottom Pt dish. Heat 1 h at 290° in electric oven or furnace with pyrometer control. Stir contents occasionally with Pt wire. Cool in desiccator. Place the anhydrous Na_2CO_3 in glass-stoppered container and store in desiccator containing efficient desiccant. Dry at 120° and cool just before weighing.

Refs.: Kolthoff & Stenger, "Volumetric Analysis," **II**, 80(1947). Ind. Eng. Chem., Anal. Ed. **9**, 141(1937). JAOAC **22**, 563(1939).

G. Standardization

Accurately weigh enough anhydrous Na_2CO_3, (**c**), to titrate ca 40 mL, transfer to 300 mL erlenmeyer, and dissolve in 40 mL H_2O. Add 3 drops methyl orange and titrate until color begins to deviate from H_2O tint (reference solution). (Equivalence point has not been reached.) Boil solution gently 2 min, and cool. Titrate until color is barely different from H_2O tint of indicator.

$$\text{Normality} = \text{g } Na_2CO_3 \times 1000/\text{mL acid} \times 52.994$$

Ref.: JAOAC **22**, 102, 563(1939).

B. Apparatus

(**a**) *Digestion rack.*—With either gas or electric heaters which will supply enough heat to 30 mL flask to cause 15 mL H_2O at 25° to come to rolling boil in ≥2 but <3 min.

(**b**) *Distillation apparatus.*—One-piece or Parnas-Wagner distillation apparatus recommended by Committee on Microchemical Apparatus, ACS.

(**c**) *Digestion flasks.*—Use 30 mL regular Kjeldahl or Soltys-type flasks (Reference: Anal. Chem. **23**, 523(1951)). For small samples, 10 mL Kjeldahl flasks may be used.

C. Determination

Weigh sample requiring 3–10 mL 0.01 or 0.02N HCl and transfer to 30 mL digestion flask. If sample weight is <10 mg, use microchemical balance (maximum weight 100 mg dry organic matter). Use charging tube for dry solids, porcelain boat for sticky solids or nonvolatile liquids, and capillary or capsule for volatile liquids. Add 1.9 ± 0.1 g K_2SO_4, 40 ± 10 mg HgO, and 2.0 ± 0.1 mL H_2SO_4. If sample weight is >15 mg, add additional 0.1 mL H_2SO_4 for each 10 mg dry organic matter >15 mg. Make certain that acid has specific gravity ≥1.84 if sample contains nitriles. (10 mL flasks and ½ quantities of reagents may be used for samples <7 mg.) Add boiling chips which pass No. 10 sieve. If boiling time for digestion rack heaters is 2–2.5 min, digest 1 h after all H_2O is distilled and acid comes to true boil; if boiling time is 2.5–3 min, digest 1.5 h. (Digest 0.5 h if sample is known to contain no refractory ring N.)

Cool, add minimum volume of H_2O to dissolve solids, cool, and place thin film of Vaseline on rim of flask. Transfer digest and boiling chips to distillation apparatus and rinse flask 5 or 6 times with 1–2 mL portions H_2O. Place 125 mL Phillips beaker or Erlenmeyer containing 5 mL saturated H_3BO_3 solution and 2–4 drops indicator under condenser with tip extending below surface of solution. Add 8–10 mL $NaOH\text{-}Na_2S_2O_3$ solution to still, collect ca 15 mL distillate, and dilute to ca 50 mL. (Use 2.5 mL H_3BO_3 and 1–2 drops indicator, and dilute to ca 25 mL if $0.01N$ HCl is to be used.) Titrate to end point. Make blank determination and calculate.

$$\%N = [(\text{mL HCl} - \text{mL blank}) \times \text{normality} \times 14.007 \times 100]/\text{mg sample}$$

References: JAOAC **32,** 561(1949); **33,** 179(1950); **43,** 689(1960).
CAS-7727-37-9 (nitrogen)

Chapter 17
Fat-Polyunsaturated

17.1   **979.19—*cis, cis*-Methylene Interrupted
Polyunsaturated Fatty Acids in Oils**
Spectrophotometric Method
First Action 1979
Final Action 1984

A. Reagents

(**a**) *Potassium borate buffer.*—1.0*M*, pH 9.0. Dissolve 61.9 g H_3BO_3 and 25.0 g KOH in ca 800 mL H_2O by stirring and heating. Cool to room temperature and adjust to pH 9.0 with 1.0*N* HCl or 1.0*N* KOH, as required. Dilute to 1 L with H_2O and mix.

(**b**) *Dilute potassium borate buffer.*—0.2*M*, pH 9.0. Dilute 200 mL 1.0*M* buffer, (**a**), to 1 L with H_2O and mix.

(**c**) *Lipoxidase solutions.*—(*1*) *Stock solution.*—Dissolve 10 mg lipoxidase, from soybean, 50,000 units/mg (ICN Pharmaceuticals Inc., Life Sciences Group, Nutritional Biochemicals Division, or equivalent), in 10 mL ice-cold dilute borate buffer, (**b**). Refrigerated solution is stable 30 days. (*2*) *Working solution.*—Mix 2.0 mL stock solution with 8.0 mL ice-cold dilute borate buffer, (**b**). If large number of analyses are to be performed, dilute 5.0 mL stock solution to 25 mL with ice-cold dilute borate buffer, (**b**). (*3*) *Inactivated solution.*—Pipet 4 mL working enzyme solution, (*2*), to 10 mL volumetric flask and hold 5 min in boiling H_2O.

(**d**) *Alcoholic potassium hydroxide solution.*—0.5*N*. Dissolve 1.40 g KOH in alcohol and dilute to 50 mL with alcohol. Prepare fresh daily.

B. Preparation of Sample

Accurately weigh ca 100 mg vegetable oil and transfer with *n*-hexane into 100 mL volumetric flask, which has just been flushed with N. Dilute to volume with *n*-hexane or acetone. Pipet 1 mL diluted solution into 100 mL volumetric flask and completely evaporate solvent under N.

C. Determination

Add 1 mL alcoholic KOH, **A**(**d**), solution to solvent-free residue in volumetric flask. Heat gently on steam bath to dissolve. Flush with N and hold stoppered, in dark, minimum of 5 h to overnight. After saponification is complete, add 20 mL 1.0*M* borate buffer, **A**(**a**), and 50 mL H_2O, and mix. Add 1 mL 0.5*N* HCl, dilute to volume with H_2O, and mix.

Pipet 3 mL saponified solution into each of four 13 × 100 mm test tubes. To 2 tubes (blanks) add 0.10 mL inactivated enzyme solution, **A**(**c**)(*3*), and mix well. To remaining duplicate tubes, add 0.10 mL working enzyme solution, **A**(**c**)(*2*). Mix by shaking vigorously 30 s immediately after adding enzyme solution, and let all tubes stand exposed to air at room temperature 30 min. Zero spectrophotometer at 234 nm with blank tubes and measure A of reacted samples.

For sample, calculate g polyunsaturated fatty acid (PUFA) as trilinolein/100 g sample $= W \times DF \times 10^{-4}$, where $W = \mu$g trilinolein/mL final solution from standard curve, and $DF =$ dilution factor.

D. Preparation of Standard Curve

Weigh 100 mg *cis,cis*-trilinolein, 99% (NuCheck Prep, PO Box 295, Elysian, MN 56028-0295, or equivalent), transfer quantitatively to 100 mL volumetric flask, and dilute to volume with *n*-hexane or acetone. Pipet 10 mL aliquot into 100 mL volumetric flask and dilute to volume with same solvent. Pipet 2, 4, 6, 8, 10 and 12 mL aliquots into separate 100 mL volumetric flasks, and evaporate each to dryness in stream of N. Pipet 1 mL alcoholic KOH, **A(d)**, into each flask, flush with N, and store stoppered in dark 5 h or overnight.

Add 20 mL 1.0M borate buffer, **A(a)**, 50 mL H$_2$O, and 1 mL 0.5N HCl to each, dilute to volume with H$_2$O, and mix. Pipet four 3 mL aliquots of each standard solution into test tubes, incubate, and proceed as in *Determination*, beginning "To 2 tubes (blanks) . . . ." Plot average A at each level against μg trilinolein/mL.

Two single determinations in 1 laboratory should not differ by >1.6%; 2 single determinations performed in 2 laboratories should not differ by >2.2%.

References: JAOAC **60,** 895(1977); **61,** 1419(1978).

17.2   957.13—Acids (Polyunsaturated) in Oils and Fats
Spectrophotometric Method
Final Action
American Oil Chemists' Society-AOAC Method

A. Principle

Natural conjugated constituents are determined by measuring UV absorption at specified wavelengths in purified solvent. Nonconjugated polyunsaturated constituents are partially conjugated by heating in KOH-glycol solution, and absorptions of conjugated constituents are redetermined. The % conjugated diene, triene, tetraene, and pentaene acids are calculated from predetermined a by simultaneous equations.

The method is applicable to determination of polyunsaturated acids, dienoic through pentaenoic, in animal and vegetable fats containing only natural or *cis* isomers, only small amounts of preformed conjugated material, and only small amounts of pigments whose absorption may undergo considerable change during the alkali isomerization. The method is not applicable, or is applicable only with specific precautions, to hydrogenated oils or other fats containing *trans* isomers of unsaturated fatty acids, to fish oils or similar fats containing acids more highly unsaturated than pentaenoic, to crude oils or samples containing pigments whose absorption undergoes changes during alkali isomerization, or to fats and oils containing large amounts of preformed conjugated fatty acids.

B. Apparatus

(a) *Isomerization apparatus.*—(*See* Fig. **957.13A.**) (*1*) *Constant temperature bath.*—180 $\pm$ 1°. Capacity sufficient to immerse 25 $\times$ 250 mm Pyrex test tubes to depth of 114 mm (4.5"). (Westinghouse, or equivalent, household deepfat fryer has been found satisfactory.) For bath liquid use Fisher Scientific Co. No. B-219 bath wax or DC 550 Fluid, Dow Corning Corp. Place bath in insulated box with insulated cover having holes for stirrer and cork supports for test tubes.

(2) *Test tubes.*—Pyrex, lipped, 25 × 250 mm.

(3) *Distributing heads.*—To fit test tubes snugly. Tubing in center of head has both ends open and 2 small holes 25 and 38 mm, respectively, from bottom. (*See* Fig. **957.13B**, right.)

(4) *Manifold.*—With 10 outlets, each connected to 50 mm long capillary tube, 1 mm bore. Cap unused outlets. (*See* Fig. **957.13B**, left.)

(5) *Nitrogen manometer.*—Construct from 6 mm od tubing bent in shape of U-tube, height ca 380 mm, width ca 30 mm. Fill manometer ca half full with H_2O containing 1 drop methyl orange and 1 drop H_2SO_4. To adjust flow of N, attach ca 90 cm rubber tubing to one of N outlets on distributing head. Fill 100 mL graduate with H_2O and invert in container of H_2O. Insert end of rubber tubing under

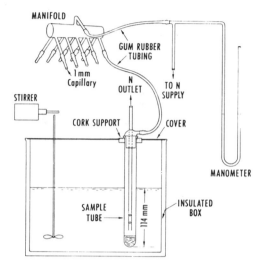

Figure **957.13A.**—Constant temperature bath and accessories.

graduate. Turn on N supply and measure rate of displacement of H_2O in graduate. Rate of flow should be 50–100 mL/min. Mark level of liquid in manometer at this flow rate.

(**b**) *Spectrophotometer.*—Covering range of 220–360 nm with wavelength scale readable to 0.1 nm. Beckman Model DU is satisfactory. Adjust H lamp with no cell in beam so meter balances at lowest possible wavelength (usually ≤211 nm). Slit widths are critical for absorption measurements at 262, 268, and 274 nm where, at final balancing, adjustments must be 0.8–0.9 mm.

(**c**) *Absorption cells.*—Quartz, matched pairs in lengths 1.000 ± 0.005 cm. When filled with H_2O or isooctane, must match within 0.01 *A* unit.

C. Reagents

(**a**) *Methanol, absolute.*—Check *A* of 1 cm layer of methyl alcohol against H_2O at 220 nm and through range of wavelengths used in analysis. *A* at 220 nm must be <0.4 and curve should be smooth in range 262–322 nm. Otherwise purify as follows, and recheck *A*:

Place 2 L methyl alcohol from new drum or glass bottles into 3 L double-neck ⊤ distilling flask; add 10 g KOH and 25 g Zn dust. Stopper one outlet and place reflux condenser in other, and reflux on steam bath 3 h. Remove from steam bath; replace reflux tube with distilling trap, 75° connecting tube, and condenser. Place flask in H_2O bath or electric heating mantle and distil, collecting distillate in 2 L erlenmeyer. Store in glass-stoppered bottle. Absolute alcohol is satisfactory if of comparable purity (as obtained or purified).

(**b**) *Isooctane (2,2,4-trimethylpentane).*—NIST certified grade or spectral grade (Phillips 66 Co., Specialty Chemicals, PO Box 968, Borger, TX 79008-0968). Hexane or cyclohexane is satisfactory if *A* requirements are met. Purify as follows: Place ca 9 cm glass wool above stopcock at lower end of 80 × 4.5 cm filter tube. Add ca 30 cm silica gel (Grade 12, 28–200 mesh, Fisher No. S-157, or equivalent). Pour isooctane

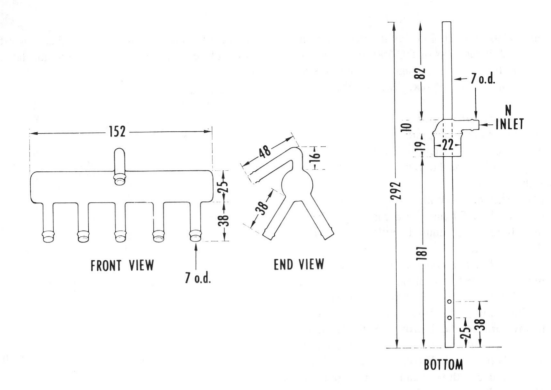

Figure 957.13B.—Right, distribution heads. Left, manifold. All dimensions are in mm.

slowly into tube, filling ca ¾ full. Insert cork stopper covered with Al foil loosely in top of tube and let isooctane filter through silica gel, collecting in 2 L erlenmeyer. Renew silica gel as often as necessary to yield isooctane conforming to A limit. Check A of 1 cm layer of the isooctane against H_2O through range of wavelengths used in analysis. A compared with H_2O set at 0 must be ≤0.070 at all wavelengths, and the resultant A versus wavelength curve must be smooth. Otherwise refilter and re-check A.

(**c**) *Potassium hydroxide-glycol solution.*—6.6% KOH for 25 min isomerization. Weigh ca 750 g ethylene glycol into 1 L round-bottom Pyrex flask. Close with hollow stopper containing short outlet tube and inlet tube reaching to bottom of flask. Connect inlet tube to O-free N supply (<0.01 % O) and bubble N through liquid during all stages of preparation to exclude all air and to agitate liquid slightly. Place in oil bath at 100–150°; raise bath temperature to 190° and hold 10 min to dry glycol. Remove bath and let bath temperature drop to 120°. Slowly and carefully add 60 g 85% KOH, keeping solution under N. Return to oil bath; reheat bath to 190° and hold at this temperature 10 min. Remove from bath, and cool. Remove hollow stopper and close with solid stopper. Store in refrigerator at ca 4° (40°F) under N.

Check KOH content by adding 10.00 g KOH-glycol solution to ca 90 mL methyl alcohol, neutralized with 1N HCl to phenolphthalein end point. Titrate with standardized 1N HCl until pink just disappears. % KOH = mL × normality × 5.61/weight solution. If % KOH is not 6.5–6.6, dry some glycol by heating under N at 190° as above, and adjust to 6.6% KOH.

(**d**) *Potassium hydroxide-glycol solution.*—21% KOH for 15 min isomerization. Prepare as in (**c**), except use 210 g 85% KOH. Titrate, and adjust to 21 ± 0.1% KOH, if necessary.

(**e**) *Nitrogen gas.*—Pre-purified grade, <0.01% O.

D. *Preparation of Sample*

Melt sample carefully on steam bath, stir thoroughly, and filter if not clear.

E. *Determination*

(The 6.6% KOH method is preferred when samples contain only linoleic and linolenic acids; the 21% KOH method is preferred when samples contain linoleic, linolenic, and arachidonic acids. When pentaenoic acids are present, 21% KOH method must be used.)

(**a**) *For conjugated polyunsaturated acids.*—Into 1 mL Pyrex cup (diameter 14 mm, height 10 mm) weigh enough sample to give A reading of ≥ 0.2 (ca 200 mg). Drop cup into 75 mL isooctane in 150 mL beaker, and rotate beaker to dissolve sample, warming if necessary. Cool to room temperature, transfer to 100 mL glass-stoppered volumetric flask, dilute to volume with solvent, and mix thoroughly. Measure A in UV region against matched cell containing solvent, diluting solution (and/or using other cell lengths if necessary so that observed A is 0.2–0.8). Also take readings on both sides of specified wavelengths to determine that maximum is present. Component is considered absent if maximum is not found in characteristic region and no further calculations are made in this region. Measure at: Dienoic, *233* nm; trienoic, 262, *268,* 274 nm; tetraenoic, 308, *315,* 322 nm; pentaenoic, *346* nm.

(**b**) *For nonconjugated polyunsaturated acids, 6.6% KOH, 25 min isomerization.*—Weigh 100 mg (to nearest 0.5 mg) sample into 1 mL Pyrex glass cup. Weigh 11.0 ± 0.1 g of the 6.6% KOH-glycol solution into 25×250 mm Pyrex test tube. Conduct ≥ 2 blank determinations with sample. Cover tube with distributing head and connect to a capillary tube on manifold. Adjust flow of N to permit ≥ 50–100 mL N to pass through tube/min. Let N sweep through tube 1 min to remove air; then immerse to depth of 114 mm in bath at $180 \pm 1°$. Check temperature frequently and standardize thermometer at frequent intervals.

After 20 min remove distributing head and drop 1 mL cup containing weighed sample into tube, note exact time, and replace head. Drop clean 1 mL cup into blanks. Keeping distributing head in place, remove tube from bath, swirl vigorously few seconds, and return to bath; after 1 min, examine solution. If clear, return to bath; if not clear, indicating incomplete saponification, swirl tube 2–3 times and return to bath. At 1 min intervals, repeat swirling until saponification is complete. Keep bath temperature at 180 $\pm 1°$.

Exactly 25 min after dropping sample into tube, remove from bath, wipe clean, and place in 3 L beaker to cool, continuing to pass N over solution. Cold H_2O bath may also be used. After cooling, remove head, and wash lower tubing with 20 mL purified methyl alcohol, collecting washings in test tube. Wash with methyl alcohol from beaker; do not use wash bottle.

Insert glass stirring rod 30 cm long with curved end at bottom into test tube and move cup up and down to mix solution. Transfer solution to 100 mL glass-stoppered volumetric flask, dilute to volume with purified methyl alcohol, and mix thoroughly. Measure A as in (**a**), using KOH-glycol blank as reference. If dilution of sample solution is required, make similar dilutions of blank. If blanks do not check, repeat tests, increasing flow of N.

(**c**) *For nonconjugated polyunsaturated acids, 21% KOH, 15 min isomerization.*—Proceed as in (**b**), except use 80 mg sample and 21 ± 0.1% KOH-glycol solution, and isomerize exactly 15 min.

F. *Spectrophotometric Readings*

If polyunsaturated fatty acid constituent is known to be absent, or its absence is confirmed during analysis (no maximum detected at its analytical wavelength), no spectrophotometeric reading is required in region of its absorption and no a at that region need be included in equations. For example, cottonseed oil is known to contain no polyunsaturated constituents more highly unsaturated than dienoic (linoleic acid).

Hence, in analysis of this oil, measurements are required only at 233 nm, and equation to calculate linoleic acid content requires a only at this wavelength.

Correction for background absorption is used only when measuring very small traces of fatty acids. When fatty acid is present in more than trace, background corrections are not required and their use may lead to erroneous results. When a of any polyunsaturated constituent after isomerization, at its analytical wavelength, is >1.0, no background correction should be made. No background corrections are to be made after isomerization with 21% KOH.

G. Calculations

(a) *Absorptivity for conjugated constituents.*—Calculate a for each wavelength recorded in determination, **957.13E(a)**, using subscripts, 233, 268, 315, 346, to designate each individual a.

Absorptivity, $a = A/bc$, where A = observed absorbance, b = cell length in cm, and c = g sample/L final dilution used for A measurement.

In following equations, subscripts 2, 3, 4, and 5 refer to diene, triene, tetraene, and pentaene constituents, respectively.

Absorptivity at 233 nm corrected for absorption by acid or ester groups = $a_2 = a_{233} - a_0$, where $a_0 = 0.07$ for esters and 0.03 for soaps and fatty acids.

Absorptivity at 268 nm corrected for background absorption = $a_3 = 2.8\,[a_{268} - \frac{1}{2}(a_{262} + a_{274})]$.

Absorptivity at 315 nm corrected for background absorption = $a_4 = 2.5\,[a_{315} - \frac{1}{2}(a_{308} + a_{322})]$.

Absorptivity at 346 nm = $a_5 = a_{346}$.

(b) *Conjugated acids.*—If quantities within brackets of a_3 or a_4 are 0 or negative, no characteristic absorption maxima are present and corresponding constituent is reported as absent. As preformed constituents are usually present in small amounts, background absorption corrections are usually required. If large amounts of preformed constituents are present, this method is not applicable. However, no background corrections are to be applied to readings in pentaenoic region, 346 nm.

$$\% \text{ Conjugated diene} = C_2 = 0.91a_2$$
$$\% \text{ Conjugated triene} = C_3 = 0.47a_3$$
$$\% \text{ Conjugated tetraene} = C_4 = 0.45a_4$$
$$\% \text{ Conjugated pentaene} = C_5 = 0.39a_5$$

(c) *Absorptivities for nonconjugated constituents, 6.6% KOH, 25 min isomerization.*—Calculate a' for each wavelength in determination, (b). $a' = A/bc$.

Absorptivity at 233 nm corrected for conjugated diene acids originally present = $a'_2 = a'_{233} - a_2 - 0.03$.

Absorptivity at 268 nm corrected for background absorption and for undestroyed conjugated triene = $a'_3 = 4.03[a'_{268} - \frac{1}{2}(a'_{262} + a'_{274})] - a_3$.

Absorptivity at 315 nm corrected for background absorption and for undestroyed conjugated tetraene = $a'_4 = 2.06[a'_{315} - \frac{1}{2}(a'_{308} + a'_{322})] - a_4$.

(d) *Nonconjugated acids, 6.6% KOH, 25 min isomerization.*—(1) Without background corrections:

$$\% \text{ Linoleic acid} = X = 1.086a'_2 - 1.324(a'_{268} - a_{268}) + 0.40(a'_{315} - a_{315})$$
$$\% \text{ Linolenic acid} = Y = 1.980(a'_{268} - a_{268}) - 4.92\,(a'_{315} - a_{315})$$
$$\% \text{ Arachidonic acid} = Z = 4.69(a'_{315} - a_{315})$$

(2) When background corrections are required:

$$\% \text{ Linoleic acid} = X = 1.086a'_2 - 1.324a'_3 + 0.40a'_4$$
$$\% \text{ Linolenic acid} = Y = 1.980a'_3 - 4.92a'_4$$
$$\% \text{ Arachidonic acid} = Z = 4.69a'_4$$

(**e**) *Absorptivities for nonconjugated constituents, 21% KOH, 15 min isomerization.*—Calculate a' for each wavelength 233, 268, 315, and 346 nm. (If no maximum is found, report component as 0 without further measurement or calculation.)

$$\text{Absorptivity at 233 nm} = a'_2 = a'_{233} - a_2$$
$$\text{Absorptivity at 268 nm} = a'_3 = a'_{268} - a_{268}$$
$$\text{Absorptivity at 315 nm} = a'_4 = a'_{315} - a_{315}$$
$$\text{Absorptivity at 346 nm} = a'_5 = a'_{346} - a_{346}$$

(**f**) *Nonconjugated acids, 21% KOH, 15 min isomerization.*—(Spectrophotometric method will not differentiate between acids with same number of double bonds but different chain length, e.g., between C_{20} and C_{22} pentaenes. First 2 sets of equations below are for samples containing C_{20} pentaene acid and for samples containing C_{22} pentaene acid, respectively. If chain length is unknown, assume that these pentaene acids are present in equal amounts, and apply third set of equations.)

(*1*) *Samples containing C_{20} pentaene acid:*

$$\% \text{ Linoleic acid} = X = 1.09a'_2 - 0.57a'_3 - 0.26a'_4 + 0.002a'_5$$
$$\% \text{ Linolenic acid} = Y = 1.10a'_3 - 0.88a'_4 + 0.31a'_5$$
$$\% \text{ Arachidonic acid} = Z = 1.65a'_4 - 1.55a'_5$$
$$\% \text{ Pentaenoic acids} = P = 1.14a'_5$$

(*2*) *Samples containing C_{22} pentaene acid:*

$$\% \text{ Linoleic acid} = X = 1.09a'_2 - 0.57a'_3 - 0.26a'_4 - 0.12a'_5$$
$$\% \text{ Linolenic acid} = Y = 1.10a'_3 - 0.88a'_4 - 0.02a'_5$$
$$\% \text{ Arachidonic acid} = Z = 1.65a'_4 - 1.86a'_5$$
$$\% \text{ Pentaenoic acids} = P = 1.98a'_5$$

(*3*) *Samples containing pentaene acids of unknown chain length (calculated as 50% C_{20}–50% C_{22} pentaenoic acids):*

$$\% \text{ Linoleic acid} = X = 1.09a'_2 - 0.57a'_3 - 0.26a'_4 - 0.03a'_5$$
$$\% \text{ Linolenic acid} = Y = 1.10a'_3 - 0.88a'_4 + 0.19a'_5$$
$$\% \text{ Arachidonic acid} = Z = 1.65a'_4 - 1.67a'_5$$
$$\% \text{ Pentaenoic acids} = P = 1.45a'_5$$

(**g**) *Total composition:*

$$\% \text{ Total conjugated polyunsaturated acids} = C_2 + C_3 + C_4 + C_5$$
$$\% \text{ Total nonconjugated polyunsaturated acids} = X + Y + Z + P$$
$$\% \text{ Oleic acid} = \{\text{I value (Wijs) of sample}$$
$$- [1.811 (C_2 + X) + 2.737(C_3 + Y) + 3.337(C_4 + Z) + 4.014^* (C_5 + P)]\}/0.899$$
$$\% \text{ Saturated acids} = \% \text{ total fatty acid} - (\% \text{ oleic acid} + \% \text{ conjugated acid} + \% \text{ nonconjugated acid})$$

(% total fatty acid of most naturally occurring oils is 95.6. To calculate to fatty acid basis, multiply the % value by 100/% total fatty acid.)

* Corresponding constant for sample containing all C_{20} pentaene acids is 4.197; for all C_{22} pentaene acids it is 3.841.

References: JAOAC **40**, 487(1957); **42**, 42, 354(1959). AOCS Method Cd 7–58.
CAS-506-32-1 (arachidonic acid)
CAS-60-33-3 (linoleic acid)
CAS-463-40-1 (linolenic acid)
CAS-112-80-1 (oleic acid)

Chapter 18
Fat-Total

18.1   960.39—Fat (Crude) or Ether Extract in Meat
Final Action

(a) Weigh 3–4 g sample by difference into thimble containing small amount of sand. Mix with glass rod, place thimble and rod in 50 mL beaker, and dry in oven 6 h at 100–102° or 1.5 h at 125°. Proceed as in **920.39C** (*see* 18.4), except dry extract to constant weight at 100°, cool, and weigh. Petroleum ether, **945.16A**, may be used instead of anhydrous ether, if desired.

> **945.16A** (Oil in Cereal Adjuncts, Petroleum Ether Extraction Method)
> *A. Reagent*
> *Petroleum ether.*—AOCS. Initial boiling temperature, 35–38°; dry-flask end point, 52–60°; ≥95% distilling at <54°, and ≤60% distilling at <40°; specific gravity at 60°F, 0.630–0.660; appearance, colorless; evaporation residue, ≤0.0011 g/100 mL; doctor test, sweet; Cu strip corrosion test, noncorrosive; only trace of unsaturated compounds permitted; residue in distilling flask, neutral to methyl orange; blotter strip odor test, odorless within 12 min; aromatic compounds, no nitrobenzene odor; saponification value, <1.0 mg KOH/100 mL.
>
> Make distillation test according to ASTM method D216-54 and make blank determination by evaporating 250 mL with ca 0.25 g stearin or other hard fat (previously brought to constant weight by heating) and drying as in actual determination. Blank must be ≤3 mg.

(b) Weigh 3–4 g sample by difference into small disposable Al dish, add sand, and mix, spreading mixture on bottom of dish with glass or Al paddle. Dry with paddle as in (a). Roll edges of dish and insert with paddle into thimble. Proceed as in **920.39C**, except dry extract to constant weight at 100°, cool, and weigh. Petroleum ether, **945.16A**, may be used in place of anhydrous ether, if desired.

18.2   976.21—Fat (Crude) in Meat
Rapid Specific Gravity Method
First Action 1976
Final Action 1979

A. Principle

Fat is extracted from sample with C_2Cl_4 in motor-driven, orbital shaker in presence of drying agent to absorb moisture. Extract is filtered and specific gravity of filtrate is measured at 37° by magnetically driven hydrometer. Digital reading is converted into fat content, using precalibrated chart.

B. Apparatus and Reagents

(a) *Foss-let fat analyzer*.—Includes orbital shaker, specific gravity readout unit, solvent dispenser, reference standard oil (specific gravity at 23° = 0.915; for periodic check of potentiometer calibration), stainless steel cup with cover and 8 mm bore brass hammer, pressure filtration device, and conversion chart (Foss Food Technology Corp.).

(b) *Drying agent*.—Plaster of Paris (available locally through paint, hardware, or building supply dealers), 8 mesh Drierite, or anhydrous $CaSO_4$.

(c) *Tetrachloroethylene*.—Technical grade C_2Cl_4 (distributed locally through dry cleaning suppliers or Fisher Scientific Co., No. C-182).

C. Determination

Prepare samples as in **983.18**. Check calibration of Foss-let potentiometer daily by using C_2Cl_4 alone to set zero point and mixture of 22.5 g reference standard oil and 120 mL C_2Cl_4 (specific gravity of mixture at 37° = 1.4763) to set 50% fat point at 850.0.

983.18 (Meat and Meat Products, Preparation of Sample)

To prevent H_2O loss during preparation and subsequent handling, do not use small samples. Keep ground material in glass or similar containers with air- and H_2O-tight covers. Prepare samples for analysis as follows:

(a) *Fresh meats, dried meats, cured meats, smoked meats, etc.*—Separate as completely as possible from any bone; pass rapidly 3 times through food chopper with plate openings ≤⅛″ (3 mm), mixing thoroughly after each grinding; and begin all determinations promptly. If any delay occurs, chill sample to inhibit decomposition.

Alternatively, use a bowl cutter for sample preparation (benchtop model, ½ HP; 14 in. bowl, 22 rpm; two 3.5 in. knives, 1725 rpm; Model 84145, Hobart Corp., 711 Pennsylvania Ave, Troy, OH 45374, or equivalent). Chill all cutter parts before preparation of each sample.

Food processor—First Action 1990.—Benchtop model, 110/120 V, 60 Hz, 1 hp, 7.5 A, 1725 rpm, fan-cooled motor, 4 qt bowl; Model R4Y, Robot Coupe, USA, Inc., Jackson, MS, or equivalent. (*Caution*: Do not remove cutter bowl lid or cutter bowl from base until motor has come to full stop. Do not put hand, finger, or any object into bowl while motor is running. Unplug appliance before servicing or cleaning.)

Precut up to 2 lb sample to maximum dimension ≤2 in., and transfer to bowl for processing. Include any separated liquid. Process 30 s, then wipe down inner side wall and bottom of bowl with spatula (use household plastic or rubber spatula with ca 2 in. by 4 in. straight-edge blade) and transfer gathered material to body of sample. Continue processing another 30 s and wipe down as before. Repeat sequence to give total of 2 min processing and 3 wipe downs.

Take particular care with certain meat types such as ground beef to assure uniform distribution of fat and connective tissue. At each wipe-down interval, reincorporate these into sample by using spatula to remove fat from inside surfaces of bowl and connective tissue from around blades. If sample consolidates as ball above blades, interrupt processing and press sample to bottom of bowl with spatula before continuing.

Ref.: JAOAC **72**, 77(1989).

(b) *Canned meats*.—Pass entire contents of can through food chopper, as in (a).

(c) *Sausages*.—Remove from casings and pass through food chopper, as in (a).

Dry portions of samples of (a), (b), and (c) not needed for immediate analysis, either *in vacuo* <60° or by evaporating on steam bath 2 or 3 times with alcohol. Extract fat from dried product with petroleum ether (bp <60°) and let petroleum ether evaporate spontaneously, finally expelling last traces by heating short time on steam bath. Do not heat sample or separated fat longer than necessary because of tendency to decompose.

Reserve fat in cool place for examination as in chapter on oils and fats and complete examination before it becomes rancid.

Reference: JAOAC **66,** 579(1983).

Using either top-load or triple-beam balance with 0.1 g sensitivity, tare Foss-let cup after setting brass hammer on its spindle. To analyze products containing ≤60% fat, weigh 45.0 g sample into cup; for products containing >60% fat, weigh 22.5 g. Add ca 80 g Plaster of Paris (or ca 60 g anhydrous $CaSO_4$). Dispense 120 mL C_2Cl_4 into cup. Press cover onto cup and install in orbital shaker. Set shaker timer for 2 min and turn unit on. While extraction proceeds, assemble pressure filtration device by placing into perforated base 7 cm filter paper to produce clear filtrate free of moisture droplets; for very wet samples, first place high retention paper, Whatman No. 50 or equivalent, and then phase separating paper, Whatman No. 1PS or equivalent. After 2 min extraction, remove cup from shaker, lift cover, and remove brass hammer from cup. Immerse cup in ice-H_2O bath ca 0.4 min while stirring contents with thermometer to cool contents from 47–52° to ca 40°. Wipe H_2O from outer surface of cup and pour contents into assembled filter. Place piston at top of filtration device and slowly press extract through measuring system. Depress drain valve button when extract appears in overflow tube and let chamber drain; then release valve button. Repeat filling and draining 2 more times until 40–50 mL extract has flowed through, retaining final 10 mL extract in measuring chamber. Remove filtration device, slide viewing lens into position, rotate control of readout potentiometer clockwise until hydrometer rises, and record reading. Establish that extract is at chamber temperature by repeating reading 3–4 times. Average readings and convert into % fat by means of conversion chart. (Multiply chart % fat by 2 if 22.5 g portion of high-fat sample was taken.)

References: JAOAC **58,** 1182(1975); **60,** 853(1977); **68,** 240(1985).

18.3 985.15—Fat (Crude) in Meat and Poultry Products
Rapid Microwave-Solvent Extraction Method
First Action 1985

A. Principle

Fat is extracted with CH_2Cl_2 from weighed, microwave-dried sample in automatic extraction system. Extract is filtered, and residue is redried to remove remaining solvent and moisture. Redried residue is weighed; weight loss due to extraction is converted to percent fat by microprocessor for digital readout.

B. Reagents and Apparatus

(**a**) *Automated solvent extractor.*—Enclosed, self-contained, thermostatically controlled fat extraction and solvent recovery system with 0.5 mg fat sensitivity and 0–100% fat measurement range (CEM Corp., PO Box 200, Matthews, NC 28106), or equivalent.

(**b**) *Methylene chloride.*—Reagent grade (Fisher Scientific Co., No. D-37), or equivalent.

(**c**) *Glass fiber pads.*—9.8 × 10.2 cm rectangular and 11 cm round (CEM Corp.), or equivalent.

(**d**) *Microwave moisture analyzer.*—0.2 mg H_2O sensitivity, moisture/solids range of 0.1–99.9%, 0.01% resolution. Includes automatic tare electronic balance, microwave drying system, and microprocessor digital computer control. Electronic balance pan is located inside drying chamber. (Balance sensitivity: 0.2 mg at 15 g capacity or 1.0 mg at 40 g capacity [CEM Corp., or equivalent].)

C. Determination

Prepare samples as in **983.18** (*see* 18.2). Place 2 rectangular and one round glass fiber pad on balance pan inside microwave moisture analyzer, and tare. Remove rectangular pads and evenly spread ca 4 g well mixed sample onto rough side of one pad, cover with second pad, and place together with round pad on balance pan. Dry sample with pads 3–5 min at 80–100% power, depending on product type. At end of drying cycle, remove dried sample and pads from balance pan. Fold rectangular pads, with dried sample, in half and place in automated solvent extractor chamber. Place round pad in recessed area at top of extractor chamber, close and latch lid. Start extraction cycle (sample and rectangular pads are blended at this time with sufficient CH_2Cl_2 to extract fat). After completion of extraction cycle, remove round pad with residue, and place on balance pan in microwave moisture analyzer. Redry pad and residue to constant weight (ca 30 s at 80–100% power) to remove residual solvent or moisture. Weight loss due to solvent extraction is converted to % fat by microprocessor and displayed on digital readout panel.

Certain product classes require addition of adjustment factors to readout for accurate results, as follows: fresh meats, pre-blends, emulsions, cured/cooked meats, factor = 0.40; cooked sausages, factor = 0.80.

Reference: JAOAC **68,** 876(1985).

18.4　　　　920.39B,C—Fat (Crude) or Ether Extract in Animal Feed
Final Action

B. Reagent

Anhydrous ether.—Wash commercial ether with 2 or 3 portions H_2O, add solid NaOH or KOH, and let stand until most of H_2O is abstracted from the ether. Decant into dry bottle, add small pieces of carefully cleaned metallic Na, and let stand until H evolution ceases. Keep ether, thus dehydrated, over metallic Na in loosely stoppered bottles. (*Caution: See Appendix* for safety notes on sodium metal and diethyl ether.)

C. Determination

(Large amounts H_2O-soluble components such as carbohydrates, urea, lactic acid, glycerol, and others may interfere with extraction of fat; if present, extract 2 g sample on small paper in funnel with five 20 mL portions H_2O prior to drying for ether extraction. *Caution: See Appendix* for safety notes on monitoring equipment, distillation, and diethyl ether.)

Extract ca 2 g sample, dried as in **934.01** or **920.36** [*see Official Methods of Analysis* (1975) 12th Ed., secs **7.006–7.007**], with anhydrous ether. Use thimble with porosity permitting rapid passage of ether. Extraction period may vary from 4 h at condensation rate of 5–6 drops/s to 16 h at 2–3 drops/s. Dry extract 30 min at 100°, cool, and weigh.

934.01 (Moisture in Animal Feed, Drying in Vacuo at 95–100°)

Dry amount sample containing ca 2 g dry material to constant weight at 95–100° under pressure ≤ 100 mm Hg (ca 5 h). For feeds with high molasses content, use temperature $\leq 70°$ and pressure ≤ 50 mm Hg. Use covered Al dish ≥ 50 mm diameter and ≤ 40 mm deep. Report loss in weight as moisture.

References: JAOAC **17,** 68(1934); **51,** 467(1968); **60,** 322(1977).

References: JAOAC **64,** 351(1981); **65,** 289(1982).

18.5   945.18A—Cereal Adjuncts
Final Action

A. Crude Fat or Ether Extract
  See **920.39B** (*see* 18.4).

18.6   945.38F—Grains
Final Action

F. Crude Fat or Ether Extract
  See **920.39C** (*see* 18.4).

18.7   933.05—Fat in Cheese
Final Action
IDF-ISO-AOAC Method

Weigh, to nearest mg, ca 1 g prepared sample, **955.30**, into small tall-form beaker; add 9 mL H_2O and, if desired, 1 mL NH_4OH. Mix until smooth; then warm mixture at low heat until casein is well softened. If NH_4OH was used, neutralize with HCl, using litmus as indicator. Add 10 mL HCl and few glass beads or other inert material, previously digested with HCl, to prevent bumping, cover with watch glass, and boil gently 5 min, or place beaker in boiling H_2O bath 20 min. Cool solution; transfer to fat-extraction flask or tube; rinse beaker successively with 10 mL alcohol, 25 mL ether, and 25 mL petroleum ether (boiling range 30–60°); transfer rinsings to flask; and mix thoroughly after adding each reagent. Proceed as in **905.02** (*see* 18.8), beginning "Centrifuge flask. . . ." Difference between duplicate determinations obtained simultaneously by same analyst should be ≤0.2 g fat/100 g product.

955.30 (Cheese, Preparation of Samples)
Cut wedge sample into strips and pass 3 times through food chopper. Grind plugs in food chopper (preferable method), or cut or shred very finely and mix thoroughly.

With creamed cottage and similar cheeses, place 300–600 g sample at <15° in 1 L (1 qt) cup of high-speed blender and blend for minimum time (2–5 min) required to obtain homogeneous mixture. Final temperature should be ≤25°. This may require stopping blender frequently after channeling and spooning cheese back into blades until blending action starts. (Use of variable transformer in line to permit slow speed at first minimizes channeling when speed is increased later.)

References: JAOAC 16, 584(1933); **31,** 300(1948); **32,** 303(1949); **52,** 240(1969).

18.8

905.02—Fat in Milk
Roese-Gottlieb Method
Final Action
Reference Method 1973
IDF-ISO-AOAC Method

(Details of this method comply with method which has been agreed upon by International Dairy Federation, International Organization for Standardization, and AOAC for publication by each organization and which is published as international standard in *FAO/WHO Code of Principles Concerning Milk and Milk Products and Associated Standards.*)

(*Caution: See Appendix* for safety notes on distillation, flammable solvents, diethyl ether, and petroleum ether.)

Prepare as in **925.21** and weigh, to nearest mg, ca 10 g sample into fat-extraction flask or tube. Add 1.25 mL NH_4OH (2 mL if sample is sour) and mix thoroughly. Add 10 mL alcohol and mix well. Add 25 mL ether (all ether must be peroxide-free), stopper with cork or stopper (synthetic rubber) unaffected by usual fat solvents, and shake very vigorously 1 min. Cool, if necessary; add 25 mL petroleum ether (boiling range 30–60°) and repeat vigorous shaking. Centrifuge flask at ca 600 rpm or let it stand until upper liquid is practically clear. Decant ether solution into suitable flask or metal dish. Wash lip and stopper of extraction flask or tube with mixture of equal parts of the 2 ethers and add washings to weighing flask or dish. Repeat extraction of liquid remaining in flask or tube twice, using 15 mL of each solvent each time and adding H_2O if necessary, but omitting rinsing with mixed solvents after final extraction. (Third extraction is not necessary with skim milk.)

> **925.21** (Preparation of Milk Sample)
>
> Bring sample to ca 20°, mix until homogeneous by pouring into clean receptacle and back repeatedly, and promptly weigh or measure test portion. If lumps of cream do not disperse, warm sample in H_2O bath to ca 38° and keep mixing until homogeneous, using policeman, if necessary, to reincorporate any cream adhering to container or stopper. Where practical and fat remains dispersed, cool warmed samples to ca 20° before transferring test portion.
>
> When Babcock method, **989.04C** (*see* 18.12), is used, adjust both fresh and composite samples to ca 38°, mix until homogeneous as above, and immediately pipet portions into test bottles.

Evaporate solvents completely on steam bath at temperature that does not cause spattering or bumping (boiling chips may be added). Dry fat to constant weight in oven at 102 ± 2° or vacuum oven at 70–75° under pressure <50 mm Hg (6.7 kPa). Weigh cooled flask or dish, without wiping immediately before weighing. Remove fat completely from container with 15–25 mL warm petroleum ether, dry, and weigh as before. Loss in weight = weight fat. Correct weight fat by blank determination on reagents used. If blank is >0.5 mg, purify or replace reagents. Difference between duplicate determinations obtained simultaneously by same analyst should be ≤0.03 g fat/100 g product.

References: Z. Nahr. Genussm. **9**, 531(1905). JAOAC **34**, 237(1951); **52**, 235(1969).

18.9   **989.05—Fat in Milk**
Modified Mojonnier
Ether Extraction Method
First Action 1989

(*Caution: See Appendix* for safety notes on distillation, ammonium hydroxide, flammable solvents, diethyl ether, ethanol, peroxides, and petroleum ether.)

A. Principle

Fat is extracted with mixture of ethers from known weight of milk. Ether extract is decanted into dry weighing dish, and ether is evaporated. Extracted fat is dried to constant weight. Result is expressed as % fat by weight.

B. Apparatus

(a) *Flask.*—Mojonnier-style ether extraction flask with volume of 21–23 mL in lower bulb plus neck at bottom of flask. Flask should have smooth, round opening at top that will seal when closed with cork (Kimble).

(b) *Weighing dishes.*—Metal, 8.5–9.5 cm diameter and 4.5–5.5 cm tall; or 250 mL glass beakers.

(c) *Calibration weights.*—Class S, standard calibration weights to verify balance accuracy within weight range to be used for weighing empty flasks and flask plus sample and weighing empty dishes and dish plus fat.

(d) *Analytical balance.*—To read to nearest 0.0001 g. Accuracy on verification within 0.0002 g. Check periodically and whenever balance is moved or cleaned. Keep record of balance calibration checks.

(e) *Desiccator.*—Room temperature. For cooling weighing dishes after preliminary and final drying. Use coarse desiccant (mesh size 6–16) that contains minimum of fine particles and that changes color when moisture is absorbed.

(f) *Tongs.*—For handling weighing dishes.

(g) *Hot plate.*—Steam bath or other heating device. For evaporation of ether at ≤100°. Carry out evaporation in hood.

(h) *Corks.*—High quality natural cork stoppers (size 5) for flasks. Soak corks in H_2O several hours to improve seal.

(i) *Vacuum or forced air oven.*—Vacuum oven capable of maintaining temperature of 70–75° at 50.8 cm (20 in.) of vacuum, or forced air oven capable of maintaining temperature of 100 ± 1°.

(j) *Water bath for tempering milk samples prior to weighing.*—With thermometer and device to maintain milk temperature of 38 ± 1°.

C. Reagents

(a) *Ethyl ether.*—ACS grade, peroxide free. No residue on evaporation.

(b) *Petroleum ether.*—ACS grade, boiling range 30–60°. No residue on evaporation.

(c) *Ammonium hydroxide.*—Concentrated, ACS grade, specific gravity 0.9.

(d) *Ethyl alcohol.*—95%. No residue on evaporation.

(e) *Distilled water.*—Free of oil and mineral residue.

(f) *Phenolphthalein indicator.*—0.5% (weight/volume) in EtOH.

D. Determination

(a) *Sample preparation.*—Prepare by tempering milk to 38° as in **925.21** (*see* 18.8). Weigh empty flask with clean, dry cork stopper. Remove stopper. Pipet ca 10 g milk into flask. Place stopper in flask. Weigh to nearest 0.1 mg. Check balance zero between samples.

(b) *Weighing dish preparation.*—Number clean weighing dishes and predry under same conditions that will be used for final drying after fat extraction. Be sure that all surfaces where weighing dishes will be placed (i.e., hot plate, desiccator, etc.) are clean and free of particulates. At end of oven drying, place pans in room temperature desiccator and cool to room temperature. On same day as fat extraction (c), weigh dishes to nearest 0.1 mg and record weights. Check balance zero after weighing each pan. Protect weighed pans from contamination with extraneous matter.

(c) *Fat extraction.*—To sample in flask add 1.5 mL NH_4OH and mix thoroughly. NH_4OH neutralizes any acid present and dissolves casein. Add 3 drops of phenolphthalein indicator to help sharpen visual appearance of interface between ether and aqueous layers during extraction. Add 10 mL ethyl alcohol, stopper with H_2O-soaked cork, and shake flask 15 s. For first extraction, add 25 mL ethyl ether, stopper with cork, and shake flask very vigorously 1 min, releasing built-up pressure by loosening stopper as necessary. Add 25 mL petroleum ether, stopper with cork, and repeat vigorous shaking for 1 min. Centrifuge flasks at ca 600 rpm for ≥30 s to obtain clean separation of aqueous (bright pink) and ether phases. Decant ether solution into suitable weighing dish prepared as in (b). When ether solution is decanted into dishes, be careful not to pour over any suspended solids or aqueous phase into weighing dish. Ether can be evaporated at ≤100° from dishes while conducting second extraction.

For second extraction, add 5 mL ethyl alcohol, stopper with cork, and shake vigorously 15 s. Next, add 15 mL ethyl ether, replace cork, and shake flask vigorously 1 min. Add 15 mL petroleum ether, stopper with cork, and repeat vigorous shaking for 1 min. Centrifuge flasks at ca 600 rpm for ≥30 s to obtain clean separation of aqueous (bright pink) and ether phases. If interface is below neck of flask, add H_2O to bring level ca half way up neck. Add H_2O slowly down inside surface of flask so that there is minimum disturbance of separation. Decant ether solution for second extraction into same weighing dish used for first extraction.

For third extraction, omit addition of ethyl alcohol and repeat procedure used for second extraction. Completely evaporate solvents in hood on hot plate at ≤100° (avoid spattering). Dry extracted fat plus weighing dish to constant weight in forced air oven at 100° ± 1° (≥30 min) or in vacuum oven at 70–75° at >0.8 cm (20 in.) of vacuum for ≥7 min. Remove weighing dishes from oven and place in desiccator to cool to room temperature. Record weight of each weighing dish plus fat.

Run pair of reagent blanks each day tests are conducted. To run reagent blank, replace milk sample with 10 mL H_2O and run test as normal. Record weight of any dry residue collected and use value in calculation. Reagent blank should be <0.0020 g residue. If reagent blanks for set of samples are negative use negative number in calculation. (*Note*: To subtract negative number [average weight blank residue] in equation below, add it to [{weight dish + fat} − weight dish].) Negative blank usually indicates that dishes were not completely dry at start of determination or that balance calibration shifted between weighing of empty pans and pans plus fat. Cause of negative blanks should be identified and corrected.

E. Calculation

Fat, % = 100 × {[(weight dish + fat) − (weight dish)] − (average weight blank residue)}/ weight milk

Maximum recommended difference between duplicates is <0.03% fat.

At 3.6% fat:

$$s_r = 0.015\% \qquad\qquad RSD_R = 0.512\%$$

$$s_R = 0.020\% \qquad r \text{ value} = 0.044\%$$
$$RSD_r = 0.396\% \qquad R \text{ value} = 0.056\%$$

Reference: JAOAC **71**, 898(1988).

18.10   938.06—Fat in Butter

A. Indirect Method
   —Final Action

IDF-ISO-AOAC Method

Take up dry butter obtained in moisture determination in which no absorbent was used, **920.116**, by macerating with 15 mL absolute ether or petroleum ether; transfer to weighed gooch or fritted glass crucible (16–40 μm) with aid of wash bottle filled with the solvent; and wash free from fat with 100 mL solvent. (Pass last 25 mL solvent through crucible without suction.) Dry crucible and contents at 100° to constant weight. Repeat washing with 25 mL solvent and dry to constant weight. Repeat operation until there is no loss in weight due to washing.

$$\% \text{ Fat} = 100 - (\% \text{ moisture} + \% \text{ residue})$$

I. **920.116** (Moisture in Butter)
IDF-ISO-AOAC Method
Weigh 1.5–2.5 g prepared sample of salted butter or 2–6 g unsalted butter, **938.05**, into weighed flat-bottom dish ≥ 5 cm diameter and dry to constant weight in oven kept at temperature of boiling H_2O. Clean, dry sand may be used if fat is not to be determined in residue by **938.06**.

II. **938.05** (Butter, Preparation of Sample)
Soften entire sample in sample container, **970.29C**, by warming in H_2O bath kept at as low temperature as practicable, $\leq 39°$. Avoid overheating, which causes visible separation of curd. Shake frequently during softening process to reincorporate any separated fat, and observe fluidity of sample. Optimum consistency is attained when emulsion is still intact but fluid enough to reveal sample level almost immediately. Remove from bath and frequently shake vigorously or place sample container in mechanical shaking machine that simulates hand shaking, with arm 23 cm (9″) long, set to oscillate at 425 ± 25 times/min through arc of 4.5 cm (1.75″). Continue shaking until sample cools to thick, creamy consistency and sample level can no longer readily be seen. Promptly weigh portion for analysis.
References: JAOAC **21**, 361(1938); **35**, 194(1952); **42**, 36(1959).

III. **970.29C** (Sampling of Butter)
C. Sample Containers
Use wide-mouth jars conforming to **968.12C(b)**. Fill jar $\geq \frac{1}{2}$ full and hermetically seal. Immediately after closure, wrap jars in paper or store in dark, if examination so requires. Do not let butter come into contact with paper or any H_2O or fat absorbing or trapping surface.

IV. **968.12** (Sampling of Dairy Products)

B. Technical Instructions

(**b**) *Sampling for bacteriological purposes.*—Clean and treat equipment by one of following methods: (*1*) Expose to hot air 2 h at 170° (may be stored if kept under sterile conditions). (*2*) Autoclave 15–20 min at 120° (may be stored if kept under sterile conditions). (*3*) Expose to steam 1 h at 100° (use equipment same day). (*4*) Immerse in H_2O 1 min at 100° (use equipment immediately). (*5*) Immerse in 70% alcohol and flame to burn off alcohol immediately before use. (*6*) Expose to hydrocarbon (propane, butane) torch flame so that all working surfaces contact flame immediately before use.

Choice of treatment depends on nature, shape, and size of equipment and on conditions of sampling. Sterilize wherever possible by method (*1*) or (*2*).

Methods (*3*), (*4*), (*5*), and (*6*) are regarded as secondary methods only.

C. Sample Containers

(**a**) *For liquids.*—Use clean and dry containers of suitable waterproof, greaseproof material (glass, stainless metal, suitable plastic material) of quality suitable for sterilization by **968.12B(b)**, if necessary, and of suitable shape and capacity for material to be sampled (as defined in each particular case).

Securely close containers either with suitable rubber or plastic stopper or by screw cap of metal or plastic having, if necessary, liquid-tight plastic liner which is insoluble, nonabsorbent, and greaseproof, and which will not influence odor, flavor, or composition of milk products.

If rubber stoppers are used, cover with nonabsorbent, flavorless material (such as suitable plastic) before pressing into sample container. Suitable plastic bags may also be used.

(**b**) *For solids or semisolids.*—Use clean and dry wide-mouth, cylindrical receptacles of suitable waterproof, greaseproof material (glass, stainless metal, suitable plastic material) of quality suitable for sterilization by **968.12B(b)**, if necessary, and of capacity suited to size of sample to be taken (as defined in each particular case). Make air-tight as in (**a**). Suitable plastic bags may also be used.

B. Direct Method
—Final Action
—Repealed First Action 1989

From dry butter obtained in determination of moisture either with or without use of absorbent, extract fat with anhydrous, alcohol-free ether or petroleum ether (bp <65°), receiving solution in weighed flask. Evaporate solvent and dry extract to constant weight at 100°.

References: JAOAC **21**, 361(1938); **35**, 194(1952); **57**, 428(1979).

18.11   920.111—Fat in Cream
Final Action
IDF-ISO-AOAC Method

A. *Roese-Gottlieb Method*

Using 5 g sample and diluting with H_2O to ca 10.5 mL, proceed as in **905.02** (*see* 18.8), beginning "Add 1.25 mL NH_4OH ... "

Babcock Method

B. *Apparatus*

(**a**) *Test bottles.*—Standard Babcock cream-test bottles are as follows:

(*1*) *50%, 9 g, short-neck, 6" cream-test bottle.*—Total height 150–165 mm (5.9–6.5"). Bottom of bottle must be flat, and axis of neck vertical when bottle stands on level surface. Amount of cream for bottle is 9 g.

Bulb.—Capacity of bulb to junction with neck is ≥45 mL. Bulb may be either cylindrical or conical. If cylindrical, od must be 34–36 mm; if conical, od of base must be 31–33 mm, and maximum diameter, 35–37 mm.

Neck.—Cylindrical and of uniform diameter from ≥5 mm below lowest graduation mark to ≥5 mm above highest. Top of neck is flared to diameter of ≥15 mm. Graduated portion of neck is ≥63.5 mm long. Total % graduation is 50. Graduations shall represent 5, 1, and ½%, respectively, from 0.0 to 50%. 5% graduations must extend at least half-way around neck to right; ½% graduations must be ≥3 mm long; and 1% graduations must be intermediate in length between 5% and ½% graduations and project 2 mm to left of 1/2% graduations. Each 5% graduation must be numbered (thus: 0, 5, 10, . . . 45, 50), number being placed to left of scale. Capacity of neck for each whole % on scale must be 0.1 mL. Maximum error in total graduation or any part thereof must not exceed volume of smallest unit of graduation.

(*2*) *50%, 9 g, long-neck, 9" cream-test bottle.*— Same specifications as in (*1*), except that total height of this bottle is 210–229 mm (8.25–9.0") and graduated portion of neck has length of ≥120 mm.

(*3*) *50%, 18 g, long-neck, 9" cream-test bottle.*— Same specifications as in (*2*), except that amount of cream for this bottle is 18 g.

Each bottle must bear on top of neck above graduations, in plain legible characters, mark denoting weight sample to be used, *viz.,* "9 g" or "18 g," as case may be.

Each bottle must be constructed so as to withstand stress to which it will be subjected in centrifuge.

(*4*) *Testing.*—Proceed as in **989.04B(a)**(*3*) (*see* 18.12).

(**b**) *Water bath for cream samples.*—Provided with thermometer and control to maintain temperature of 38°.

(**c**) *Cream weighing scales.*—With sensibility reciprocal of 30 mg, *i.e.,* addition of 30 mg to either pan of scale, when loaded to capacity, causes deflection of ≥1 subdivision of graduation. Set scales level upon support and protect from drafts.

(**d**) *Weights.*—9 g and 18 g, respectively, and plainly marked "9 g" or "18 g," as case may be. Must be made of material capable of resisting corrosion or other injury, and preferably of low squat shape, with rounded edges. Verify them at frequent intervals by comparison with standardized weights.

(**e**) *Acid measure.*—See **989.04B(c)**.

(**f**) *Centrifuge or "tester."*—See **989.04B(d)**.

(g) *Dividers or calipers.—See* **989.04B(e)**.

(h) *Water bath for test bottles.—See* **989.04B(f)**.

C. Determination

Weigh 9 g prepared sample, **925.26**, directly into 9 g cream-test bottle, or 18 g into 18 g bottle, and proceed by one of following methods.

> **925.26** (Cream, Preparation of Sample)
>
> Immediately before withdrawing test portions, mix sample by shaking, pouring, or stirring (or use hand homogenizer) until it pours readily and uniform emulsion forms. If sample is very thick, warm to 30–35° and mix. In case lumps of butter have separated, heat sample to ca 38° by placing in warm H_2O bath. (Temperature appreciably $>38°$ may cause fat to "oil off," especially in case of thin cream.) Thoroughly mix portions for analysis and weigh immediately. (In commercial testing for fat by Babcock method, it may be advisable to warm all samples to ca 38° in H_2O bath previous to mixing.)

(a) *Method 1.*—After weighing cream into test bottle, add 8–12 mL H_2SO_4 (specific gravity 1.82–1.83 at 20°) to 9 g bottle; or 14–17 mL to 18 g bottle; or add acid until mixture of cream and acid, after shaking, is chocolate-brown. Shake until all lumps completely disappear and add 5–10 mL soft H_2O at 60° or above. Transfer bottle to centrifuge, counterbalance it, and after proper speed is reached, centrifuge 5 min. Fill bottle to neck with hot H_2O and centrifuge 2 min. Add hot H_2O until liquid column approaches top graduation of scale; then centrifuge 1 min longer at 55–60°. Adjust temperature as in **989.04C**, and with aid of dividers or calipers measure fat column, in terms of % by weight, from lower surface to bottom of upper meniscus.

(b) *Method 2.—For 9 g bottle only.*—After weighing cream into test bottle, add 9 mL soft H_2O and mix thoroughly; add ca 17.5 mL of the H_2SO_4 and shake until all lumps completely disappear. Transfer bottle to centrifuge, counterbalance it, and after proper speed is reached, centrifuge 5 min. Fill bottle to neck with hot H_2O and centrifuge 2 min. Add hot H_2O until liquid column approaches top graduation of scale, and centrifuge 1 min longer at 55–60°. Adjust temperature and measure fat column as in (a).

Whichever method is followed, fat column, at time of reading, should be translucent, golden yellow to amber, and free from visible suspended particles. Reject all tests in which fat column is milky or shows presence of curd or of charred matter, or in which reading is indistinct or uncertain; repeat test, adjusting amount of H_2SO_4 added.

If desired, add glymol or pure white mineral oil (specific gravity ≤ 0.85 at 20°). Introduce only few drops into bottle just before reading is made, letting it flow down inside of neck. For purpose of measurement, surface separating glymol and fat is regarded as representing upper limit of column. Oil-soluble artificial color may be added to the white mineral oil.

18.12   **989.04—Fat in Raw Milk**
Babcock Method
Final Action 1920
Revised First Action 1989

(*Caution: See Appendix* for safety notes on centrifuges, sulfuric acid, and mercury.)

A. *Principle*

Known weight of milk is delivered into Babcock bottle, and heat generated by addition of H_2SO_4 releases fat. Centrifuging and H_2O addition isolates fat for quantitation in graduated portion of Babcock bottle. Result is expressed as % fat by weight.

B. *Apparatus*

(**a**) *Standard Babcock milk-test bottle.*—8%, 18 g, milk-test bottle, total height 160–170 mm (6.3–6.7 in.). Bottom of bottle is flat, and axis of neck is vertical when bottle stands on level surface. Quantity of milk for bottle is 18 g. (Available from Kimble).

(*1*) *Bulb.*—Capacity of bulb to junction with neck must be ≥45 mL. Shape of bulb may be either cylindrical or conical. If cylindrical, od of base must be between 34 and 36 mm; if conical, od of base must be between 31 and 33 mm, and maximum diameter must be between 35 and 37 mm.

(*2*) *Neck.*—Cylindrical and of uniform diameter from ≥5 mm below lowest graduation mark to ≥5 mm above highest mark. Top of neck is flared to diameter of ≥10 mm. Graduated portion of neck has length ≥75.0 mm and is graduated in whole %, 0.5%, and 0.1%, respectively, from 0.0 to 8.0%. Graduations may be etched, with black or dark pigment annealed to graduation, or may be unetched black or dark lines permanently annealed to glass. Graduation line widths ≤0.2 mm. Tenths % graduations are ≥3 mm long; 0.5% graduations are ≥4 mm long and project 1 mm to left; and whole % graduations extend at least halfway around neck to right but no more than three-quarters of way around and project ≥2 mm to left of tenths % graduations. Each whole % graduation is numbered, with number placed to left of scale. Vertical line may be etched and annealed with black or dark pigment or may be an unetched black or dark line permanently annealed to glass located 1 mm to right of 0.1% graduation marks and extends ≥1 mm above 8% line and ≥1 mm below 0% line. Zero line must be etched and annealed with black or dark pigment, and must be ≤0.2 mm wide. Capacity of neck for each whole % on scale is 0.200 mL. Maximum error of total graduation or any part thereof must not exceed 0.008 mL (0.04% fat).

Each bottle must be constructed so as to withstand stress to which it will be subjected in centrifuge.

(*3*) *Testing.*—Accuracy of each bottle shall be determined. Bottle calibration accuracy is determined by placing bottle upside down on Babcock bottle calibration apparatus (modified Nafis tester) that is capable of delivering known volumes of Hg into Babcock bottle neck. Bottle calibration apparatus delivery is calibrated and volume of Hg contained between 8 and 4% (0.800 mL), 4 and 0% (0.800 mL), and 8 and 0% (1.600 mL) marks is determined. Accuracy of any bottle can also be determined by calibration with Hg (13.5471 g clean, dry Hg at 20° to be equal to 5% on scale of 18 g milk bottle and 10% on scale of 9 g cream bottle, **920.111B(a)** (*see* 18.11), bottle having been previously filled to 0 mark with Hg. Accuracy should be ≤ ±0.04% on scale of 18 g milk-test bottle. Calibrated bottles are available from Kimble.

(**b**) *Pipet.*—Standard milk pipet conforms to following specifications:

	mm
Total length	≤330
Od of suction tube	6–8
Length of suction tube	130
Od of delivery tube (must fit into bottle [**a**])	4.5–5.0
Length of delivery tube	100–120
Distance of graduation mark above bulb	15–45

Nozzle parallel with axis of pipet, but slightly constricted so as to discharge in 5–8 s when filled with H_2O.
Graduation, marked to contain 17.6 mL H_2O at 20° when bottom of meniscus coincides with mark on suction tube.
Maximum error in graduation, ≤0.05 mL.

To test pipet, place tip of pipet against firm rubber surface, clamp pipet in vertical position, and use buret (Class A—graduations ≤0.05 mL) to fill to pipet to graduation mark with H_2O (at 20°).

(**c**) *Acid measure.*— Device used to measure H_2SO_4 should deliver in range from 10 to 20 mL. Use device that can be set to consistently deliver appropriate amount of acid to obtain desired milk acid reaction temperature in *Determination.*

(**d**) *Centrifuge or "tester."*—Standard centrifuge, however driven, must be constructed throughout and so mounted as to be capable, when filled to capacity, of rotating at necessary speed with minimum vibration and without liability of causing injury or accident. Centrifuge must be heated, electric or otherwise, to temperature of 55–60° during centrifuging. It must be provided with speed indicator, permanently attached, if possible. Proper rate of rotation may be determined by reference to table below. Rotation speed with full centrifuge should be checked periodically with tachometer. "Diameter of wheel" means distance between inside bottoms of opposite cups measured through center of rotation of centrifuge wheel while cups are horizontally extended.

Diam. of wheel, in.	rpm
14	909
16	848
18	800
20	759
22	724
24	693

(**e**) *Dividers or calipers.*—For measuring fat column.
(**f**) *Water bath for test bottles.*—Provided with thermometer and device to maintain temperature of fat column at 57.5 ± 1°.
(**g**) *Water bath for tempering milk samples prior to pipetting.*—Provided with thermometer and device to maintain temperature of milk at 38 ± 1°.
(**h**) *Water bath for addition of water after 1st and 2nd centrifugation.*—Provided with thermometer, device to maintain temperature of soft H_2O at 59–61°, and device to deliver H_2O into Babcock bottles.
(**i**) *Bottle shaker.*—Variable speed and matched to maximum capacity of centrifuge.

(**j**) *Digital thermometer for measurement of milk-acid reaction temperature.*—To read to nearest degree in range of 100–120°. Use acid-resistant probe, with small diameter (≤0.5 mm) to ensure rapid response time. Length of probe should be such that its tip is ca 1 cm above bottom of bottle when fully inserted.
(**k**) *Reading light.*—As background when measuring fat columns. Light should be diffused (soft white color) and provide illumination from angles above and below level of fat column. Magnification device must be used to aid reading.

C. Determination

(**a**) *Sample preparation and temperature adjustment.*—With pipet, *Apparatus* (**b**), transfer 17.60 ± 0.05 mL prepared sample, at 38°, **925.21** (*see* 18.8), to milk-test bottle. Blow out milk in pipet tip ca 30 s after free outflow ceases. Adjust milk in test bottles to 20–22°. Adjust H_2SO_4 (sp gr 1.82–1.83 at 20°) to 20–22°. Pipet some additional milk samples for use as temperature control samples.

(**b**) *Measurement of milk-acid reaction temperature and determination of amount of H_2SO_4 to use.*—Prior to testing group of samples, determine correct amount of acid to be used by measuring milk-acid reaction temperature. Start by adding 17.5 mL 20–22° Babcock H_2SO_4 to bottle containing 18 g milk of same temperature; add 17.5 mL portion of acid in 1 delivery that washes all traces of milk into bulb and cleanly layers acid under milk. Fully insert digital thermometer probe down bottle neck, and immediately shake by hand rotation until all traces of curd disappear. Peak reaction temperature should be 108 ± 2°. Adjust amount of H_2SO_4 added until reaction temperature is within this range and fat column is translucent golden-yellow to amber. Amount of acid required may be different for different technicians and different batches of acid.

(**c**) *Testing milk samples.*—Add appropriate amount of H_2SO_4 (as determined in (**b**)) by delivering acid in 1 addition that washes all traces of milk into bulb and cleanly layers acid under milk. Immediately shake by hand rotation (as in (**b**)) until all traces of curd disappear. Place bottle in Babcock bottle shaker set at medium speed. Continue to add acid to all samples to be tested, and then shake full set 1 additional min. Temperature of milk plus acid in first bottle should not be less than 60° at time bottles are transferred to centrifuge. Place bottles in heated centrifuge, counter-balance, and, after proper speed is reached, centrifuge 5 min. Add soft H_2O at 59–61° until bulb of bottle is filled. Centrifuge 2 min. Add soft H_2O at 59–61° until top of fat column approaches 7% mark of bottle calibration. Centrifuge 1 min longer at ca 60°. Transfer bottle to warm H_2O bath kept at 57.5 ± 1°, immerse bottle to level slightly above top of fat column, and leave until column is in equilibrium and lower fat surface assumes final convex form (≥5 min). Remove 1 bottle from bath, wipe it, and with aid of reading light and magnification (**k**), use dividers or calipers to quickly measure fat column (before it begins to cool and contract). Place caliper points in vertical line on neck of bottle, with 1 point at lowest surface of *lower* meniscus and other point at *top* of upper meniscus. Without changing distance between 2 points on calipers, move calipers down bottle neck until lower point rests in etched horizontal graduation mark at 0%. Place upper point of calipers against bottle graduation and read test in % by weight to nearest 0.05%. Repeat for each bottle.

Fat column, at time of measurement, should be translucent, golden-yellow or amber, and free from visible suspended particles. Reject all tests in which fat column is milky or shows presence of curd or charred matter, or in which meniscus is indistinct or distorted; repeat test, adjusting volume H_2SO_4 added to obtain proper color and milk-acid reaction temperature.

Maximum recommended difference between duplicates is 0.1% fat.
At 3.6% fat:

$s_r = 0.029$	$RSD_R = 1.014\%$
$s_R^1 = 0.037$	r value $= 0.081\%$
$RSD_r = 0.742\%$	R value[1] $= 0.104\%$

[1]Using regression equations for milk containing 3.6% fat:

$$s_R = (0.0080 \times 3.6\%) + 0.0080$$
$$R \text{ value} = (0.0227 \times 3.6\%) + 0.0226$$

D. Alternative Apparatus—First Action 1986

(a) *Gercock-style milkfat test bottle.*—5%, 162 ± 3 mm high. Bottom of bottle is flat, and axis of flat graduated tube is vertical when bottle stands on level surface. Quantity of milk charge is 18 g; 18 g is acid-etched and pigmented in clear space above 5% graduated line. Specifications:

(1) *Bulb.*—Capacity of bulb to junction with neck must be ≥ 45 mL. Shape of bulb is cylindrical, 36 ± 0.5 mm od. Wall thickness 1.4 ± 0.2 mm. Word "Sealed", manufacturer's number or name, and matted marking spot must be legibly and permanently marked on surface.

(2) *Side filling tube.*—8 mm od, 0.1 mm wall thickness. To enter bulb below junction of bulb and neck of flat graduated tube along curved portion of bulb and with minimum angle extend to center of bulb and maintain vertical axis for 40 mm to height of 3 ± 2 mm above bottom of bottle.

(3) *Neck.*—Graduated portion of flat tube is uniform cross section ≥ 4 mm beyond extremes of graduated scale. Length of graduated portion of flat neck ≥ 75 mm. Graduated at whole %, 0.5%, 0.1%, and 0.05%. Graduations are acid-etched, with black pigment annealed to graduation. Graduation widths ≥ 0.2 mm. Each whole % and 0.5% line is numbered on left above line and these lines extend across flat surface. Smallest graduated line is ≥ 2.5 mm. Intermediate graduation line extends 1 ± 0.2 mm equally on both sides of smallest graduated line.

(4) *Vertical line.*—Vertical line is acid-etched and pigmented on right side of graduated flat tube. This line touches intermediate lines at their extreme right end and extends beyond 0 and 0.5% lines ≥ 3 mm. Width of vertical lines ≤ 0.2 mm.

(5) *Error.*—Maximum error of total graduation or any part thereof must not exceed volume of smallest unit of graduation ($=0.01$ mL).

(b) *Gercock-style pipet—raw milk.*—To conform to following specifications:

Total length	≤ 280 nm
Suction tube diameter	7 ± 0.2 mm od
Wall thickness	0.9 ± 0.04 mm
Suction tube length	130 mm
Delivery tube diameter	5 ± 0.2 mm od
Distance of graduation mark above bulb	15–45 mm
Length of nozzle	15–20 mm
Delivery time	5–8 s
Graduation	To deliver 17.6 mL at 20° when bottom of meniscus coincides with mark on suction tube
Maximum error	≤ 0.05 mL
Permanent markings on bulb	"Sealed," mfgr's No. or name, TD 17.6 mL at 20°, tolerance 0.05 mL, 5–8 s

(**c**) *Gercock-style pipet—processed milk.*—To conform to following specifications:

Total length	≥280 mm
Suction tube diameter	7 ± 0.2 mm od
Wall thickness	0.9 ± 0.04 mm
Length of suction tube	130 mm
Delivery tube diameter	5 ± 0.2 mm od
Distance of graduation mark above bulb	15–45 mm
Length of nozzle	15–20 mm
Delivery time	5–8 s
Graduation	To deliver 17.6 mL at 38° when bottom of meniscus coincides with mark on suction tube
Maximum error	≤0.05 mL
Permanent markings on bulb	"Sealed," mfgr's No. or name, TD 17.6 mL at 38°, tolerance 0.05 mL, 5–8 s

(Glassware is available from Forcoven Products, Inc., PO Box 1556, Humble, TX 77347.)

References: JAOAC **8,** 4(1924); **8,** 471,(1925); **56,** 1401(1973); **58,** 949(1975); **69,** 831(1986); **71,** 898(1988).

18.13   952.06—Fat in Ice Cream and Frozen Desserts
Roese-Gottlieb Method
Final Action
IDF-ISO-AOAC Method

Accurately weigh 4–5 g thoroughly mixed sample directly into fat-extraction flask or tube, using free-flowing pipet; dilute with H_2O to ca 10 mL, working sample into lower chamber and mix by shaking. Add 2 mL NH_4OH, mix thoroughly, and heat in H_2O bath 20 min at 60° with occasional shaking. Cool, and proceed as in **905.02** (*see* 18.8), beginning "Add 10 mL alcohol and mix well."

Reference: JAOAC **35,** 212(1952).

18.14   945.48—Evaporated Milk (Unsweetened)
Final Action

B. Preparation of Sample—Procedure
IDF-ISO-AOAC Method
(**a**) Temper unopened can in H_2O bath at ca 60°. Remove and vigorously shake can every 15 min. After 2 h remove can and let cool to room temperature. Remove entire lid and thoroughly mix by stirring contents in can with spoon or spatula. (If fat separates, sample is not properly prepared.)
References: JAOAC **28,** 207(1945); **52,** 239(1969).

G. Fat—Roese-Gottlieb Method

IDF-ISO-AOAC Method

Weigh, to nearest mg, 4–5 g undiluted sample, **945.48B(a)**, into fat-extraction flask or tube; dilute with ca 7 mL H_2O to ca 10.5 mL and shake with slight warming (40–50°) until sample is completely dispersed. Proceed as in **905.02** (*see* 18.8), beginning "Add 1.25 mL NH_4OH. . . ." Some evaporated milks may require centrifuging as long as 20 min at 600 rpm for complete separation of emulsion. Difference between duplicate determinations obtained simultaneously by same analyst should be ≤0.05 g fat/100 g product. References: JAOAC **28,** 207(1945); **52,** 239(1969).

18.15   932.06—Fat in Dried Milk
Roese-Gottlieb Method
Final Action
IDF-ISO-AOAC Method

A. Preparation of Solution

Proceed as in one of following methods:

(**a**) Quickly weigh to nearest mg ca 1 g well-mixed sample into small beaker. Add 1 mL H_2O and rub to smooth paste. Add 9 mL additional H_2O and 1–1.25 mL NH_4OH, and warm on steam bath. Transfer to fat-extraction flask or tube. Cool, and proceed as in **932.06B**, rinsing beaker successively with the alcohol and ethers used in first extraction.

(**b**) Quickly weigh to nearest mg ca 1 g well mixed sample and transfer to fat-extraction flask or tube. Add 10 mL H_2O and shake until homogeneous, warming if necessary. Add 1–1.25 mL NH_4OH and heat in H_2O bath 15 min at 60–70°, shaking occasionally. Cool, and proceed as in **932.06B**.

B. Determination

Add 10 mL alcohol to sample and mix. Extract with ether and petroleum ether as in **905.02** (*see* 18.8). For second extraction add 4 mL alcohol, and again extract as in **905.02**. With whole milk and cream powders make third extraction, using 15 mL of each solvent after adding, if necessary, enough H_2O to bring aqueous layer in tube to original volume.

      Difference between duplicate determinations obtained simultaneously by same analyst should be ≤0.2 g fat/100 g product.

References: JAOAC **15,** 524(1932); **52,** 240(1969).

18.16   948.15—Fat (Crude) in Seafood
Acid Hydrolysis Method
Final Action

A. Preparation of Sample

Prepare sample according to type of pack as in **937.07** and keep ground material in sealed jar. If jar has been chilled, let sample come to room temperature and shake jar so that any separated liquid is absorbed by fish. Open jar and stir contents with spatula, thoroughly scraping sides and lid so as to incorporate any separated liquid or fat.

937.07 (Fish and Marine Products, Treatment and Preparation of Sample)

To prevent loss of H_2O during preparation and subsequent handling, use samples as large as practicable. Keep ground material in container with air-tight cover. Begin all determinations as soon as practicable. If any delay occurs, chill sample to inhibit decomposition. In general, prepare sample of fish as it is usually prepared by consumer, by including skin and discarding bones, but subject to overall rule of edibility, e.g., inedible catfish skin is discarded; softened canned salmon bones are included; sardines are examined whole. Instructions may be modified in accordance with purpose of specific examination. Prepare samples for analysis as follows:

(a) *Fresh fish.*—Clean, scale, and eviscerate fish. In case of small fish ≤15 cm (6"), use 5–10 fish. In case of large fish, from each of ≥3 fish cut 3 cross-sectional slices 2.5 cm (1") thick, 1 slice from just back of pectoral fins, 1 slice halfway between first slice and vent, and 1 slice just back of vent. Remove bone. For intermediate-size fish, remove and discard heads, scales, tails, fins, guts, and inedible bones; fillet fish to obtain all flesh and skin from head to tail and from top of back to belly on both sides. For determination of fat and fat-soluble components, skin must be included, since many fish store large amounts of fat directly beneath skin.

Pass sample rapidly through meat chopper 3 times. Remove unground material from chopper after each grinding and mix thoroughly with ground material. Meat chopper should have holes as small as practicable (1.5–3 mm (1/16–1/8") diameter) and should not leak around handle end. As alternative for soft fish, high-speed blender may be used. Blend several minutes, stopping blender frequently to scrape down sides of cup.

(b) *Canned fish, shellfish, and other canned marine products.*—Place entire contents of can (meat and liquid) in blender and blend until homogeneous or grind 3 times through meat chopper. For large cans, drain meat 2 min on No. 8–12 sieve and collect all liquid. Determine weight of meat and volume of liquid. Recombine portion of each in proportionate amounts. Blend recombined portions in blender (or grind) until homogeneous.

(c) *Canned marine products packed in oil, sauce, broth, or water.*—Drain 2 min on No. 8 sieve. Prepare solid portion as in (b). Liquid may be analyzed separately, if desired, or reincorporated with solids. H_2O is usually discarded.

(d) *Fish packed in salt or brine.*—Drain and discard brine and rinse off adhering salt crystals with saturated NaCl solution. Drain again 2 min and proceed as in (a).

(e) *Dried smoked or dried salt fish.*—Proceed as in (a).

(f) *Frozen fish.*—Let thaw at room temperature, and discard draining. *(1) Fillet.*—Use entire piece. (2) *Whole fish.*—Proceed as in (a).

(g) *Shellfish other than oysters, clams, and scallops.*—If sample is received in shell, wash as in (h) and separate edible portions in usual way. Prepare edible portion for analysis as in (a).

(h) *Shell oysters, shell clams, and scallops.*—Wash shells in potable H_2O to remove all loose silt and dirt, and drain well. Shuck enough oysters or clams into clean dry container to yield ≥500 mL (1 pt) drained meats. Transfer shellfish meats to skimmer, **953.11A**, pick out pieces of shell, drain 2 min on skimmer, and proceed as in (**i**) or (**j**).

953.11A (Drained Liquid from Shucked Oysters)

A. Apparatus

Skimmer or strainer.—Flat-bottom metal pan or tray with ca 5 cm (2″) sides, with area of ≥1900 cm² (300 square inches) for each gal. of oysters to be poured on tray, and with perforations 0.6 cm (0.25″) diameter and 3.2 cm (1.25″) apart in square pattern, or perforations of equivalent area and distribution. Support skimmer over slightly larger solid tray so that liquid drains into solid tray.

(**i**) *Shucked clams or scallops.*—Prepare as in (**b**).

(**j**) *Shucked oysters.*—Blend meats, including liquid, 1–2 min in high-speed blender.

(**k**) *Breaded fish, raw or cooked.*—Do not remove breading or skin. Proceed as in (**a**).

References: JAOAC **20,** 70(1937); **21,** 85(1938); **35,** 218(1952); **36,** 608(1953); **38,** 194(1955); **59,** 312(1976).

B. Determination

Weigh 8 g well-mixed sample into 50 mL beaker and add 2 mL HCl. Using stirring rod with extra large flat end, break up coagulated lumps until mixture is homogeneous. Add additional 6 mL HCl, mix, cover with watch glass, and heat on steam bath 90 min, stirring occasionally with rod. Cool solution and transfer to Mojonnier fat-extraction flask. Rinse beaker and rod with 7 mL alcohol, add to extraction flask, and mix. Rinse beaker and rod with 25 mL ether, added in 3 portions; add rinsings to extraction flask, stopper with cork or stopper of synthetic rubber unaffected by usual fat solvents, and shake vigorously 1 min. Add 25 mL petroleum ether (bp <60°) to extraction flask and repeat vigorous shaking. Centrifuge Mojonnier flask 20 min at ca 600 rpm and proceed as in **922.06**, beginning "Draw off as much as possible of ether-fat solution. . . ."

Drying to constant weight takes ca 40 min for fish. Long heating periods may increase weight of fat. If centrifuge is not available, extraction can generally be made by letting Mojonnier flask stand until upper liquid is practically clear, then swirling flask and again letting stand until clear. If troublesome emulsion forms, let stand, pour off as much of ether-fat solution as possible, add 1–2 mL alcohol to Mojonnier flask, swirl, and again let mixture separate.

922.06 (Fat in Flour, Acid Hydrolysis Method)

(*Caution: See Appendix* for safety notes on distillation, diethyl ether, and petroleum ether.)

Place 2 g sample in 50 mL beaker, add 2 mL alcohol, and stir to moisten all particles to prevent lumping on addition of acid. Add 10 mL HCl (25 + 11), mix well, set beaker in H$_2$O bath held at 70–80°, and stir at frequent intervals during 30–40 min. Add 10 mL alcohol and cool.

Transfer mixture to Mojonnier fat-extraction apparatus. Rinse beaker into extraction tube with 25 mL ether, added in 3 portions; stopper flask (with glass, cork, Neoprene, or other synthetic rubber stopper not affected by solvents) and shake vigorously 1 min. Add 25 mL redistilled petroleum ether (bp <60°) and again shake vigorously 1 min. Let stand until upper liquid is practically clear, or centrifuge 20 min at ca 600 rpm.

Draw off as much as possible of ether-fat solution through filter consisting of cotton pledget packed just firmly enough in funnel stem to let ether pass freely into weighed 125 mL beaker-flask containing porcelain chips or broken glass. Before weighing beaker-flask, dry it and similar flask as counterpoise in oven at 100°; then let stand in air to constant weight.

Re-extract liquid remaining in tube twice, each time with only 15 mL of each ether. Shake well on addition of each ether. Draw off clear ether solutions through filter into same flask as before and wash tip of spigot, funnel, and end of funnel stem with few mL of mixture of the 2 ethers in equal volumes, free from suspended H_2O. Evaporate ethers slowly on steam bath; then dry fat in oven at 100° to constant weight (ca 90 min). Remove flask and counterpoise from oven, let stand in air to constant weight (ca 30 min), and weigh. (Owing to size of flask and nature of material, there is less error by cooling in air than by cooling in desiccator.) Correct this weight by blank determination on reagents used. Report as % fat by acid hydrolysis.

References: JAOAC **6,** 508(1922); **9,** 41, 429(1926).

Reference: JAOAC **31,** 334(1948).

18.17   986.25—Proximate Analysis of Milk-Based Infant Formula
First Action 1986
Final Action 1988

B. Fat

See **945.48B(a)** (*see* 18.14); **945.48G**; and **925.25**, using sample size 4–5 g.

I. **925.25** (Cream, Collection of Sample)
(*See* also **968.12** and **970.26**.)

Proceed as in **925.20**. Promptly analyze sample, preferably within 3 days after collection.

II. **925.20** (Collection of Milk Sample)
(*See* also **968.12** and **970.26**.)

Sample size necessary varies with analyses required. For usual analysis collect 250–500 mL (½–1 pt) sample; for fat determination only, collect 50–60 mL (ca 2 fl oz).

For bottled milk, collect ≥1 container as prepared for sale. Thoroughly mix bulk milk by pouring from one clean vessel into another 3 or 4 times or stir ≥30 s with utensil reaching to bottom of container. If cream has formed, detach all of it from sides of vessel and stir until liquid is evenly emulsified or use hand homogenizer.

Place in nonabsorbent, air-tight containers and keep cold, but above freezing temperature, until examined. When transporting samples, completely fill containers, stopper tightly, and identify. Tablets containing $HgCl_2$, $K_2Cr_2O_7$, or other suitable preservative, ≥0.5 g active ingredient per tablet for each 8 fl oz (250 mL) milk, but total weight of such tablet ≤1 g, or 36%

solution of HCHO, 0.1 mL (2 drops) per fl oz (30 mL), may be used unless presence of preservative is objectionable in physical or chemical tests to be made in addition to determination of fat. If phosphatase test is to be made, only $CHCl_3$ can be used as preservative, and stoppers must be of phenol-free material such as red rubber.

III. **970.26** (Sampling of Milk and Liquid Milk Products)
(Not applicable to evaporated and sweetened condensed milk)
A. Sampling Equipment
(a) *Plungers or agitators, necessary for mixing liquids in bulk.*—Use equipment, **970.27A(a)**, of sufficient area to produce adequate agitation of product and light enough in weight for operator to be able to move it rapidly through liquid. Mix contents of large vessels by mechanical stirring.

> **970.27A(a)** (Sampling of Condensed Milk and Evaporated Milk)
> *A. Bulk Containers (Barrels, Drums, Etc.)*
> (a) *Sampling equipment.*—Broad-bladed metal stirrer fitted with wide perforated disk at bottom and long enough to reach bottom of container.

(b) *Dipper of suitable size, for collecting sample.*— When sample is required for bacteriological examination, sterilize sampling equipment as in **968.12B(b)**.

B. Sampling Technique
Thoroughly mix all liquids by pouring from one vessel to another, by plunging, or by mechanical stirring. With large containers, continue agitation until liquid is thoroughly mixed. In case of cream, plunge sufficient number of times to ensure thorough mixing. Move submerged plunger from place to place with special care to avoid foaming, whipping, and churning. Take sample with dipper immediately after mixing. If obtaining perfect homogeneity presents difficulties, take sample from different positions of container totaling ≥200 mL.
(For additional instructions, *see* **925.20** for milk and **925.25** for cream.)

IV. **968.12** (Sampling of Dairy Products)
A. Instructions of Administrative Character
(This section is usually prescribed by specific regulatory agency. It is included for completeness.)
Sampling should be performed by authorized or sworn independent agent, properly trained in appropriate technique. Agent should be free from any infectious disease. If possible, representatives of parties concerned should be given opportunity to be present when sampling is performed.
Samples should be accompanied by report, signed by sworn or authorized sampling agent and countersigned by any witnesses present. Report should give particulars of place, date, and time of sampling; name and designation of agent and of any witnesses; precise method of sampling which is followed if this deviates from prescribed standard method; nature and number of units constituting consignment together with their batch code markings, where available; number of samples duly identified as to batches from which they are drawn; and place to which the samples will be sent.
When appropriate, report should also include any relevant conditions or circumstances, e.g., condition of packages and their surroundings, temperature and humidity of atmosphere,

method of sterilization of sampling equipment, whether preservative has been added to samples, and any other special information relating to material being sampled.

Each sample should be sealed and labeled to give nature of product, identification number, and any code markings of batch from which sample has been taken, date of sampling, and name and signature of sampling agent. When necessary, additional information may be required, for example, weight of sample and unit from which it was taken.

All samples should be taken at least in duplicate, one set being held, if necessary, in cold storage and put at disposal of second party as soon as possible. Precise method of sampling and weight or volume of product to be taken as sample vary with nature of product and purpose for which sampling is required and are defined for each particular case.

When previously agreed between parties, take additional sets of samples and retain for independent arbitration, if necessary. Send samples to testing laboratory immediately after sampling.

B. Technical Instructions

(*See* sampling equipment specifications laid down for each product to be sampled.)

(**a**) *Sampling for chemical purposes.*—Clean and dry all equipment.

(**b**) *Sampling for bacteriological purposes.*—Clean and treat equipment by one of following methods: (*1*) Expose to hot air 2 h at 170° (may be stored if kept under sterile conditions). (*2*) Autoclave 15–20 min at 120° (may be stored if kept under sterile conditions). (*3*) Expose to steam 1 h at 100° (use equipment same day). (*4*) Immerse in H_2O 1 min at 100° (use equipment immediately). (*5*) Immerse in 70% alcohol and flame to burn off alcohol immediately before use. (*6*) Expose to hydrocarbon (propane, butane) torch flame so that all working surfaces contact flame immediately before use.

Choice of treatment depends on nature, shape, and size of equipment and on conditions of sampling. Sterilize wherever possible by method (*1*) or (*2*).

Methods (*3*), (*4*), (*5*), and (*6*) are regarded as secondary methods only.

(**c**) *Sampling for organoleptic purposes.*—Use equipment as in (**a**) or (**b**), or as specified for specific product. Equipment should not impart any flavor or odor to product.

C. Sample Containers

(**a**) *For liquids.*—Use clean and dry containers of suitable waterproof, greaseproof material (glass, stainless metal, suitable plastic material) of quality suitable for sterilization by **968.12B(b)**, if necessary, and of suitable shape and capacity for material to be sampled (as defined in each particular case).

Securely close containers either with suitable rubber or plastic stopper or by screw cap of metal or plastic having, if necessary, liquid-tight plastic liner which is insoluble, nonabsorbent, and greaseproof, and which will not influence odor, flavor, or composition of milk products.

If rubber stoppers are used, cover with nonabsorbent, flavorless material (such as suitable plastic) before pressing into sample container. Suitable plastic bags may also be used.

(**b**) *For solids or semisolids.*—Use clean and dry wide-mouth, cylindrical receptacles of suitable waterproof, greaseproof material (glass, stainless metal, suitable plastic material) of quality suitable for sterilization by **968.12B(b)**, if necessary, and of capacity suited to size of sample to be taken (as defined in each particular case). Make air-tight as in (**a**). Suitable plastic bags may also be used.

(**c**) *Small retail containers.*—Contents of intact and unopened containers constitute samples.

D. Preservation of Samples

To samples of liquid products or cheese intended for chemical analysis, suitable preservative may be added. Such preservative should not interfere with subsequent analysis. Indicate nature and amount of addition on label and in any reports.

Do not add preservatives to samples of semisolid, solid (except cheese), or dried products intended for chemical analysis. Rapidly cool and store samples in refrigerator at 0–5°. Dried milks may be kept at room temperature.

Do not add preservatives to samples intended for bacteriological or organoleptic examination. Hold at 0–5°, except for condensed (conserved) milk products when sample comprises unopened hermetically sealed containers in which products are sold. Keep liquid products and butter cold. Start bacteriological examination of liquid products as soon as possible and never >24 h after sampling.

E. Transport of Samples

Transport samples to laboratory as quickly as possible after sampling. Take precautions to prevent, during transit, exposure to direct sunlight, or to temps <0° or >10° in case of perishable products. For samples intended for bacteriological examination, use insulated transport container capable of maintaining temperature at 0–5°, except for samples of condensed (conserved) milk products in unopened containers, or in case of very short journeys.

Maintain samples of cheese under such conditions as to avoid separation of fat or moisture. Maintain soft cheese at 0–5°.

References: JAOAC **49,** 58(1966); **50,** 531(1967).

18.18   925.32—Fat in Eggs
Acid Hydrolysis Method
Final Action

A. Preparation of Solution

(**a**) *Liquid eggs.*—From well-mixed sample, **925.29**(**a**) or (**b**), accurately weigh, by difference, into Mojonnier fat-extraction tube ca 2 g yolks, 3 g whole eggs, or 5 g whites. Slowly, with vigorous shaking, add 10 mL HCl, set tube in H_2O bath heated to 70°, bring to boiling, and continue heating at bp 30 min, shaking tube carefully every 5 min. Remove tube, add H_2O to nearly fill lower bulb of tube, and cool to room temperature.

I. **925.29** (Sampling of Eggs, Collection and Preparation of Sample)

No simple rules can be made for collection of sample representative of average of any particular lot of egg material, as conditions may differ widely. Experienced judgment must be used in each instance. For large lots, preferably draw several samples for separate analyses rather than attempt to get one composite representative sample. Sampling for microbiological examination, if required, should be performed first; *see Official Methods of Analysis* (1990) 15th Ed., sec. **939.14A–B.**

(a) *Liquid eggs.*—Obtain representative container or containers. Mix contents of container thoroughly and draw ca 300 g. (Long-handle dipper or ladle serves well.) Keep sample in hermetically sealed jar in freezer or with solid CO_2. Report odor and appearance.

(b) *Frozen eggs.*—Obtain representative container or containers. Examine contents as to odor and appearance. (Condition of contents can be determined best by drilling to center of container with auger and noting odor as auger is withdrawn. If impossible to secure individual containers, samples may consist of composite of borings from contents of each container.) Take borings diagonally across can from ≥ 3 widely separated parts, starting 2–5 cm in from edge and extending to opposite side as near to bottom as possible. Pack shavings tightly into sample jar and fill it completely to prevent partial dehydration of sample. Seal jar tightly and store in freezer or with solid CO_2. Before analyzing, warm sample in bath held at $<50°$, and mix well.

B. Determination

To extraction tube containing treated sample, **925.32A**, add 25 mL ether and mix. Add 25 mL redistilled petroleum ether (bp $<60°$), mix, and let stand until solvent layer is clear. Proceed as in **922.06** (*see* 18.16), beginning "Draw off as much as possible . . ." but omitting filtration.

References: JAOAC **8**, 601(1925); **16**, 298(1933); **58**, 314(1975).

18.19   948.22—Fat (Crude) in Nuts and Nut Products
Gravimetric Methods
First Action

(*Caution: See Appendix* for safety notes on distillation, flammable solvents, and diethyl ether.)

(a) *Direct method.*—If large amounts of soluble carbohydrates interfere with complete extraction of fat, extract with H_2O before making determination. Extract ca 2 g sample 16 h in Soxhlet-type extractor with ether, dried as follows: Wash commercial ether with 2 or 3 portions H_2O, add solid NaOH or KOH, and let stand until most H_2O is abstracted from ether. Decant into dry bottle, add small pieces of carefully cleaned metallic Na, and let stand until H evolution ceases. Keep ether thus dehydrated, over metallic Na in loosely stoppered bottles. Evaporate ether, dry residue 30 min at 95–100°, cool in desiccator, and weigh; continue this alternate drying and weighing at 30 min intervals to constant weight (1–1.5 h is usually required).

(b) *Indirect method.*—Proceed as in **925.40**; then extract dried substance 16 h as in (a), and dry as in (a). Report loss in weight as ether extract.

> **925.40** (Moisture in Nuts and Nut Products)
> (Not applicable to high sugar products or products containing glycerol or propylene glycol)
> Dry sample representing ca 2 g dry material to constant weight (ca 5 h) at 95–100° under pressure ≤ 100 mm Hg (13.3 kPa). Report loss in weight as moisture.
> References: JAOAC 8, 295(1925); **31**, 521(1948); **32**, 527(1949); **33**, 753(1950); **34**, 357(1951); **37**, 845(1954).

References: JAOAC **31**, 521(1948); **33**, 753(1950); **34**, 357(1951); **37**, 845(1954).

18.20 950.54—Fat (Total) in Food Dressings
Final Action

(*Caution: See Appendix* for safety notes on distillation, flammable solvents, diethyl ether, and petroleum ether.)

Thoroughly mix sample, and accurately weigh ca 1 g, by difference, into Mojonnier tube. Add 10 mL HCl, shake, set tube in H_2O bath heated to 70°, and bring to bp. Boil 30 min, shaking tube thoroughly every 5 min. Remove from H_2O bath, add H_2O to fill lower bulb of tube (but not neck), and cool to room temperature.

To mixture in Mojonnier tube add 25 mL ether and shake vigorously ≥1 min. Add 25 mL petroleum ether and again shake vigorously ≥1 min. To break emulsion centrifuge 5–10 min at ca 300 rpm. Decant ether-fat solution into flask, containing porcelain chips or glass beads, that has been dried at 100°, allowed to cool in air to constant weight, and weighed against similar flask similarly treated as counterpoise. Rinse off mouth of tube with small volume ether after each decantation, letting ether run into flask. Repeat ether extractions twice, using only 15 mL of each ether for second and third extractions. Again shake vigorously after addition of each ether and centrifuge. If necessary in order to decant all ether-fat solution after first extraction, add more H_2O prior to second decantation.

Slowly evaporate combined ether solutions in flask, dry ca 90 min at 100° (placing counterpoise in oven at same time), cool in air to constant weight, and weigh.

18.21 945.44—Fat in Fig Bars and Raisin-Filled Crackers
Ether Extraction Method
Final Action

(*Caution: See Appendix* for safety notes on distillation, diethyl ether, and petroleum ether.)

Accurately weigh ca 2 g well-mixed sample, prepared by grinding twice through food chopper, and transfer to Mojonnier tube. Add 2 mL alcohol, warm to 60–70°, and shake gently until sample is thoroughly disintegrated and mixed with alcohol. Add 10 mL HCl (25 + 11). Place tube in H_2O bath held at 70–80° and shake frequently until sample is thoroughly digested (40–80 min).

If weighed sample cannot be transferred to tube directly, digest in 50 mL beaker. Transfer digested mixture to tube as completely as possible by draining from lip of beaker down small stirring rod. Rinse beaker thoroughly with 10 mL alcohol, transfer to tube, mix thoroughly, and cool. Rinse beaker with portions of first 25 mL ether added for first extraction. Repeat rinsing with portions of petroleum ether (bp <60°) as it is added for first extraction. Rinse thoroughly so that all fat is transferred to extraction tube. (After digestion, all particles should be completely disintegrated, except hard seeds (in fig fillers) and strong fibers. Very small amount of fat may be retained by such particles after digestion, but in analysis of biscuits and crackers this loss will be within experimental error.)

When digesting in extraction tube, add 10 mL alcohol to digested charge and cool. (Level of liquid should be in neck of Mojonnier tube just below pour-off level.) Add 25 mL ether, stopper flask with cork, Neoprene, or other synthetic rubber stopper not affected by solvents, and shake thoroughly ca 1 min. Carefully release pressure so that none of solvent containing fat is lost. Wash adhering solvent and fat from stopper into extraction tube with few mL petroleum ether. (Glass wash bottle producing fine jet is convenient.) Let mixture stand few minutes; then add 25 mL petroleum ether (bp <60°), stopper tube tightly, and again shake thoroughly ca 1 min. Carefully release pressure, remove stopper, and again wash adhering solvent and fat into tube with few mL of petroleum ether. Let mixture stand until ether layer is clear (10–20 min), or centrifuge 20 min at ca 600 rpm.

Pour off as much as possible of clear ether-fat solution through small, fast filter by tilting tube gradually. (Plug of ether-extracted cotton packed just firmly enough in stem of funnel to let ether pass freely makes excellent filter for these extractions.) Catch ether-fat solutions from extractions in clean 250 mL beaker or flask. Re-extract digested sample remaining in tube 3 times more as for first extraction. (Volume of ether may be reduced to 15 or 20 mL for last 3 extractions.) Wash mouth of tube each time after draining ether-fat solution, and filter this ether through funnel into receptacle.

Evaporate combined ethers from extractions with air current or suction. After ethers are practically off, heat ca 10 min on hot H_2O or steam bath to drive off most of alcohol and H_2O carried over with ethers. Transfer beaker to 100° oven, dry 1 h, remove, and let cool. Redissolve dried fat in 15–20 mL mixture of equal parts of ether and petroleum ether, and filter through small fat-free paper into beaker or flask previously dried at 100°, cooled in desiccator, and weighed.

Wash all traces of fat from first receptacle, filter paper, and funnel into the tared beaker or flask with jet of petroleum ether from wash bottle. Evaporate ethers from tared receptacle with air current or suction and dry purified fat to constant weight in 100° oven (1–1.5 h). Cool in desiccator and weigh as soon as room temperature is attained. Make blank determinations on reagents.

Notes: Good quality rubber stoppers thoroughly cleaned with alcohol are satisfactory for stoppering extraction tubes. Remove stoppers from tubes after each shaking period and do not allow to remain in contact with solvents longer than necessary. Solvent may have some action on rubber. Very fine grain cork stoppers washed with alcohol and ether are also satisfactory for stoppering extraction tubes, provided leakage of solvents can be prevented during shaking.

If trouble is experienced in releasing pressure after shaking extraction tube containing ethers, cool tube slightly by holding it under stream of cold H_2O before removing stopper.

Al beakers are very satisfactory for weighing purified fat; they are light weight and cool to room temperature rapidly.

References: JAOAC **26**, 305(1943); **28,** 497(1945).

18.22   963.15—Fat in Cacao Products
Soxhlet Extraction Method
Final Action 1973
Office International du Cacao et du Chocolat-AOAC Method

(Applicable to cacao products with or without milk ingredients or to products prepared by cooking
with sugar and H_2O, and drying)

A. Apparatus and Reagents

     (a) *Soxhlet apparatus.*—With **T** joints, siphon capacity ca 100 mL (33 × 80 mm thimble), 250 mL erlenmeyer, and regulated heating mantle.

     (b) *Petroleum ether.*—Distilled in glass, bp 30–60°.

B. Determination

Prepare sample as in **970.20(b)**(*1*) (*see* 18.23). Accurately weigh 3–4 g chocolate liquor, 4–5 g cocoa, 4–5 g sweet chocolate, or 9–10 g milk chocolate into 300–500 mL beaker. Add slowly, while stirring, 45 mL boiling H_2O to give homogeneous suspension. Add 55 mL ca 8*N* HCl (2 + 1) and few defatted SiC chips or other antibumping agent, and stir. Cover with watch glass, bring slowly to boil, and boil gently 15 min. Rinse watch glass with 100 mL H_2O. Filter digest through 15 cm S&S 589 medium fluted paper, or equivalent, rinsing beaker 3 times with H_2O. Continue washing until last portion of filtrate is Cl-free as determined by addition of 0.1*N* $AgNO_3$. Transfer wet paper and sample to defatted extraction thimble and dry 6–18 h in small beaker at 100°. Place glass wool plug over paper.

Add few defatted antibumping chips to 250 mL erlenmeyer and dry 1 h at 100°. Cool to room temperature in desiccator and weigh. Place thimble containing dried sample in soxhlet, supporting it with spiral or glass beads. Rinse digestion beaker, drying beaker, and watch glass with three 50 mL portions petroleum ether, and add washings to thimble. Reflux digested sample 4 h adjusting heat so that extractor siphons ≥30 times. Remove flask, and evaporate solvent on steam bath. Dry flask at 100–101° to constant weight (1.5–2 h). Cool in desiccator to room temperature and weigh. Constant weight is attained when successive 1 h drying periods show additional loss of <0.05% fat. % Fat = g fat × 100/g sample. Duplicate determinations should agree within 0.1% fat.

References: JAOAC **28,** 482(1945); **33,** 342(1950); **34,** 442(1951); **53,** 490(1970). Analytical Methods of the OICC (Ref. *2*), page 8a-E/1963.

18.23   925.07—Fat in Cacao Products
Knorr Tube Method
Final Action

(*Caution:* Asbestos is a carcinogen. Also, *see Appendix* for safety notes on distillation, flammable solvents, and petroleum ether.)

Use filter tube of Knorr extraction tube style, ca 20 mm id, with body ca 11 cm long and stem 6–8 mm od, ca 10 cm long, provided with removable, close fitting perforated Ni, monel metal, glass, or porcelain disk at bottom of larger tube. Prepare 6 mm tightly packed matt of asbestos, purified by placing 60 g fiber in blender, adding 800 mL H_2O, and blending 1 min at low speed; carefully remove any coarse pieces. (Not applicable to cacao products containing milk ingredients or to products prepared by cooking with sugar and water, and drying; cacao nibs must be finely ground. *All* petroleum ether used in this determination must be redistilled at <60°.)

(Allihn type filter tube with coarse fritted disk such as Ace Glass Inc. No. 7195 is also satisfactory.) Wash filter with alcohol, ether, and little petroleum ether. Weigh 2–3 g prepared sample, **970.20,** into tube and insert tube into rubber stopper in filtering bell jar connected to suction through 2-way stopcock, taking care that no rubber particles adhere to tip of stem. Place weighed 200 mL erlenmeyer at such height that tube stem passes through neck into flask. (Lengthen stem of tube if necessary.) Fill tube to ca ⅔ capacity with petroleum ether, and stir sample thoroughly with flat-end rod, crushing all lumps. Let stand 1 min and drain by suction. Regulate suction so that collected solvent will not boil violently. Release vacuum after each draining before adding more solvent. Add solvent from wash bottle while turning tube between thumb and finger so that sides of tube are washed down by each addition. Repeat extractions, with stirring, until fat is removed (usually 10 extractions). Remove tube with stopper from bell jar, wash traces of fat from end of stem with petroleum ether, evaporate solvent, and dry to constant weight at 100°.

I. **970.20** (Cacao Products, Preparation of Sample)

(**a**) *Powdered products.*—Mix thoroughly and preserve in tightly stoppered bottles.

(**b**) *Chocolate products.*—(*1*) Chill ca 200 g sweet or bitter chocolate until hard, and grate or shave to fine granular condition. Mix thoroughly and preserve in tightly stoppered bottle in cool place. Alternatively—

(*2*) Melt ca 200 g bitter, sweet, or milk chocolate by placing in suitable container and partly immersing container in bath at ca 50°. Stir frequently until sample melts and reaches temperature of 45–50°. Remove from bath, stir thoroughly, and while still liquid, remove portion for analysis, using glass or metal tube, 4–10 mm diameter, provided with close-fitting plunger to expel sample from tube, or disposable plastic syringe.

Reference: JAOAC **53,** 388(1970).

References: JAOAC **8,** 705(1925); **9,** 469(1926).

18.24 920.177—Ether Extract of Confectionery
First Action

(*Caution: See Appendix* for safety notes on distillation, flammable solvents, diethyl ether, petroleum ether, and asbestos.)

A. Continuous Extraction Method

Measure 25 mL 20% mixture or solution into very thin, readily breakable glass evaporating shell, or thin Pb or Sn foil containing 5–7 g freshly ignited asbestos fiber, or, if possible to obtain uniform sample, weigh 5 g mixed, finely divided sample into dish and wash with H_2O onto asbestos in evaporating shell, using small portion of asbestos fiber on stirring rod to transfer last traces of sample from dish to shell.

Dry to constant weight at 100°, cool, wrap glass dish loosely in smooth paper, crush into rather small fragments between fingers, and carefully transfer crushed mass, including paper, to extraction tube or fat extraction cartridge. If metal dish is used, cut into small pieces and place in extraction tube. Extract with anhydrous ether or petroleum ether (bp 45–60° and without weighable residue) in continuous extraction apparatus ≥25 h. In most cases it is advisable to remove substance from extractor after first 12 h, grind with sand to fine powder, and re-extract remaining 13 h. Transfer extract to weighed flask, evaporate solvent, and dry to constant weight at 100°.

B. Roese-Gottlieb Method

Introduce 4 g sample, or amount of uniform solution equivalent to this weight dry substance, into Mojonnier fat extraction tube or similar apparatus; dilute to 10 mL with H_2O, add 1.25 mL NH_4OH, and mix thoroughly. Add 10 mL alcohol and mix; then add 25 mL ether and shake vigorously ca 30 s; and finally add 25 mL petroleum ether (bp <60°) and shake again ca 30 s. Let stand 20 min or until separation of liquids is complete.

Draw off as much as possible of ether-fat solution (usually 0.5–0.8 mL is left) into weighed flask through small, rapid filter. (Weigh flask with similar one as counterpoise.) Again extract liquid remaining in tube, this time with 15 mL each of ether and petroleum ether; shake vigorously ca 30 s with each solvent and let settle. Proceed as above, washing mouth of tube and filter with few mL of mixture of equal parts of the 2 solvents (previously mixed and freed from deposited H_2O).

For greater degree of accuracy, repeat extraction. If previous solvent-fat solutions have been drawn off closely, third extraction usually yields ≤ 1 mg fat, or ca 0.02% with 4 g sample. Slowly evaporate solvent on steam bath and then dry fat in 100° oven to constant weight. Test purity of fat by dissolving in little petroleum ether. If residue remains, wash fat out completely with petroleum ether, dry residue, weigh, and deduct weight.

18.25　　　920.172—Ether Extract of Prepared Mustard
Gravimetric Method
Final Action

(*Caution: See Appendix* for safety notes on monitoring equipment, distillation, flammable solvents, and diethyl ether.)

Weigh 10 g sample into SiO_2, Al, or porcelain drying dish and mix with ca 30 g sand. Heat on H_2O bath until mixture appears dry; then finish drying in oven at 100°. Grind until all lumps are broken up, and determine ether extract by extracting 16 h with anhydrous ether in Soxhlet extractor with Whatman single thickness or other close-texture thimble. Dry extract 30 min at 100°, cool, and weigh.

18.26　　　963.22—Methyl Esters of Fatty Acids in Oils and Fats
Gas Chromatographic Method
First Action 1963
Final Action 1984
AOAC-IUPAC Method

A. Principle
Methyl esters of fatty acids from animal and vegetable fats having 8–24 C atoms are separated and determined by gas chromatography. Method is not applicable to epoxy, oxidized, or polymerized fatty acids.

B. Apparatus
The following conditions are for use with flame ionization detector:
(a) *Gas chromatograph*.—With minimum dead space in injection system, which is maintained at 20–50° higher than column temperature. Maintain column temperature within $\pm$ 1° to at least 220°. If programmed heated, dual columns are recommended.

(b) *Columns.*—1–3 m × 2–4 mm id glass or stainless steel (do not use stainless steel with polyunsaturated components with >3 double bonds). Use short column when long-chain (>20 C atoms) acids are present.

(c) *Packing.*—Acid-washed and silanized diatomaceous earth, with narrow range (25 μm) grain size between 125–250 μm (No. 60–120). Average grain size is inversely related to id and directly related to column length. Coat with 5–20% polyester type polar liquid stationary phase (diethylene glycol polysuccinate, butanediol polysuccinate, ethylene glycol polyadipate, etc.) or other liquid (e.g., cyanosilicones) meeting efficiency and resolution specifications. Nonpolar phase can be used for certain separations.

Condition column while disconnected from detector at 185° with current of inert gas at 20–60 mL/min for ≥16 h and for additional 2 h at 195°. Conditioning temperature may vary with specific liquid phase.

(d) *Syringe.*—Maximum volume 10 μL, graduated to 0.1 μL.

(e) *Recorder.*—0–2.5 or 5.0 mv range, <1.5 s response rate (time for pen to pass from 0 to 90% following momentary introduction of 100% signal), 25 cm minimum paper width, and 25–100 cm/h paper speed, with attenuator switch to change range. If integrator is used, it must have linear response with adequate sensitivity and satisfactory baseline correction.

If thermal conductivity detector is used, conditions must be modified as follows: Column, 2–4 m × 4 mm id; support, grain size 150–250 μm (No. 60–100); stationary phase, 15–25%; carrier gas, He or H; no auxiliary gas; temperatures: column 180–200°, injector 40–60° above that of column; carrier gas flow, 60–80 mL/min; recorder, 0–1 mv range; and amount sample injected, 0.5–2 μL. Correction factors must be used.

C. Reagents

(a) *Carrier gas.*—N, He, Ar dried and containing <10 mg O/kg.

(b) *Other gases.*—H, 99.9+%, free from organic impurities. Air or O, free from organic impurities (<2 ppm hydrocarbons equivalent to CH_4).

(c) *Reference standards.*—Known mixtures of methyl esters or methyl esters of oil of known composition, preferably similar to that of material to be analyzed.

D. Operating Conditions

The following variables are involved in selecting appropriate test conditions: length and id of column, temperature of column, carrier gas flow, resolution required, size of sample, and time of analysis. Size of sample should be such that linear response of detector and electrometer is obtained. In general, following conditions will elute methyl stearate within ca 15 min at ≥2000 theoretical plates:

Column id, mm	Carrier gas flow, mL/min	Concentration of stationary phase, %	Column temperature, °C
2	15–25	5	175
3	20–40	10	180
4	40–60	15	185
		20	185

If apparatus permits, injector should be at ca 200° and detector at temperature above that of column. Flow of H to detector should be ca half that of carrier gas (H flow may be equal to carrier gas flow with N and 2 mm id column); flow of O ca 5–10 times that of H.

E. Performance Specifications

Perform analysis on mixture of methyl stearate and methyl oleate in ca equal proportions (e.g., methyl esters from cocoa butter). Adjust sample size, column temperature, and carrier gas flow so that methyl stearate peak is recorded ca 15 min after solvent peak, ca ¾ full scale. Measure base widths in mm of methyl stearate (w_1) and methyl oleate (w_2) between points of intersection with baseline of tangents drawn to inflection points of curves. Also measure retention distance in mm (S) from start to peak maximum for methyl stearate and distance in mm between peak maximum for methyl stearate and methyl oleate, Y. Calculate theoretical plates, n (efficiency), and resolution, R:

$$n = 16(S/w_1)^2$$
$$R = 2Y/(w_1 + w_2)$$

Select conditions to obtain $n \geq 2000$ and $R \geq 1.25$. In addition, linolenic acid (18:3) methyl ester should be separated from arachidic acid (20:0) and gadoleic acid (20:1) esters. Columns will show gradual loss in R with use; when value becomes ≤ 1.25, replace.

F. Determination

With apparatus showing stable baseline, inject 0.1–2 μL 5–10% heptane solution of methyl esters, **969.33A**. If trace components are desired, sample may be increased $\leq 10\times$. Pierce septum of inlet port and quickly discharge sample. Withdraw needle and note on chart small peak due to air or solvent, marking start reference point. Adjust sample size so major peak is not attenuated $>8\times$, preferably less. Change setting of attenuator as necessary to keep peaks on chart paper. Mark attenuator setting on chart.

969.33 (Fatty Acids in Oils and Fats, Preparation of Methyl Esters)

A. Principle

Glycerides and phospholipids are saponified, and fatty acids are liberated and esterified in presence of BF$_3$ catalyst for further analysis by IR, **965.34E** (*Official Methods of Analysis* [1990] 15th Ed.), or GC, **963.22F**.

Method is applicable to common animal and vegetable oils and fats, and fatty acids. Unsaponifiables are not removed, and if present in large amounts, may interfere with subsequent analyses.

Method is not suitable for preparation of methyl esters of fatty acids containing major amounts of epoxy, hydroperoxy, aldehyde, ketone, cyclopropyl, and cyclopropenyl groups, and conjugated polyunsaturated and acetylenic compounds because of partial or complete destruction of these groups.

For determination of acids $<C_{12}$, lower column temperature is needed; for $>C_{20}$, higher. Temperature programming is useful in such cases, e.g., with acids $<C_{12}$, inject at 100° and raise temperature 4–8°/min to optimum, or program up to a fixed temperature and continue at constant temperature until all components are eluted. If apparatus does not use programmed heating, operate at 2 fixed temperatures between 100 and 195°.

G. Identification

Analyze reference standard mixtures under same operating conditions as for sample. Measure retention distances (S) for known esters. Plot log S as function of no. of C atoms of acids. Under isothermal conditions, graphs of straight chain esters of same degree of unsaturation should be straight lines, approximately parallel. Identify peaks from sample from these graphs, interpolating if necessary. Avoid conditions which permit "masked peaks," i.e., which are not sufficiently resolved.

Esters appear in order of increasing no. of C atoms and of increasing unsaturation for same no. of C atoms. C_{16} is ahead of C_{18}, and C_{18} methyl esters appear in order: stearate (18:0), oleate (18:1), linoleate (18:2), and linolenate (18:3). C_{20} saturated ester (arachidic, 20:0) usually appears before 18:3 ester, but may be reversed on some columns, or positions may change with column use.

H. Calculations

Use method of normalization, which assumes all components of sample are represented on chromatogram, so that sum of areas under peaks represents 100% of constituents (total elution).

If instrument is equipped with integrator, use figures shown. If not, use triangulation: Draw lines for each peak tangent to sides and intersecting baseline. Calculate area of resulting triangle by multiplying height (corrected for any change in attenuation) by ½ base. For automatically attenuated peak, obtain peak width by drawing tangents to outer sides of peak (these must be full chart span, and upper ⅔ of peak must be used) and intersecting baseline. Calculate area by multiplying height (corrected for attenuation) by ½ base.

If significant amounts of components with < 12 C atoms are absent, calculate % by weight of each component, expressed as methyl ester:

$$C_i = G_i \times 100/\Sigma\, G_i$$

where G_i = area of peak corresponding to component i, and $\Sigma\, G_i$ = sum of areas under all peaks.

In certain cases, e.g., in presence of components with < 12 C atoms, large differences in molecular weights, and presence of secondary groups, correction factors must be used to convert peak areas into weight %. Determine correction factors by analyzing known reference standards of methyl esters of composition similar to that of sample under identical operating conditions. For reference standard:

$$\text{\% by weight component i} = B_i \times 100/\Sigma\, B_i$$

where B_i = weight of component i in reference standard, and $\Sigma\, B_i$ = total weight of all components in reference standard. Calculate from chromatogram:

$$\text{\% (area/area) of component i} = G_i \times 100/\Sigma\, G_i$$

from which calculate correction factor for each component:

$$K_i = (B_i/\Sigma\, B_i) \times (\Sigma\, C_i/C_i)$$

Determine correction factors relative to palmitic acid, $K_{16} = 1$, so that

$$K' = K_i/K_{16}$$

Then to calculate % of each component (as methyl esters), multiply its area by appropriate correction factor, and sum corrected areas:

$$\text{\% by weight component i} = (K'_i \times G_i) \times 100/\Sigma\, (K'_i \times G_i)$$

In certain cases, e.g., when all components are not eluted, use internal standard, S, such as C_{15} or C_{17} methyl ester, and determine its correction factor. Then:

$$\text{\% by weight of component i as methyl ester} = (w_S/w) \times (K'_i/K'_S) \times (G_i/G_S) \times 100$$

where w_S = mg internal standard and w = total mg sample, and subscript S refers to internal standard component.

Report results to following significant figures, with 1 figure beyond decimal point in all cases: 3 for >10%, 2 for 1–10%, and 1 for <1%.

I. Precision

(a) *Repeatability.*—Two single determinations performed on same day by same operator with same apparatus on same sample for major components (>5%) should not differ by >3% relative, with an absolute value of 1%.

(b) *Reproducibility.*—Two single determinations performed in different laboratories for major components should not differ by >10% relative, with an absolute value of 3%.

References: IUPAC 2.302, 6th Ed. JAOAC **46,** 146(1963); **50,** 216(1967); **57,** 336(1970); **62,** 709(1979).

18.27 979.19—*cis, cis*-Methylene Interrupted Polyunsaturated Fatty Acids in Oils
Spectrophotometric Method
First Action 1979
Final Action 1984

A. Reagents

(a) *Potassium borate buffer.*—1.0M, pH 9.0. Dissolve 61.9 grams H_3BO_3 and 25.0 g KOH in ca 800 mL H_2O by stirring and heating. Cool to room temperature and adjust to pH 9.0 with 1.0N HCl or 1.0N KOH, as required. Dilute to 1 L with H_2O and mix.

(b) *Dilute potassium borate buffer.*—0.2M, pH 9.0. Dilute 200 mL 1.0M buffer, **(a)**, to 1 L with H_2O and mix.

(c) *Lipoxidase solutions.*—(*1*) *Stock solution.*—Dissolve 10 mg lipoxidase, from soybean, 50,000 units/mg (ICN Pharmaceuticals Inc., Life Sciences Group, Nutritional Biochemicals Division, or equivalent), in 10 mL ice-cold dilute borate buffer, **(b)**. Refrigerated solution is stable 30 days. (*2*) *Working solution.*—Mix 2.0 mL stock solution with 8.0 mL ice-cold dilute borate buffer, **(b)**. If large no. of analyses are to be performed, dilute 5.0 mL stock solution to 25 mL with ice-cold dilute borate buffer, **(b)**. (*3*) *Inactivated solution.*—Pipet 4 mL working enzyme solution, (*2*), to 10 mL volumetric flask and hold 5 min in boiling H_2O.

(d) *Alcoholic potassium hydroxide solution.*—0.5N. Dissolve 1.40 g KOH in alcohol and dilute to 50 mL with alcohol. Prepare fresh daily.

B. Preparation of Sample

Accurately weigh ca 100 mg vegetable oil and transfer with *n*-hexane into 100 mL volumetric flask, which has just been flushed with N. Dilute to volume with *n*-hexane or acetone. Pipet 1 mL diluted solution into 100 mL volumetric flask and completely evaporate solvent under N.

C. Determination

Add 1 mL alcoholic KOH, **(d)**, solution to solvent-free residue in volumetric flask. Heat gently on steam bath to dissolve. Flush with N and hold stoppered, in dark, minimum of 5 h to overnight. After saponification is complete, add 20 mL 1.0M borate buffer, **(a)**, and 50 mL H_2O, and mix. Add 1 mL 0.5N HCl, dilute to volume with H_2O, and mix.

Pipet 3 mL saponified solution into each of four 13 × 100 mm test tubes. To 2 tubes (blanks) add 0.10 mL inactivated enzyme solution, **(c)**(*3*), and mix well. To remaining duplicate tubes, add 0.10 mL working enzyme solution, **(c)**(*2*). Mix by shaking vigorously 30 s immediately after adding enzyme solution, and let all tubes stand exposed to air at room temperature 30 min. Zero spectrophotometer at 234 nm with blank tubes and measure A of reacted samples.

For sample, calculate g polyunsaturated fatty acid (PUFA) as trilinolein/100 g sample $= W \times DF \times 10^{-4}$, where $W = \mu$g trilinolein/mL final solution from standard curve, and $DF =$ dilution factor.

D. Preparation of Standard Curve

Weigh 100 mg *cis,cis*-trilinolein, 99% (NuCheck Prep, PO Box 295, Elysian, MN 56028-0295, or equivalent), transfer quantitatively to 100 mL volumetric flask, and dilute to volume with *n*-hexane or acetone. Pipet 10 mL aliquot into 100 mL volumetric flask and dilute to volume with same solvent. Pipet 2, 4, 6, 8, 10 and 12 mL aliquots into separate 100 mL volumetric flasks, and evaporate each to dryness in stream of N. Pipet 1 mL alcoholic KOH, (**d**), into each flask, flush with N, and store stoppered in dark 5 h or overnight.

Add 20 mL 1.0*M* borate buffer, (**a**), 50 mL H_2O, and 1 mL 0.5*N* HCl to each, dilute to volume with H_2O, and mix. Pipet four 3 mL aliquots of each standard solution into test tubes, incubate, and proceed as in determination, beginning "To 2 tubes (blanks). . . ." Plot average A at each level against μg trilinolein/mL.

Two single determinations in 1 laboratory should not differ by $>1.6\%$; 2 single determinations performed in 2 laboratories should not differ by $>2.2\%$.

References: JAOAC **60,** 895(1977); **61,** 1419(1978).

Chapter 19
Folacin

19.1

960.46—Vitamin Assays
Microbiological Methods
Final Action

See Chapter 15.1.

19.2   ## 944.12—Folic Acid (Pteroylglutamic Acid) in Vitamin Preparations
Microbiological Methods
Final Action 1960

(Applicable only to materials containing free forms of folic acid)

A. Basal Medium Stock Solution

Using ingredients in amounts prescribed for folic acid, Table **960.46(b)** (*see* Chapter 15.1), proceed as directed below.

Using solutions prepared as in **960.46A** (*see* Chapter 15.1) add, with mixing, and in following order: acid-hydrolyzed casein solution, (**a**); tryptophan solution, (**k**); adenine-guanine-uracil solution, (**b**); xanthine solution, (**r**); asparagine solution, (**c**); vitamin solution III, (**n**); and salt solution B, (**j**). Add ca 50 mL H_2O, and add, with mixing, cysteine, anhydrous glucose, Na citrate dihydrate, anhydrous K_2HPO_4, and glutathione. When solution is complete, adjust to pH 6.8 with NaOH solution, add, with mixing, polysorbate 80 solution, (**h**), and $MnSO_4$ solution, (**f**), and dilute with H_2O to 250 mL.

Titrimetric Method

B. Folic Acid Standard Solutions

(Do not shake standard solutions stored under toluene.)

(**a**) *Stock solution.*—100 µg/mL. Accurately weigh, in closed system, USP Folic Acid Reference Standard, equivalent to 50–60 mg folic acid, that has been dried to constant weight and stored in dark over P_2O_5 in desiccator. Dissolve in ca 30 mL 0.01N NaOH, add ca 300 mL H_2O, adjust to pH 7–8 with HCl solution, and dilute with additional H_2O to make folic acid concentration exactly 100 µg/mL. Store under toluene in dark at ca 10°.

(**b**) *Intermediate solution I.*—1 µg/mL. To 10 mL stock solution, (**a**), add ca 500 mL H_2O, adjust to pH 7–8, and dilute with additional H_2O to 1 L. Store under toluene in dark at ca 10°.

(**c**) *Intermediate solution II.*—100 ng/mL. To 100 mL intermediate solution I, (**b**), add ca 500 mL H_2O, adjust to pH 7–8, and dilute with additional H_2O to 1 L. Store under toluene in dark at ca 10°.

(d) *Working solution*.—Dilute suitable volume intermediate solution II (c), with H_2O to measured volume such that after incubation as in **960.46D** and **E**, response at 5.0 mL level of this solution is equivalent to titration (as described in **960.46E**) of ca 8–12 mL. Designate this as standard solution. (This concentration is usually 1.0–4.0 ng folic acid/mL standard solution.) Prepare fresh standard solution for each assay.

C. Inoculum

Make transfer of cells from stock culture of *Streptococcus faecalis*, **960.46C(b)**, to sterile tube containing 10 mL liquid culture medium, **960.46B(a)**. Incubate 6–24 h at any selected temperature between 30 and 40° held constant to within ±0.5°. Under aseptic conditions, centrifuge culture and decant supernate. Wash cells with 3 ca 10 mL portions sterile 0.9% NaCl solution or sterile suspension medium, **960.46B(c)**. Resuspend cells in 10 mL sterile 0.9% NaCl solution or sterile suspension medium. Cell suspension so obtained is inoculum.

D. Assay Solution

Place measured amount of sample in flask and add volume H_2O equal in mL to ≥10 times dry weight sample in grams; resulting solution must contain ≤1.0 mg folic acid/mL. Add equivalent of 2 mL NH_4OH (2 + 3)/100 mL liquid. If sample is not readily soluble, comminute to disperse it evenly in liquid; then agitate vigorously and wash down sides of flask with 0.1N NH_4OH.

Autoclave mixture 15 min at 121–123° and cool. If lumping occurs, agitate mixture until particles are evenly dispersed. Dilute mixture to measured volume with H_2O, and let any undissolved particles settle, or filter or centrifuge if necessary. Take aliquot of clear solution, add H_2O, adjust to pH 6.8, and dilute with additional H_2O to measured volume containing, per mL, folic acid ca equivalent to that of standard solution, **944.12B(d)**. Designate this as assay solution.

E. Assay

Using standard solution, **944.12B(d)**; assay solution, **944.12D**; basal medium stock solution, **944.12A**; and inoculum, **944.12C**; proceed as in **960.46D**, **E**, and **H**.

Turbidimetric Method

F. Folic Acid Standard Solution

Dilute suitable volume folic acid intermediate solution II, **944.12B(c)**, with H_2O to measured volume such that after incubation as in **960.46D** and **960.46G**, with inoculated blank set at 100% T, % T at 5.0 mL level of this solution is equivalent to that for dried cell weight (as described in **960.46F**) of ≥1.25 mg. Designate this as standard solution. (This concentration is usually 0.5–2.0 ng folic acid/mL standard solution.) Prepare fresh standard solution for each assay.

G. Assay Solution

Proceed as in **944.12D**, except that where reference is made to folic acid concentration ca equivalent to that of standard solution, **944.12B(d)**, replace by folic acid concentration ca equivalent to that of standard solution, **944.12F**. Designate solution so obtained as assay solution.

H. Assay

Using standard solution, **944.12F**, assay solution, **944.12G**, basal medium stock solution, **944.12A**, and inoculum, **944.12C**, proceed as in **960.46D**, **G**, and **H**.

References: Science **100**, 295(1944). J. Biol. Chem. **157**, 303(1945); **163**, 447, 449(1946). Ann. N.Y. Acad. Sci. **48**, 261(1946). Analyst **72**, 84(1947). JAOAC **31**, 466(1948); **32**, 464(1949); **33**, 633(1950); **39**, 172(1956); **40**, 855, 856(1957); **41**, 61, 587, 591(1958); **42**, 529(1959).
CAS-59-30-3 (folic acid)

19.3   992.05—Folic Acid (Pteroylglutamic Acid) in Infant Formula
Microbiological Methods
First Action 1992

(Applicable only to free form of folic acid)

Method Performance (milk-based liquid, ready-to-feed):

Mean recovery = 173.1 μg folic acid/L infant formula

s_r = 16.2; s_R = 44.0; RSD$_r$ = 9.35%; RSD$_R$ = 25.44%

A. Principle

Folic acid content of infant formula samples is estimated from acidimetric response of *Lactobacillus casei*.

B. Apparatus

(a) *Incubator.*—Forced-draft incubator or circulating H_2O bath, capable of maintaining within $\pm$ 0.5° temperatures between 28 and 40°.

(b) *Centrifuge.*—Capable of operating at 3000 rpm for $\geq$3 min, with adapters to hold culture tubes.

(c) *Mechanical shaker.*—Capable of operating 72 h at 100–200 horizontal strokes per min; minimum capacity 100 tubes; if shaker cannot be placed inside **(a)**, shaker itself must maintain temperature specified in **(a)**.

C. Basal Medium Preparation

(Store all solutions in dark at ca 10°. Store all solutions except those containing alcohol under toluene. Proportionate amounts may be prepared.)

(a) *Acid-hydrolyzed casein solution.*—Mix 400 g vitamin-free casein with 2 L HCl (1 + 1), and heat at reflux temperature 8 h. Remove HCl by distillation under reduced pressure until thick paste remains. Dissolve paste in H_2O and transfer to 4 L beaker using total of 1500 mL H_2O. Adjust to pH 3.5 $\pm$ 0.1 with ca 200 mL 40% NaOH (400 g NaOH/L H_2O). Transfer solution to 2 L mixing cylinder and dilute to volume with H_2O. Pour solution into 6 L Erlenmeyer flask. Add additional 2 L H_2O. Add 80 g activated charcoal (Norit A is suitable), stir 1 h, and filter through fluted paper. Repeat treatment with activated charcoal. Add 35 mL toluene, shake well, and store at 10°. If precipitate forms in storage, filter before use.

(b) *Adenine-guanine-uracil solution.*—Add 1.0 g each of adenine sulfate, guanine HCl, and uracil to 50 mL hot (90°) HCl (1 + 1) in 150 mL beaker. Heat at 90° until solids are dissolved. Cool and transfer solution quantitatively to 1 L volumetric flask using H_2O. Dilute to volume with H_2O and mix thoroughly. Add 10 mL toluene, mix well, and store at 10°. Prepare fresh every 3 months.

(c) *Cystine solution.*—Weigh 1.25 g L-cystine; suspend in 40 mL H_2O. Add concentrated HCl dropwise with stirring (ca 2 mL required) until L-cystine dissolves. Transfer to 50 mL volumetric flask and dilute to volume with H_2O.

(d) *Salt solution II.*—Dissolve 10 g $MgSO_4 \cdot 7H_2O$, 0.5 g NaCl, 0.5 g $FeSO_4 \cdot 7H_2O$, 1.5 g $MnSO_4 \cdot H_2O$, and 1 mL concentrated HCl in 250 mL H_2O. Add 2 mL toluene and store at 10°. Make fresh every 3 months.

(e) *Xanthine solution.*—Suspend 1.0 g xanthine in 200 mL H_2O in 400 mL beaker. Heat to 70°. Add 30 mL NH_4OH (2 + 3) and stir until dissolution is complete. Quantitatively transfer solution to 1 L volumetric flask, using H_2O. Dilute to volume with H_2O and mix thoroughly. Store under toluene at 10°. Prepare fresh every 3 months.

(f) *Basal medium stock solution.*—To 700 mL H_2O in 1 L beaker, add 127 mL acid-hydrolyzed casein solution, **(a)**; 20 mL adenine-guanine-uracil solution, **(b)**; 16 mL cystine solution, **(c)**; 10 mL salt solution II, **(d)**; and 10 mL xanthine solution, **(e)**. Mix. Using pH meter, adjust to pH 6.4–6.5 by adding 1.0N NaOH and dilute to 1 L in glass-stoppered graduated cylinder. Dispense 200 mL portions into 16 oz polyethylene bottles, cap, and freeze (use within 2 months).

D. Other Solutions

(a) *Salt solution I.*—Dissolve 50 g K_2HPO_4 and 50 g KH_2PO_4 in 500 mL H_2O. Add 10 mL toluene and store at 10°. Make fresh every 3 months.

(b) *Polysorbate 80 solution.*—Dissolve 25 g polysorbate 80 (polyoxyethylene sorbitan monooleate) in ethanol to make 250 mL solution.

(c) *Clarified skim milk.*—Add 10 g spray-dried skim milk powder to 80 mL H_2O. Mix thoroughly. Using pH meter, adjust pH to 4.2 with HCl (1 + 1). Centrifuge mixture 15 min at 3000 rpm to obtain clear supernate. Decant supernate into 150 mL beaker. Adjust pH to 7.0 by addition of NaOH solution. Centrifuge 15 min at 3000 rpm to obtain clear supernate. Decant supernate into 100 mL cylinder and dilute to 100 mL with H_2O.

(d) *Phosphate buffer solution.*—0.05M. Dissolve 5.85 g KH_2PO_4 and 1.22 g K_2HPO_4 in H_2O and dilute to 1 L. Prepare fresh daily.

(e) *Bromthymol blue indicator solution.*—Weigh 0.1 g bromthymol blue into small beaker. Dissolve in few mL ethanol, add 1.6 mL 0.1N NaOH, and dilute with H_2O to 250 mL.

(f) *Isotonic salt solution.*—Weigh 0.9 g NaCl and transfer to 100 mL volumetric flask. Dilute to volume with H_2O and shake until salt has dissolved. Transfer 10 mL portions to culture tubes, plug with cotton or cap with stainless steel caps and sterilize 20 min at 121°. Prepare fresh weekly.

(g) *Biotin solution.*—Weigh 50 mg biotin into 1 L volumetric flask and add 10 mL 0.2N NaOH. When biotin is dissolved, dilute to volume with H_2O and mix well. Store at 10°. Prepare fresh every 6 months.

(h) *Vitamin solution.*—Dissolve 50 mg niacin, 71.4 mg sodium riboflavin-5-phosphate (equivalent to 50 mg ribloflavin), 50 mg thiamine hydrochloride, 50 mg calcium pantothenate, 10 mg *p*-aminobenzoic acid, and 10 mL biotin solution, **D(g)**, in 150 mL H_2O and dilute to 200 mL. Add 6 mL toluene, mix well, and store at 10°. Prepare fresh every 2 months.

(i) *Pyridoxamine solution.*—Dissolve 14.3 mg pyridoxamine dihydrochloride in H_2O and dilute to 100 mL. Add 3 mL toluene, mix well, and store at 10°.

(j) *Chick pancreas preparation.*—Weigh 100 mg desiccated chick pancreas (Difco Laboratories, Cat. No. 0459-12-2), add 20 mL H_2O, and stir 15 min. Centrifuge 10 min at 3000 rpm and use clear supernate.

Prepare fresh daily.

(k) *Phosphate buffer (0.05M)–ascorbic acid solution.*—Dissolve 50 mg ascorbic acid in 100 mL 0.05M phosphate buffer solution, **D(d)**. Prepare just prior to use.

E. Culture and Maintenance Media

(a) *Maintenance medium.*—Add 10 g tryptone; 10 g anhydrous dextrose; 2 g K_2HPO_4; 3 g $CaCO_3$; 1 g Liver Concentrate NF (Pharmaceutical Division, Wilson & Co, Chicago, IL is suitable); 5 mL salt solution I, **D(a)**; 5 mL salt solution II, **C(d)**; and 15 g agar to 990 mL H_2O. Bring mixture to boil and stir until agar is dissolved. Continue stirring while dispensing 10 mL portions into 18×150 mm hard glass culture tubes. Plug tubes with polyurethane or cotton plugs and sterilize 15 min at 121°. Cool to room temperature in upright position. Maintenance medium will keep indefinitely in closed container stored at 10°.

(b) *Culture medium.*—Add 9.6 g riboflavin assay medium (Bacto-Riboflavin Assay Medium, Difco Laboratories is suitable) to 360 mL boiling H_2O and stir until dissolved. Cool to room temperature, add 40 mL clarified skim milk, **D(c)**, and mix well. Dispense 10 mL portions into 18×150 mm test tubes, cap with stainless steel caps, and sterilize 15 min at 121°. Cool and store at 10°. Make fresh after 3 months.

F. Stock Cultures of Test Organisms

Inoculate, by stab, 3 tubes of maintenance medium, **E(a)**, from pure culture of *Lactobacillus casei* (ATCC No. 7469). Incubate 24 h at 37°, label as monthly cultures, and store at 10°. From 1 of monthly cultures, inoculate 4 tubes of maintenance medium, incubate 24 h at 37°, and label as weekly cultures. Each week, inoculate 4 or 5 tubes of maintenance medium from weekly culture, incubate 24 h at 37°, and label as daily cultures. Use daily culture to prepare inoculum. At beginning of next month, inoculate 3 new monthly cultures from unused monthly culture from fresh stock.

Titrimetric Method

G. Folic Acid Standard Solutions

(Do not shake standard solutions stored under toluene.)

(a) *Stock standard solution.*—500 μg/mL. Accurately weigh USP Folic Acid Reference Standard, equivalent to 55–56 mg folic acid, dried to constant weight and stored in dark over P_2O_5 in desiccator. Using 50 mL H_2O, quantitatively transfer to 100 mL volumetric flask. Add 2 mL NH_4OH (2 + 3). When completely dissolved, dilute to volume with H_2O, and add, by pipet, additional H_2O needed for final volume, calculated as follows, to bring stock standard solution to 500 μg/mL folic acid:

$$V_f = (W_s \times P_s \times 1000)/(100 \times 500) = (W_s \times P_s)/50$$

where V_f = final volume, mL, stock solution; W_s = weight, mg, folic acid standard; and P_s = purity, %, folic acid standard (from label).

Mix well. Store in red or amber bottle at 10°. Prepare fresh after 4 months.

(b) *Intermediate standard solution.*—50 μg/mL. Accurately pipet 10 mL stock standard solution, **(a)**, into 100 mL amber or red volumetric flask, dilute to volume with H_2O, and mix thoroughly. Store at 10°. Make fresh after 1 month.

(c) *Working standard solution.*—0.1 ng/mL. Pipet 1 mL intermediate standard solution, **(b)**, into amber or red 100 mL volumetric flask, dilute to volume with H_2O and mix. Pipet 1 mL this first solution into another 100 mL amber or red volumetric flask, dilute to volume, and mix. Pipet 5 mL this second solution into 250 mL amber or red volumetric flask, dilute to volume with phosphate buffer solution, **D(d)**, and mix. Label this as standard solution (0.0001 μg/mL or 0.1 ng/mL). Prepare fresh for each assay.

H. Inoculum

Inoculate tube of culture medium, **E(b)**, with cells from daily culture, **F**, and incubate 16–20 h at 37°. Under aseptic conditions, centrifuge culture 10 min at 2000 rpm to obtain clear supernate, discard supernate, and resuspend cells by shaking or swirling in 10 mL isotonic salt solution, **D(f)**. Repeat from "centrifuge culture 10 min ..." 2×. Add 1 mL of final suspension to 10 mL isotonic salt solution, **D(f)**, and swirl to form uniform suspension. Use as inoculum.

I. Assay Solution

For powder samples, accurately weigh sample containing ca 5 μg folic acid into 100 mL beaker. Reconstitute in 25–30 mL H_2O and quantitatively transfer to 100 mL volumetric flask. Dilute to volume with H_2O.

For liquid samples, pipet volume containing ca 5 μg folic acid into 100 mL volumetric flask. Dilute to volume with H_2O. (Sample solutions contain ca 0.05 μg [50 ng] folic acid/mL.)

Pipet 1 mL diluted sample and 1 mL chick pancreas preparation, **D(j)**, into 18 × 150 mm screw top culture tube, and mix well. Add 18 mL 0.05M phosphate buffer–ascorbic acid solution, **D(k)**, and 1 mL toluene. Mix.

For enzyme and reagent blank, pipet 1 mL H_2O and 1 mL chick pancreas preparation into 18 × 150 mm screw top culture tube and mix. Add 18 mL 0.05M phosphate buffer–ascorbic acid solution and 1 mL toluene. Mix.

Incubate sample and blank tubes 16 h at 37°. Sterilize 10 min at 121°, and centrifuge 10 min at 2000 rpm to obtain clear supernate. Dilute supernates with 0.05M phosphate buffer–ascorbic acid solution to volume, V_f, **G(a)**. Label as assay solution.

J. Assay Tubes

Meticulously cleanse by suitable means (Na Lauryl Sulfate USP has been found satisfactory as detergent), hard glass tubes and other necessary glassware. (Test organisms are highly sensitive to minute amounts of growth factors and to many cleansing agents. Therefore, it may be preferred to follow cleansing by heating glassware 1–2 h at ca 250°.)

Prepare tubes containing standard solution, **G(c)**, as follows: To tubes (in duplicate or replicate) add: 0.0 (for uninoculated blanks), 0.0 (for inoculated blanks), 1.0, 2.0, 3.0, and 4.0 mL standard solution, respectively.

Prepare tubes containing assay solution, **I**, as follows: To similar tubes (in duplicate or replicate) add 1.0, 2.0, 3.0, and 4.0 mL assay solution, respectively.

To each tube, standard and assay solutions, add phosphate buffer solution, **D(d)**, to make 5.0 mL. To bottle containing 200 mL basal medium stock solution, **C(f)**, add 1.0 mL vitamin solution, **D(h)**, and 0.8 mL pyridoxamine solution, **D(i)**, and mix well. Add 5.0 mL this medium to each standard and sample tube. Cover tubes suitably to prevent bacterial contamination, and sterilize 10 min at 121°. Cool as rapidly as practicable to minimize color formation. Take precautions to keep sterilizing and cooling conditions uniform throughout assay. Too close packing of tubes in autoclave, or overloading autoclave, may cause variation in heating rate.

Aseptically inoculate each tube, except 1 set of duplicate or replicate tubes containing 0.0 mL standard solution (uninoculated blanks), with 1 drop inoculum. Incubate 60–72 h, at temperature between 28 and 40°, maintained within ± 0.5°. Contamination of assay tubes with any foreign organism invalidates assay.

K. Determination

Prior to determination of response, visually inspect each set of tubes. Uninoculated blanks should be clear; standards and samples should be free of growth other than test organism. Titrate contents of each tube with 0.1N NaOH, using bromthymol blue indicator, **D(e)**, or using pH meter to pH 6.8. When determining pH, read pH values to nearest 0.01 pH unit after incubation. pH at 5.0 mL level of standard solution is normally 1.0–1.5 pH units below inoculated blank. Disregard results of assay if titer of inoculated blank is more than 1.5 mL greater than titer of uninoculated blank. Titer at 5.0 mL level of standard solution should be 8–12 mL.

Prepare standard concentration-response curve by plotting titration values, expressed in mL 0.1N NaOH for each level of standard solution used, against amount of reference standard contained in respective tubes.

Determine amount of folic acid for each level of assay solution by interpolation from standard curve. Discard results of any sample with titer of <0.5 mL or >4.5 mL.

L. Calculation

For each level of assay solution used, calculate folic acid content/mL assay solution. Calculate average values from tubes that do not vary by $\geq 15\%$ from this average. If number of acceptable values remaining is <2/3 original number of tubes used in 4 levels of assay solution, data are insufficient. If number of acceptable values remaining is $\geq 2/3$ original number of tubes, calculate folic acid concentration ($\mu g/100$ mL "as fed" formula) in sample from the average.

$$\text{Folic acid} = [(X \times D) - EB] \times [(100 \times R)/1000\ Q)]$$

where X = average value of folic acid per mL of assay solution, ng; D = dilution factor based on 1 mL sample dilution incubated with enzyme preparation, mL; EB = folic acid value found in enzyme blank, ng/mL enzyme preparation; Q = sample weight or volume, g or mL; and R = reconstitution value of sample required to make 100 mL of "as fed" formula, expressed as weight or volume.

Turbidimetric Method

(Not applicable in presence of extraneous turbidity or color in amount that interferes with turbidimetric measurements)

M. Folic Acid Standard Solutions

Proceed as in **G**.

N. Inoculum

Proceed as in **H**.

O. Assay Solution

Proceed as in **I**.

P. Assay Tubes

Proceed as in **J**.

Q. Calibration of Photometer

See **960.46F**, Chapter 15.1.

271

R. Determination
>   *See* **960.46G**.

S. Calculation
>   Proceed as in **L**.

Ref.: J. AOAC Int. **76**, 398(1993).
CAS-59-30-3 (folic acid)

Chapter 20
Iodine

20.1   **992.22—Iodine (as Iodide) in Pasteurized Liquid Milk**
and Skim Milk Powder
Liquid Chromatographic Method
First Action 1992

(Applicable to determination of iodine, as iodide, in liquid and powdered milk)

(*Caution*: Observe common safety procedures for operating centrifuge. Acetonitrile is extremely flammable and
skin irritant. If skin contact occurs, immediately flush affected area with large amounts of water.)

Method Performance:
  Iodine, 303, 308 μg/L, in liquid milk
  Mean recovery of total iodine = 87%
  s_r = 22; s_R = 22; RSD_r = 8.2%; RSD_R = 8.3%
  Iodine, 0.5–4.6 μg/g, in powdered skim milk
  Mean recovery of total iodine = 91%
  s_r = 0.14; s_R = 0.22; RSD_r = 9.0%; RSD_R = 12.7%

A. Principle

Iodine in milk samples is measured only in form of iodide (I^-). Protein and insoluble material in liquid milk
samples are removed by passing through 25,000 MW cutoff membrane. Iodide in clear filtrate is separated
using reversed-phase ion pair liquid chromatography (LC) and is selectively detected electrochemically with
silver working electrode at 0 to +50 mV applied potential. Iodide is quantitated against external iodide
standards.

B. Apparatus

(**a**) *Membrane cones.*—25,000–30,000 MW cutoff (Amicon CENTRIFLO, CF–25, Amicon Corp.,
Danvers, MA or Millipore Ultrafree PF, Bedford, MA, is suitable).
(**b**) *Conical membrane support.*—To support membrane cone in centrifuge tube (Amicon No. CS1A is
suitable).
(**c**) *Guard column (optional).*—C_{18} cartridge, 15 × 3.2 mm.
(**d**) *Analytical column.*—5 μm C_{18} to yield acceptable k' and column efficiency (see **E**) (PARTISPHERE
C_{18}, 110 × 4.7 mm, Whatman Inc., Clifton, NJ is suitable).
(**e**) *Membrane filters.*—47 mm, NYLON-66 1.2 μm, 0.5 μm.
(**f**) *Centrifuge tubes.*—50 mL, 27 mm id, conical, disposable plastic, with screw cap.

(**g**) *Centrifuge.*—Capable of holding 50 mL centrifuge tubes and delivering 1000 rcf centrifugal force (rcf = 0.0000118 × radius (cm) × rpm × rpm). Lower rcf force can be used if centrifugation time is increased.

(**h**) *LC system.*—LC pump capable of 5000 psi and 5 mL/min flow rate; valve injector capable of 50–200 μL injections; electrochemical LC detector with silver working electrode at 0 to +50 mV potential (BAS LC-4B, Bioanalytical Systems, Inc., West Lafayette, IN is suitable) or pulsed amperometric detector (PAD) (Dionex Corp., Sunnyvale, CA is suitable) may be used with solvent compatible silver electrode kit; strip chart recorder or electronic integrator/plotter.

C. Reagents

(*Note*: Iodide is unstable in light, store all iodide solutions away from extended exposure to white light.)

(**a**) *Iodide reference standard solution.*—0.100 ± 0.001M sodium or potassium iodide solution (12.69 g iodide/L), recommend standardization traceable to certified reference material. Discard 12 months after standardization or 6 months after opening container. (Iodide reference standard traceable to NIST Standard Reference Material is available on special order from Ricca Chemical Co, Arlington, TX).

(**b**) *Reagent-grade chemicals.*—Dibasic sodium phosphate, 85% phosphoric acid, *n*-amyl alcohol (octanol may be substituted) and reagent alcohol (90% ethanol, 5% methanol, 5% propanol) (pure ethanol or 2-propanol may be substituted).

(**c**) *Acetonitrile.*—LC grade.

(**d**) *Hexadecyltrimethylammonium chloride solution.*—25% in H_2O (0.78M) hexadecyltrimethylammonium chloride (cetyltrimethylammonium chloride) (Aldrich Chemical, Milwaukee, WI is suitable supplier).

(**e**) *LC mobile phase.*—10.0mM dibasic sodium phosphate, 1.0mM cetyltrimethylammonium chloride, 32% acetonitrile, pH = 6.8. Dissolve 1.42 ± 0.05 g dibasic sodium phosphate in ca 600 mL H_2O in 1 L beaker. Add 1.3 mL hexadecyltrimethylammonium chloride solution and mix. Add 320 mL acetonitrile and mix well. Adjust pH of mobile phase to 6.8 ± 0.1 with phosphoric acid solution. Dilute to 1 L with H_2O and mix well. Filter solution through 0.5 μm NYLON-66 membrane filter. (Mobile phase may be slightly cloudy before filtration. Pre-filtering through 1.2 μm filter aids significantly in filtration through 0.5 μm filter.) Dilute mobile phase slightly with H_2O or acetonitrile to adjust to desired iodide retention time.) Store in tightly capped container. Discard after 1 year.

(**f**) *50% acetonitrile solution.*—Add 500 mL acetonitrile to 1 L volumetric flask. Dilute to volume with H_2O and mix well. Store in stoppered glass container. Discard after 2 years.

(**g**) *20% alcohol solution.*—Add 200 mL reagent alcohol to 800 mL H_2O; mix well.

(**h**) *Stock iodide standard solution.*—101.5 mg/L. Pour ca 10 mL iodide reference standard solution, (**a**), into 50 mL beaker. Pipet 8.00 mL iodide standard into 1 L volumetric flask. Dilute to volume with H_2O; mix well. Store at room temperature and protect from white light. Discard after 30 days.

(**i**) *Intermediate iodide standard solution.*—1015 μg/L. Dilute 10.00 mL stock iodide standard solution, (**h**), to 1 L with H_2O. Mix well. Protect from white light. Discard after 7 days.

(**j**) *Working iodide standard solutions.*—254, 152, 102, and 20.3 μg/L. Dilute 25.00, 15.00, 10.00, and 2.00 mL of intermediate standard solution, (**i**), to 100 mL with H_2O in separate volumetric flasks. Mix well. Protect from white light. Discard after 7 days.

D. Preparation of Sample

Soak new membrane cones in 20% alcohol solution ≥1 h. Remove cone from alcohol solution, drain, mount in support, and place in 50 mL centrifuge tube. Centrifuge 5–10 min at 900–1000 rcf to remove excess liquid from membranes. Invert and drain cone to confirm that no appreciable amount of liquid remains in cone before use. Place prepared cones into membrane supports mounted in clean, labeled centrifuge tubes for sample analysis.

For powdered milk samples.—Accurately weigh 4–4.5 g milk powder to nearest 0.01 g. Place in beaker containing 70–80 mL H$_2$O. Stir briskly 5–10 min to fully wet and mix milk powder. Visually verify complete wetting and mixing of powder. Transfer sample quantitatively to 100 mL volumetric flask, add 1 drop *n*-amyl alcohol to reduce foaming, and dilute to volume with H$_2$O. Mix well.

For liquid milk samples.—Dilute 10 mL sample with 10 mL H$_2$O and mix well. Prepare 2 cones/sample. Fill membrane cone with diluted powdered or liquid sample,

Figure 992.22.—Typical liquid chromatograms of iodide in iodide standard solution and powdered milk sample.

above, to within 5 mm of cone top. Centrifuge samples at 900–1000 rcf 15–20 min (if centrifuge will not attain 900 rcf, use highest rcf available and increase time to attain enough filtrate for LC analysis). Inject filtrate from each cone separately on LC system. Soak used membrane cones and supports immediately in hot water. Flush cones well with stream of hot water to remove sample residue. Store in 20% alcohol solution. Membrane cones may be re-used several times.

E. LC Analysis

For new LC column, wash column with ca 50 mL 50% acetonitrile solution. Pump 30 mL mobile phase through column, discarding eluent. Turn on working electrode of detector and verify proper applied potential. Begin re-cycling mobile phase and pump mobile phase through system at 2 mL/min until stable baseline is obtained (1 h minimum). Stable retention time and peak area or height reproducibility of 3% for consecutive injections of 254 µg/L standard iodide solution indicates equilibrated and properly operating system.

Iodide peak capacity factor (k') should be 3–10 and column effiency should allow quantitation of 20.3 µg/L working iodide standard solution. If using integrator, adjust parameters for proper integration of iodide peak, but do not integrate negative "tail" of iodide peak (*see* Fig. **992.22**; LC conditions: analyzed on 110 × 4.7 mm id PARTISPHERE C$_{18}$ 5 µm, 2 mL/min flow rate, 60 µL injection, BAS LC-4B detector, 10 nA full scale, +50 mV). If using manual peak heights, adjust injection volume or detector sensitivity for ≥70% full scale peak height for 254 µg/L working iodide standard solution. Adjust applied potential to EC detector working silver electrode within 0 to +50 mV to optimize peak shape and sensitivity.

When LC system is equilibrated, inject working iodide standard solutions and samples. Wait ≥5 min after iodide peak elutes before next injection. Distribute working iodide standard solution injections throughout run to assure adequate quantitation of samples and to acount for any drift in system. (*Note*: Recommend inject all 4 working iodide standard solutions every 6–8 sample injections.)

Mobile phase may be recycled between sample analyses or when standard solutions alone are being injected. However, when samples are being injected, do not recycle column eluent because this can reduce column life and may lead to interfering peaks and gradually drifting baseline. During extended intervals between use, flush column and system with 50% acetonitrile solution and reequilibrate column with mobile phase before next use. In routine use, recycle mobile phase at low flow rate (0.2 mL/min) to maintain system readiness.

F. Calculations

(*Note*: Silver electrode may yield negative tailing on iodide peak; *see* Fig. **992.22**). Measure peak heights from baseline extended from baseline immediately before iodide peak. To accomplish this when using integrator equipped with negative peak function, activate negative peak function ca 1 min before iodide peak elutes and deactivate shortly before end of run.

Measure peak responses (areas or heights) of iodide peaks in chromatograms of working standards. (Peak area is preferred to peak height because peak shape can vary during run. Visually verify that each iodide peak is being detected reasonably well.) Perform linear least-squares analysis on relationship between standard concentration (μg/L) vs. peak area (height) to obtain calibration line. [Use only the 4 working iodide standard solutions for calibration line; do not use zero (0,0).] Correlation coefficient (r) of line should be ≥ 0.99.

For each sample injection, calculate iodide concentration, C, in μg/L, in sample filtrate from sample peak response and calibration line.

Calculate iodide level, I_L, in original liquid sample:

$$I_L, \mu g/L = C \times 2$$

where 2 = dilution factor of original sample.

Calculate iodide level, I_P, in original powdered milk sample:

$$I_P, \mu g/g = C \times 0.100 L/W$$

where W = sample weight, g, and 0.100L = volume of diluted powdered milk.

Calculate mean of single determinations for filtrate from each membrane cone for each sample; round mean to 3 significant figures.

Ref.: J. AOAC Int. (1993) **76** July/August issue.

Chapter 21
Iron

21.1

968.08—Minerals in Animal Feed
Atomic Absorption Spectrophotometric Method
First Action 1968
Final Action 1969

See Chapter 12.1.

21.2

975.03—Metals in Plants
Atomic Absorption Spectrophotometric Method
First Action 1975
Final Action 1988

See Chapter 12.2.

21.3

980.03—Metals in Plants
Direct Reading Spectrographic Method
Final Action 1988

See Chapter 12.3

21.4

965.09—Nutrients (Minor) in Fertilizers
Atomic Absorption Spectrophotometric Method
First Action 1965
Final Action 1969

See Chapter 12.4.

21.5   953.01—Metals in Plants
General Recommendations for Emission Spectrographic Methods
First Action 1988

See Chapter 12.5.

21.6   945.40—Iron in Bread
Preparation of Sample
Final Action

Slice bread, let air dry until in equilibrium with air, and crush to ca 20-mesh size on wooden surface with wooden rolling pin. (Grinding may be done in mill if tests show no increase in Fe due to grinding of particular material under examination. In general, grinding in mills increases Fe content.)

Proceed as in **944.02B** (*see* 21.8).

21.7   950.39—Iron in Macaroni Products
Final Action

Proceed as in **944.02C** (*see* 21.8)

21.8   944.02—Iron in Flour
Spectrophotometric Method
Final Action

(Applicable to enriched, enriched self-rising, and phosphated flours. Rinse all flasks, beakers, funnels, etc., with H_2O before use, and filter all reagents to remove suspended matter.)

A. Reagents

(a) *Orthophenanthroline solution.*—Dissolve 0.1 g *o*-phenanthroline in ca 80 mL H_2O at 80°, cool, and dilute to 100 mL.

(b) *Alpha,alpha-dipyridyl solution.*—Dissolve 0.1 g α,α-dipyridyl in H_2O and dilute to 100 mL.

(Reagents (a) and (b) kept in cool, dark place will remain stable several weeks.)

(c) *Iron standard solution.*—0.01 mg Fe/mL. (*1*) Dissolve 0.1 g anhydrous grade Fe wire in 20 mL HCl and 50 mL H_2O, and dilute to 1 L. Dilute 100 mL of this solution to 1 L. Or—(*2*) Dissolve 3.512 g $Fe(NH_4)_2(SO_4)_2 \cdot 6H_2O$ in H_2O, add 2 drops HCl, and dilute to 500 mL. Dilute 10 mL of this solution to 1 L.

(d) *Hydroxylamine hydrochloride solution.*—Dissolve 10 g $H_2NOH \cdot HCl$ in H_2O and dilute to 100 mL.

(e) *Magnesium nitrate solution.*—Dissolve 50 g $Mg(NO_3)_2 \cdot 6H_2O$ in H_2O and dilute to 100 mL.

(f) *Acetate buffer solution.*—Dissolve 8.3 g anhydrous NaOAc (previously dried at 100°) in H_2O, add 12 mL CH_3COOH, and dilute to 100 mL. (It may be necessary to redistil the CH_3COOH and recrystallize the NaOAc from H_2O, depending on amount of Fe present.)

(g) *Sodium acetate solution.*—2M. Dissolve 272 g $NaOAc \cdot 3H_2O$ in H_2O and dilute to 1 L.

(h) *Buffer solution, pH 3.5.*—Dilute 6.4 mL 2M NaOAc solution, (g), and 93.6 mL 2M CH_3COOH (120 g/L) to 1 L with H_2O.

B. Preparation of Standard Curve

Prepare 11 solutions containing 0.0, 2.0, 5.0, 10.0, 15.0, 20.0, 25.0, 30.0, 35.0, 40.0, and 45.0 mL, respectively, of the final diluted Fe standard solution, plus 2.0 mL HCl, in 100 mL. Using 10 mL of each of these solutions, proceed as in **944.02C**, beginning " ... add 1 mL $H_2NOH \cdot HCl$ ... " Plot concentration against scale reading.

C. Determination

(a) *By dry ashing.*—Ash 10.0 g flour in Pt, SiO_2, or porcelain dish (ca 60 mm diameter, 35 mL capacity) as in **923.03**. (Porcelain evaporating dishes of ca 25 mL capacity are satisfactory. Do not use flat-bottom dishes of diameter >60 mm.) Cool, and weigh if % ash is desired. Continue ashing until practically C-free. To diminish ashing time, or for samples that do not burn practically C-free, use one of following ash aids:

Moisten ash with 0.5–1.0 mL $Mg(NO_3)_2$ solution or with redistilled HNO_3. Dry and carefully ignite in furnace, avoiding spattering. (White ash with no C results in most cases.) Do not add these ash aids to self-rising flour (products containing NaCl) in Pt dish because of vigorous action on dish. Cool, add 5 mL HCl, letting acid rinse upper portion of dish, and evaporate to dryness on steam bath. Dissolve residue by adding 2.0 mL HCl, accurately measured, and heat 5 min on steam bath with watch glass on dish. Rinse watch glass with H_2O, filter into 100 mL volumetric flask, cool, and dilute to volume.

Pipet 10 mL aliquot into 25 mL volumetric flask, and add 1 mL $H_2NOH \cdot HCl$ solution; in few min add 5 mL buffer solution, (f), and 1 mL *o*-phenanthroline or 2 mL dipyridyl solution, and dilute to volume. Determine *A* in spectrophotometer or photometer at ca 510 nm. From reading, determine Fe concentration from equation of line representing standard points or by reference to standard curve for known Fe concentration. Determine blank on reagents and make correction. Calculate Fe in flour as mg/lb.

923.03 (Ash of Flour, Direct Method)

Weigh 3–5 g well mixed sample into shallow, relatively broad ashing dish that has been ignited, cooled in desiccator, and weighed soon after reaching room temperature. Ignite in furnace at ca 550° (dull red) until light gray ash results, or to constant weight. Cool in desiccator and weigh soon after reaching room temperature. Reignited CaO is satisfactory drying agent for desiccator.

Reference: JAOAC 7, 132(1923).

(b) *By wet digestion.*—(*Caution: See Appendix* for safety notes on distillation, wet oxidation, nitric acid, and sulfuric acid.) Transfer 10.00 g flour to 800 mL Kjeldahl flask, previously rinsed with dilute acid, then with H_2O; add 20 mL H_2O and mix; pipet 5 mL H_2SO_4 into flask and mix; add 25 mL HNO_3 and mix well. After few minutes, heat flask very gently at brief intervals (to avoid foaming out of flask) until heavy evolution of NO_2 fumes ceases. Continue to heat gently until material begins to char; then add few mL

HNO_3 cautiously at intervals until SO_3 fumes evolve and colorless or very pale yellow liquid is obtained (60–65 mL HNO_3 total in ca 2 h). Cool, add 50 mL H_2O and 1 Pyrex glass bead, and heat to SO_3 fumes; cool, add 25 mL H_2O, and filter quantitatively through 11 cm paper into 100 mL volumetric flask; cool, and dilute to volume.

Pipet 10 mL into 25 mL volumetric flask, add 1 mL $H_2NOH\cdot HCl$ solution, rotate flask, and let stand few min. Add 9.5 mL $2M$ NaOAc solution, (g), and 1 mL o-phenanthroline solution, dilute to volume, and mix. Let stand ≥ 5 min and determine A in spectrophotometer or photometer at ca 510 nm.

With self-rising flour, the 9.5 mL $2M$ NaOAc solution, (g), may be reduced to 8.0 mL. To determine exact amount of buffer solution, (g), needed to adjust each digest to most desirable pH range, mix 10 mL aliquot of sample with measured amount of buffer solution, (g), dilute with H_2O to 25 mL, and determine pH either potentiometrically or colorimetrically.

For colorimetric determination, add 5 drops bromophenol blue indicator (grind 0.1 g powder with 1.5 mL $0.1N$ NaOH and dilute to 25 mL) to solution and compare color with that of equal volume of pH 3.5 buffer solution, (h), also treated with 5 drops indicator. Although color develops from pH 2–9, avoid pH <3.0 and preferably work at pH 3.5–4.5. With cereal products, 9.5 mL buffer solution, (g), is satisfactory. With samples high in Fe, aliquot of 5 mL instead of 10 mL may be used with 4.8 mL buffer solution, (g).

Conduct digestion so as to avoid contamination with Fe, and determine blank. After correction for blank, calculate as mg Fe/lb.

References: JAOAC **27**, 86, 396(1944); **28**, 77(1945).
CAS-7439-89-6 (iron)

21.9 984.27—Calcium, Copper, Iron, Magnesium, Manganese, Phosphorus, Potassium, Sodium, and Zinc in Infant Formula
Inductively Coupled Plasma Emission Spectroscopic Method
First Action 1984
Final Action 1986

See Chapter 12.13.

21.10 985.35—Minerals in Ready-to-Feed Milk-Based Infant Formula
Atomic Absorption Spectrophotometric Method
First Action 1985
Final Action 1988

See Chapter 12.14.

21.11   **990.05—Copper, Iron, and Nickel in Edible Oils and Fats**
Direct Graphite Furnace
Atomic Absorption Spectrophotometric Method
First Action 1990
IUPAC-AOAC Method

See Chapter 14.11.

Chapter 22
Magnesium

22.1

975.03—Metals in Plants
Atomic Absorption Spectrophotometric Method
First Action 1975
Final Action 1988

See Chapter 12.2.

22.2

980.03—Metals in Plants
Direct Reading Spectrographic Method
Final Action 1988

See Chapter 12.3.

22.3

965.09—Nutrients (Minor) in Fertilizers
Atomic Absorption Spectrophotometric Method
First Action 1965
Final Action 1969

See Chapter 12.4.

22.4

953.01—Metals in Plants
General Recommendations for Emission Spectrographic Methods
First Action 1988

See Chapter 12.5.

22.5   **985.01—Metals and Other Elements in Plants**
Inductively Coupled Plasma Spectroscopic Method
First Action 1985
Final Action 1988

See Chapter 12.6.

22.6   **991.25—Calcium, Magnesium, and Phosphorus in Cheese**
Atomic Absorption Spectrophotometric and Colorimetric Methods
First Action 1991

See Chapter 12.12.

22.7   **984.27—Calcium, Copper, Iron, Magnesium,**
Manganese, Phosphorus, Potassium, Sodium,
and Zinc in Infant Formula
Inductively Coupled Plasma Emission Spectroscopic Method
First Action 1984
Final Action 1986

See Chapter 12.13.

22.8   **985.35—Minerals in Ready-to-Feed Milk-Based Infant Formula**
Atomic Absorption Spectrophotometric Method
First Action 1985
Final Action 1988

See Chapter 12.14.

Chapter 23
Moisture

23.1   925.04—Moisture in Animal Feed by Distillation with Toluene
Final Action

A. Apparatus

Connect 250 mL flask of Pyrex or other resistant glass by means of Bidwell-Sterling moisture receiver to 500 mm Liebig condenser. Calibrate receiver, 5 mL capacity, by distilling known amounts H_2O into graduated column, and estimating column of H_2O to 0.01 mL. Clean tube and condenser with chromic acid cleaning mixture, rinse thoroughly with H_2O, then alcohol, and dry in oven to prevent undue amount H_2O from adhering to inner surfaces during determination.

B. Determination

If sample is likely to bump, add dry sand to cover bottom of flask. Add enough toluene to cover sample completely (ca 75 mL). Weigh and introduce enough sample into toluene to give 2–5 mL H_2O and connect apparatus. Fill receiving tube with toluene, pouring it through top of condenser. Bring to boil and distil slowly, ca 2 drops/s, until most of the H_2O passes over; then increase rate of distillation to ca 4 drops/s.

When all H_2O is apparently over, wash down condenser by pouring toluene in at top, continuing distillation short time to see whether any more H_2O distils over; if it does, repeat washing-down process. If any H_2O remains in condenser, remove by brushing down with tube brush attached to Cu wire and saturated with toluene, washing down condenser at same time. (Entire process is usually completed within 1 h.) Let receiving tube come to room temperature. If any drops adhere to sides of tube, force them down, using Cu wire with end wrapped with rubber band. Read volume H_2O and calculate to %.

References: JAOAC **8**, 295(1925); **9**, 30(1926).

23.2   986.21—Moisture in Spices
Distillation Method
First Action 1986
Final Action 1988

A. Apparatus

Connect 500 or 1000 mL short-neck round-bottom flask by means of Bidwell-Sterling 5 mL capacity moisture receiver to 400 mm West-type condenser. Clean distilling tube receiver and condenser with chromic acid solution, rinse thoroughly with H_2O and then with ca 0.5N alcoholic KOH, and drain 10 min.

If alcoholic KOH solution contains carbonates, follow with alcoholic rinse. Calibrate receiver by distilling 1 ± 0.01 mL H_2O with 100 mL solvent into receiver. Cool; repeat until calibration is complete.

B. Reagents

(a) *Toluene.*—For most spices.

(b) *Hexane.*—For capsicums, onions, garlic, and other spices containing large amounts of sugar.

C. Determination

Place 40 g spice (or enough to yield 2–5 mL H_2O) in distilling flask. Add enough solvent to cover sample completely (never <75 mL). Fill receiving tube with solvent, pouring through top of condenser. Insert loose cotton plug in top of condenser to prevent condensation of atmospheric moisture in tube. Bring to boil and distil slowly, ca 2 drops/s, until most of H_2O distils over; then increase rate of distillation to ca 4 drops/s. Continue distilling until 2 consecutive readings 15 min apart show no change. Dislodge any H_2O held up in condenser with brush or wire loop. Rinse condenser carefully with ca 5 mL toluene. Continue distillation 3–5 min; cool receiver to room temperature (ca 25°), allowing it to stand in air or immersing it in H_2O. Solvent and H_2O layers should now be clear; if not, let stand until clearing occurs. Read volume of H_2O, estimating to nearest 0.01 mL, and calculate to percent.

Reference: JAOAC **69**, 834(1986).

23.3   972.20—Moisture in Prunes and Raisins
Moisture Meter Method
First Action 1972
Final Action 1980

A. Apparatus

Dried fruit moisture tester meter.—Type A series (DFA of California, PO Box 270A, Santa Clara, CA 95052); *see* Fig. **972.20** for electric circuit.

B. Determination

Grind sample 3 times through food chopper, using cutter with 16 teeth. If testing hot fruit from processor, cool fruit as follows: Mix ca 60 g chopped solid CO_2 with fruit and then grind mixture 3 times before taking moisture reading. Pack ground sample into Bakelite cylinder with fingers, making certain that it is packed tightly around bottom electrode. Fill cylinder completely with tightly packed sample, and level.

Lower top electrode and press it into sample until top electrode lever is against stop. Insert thermometer into ground sample until thermometer bulb is ca halfway between electrodes.

Select correct table for type and condition of fruit being tested (Table **972.20A**: natural or low moisture, tap 6 setting; Table **972.20B**: processed, tap 3 setting). Set switch (S2) to number given on table selected.

Plug tester into 110 v ac outlet and put switch to "on". (Red light indicates current.) Keep push button down and turn dial so that meter needle moves toward 0. Adjust dial so that needle is at its lowest, or turning, point. After making fine adjustment of dial to meter 0 or turning point, read dial and then read thermometer.

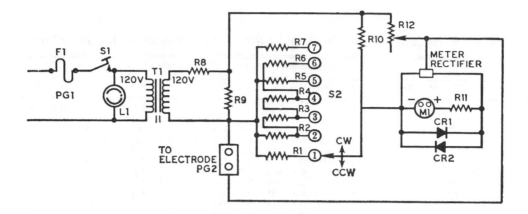

Figure 972.20.—Electrical circuit diagram for dried fruit moisture tester.

Explanation to Figure 972.20:

Item	Item	Value	Tolerance, %	Power Rating, w
F1—Fuse 3AG 2A, 125 v	R1	10K	1	1
S1—Push-button switch	R2	200K	1	½
L1—Neon light	R3	1K	1	1
T1—Isolating transformer 1-1, 120 v, 50 ma	R4	100K	1	½
PG1—Plug, 120 v	R5	40K	1	½
PG2—Plug to electrode	R6	20K	1	½
M1—Microammeter rectifier, type 0-100 ma meter rectifier	R7, R10	3K	1	1
CR1—Rectifier F4 (5M2483)	R8	2.5K	-	10
CR2—Rectifier F4 (5M2483)	R9	5K	-	10
S2—2 Wafer 7-point tap switch	R11	1.5K	10	½
	R12	10K	±5	(wire-wound)

C. Use of Tables

Choose temperature column of appropriate table nearest to sample temperature. Read down this column to figure closest to dial reading, then read across to "% Moisture" column.

D. Example

Examination of processed raisin sample gave following data: dial setting 76 and temperature 74°F, on tap 3. Looking down 74° column (Table **972.20B**), obtain 75.2 at 18.5% moisture and 78.4 at 19.0% moisture. Since reading is nearer to 18.5 than 19.0%, report sample as containing 18.5% moisture, or interpolate.

Table 972.20A.—Conductance-Temperature Correlation for Natural or Low Moisture Raisins; Switch Setting, Tap 6

	Conductance Readings at Temperatue (°F):																							
M^a	56	58	60	62	64	66	68	70	72	74	76	78	80	82	84	86	88	90	92	94	96	98	100	102
9.0																9.0	15.0	21.0	25.0	29.0	33.0	36.0	39.0	42.0
9.5													4.0	11.0	17.5	22.5	27.0	32.5	37.0	40.5	44.0	47.0	49.0	51.5
10.0									1.0	7.0	13.5	17.5	23.0	28.5	34.0	38.0	41.5	45.5	49.0	52.0	54.5	57.0	59.0	61.5
10.5							7.5	13.0	18.0	24.0	29.5	35.0	40.0	44.5	49.0	51.5	54.0	57.0	60.0	62.0	64.0	66.0	68.0	70.0
11.0					8.5	16.0	22.5	28.0	34.0	39.0	44.0	48.5	53.0	56.0	59.0	61.5	64.0	66.0	68.5	70.5	72.5	73.8	75.3	76.8
11.5			9.0	18.0	26.0	31.0	36.0	42.0	47.5	51.5	55.5	58.7	62.5	64.7	67.5	69.5	71.0	73.0	75.0	76.5	78.3	79.6	81.0	82.5
12.0			23.5	30.5	37.5	42.5	47.0	52.0	56.5	60.0	63.3	66.5	69.0	71.0	73.0	74.5	76.0	78.0	79.7	81.0	82.0	83.8	85.2	86.5
12.6	16.5	27.0	34.5	40.0	46.0	50.5	55.0	59.0	63.0	65.8	68.6	71.0	73.3	75.0	76.6	78.0	79.7	81.3	82.6	84.0	85.4	86.7	88.0	89.3
13.0	30.5	37.2	42.5	48.0	52.3	56.5	60.5	64.3	67.7	70.0	72.5	74.8	76.7	78.3	79.7	81.2	82.6	83.8	85.2	86.5	87.8	89.2	90.5	91.3
13.5	40.0	45.0	49.7	54.0	58.0	61.5	65.0	68.5	71.3	73.4	75.4	77.5	79.4	80.7	82.0	83.5	85.0	86.2	87.3	88.5	89.8	91.0	92.2	93.0
14.0	48.3	52.5	56.5	60.0	63.0	66.0	69.2	72.0	74.5	76.4	78.0	80.0	81.7	83.0	84.4	85.6	87.0	88.0	89.3	90.3	91.5	92.6	93.8	94.6
14.5	55.3	59.0	62.3	65.0	67.6	70.4	72.7	75.0	77.0	78.7	80.4	82.0	83.7	85.0	86.2	87.3	88.7	89.7	90.8	91.8	93.0	94.0	95.0	95.8
15.0	61.6	64.5	67.7	70.8	72.4	74.3	76.0	78.0	79.7	81.1	82.6	84.0	85.6	86.7	87.9	89.1	90.3	91.4	92.5	93.5	94.5	95.5	96.4	97.0

^{a} M = % moisture.

Table 972.20B.—Conductance-Temperature Correlation for Processed Raisins; Switch Setting, Tap 3

	Conductance Readings at Temperature (°F):																							
M^a	56	58	60	62	64	66	68	70	72	74	76	78	80	82	84	86	88	90	92	94	96	98	100	102
13.0											0.0	6.7	12.8	18.0	22.2	26.8	31.4	35.4	39.5	43.7	48.0	52.2	55.8	59.0
13.5										2.5	9.0	15.4	21.0	25.2	29.4	34.0	38.3	42.7	46.5	50.5	54.3	58.0	61.5	64.8
14.0									5.7	11.7	17.0	23.0	27.5	32.4	36.6	40.8	44.2	48.3	52.6	56.2	59.6	62.8	66.3	69.2
14.5							1.0	7.5	14.0	19.0	24.3	29.4	34.2	39.0	42.8	46.7	50.9	54.4	57.5	60.8	64.2	67.2	70.3	73.0
15.0						2.5	9.3	15.5	21.7	27.0	31.6	36.3	40.9	45.5	49.2	53.0	56.8	59.7	62.7	65.4	68.2	70.9	73.6	76.1
15.5					4.0	11.0	17.7	23.1	29.7	34.0	38.2	42.7	47.3	51.6	55.2	58.5	62.1	64.9	67.2	69.7	72.0	74.2	76.6	78.7
16.0					13.5	20.0	25.3	31.0	36.0	41.0	45.5	50.0	54.0	58.0	61.6	64.5	67.4	69.6	72.0	73.7	75.5	77.3	79.3	81.0
16.5			13.0	20.5	26.5	32.0	36.6	42.0	46.5	50.7	54.8	58.5	62.0	65.5	68.8	71.0	73.0	75.2	77.0	78.4	79.7	81.3	82.8	84.3
17.0	13.5	22.0	28.4	34.0	39.0	43.5	47.2	51.7	55.7	59.4	62.6	66.0	68.8	71.5	74.1	76.0	77.8	79.4	80.9	82.0	83.2	84.2	85.5	86.7
17.5	31.0	36.0	41.0	45.0	49.0	52.5	56.0	59.5	63.0	66.0	69.0	71.6	74.0	76.2	78.4	80.0	81.5	82.6	83.9	84.8	85.8	86.8	87.8	88.7
18.0	43.0	47.0	50.0	53.5	57.0	59.7	62.7	64.8	69.0	71.5	73.8	76.0	78.0	79.8	81.6	82.7	84.0	85.0	86.0	86.8	87.7	88.5	89.5	90.2
18.5	50.5	53.3	56.0	59.4	62.5	65.0	67.7	70.4	73.0	75.2	77.3	79.2	81.0	82.4	83.8	84.8	85.8	86.7	87.7	88.4	89.0	89.9	90.7	91.3
19.0	56.0	58.5	61.2	64.0	66.8	69.2	71.6	74.0	76.4	78.4	80.2	81.7	83.3	84.5	85.7	86.7	87.6	88.5	89.3	89.8	90.4	91.0	91.7	92.3
19.5	60.7	63.0	65.5	68.3	70.5	72.7	74.7	77.2	79.2	80.8	82.5	83.9	85.2	86.2	87.2	88.0	88.8	89.5	90.3	90.9	91.4	91.9	92.5	93.0
20.0	65.0	67.5	69.6	71.8	74.0	76.0	77.9	79.8	81.7	83.1	84.6	85.7	87.0	87.8	88.7	89.5	90.1	90.7	91.4	91.8	92.3	92.8	93.4	93.9
20.5	69.2	71.3	73.3	75.2	77.2	78.6	80.6	82.4	83.9	85.3	86.4	87.4	88.4	89.3	90.0	90.6	91.2	91.8	92.5	92.9	93.3	93.8	94.3	94.7

^{a} M = % moisture.

References: JAOAC **52**, 858(1969); **54**, 219(1971); **55**, 202(1972); **59**, 331(1976).

23.4   977.10—Moisture in Cacao Products
Karl Fischer Method
First Action 1977
Final Action 1979

(Applicable to milk chocolate and confectionary coatings)

A. Apparatus and Reagents

(**a**) *Karl Fischer titration assembly.*—Manual or automatic, with stirrer.

(**b**) *Syringes.*—1 mL with needle end cap (0–40 unit insulin type is satisfactory) and 10 mL without needle (disposable plastic type is satisfactory).

(**c**) *Karl Fischer reagent.*—Stabilized, with H_2O equivalent of ca 5 mg H_2O/mL reagent. Available commercially or prepare as follows: Dissolve 133 g I in 425 mL dry pyridine in dry glass-stoppered bottle. Add 425 mL dry ethylene glycol monomethyl ether. Cool to 4° in ice bath and bubble in 102–105 g SO_2. Mix well and let stand 12 h. Reagent is reasonably stable, but restandardize for each series of determinations. Place 50 mL formamide, practical grade, into 200 mL Berzelius beaker containing magnetic stirrer. Place in titrimeter and titrate. (Titrate slowly near end point until 0.1 mL addition causes meter to deflect to right of 0 and remain 60 s.) Quickly add accurately weighed amount (0.250–0.350 g) disodium tartrate·$2H_2O$. Titrate immediately to same end point. Repeat determination and calculate average.

$$\text{mg } H_2O/\text{mL reagent} = (\text{mg Na}_2\text{C}_4\text{H}_4\text{O}_6 \cdot 2H_2O \times 0.1566)/\text{mL reagent}$$

(**d**) *Karl Fischer solvent.*—Mix equal volumes anhydrous methyl alcohol and $CHCl_3$.

B. Determination

Standardize reagent, (**c**), by accurately weighing ca 125 mg H_2O from 1 mL syringe (5 units) into 30–50 mL pretitrated solvent. (Keep needle capped except while delivering H_2O, to eliminate evaporation.) Titrate with reagent, (**c**), until near end point; then add in 0.1 mL increments until end point remains 1 min (usually >50 μamp). Calculate C = g H_2O/mL reagent. Duplicates must agree within 0.1 mg H_2O/mL reagent.

Melt sample in closed Whirl-Pak bag supported in 400 mL beaker ≤2 h in oven at 40 ± 2°. Mix thoroughly by first gently squeezing bag and then stirring ca 1 min with glass rod or spatula. Remove portion with 10 mL syringe, weigh, add portion containing ca 100 mg H_2O to 30–50 mL pretitrated reagent, and reweigh. Titrate as in standardization.

$$\% H_2O = \text{mL reagent} \times C \times 100/\text{g sample}$$

Reference: JAOAC **60**, 654(1977).

23.5 984.20—Moisture in Oils and Fats
Karl Fischer Method
First Action 1984
Final Action 1985
ISO/TC34/SC11/N99-AOAC Method

(Applicable to oils and fats except for alkaline or oxidized samples)

A. Apparatus and Reagents

(a) *Karl Fischer titration assembly.*—Manual or automated, with stirrer.

(b) *Karl Fischer reagent.—Stabilized,* with H_2O equivalent of ca 5 mg H_2O/mL reagent. Available commercially or prepare as follows: Dissolve 133 g I in 425 mL dry pyridine in dry glass-stoppered bottle. Add 425 mL dry ethylene glycol monomethyl ether. Cool to $<4°$ in ice bath and bubble in 102–105 g SO_2. Mix well and let stand 12 h. Reagent is reasonably stable, but restandardize for each series of determinations. Standardize daily with Na tartrate·$2H_2O$ (1 mg Na tartrate·$2H_2O$ = 0.1566 mg H_2O). Alternatively, standardize with weighed H_2O in methyl alcohol as follows: Transfer accurately weighed amount (50 mg) H_2O to titration vessel and titrate to electrometric end point. Calculate C = mg H_2O/mL reagent.

(c) *Karl Fischer reagent diluent.*—2 Methoxyethanol-pyridine (4 + 1).

(d) *Sample solvent*—Anhydrous $CHCl_3$–methyl alcohol (1 + 1 or 2 + 1).

B. Determination

Weigh, to nearest 0.01 g, 5–25 g prepared sample, containing ≤ 100 mg H_2O, into titration vessel, dissolve in anhydrous $CHCl_3$–methyl alcohol. Titrate with undiluted or diluted (1 + 1) Karl Fischer reagent to electrometric end point. Carry out blank test using same amounts of reagent, diluent, and solvents. Subtract blank titer.

$$\% \ H_2O = (\text{mL reagent} \times C)/(\text{g sample} \times 10)$$

Reference: JAOAC **67,** 299(1984).

23.6 920.116—Moisture in Butter
Final Action
IDF-ISO-AOAC Method

Weigh 1.5–2.5 g prepared sample of salted butter or 2–6 g unsalted butter, **938.05**, into weighed flat-bottom dish ≥ 5 cm diameter and dry to constant weight in oven kept at temperature of boiling H_2O. Clean, dry sand may be used if fat is not to be determined in residue by **938.06** (*see* Chapter 18.10).

I. **938.05** (Butter, Preparation of Sample)

Soften entire sample in sample container, **970.29C**, by warming in H_2O bath kept at as low temperature as practicable, $\leq 39°$. Avoid overheating, which causes visible separation of curd. Shake frequently during softening process to reincorporate any separated fat, and observe fluidity of sample. Optimum consistency is attained when emulsion is still intact but fluid enough to reveal sample level almost immediately. Remove from bath and frequently shake vigorously or place sample container in mechanical shaking machine that simulates hand shaking, with arm 23 cm (9″) long, set to oscillate at 425 ± 25 times/min through arc of 4.5 cm (1.75″). Continue shaking until sample cools to thick, creamy consistency and sample level can no longer readily be seen. Promptly weigh portion for analysis.

References: JAOAC **21,** 361(1938); **35,** 194(1952); **42,** 36(1959).

II. **970.29C** (Sampling of Butter)

C. Sample Containers

Use wide-mouth jars conforming to **968.12C(b)**. Fill jar ≥½ full and hermetically seal. Immediately after closure, wrap jars in paper or store in dark, if examination so requires. Do not let butter come into contact with paper or any H_2O or fat absorbing or trapping surface.

III. **968.12** (Sampling of Dairy Products)

B. Technical Instructions

(**b**) *Sampling for bacteriological purposes.*—Clean and treat equipment by one of following methods: (*1*) Expose to hot air 2 h at 170° (may be stored if kept under sterile conditions). (*2*) Autoclave 15–20 min at 120° (may be stored if kept under sterile conditions). (*3*) Expose to steam 1 h at 100° (use equipment same day). (*4*) Immerse in H_2O 1 min at 100° (use equipment immediately). (*5*) Immerse in 70% alcohol and flame to burn off alcohol immediately before use. (*6*) Expose to hydrocarbon (propane, butane) torch flame so that all working surfaces contact flame immediately before use.

Choice of treatment depends on nature, shape, and size of equipment and on conditions of sampling. Sterilize wherever possible by method (*1*) or (*2*).

Methods (*3*), (*4*), (*5*), and (*6*) are regarded as secondary methods only.

C. Sample Containers

(**a**) *For liquids.*—Use clean and dry containers of suitable waterproof, greaseproof material (glass, stainless metal, suitable plastic material) of quality suitable for sterilization by **968.12B(b)**, if necessary, and of suitable shape and capacity for material to be sampled (as defined in each particular case).

Securely close containers either with suitable rubber or plastic stopper or by screw cap of metal or plastic having, if necessary, liquid-tight plastic liner which is insoluble, nonabsorbent, and greaseproof, and which will not influence odor, flavor, or composition of milk products.

If rubber stoppers are used, cover with nonabsorbent, flavorless material (such as suitable plastic) before pressing into sample container. Suitable plastic bags may also be used.

(**b**) *For solids or semisolids.*—Use clean and dry wide-mouth, cylindrical receptacles of suitable waterproof, greaseproof material (glass, stainless metal, suitable plastic material) of quality suitable for sterilization by **968.12B(b)**, if necessary, and of capacity suited to size of sample to be taken (as defined in each particular case). Make air-tight as in (**a**). Suitable plastic bags may also be used.

23.7   925.10—Solids (Total) and Moisture in Flour
Air Oven Method
Final Action

[Results closely approximate those obtained by **925.09B** (*see* 23.27).]

In cooled and weighed dish (provided with cover), **925.09A(a)**, previously heated to 130 ± 3°, accurately weigh ca 2 g well-mixed sample. Uncover sample, and dry dish, cover, and contents 1 h in oven provided with opening for ventilation and maintained at 130 ± 3°. (One hour drying period begins when oven temperature is actually 130°.) Cover dish while still in oven, transfer to desiccator, and weigh soon after reaching room temperature. Report flour residue as total solids and loss in weight as moisture (indirect method).

References: JAOAC **8,** 665(1925); **9,** 40(1926).

23.8   925.23—Solids (Total) in Milk
IDF-ISO-AOAC Method

A. Method I—Final Action

Weigh 2.5–3 g prepared sample, **925.21**, into weighed flat-bottom dish ≥5 cm diameter; use ca 5 g and Pt dish if ash is to be determined on same portion. Heat on steam bath 10–15 min, exposing maximum surface of dish bottom to live steam; then heat 3 h in air oven at 98–100°. Cool in desiccator, weigh quickly, and report % residue as total solids.

925.21 (Preparation of Milk Sample, Procedure)

Bring sample to ca 20°, mix until homogeneous by pouring into clean receptacle and back repeatedly, and promptly weigh or measure test portion. If lumps of cream do not disperse, warm sample in H_2O bath to ca 38° and keep mixing until homogeneous, using policeman, if necessary, to reincorporate any cream adhering to container or stopper. Where practical and fat remains dispersed, cool warmed samples to ca 20° before transferring test portion.

When Babcock method, **989.04C** (*see* Chapter 18.12), is used, adjust both fresh and composite samples to ca 38°, mix until homogeneous as above, and immediately pipet portions into test bottles.

B. Method II (Approximate)—Procedure

Determine specific gravity of milk with Quévenne lactometer (reading top of meniscus), observe temperature, and correct reading L to 60°F by **921.14** (*Official Methods of Analysis* [1990] 15th Ed.). Calculate total solids either from formula $0.25 L + 1.2 F$, in which F = % fat in milk, or from **945.101** (*Official Methods of Analysis* [1990] 15th Ed.).

C. Infrared Method—First Action

See **972.16J** (*see* 23.33).

23.9   **930.15—Moisture in Animal Feed**
Drying at 135°
Final Action

(Not to be used when fat determination is to be made on same sample)

Regulate air oven to 135 ± 2°. Using low, covered Al dishes, **934.01** (*see* 23.23), weigh ca 2 g sample into each dish and shake until contents are evenly distributed. With covers removed, place dishes and covers in oven as quickly as possible and dry samples 2 h. Place covers on dishes and transfer to desiccator to cool. Weigh, and calculate loss in weight as H_2O.

References: JAOAC **13**, 173(1930); **14**, 152(1931); **17**, 178(1934); **18**, 80(1935).

23.10   **931.04—Moisture in Cacao Products**
Gravimetric Method
First Action

Dry 2 g prepared sample, **970.20**, to constant weight in Pt dish in air oven at 100°. (Al dish may be used when ash is not determined on same sample.) Report loss in weight as H_2O.

> **970.20** (Cacao Products, Preparation of Sample)
> (**a**) *Powdered products.*—Mix thoroughly and preserve in tightly stoppered bottles.
> (**b**) *Chocolate products.*—(*1*) Chill ca 200 g sweet or bitter chocolate until hard, and grate or shave to fine granular condition. Mix thoroughly and preserve in tightly stoppered bottle in cool place. Alternatively—
> (*2*) Melt ca 200 g bitter, sweet, or milk chocolate by placing in suitable container and partly immersing container in bath at ca 50°. Stir frequently until sample melts and reaches temperature of 45–50°. Remove from bath, stir thoroughly, and while still liquid, remove portion for analysis, using glass or metal tube, 4–10 mm diameter, provided with close-fitting plunger to expel sample from tube, or disposable plastic syringe.
> Reference: JAOAC **53**, 388(1970).

Reference: JAOAC **14**, 529(1931).

23.11   935.29—Moisture in Malt
Gravimetric Method
Final Action

A. Apparatus

(a) *Weighing dish.*—Use glass bottle or Al dish, with tight-fitting cover, ca 40 mm diameter for 5 g sample, or 55 mm for 10 g sample.

(b) *Oven.*—With automatic control holding temperature within $\pm 0.5°$, and large enough to hold all samples on 1 shelf in such manner that no sample is outside area indicated by test to give comparable results in duplicate samples. Standardize oven as follows: Place weighed duplicate samples in oven at 103–104° and dry 3 h. Weigh, and redry 1 h longer. If loss of moisture is >0.1%, raise temperature 1° and again test with new duplicate samples. Take, as standard, lowest temperature <106° giving moisture content that, after 3 h of drying, is within 0.1% of value attainable at same temperature within 4 h. Keep ventilators of oven open during entire drying period, and do not open door during the 3 h of drying.

B. Preparation of Sample

(a) *If extract determination is to be made.*—Grind sample as in **982.12A**, and transfer in one continuous operation. When many samples are to be analyzed, grind first sample, remove beaker, and grind second sample while adjusting weight of first sample. Remove second sample, insert third sample, and repeat operation.

982.12 (*N*-Nitrosodimethylamine in Beer, Gas Chromatographic Method)

A. Principle

Sample is treated with sulfamic acid and HCl, and *N*-nitrosodipropylamine (NDPA) is added as internal standard. Solution is made alkaline, and NDMA is separated by distillation and determined by GC with thermal energy analyzer (TEA) detector.

Caution: N-Nitrosamines are potent carcinogens; take adequate precaution to avoid exposure. Carry out all steps, whenever possible, in well-ventilated fume hood and wear protective gloves while handling nitrosamine standards. Use mechanical pipetting aids for measuring all solutions. Use separate pipetting device for measuring standards and mark it appropriately; do not use it for pipetting other reagents. Because these compounds are highly photolabile, all work should be carried out under subdued light. Destroy all nitrosamine standards by boiling with HCl, KI, and sulfamic acid before disposal.

(b) *If extract determination is not to be made.*— Have sample of same fineness as finely ground malt used to determine extract. Weigh ca 5 g whole malt (or 10 g if 55 mm diameter weighing bottle is used) and grind through clean dry mill directly into weighing bottle. Brush all malt from mill into weighing bottle and cover immediately.

C. Determination

Weigh sample to 1 mg and place in oven previously heated to standard temperature. Remove cover of weighing bottle and heat exactly 3 h at standard temperature. Replace cover, transfer to desiccator, cool to room temperature, and weigh to 1 mg. Report moisture to nearest 0.1%.

23.12   941.08—Total Solids in Ice Cream and Frozen Desserts
Gravimetric Method
Final Action

Into round, flat-bottom dish ≥5 cm diameter, quickly weigh 1–2 g sample. (Sample may be weighed by means of short, bent, 2 mL measuring pipet.) Heat on steam bath 30 min and then in air oven 3.5 h at 100°. Cool in desiccator and weigh quickly to avoid absorption of moisture.

Reference: JAOAC **24,** 575(1941).

23.13   948.12—Moisture in Cheese
Method II (Rapid Screening Method)
First Action

Weigh 2–3 g prepared sample into moisture dish with tight-fit cover. Partially dry on steam bath with lid removed and then insert in forced-draft oven that has come to equilibrium at 130 ± 1°. Dry 1.25 h (with cover entirely off), cover tightly, remove from oven, cool, and weigh.

References: JAOAC **31,** 300(1948); **32,** 303(1949).

23.14   952.08—Solids (Total) in Seafood
Gravimetric Method
Final Action 1961

A. *For All Marine Products Except Raw Oysters*
(*Caution: See Appendix* for safety notes on asbestos.)
Cut into short lengths ca 2 g asbestos fibers of type used in preparing gooches. Place cut fibers and glass stirring rod ca 8 cm long with flat end into flat-bottom metal weighing dish, ca 9 cm diameter, with cover. Dry dish, asbestos, and rod in oven 1 h at 100°, cool, and weigh. Quickly weigh into dish, to nearest mg, 9.5–10.5 g prepared sample. Add 20 mL H_2O and mix sample thoroughly with asbestos. Support end of rod on edge of dish and evaporate just to dryness on steam bath, stirring once while still moist. Drop rod into dish and heat 4 h in oven at 100°, or in preheated forced-draft oven set for full draft, 1 h at 100°. Cover dish, cool in desiccator, and weigh promptly.
References: JAOAC **35,** 216(1952); **37,** 602(1954).

B. *For Raw Oysters Only*
Quickly weigh, to nearest mg, 9.5–10.5 g prepared sample into weighed, flat-bottom metal dish ca 9 cm diameter and 2 cm high with cover. Spread sample evenly over bottom of dish. Then:
(a) Evaporate just to dryness on steam bath and dry 3 h in oven at 100°; or—

(b) Insert directly into preheated forced-draft oven set at full draft and dry 1.5 h at 100°.
Cover, cool in desiccator, and weigh promptly.

References: JAOAC **20**, 71(1937); **35**, 218(1952); **36**, 608(1953); **37**, 607(1954); **44**, 276(1961); **46**, 744(1963).

23.15 984.25—Moisture (Loss of Mass on Drying) in Frozen French-Fried Potatoes
Convection Oven Method
First Action 1984

(Applicable to quick-frozen french fried potatoes)

A. *Principle*

Loss of mass on drying is determined under specified conditions. Species other than moisture may be lost.

B. *Determination*

Thoroughly homogenize frozen sample in blender and weigh ca 10 g in duplicate, using balance accurate to 0.1 mg. Use desiccated, tared weighing dishes, preferably made of Ni, Al, stainless steel, or glass, 60–80 mm diameter and 25 mm deep, with well fitting but easily removable lids.

Place uncovered dish containing samples, with lid, in convection drying oven at 103 ± 2° for 16 h. Replace lid and transfer to desiccator to cool. When cool, weigh as quickly as possible to 0.1 mg. Uncover and replace dish and lid in oven additional 2 h. Replace lid, cool in desiccator, and re-weigh. Repeat 2 h drying, desiccation, and weighing steps until decrease in mass between successive weighings does not exceed 0.5 mg or until increase in mass is recorded.

C. *Calculation*

$$\% \text{ Moisture} = [(M_1 - M_2)/(M_1 - M_0)] \times 100$$

(report to 2 decimal places)

where M_0 = mass in grams of dried, tared dish and lid; M_1 = mass in grams of dried, tared dish, lid, and undried sample; M_2 = (lowest) mass in grams of dried, tared dish, lid, and dried sample.

Reference: JAOAC **67**, 635(1984).

23.16   985.14—Moisture in Meat and Poultry Products
Rapid Microwave Drying Method
First Action 1985

A. Principle

Moisture is removed (evaporated) from sample by using microwave energy. Weight loss is determined by electric balance readings before and after drying and is converted to moisture content by microprocessor with digital percent readout.

B. Apparatus

(a) *Microwave moisture analyzer.*—0.2 mg H_2O sensitivity, moisture/solids range of 0.1–99.9%, 0.1% resolution. Includes automatic tare electronic balance, microwave drying system, and microprocessor digital computer control. Electronic balance pan is located inside drying chamber. Balance sensitivity: 0.2 mg at 15 g capacity or 1.0 mg at 40 g capacity. (CEM Corp., PO Box 200, Matthews, NC, 28106), or equivalent.

(b) *Glass fiber pads.*—9.8 × 10.2 cm rectangular glass fiber pads (CEM Corp.), or equivalent.

C. Determination

Prepare samples as in **983.18**. Place 2 rectangular glass fiber pads on balance pan in microwave moisture analyzer drying chamber, and tare. Remove pads from chamber, rapidly and evenly deposit ca 4 g well-mixed sample on rough side of one pad. Place second pad over sample and replace pads and sample on balance pan. Dry sample with pads 3–5 min at 80–100% power, depending on product type. At completion of microwave drying cycle, read percent moisture displayed on digital readout panel.

> **983.18** (Meat and Meat Products, Preparation of Sample)
>
> To prevent H_2O loss during preparation and subsequent handling, do not use small samples. Keep ground material in glass or similar containers with air- and H_2O-tight covers. Prepare samples for analysis as follows:
>
> (a) *Fresh meats, dried meats, cured meats, smoked meats, etc.*—Separate as completely as possible from any bone; pass rapidly 3 times through food chopper with plate openings ≤⅛″ (3 mm), mixing thoroughly after each grinding; and begin all determinations promptly. If any delay occurs, chill sample to inhibit decomposition.
>
> Alternatively, use a bowl cutter for sample preparation (benchtop model, ½ HP; 14 in. bowl, 22 rpm; two 3.5 in. knives, 1725 rpm; Model 84145, Hobart Corp., 711 Pennsylvania Ave, Troy, OH 45374, or equivalent). Chill all cutter parts before preparation of each sample.
>
> (b) *Canned meats.*—Pass entire contents of can through food chopper, as in (a).
>
> (c) *Sausages.*—Remove from casings and pass through food chopper, as in (a).
>
> Dry portions of samples of (a), (b), and (c) not needed for immediate analysis, either *in vacuo* <60° or by evaporating on steam bath 2 or 3 times with alcohol. Extract fat from dried product with petroleum ether (bp <60°) and let petroleum ether evaporate spontaneously, finally expelling last traces by heating short time on steam bath. Do not heat sample or separated fat longer than necessary because of tendency to decompose. Reserve fat in cool place for examination as in chapter on oils and fats and complete examination before it becomes rancid.
>
> Reference: JAOAC **66**, 579(1983).

Certain product classes require addition of adjustment factor to readout for accurate results, as follows: cooked sausage, preblends/emulsions, cured/cooked meats, factor = 0.55%.

Reference: JAOAC **68,** 876(1985).

23.17 950.46B—Moisture in Meat

B. Air Drying
—First Action
(a) With lids removed, dry sample containing ca 2 g dry material 16–18 h at 100–102° in air oven (mechanical convection preferred). Use covered Al dish ≥50 mm diameter and ≤40 mm deep. Cool in desiccator and weigh. Report loss in weight as moisture.

(b) With lids removed, dry sample containing ca 2 g dry material to constant weight (2–4 h depending on product) in mechanical convection oven or in gravity oven with single shelf at ca 125°. Use covered Al dish ≥50 mm diameter and ≤40 mm deep. Avoid excessive drying. Cover, cool in desiccator, and weigh. Report loss in weight as moisture. (Dried sample is not satisfactory for subsequent fat determination.)

References: JAOAC **33,** 749(1950); **36,** 279(1953).

23.18 920.151—Solids (Total) in Fruits and Fruit Products
Final Action 1980

A. Insoluble Matter Present
Fresh and canned fruits, jams, marmalades, and preserves.—Accurately weigh, into large flat-bottom dish, 20 g pulped fresh fruit, or weight of fruit products that will give ≤3–4 g dry material. If necessary to secure thin layer of material, add few mL H_2O and mix thoroughly. Dry at 70° under pressure ≤100 mm Hg (13.3 kPa) until consecutive weighings made at 2 h intervals vary ≤3 mg.

B. Insoluble Matter Absent
Fruit juices, jellies, and sirups.—Proceed as in **925.45C** (*see* 23.30), **925.45D**, **932.14A** (*see Official Methods of Analysis* [1990] 15th Ed.), **932.14B**, or **932.14C**, using sample prepared as in **920.149(a)** or **(b)**.

920.149 (Preparation of Fruit Sample)
Transfer samples received in open packages (i.e., not sterile) without delay to glass-stoppered containers and keep in cool place. To avoid effects of fermentation, make prompt determinations of alcohol, total and volatile acids, solids, and sugars, particularly in case of fruit juices and fresh fruits. (Portions for determination of sucrose and reducing sugars may be weighed and kept several days without fermenting if the slight

excess of neutral Pb(OAc)$_2$ solution required in determination is added. *Note:* Pb(OAc)$_2$ is toxic. Label samples to show its addition.) Prepare various products for analysis as follows:

(**a**) *Juices.*—Mix thoroughly by shaking to ensure uniform sample, and filter through absorbent cotton or rapid paper. Prepare fresh juices by pressing well-pulped fruit and filtering. Express juice of citrus fruits by commercial device, and filter.

(**b**) *Jellies and sirups.*—Mix thoroughly to ensure uniform sample. Prepare solution by weighing 300 g thoroughly mixed sample into 2 L flask and dissolve in H$_2$O, heating on steam bath if necessary. Apply as little heat as possible to minimize inversion of sucrose. Cool, dilute to volume, mix thoroughly by shaking, and use aliquots for the various determinations. If insoluble material is present, mix thoroughly and filter first.

23.19   925.40—Moisture in Nuts and Nut Products
First Action

(Not applicable to high sugar products or products containing glycerol or propylene glycol)

Dry sample representing ca 2 g dry material to constant weight (ca 5 h) at 95–100° under pressure ≤100 mm Hg (13.3 kPa). Report loss in weight as moisture.

References: JAOAC **8,** 295(1925); **31,** 521(1948); **32,** 527(1949); **33,** 753(1950); **34,** 357(1951); **37,** 845(1954).

23.20   926.08—Moisture in Cheese
Method I
Final Action

Weigh 2–3 g prepared sample, **955.30,** into weighed round, flat-bottom metal dish, ≥5 cm diameter and provided with tight-fit, slip-in cover. In case of soft cheese and process cheese of high moisture content, weigh 1–2 g and partially dry on steam bath. Place loosely covered dish on metal shelf (dish resting directly on shelf) in vacuum oven, kept at 100°. Dry to constant weight (ca 4 h) under pressure ≤100 mm Hg (13.3 kPa). During drying admit into oven slow current of air (ca 2 bubbles/s) dried by passing through H$_2$SO$_4$. Stop vacuum pump and carefully admit air into oven. Press cover tightly into dish, remove dish from oven, cool, and weigh. Express loss in weight as moisture.

      955.30 (Cheese, Preparation of Samples)

            Cut wedge sample into strips and pass 3 times through food chopper. Grind plugs in food chopper (preferable method), or cut or shred very finely and mix thoroughly.

            With creamed cottage and similar cheeses, place 300–600 g sample at <15° in 1 L (1 qt) cup of high-speed blender and blend for minimum time (2–5 min) required to obtain homogeneous mixture. Final temperature should be ≤25°. This may require stopping blender frequently after channeling and spooning cheese back into blades until blending action starts. (Use of variable transformer in line to permit slow speed at first minimizes channeling when speed is increased later.)

References: JAOAC 9, 44(1926); **18,** 57(1935).

23.21   926.12—Moisture and Volatile Matter in Oils and Fats
Vacuum Oven Method
Final Action

Soften sample, if necessary, by gentle heat, taking care not to melt it. When soft enough, mix thoroughly with effective mechanical mixer.

Weigh 5 ± 0.2 g prepared sample into Al moisture dish ca 5 cm diameter and 2 cm deep with tight-fit slip-over cover. Dry to constant weight in vacuum oven at uniform temperature 20–25° above bp of H_2O at working pressure, which should be ≤100 mm Hg (13.3 kPa). Cool in efficient desiccator 30 min and weigh. Constant weight is attained when successive 1 h drying periods show additional loss of ≤0.05%. Report % loss in weight as moisture and volatile matter.

References: Ind. Eng. Chem. **18,** 1347(1926). JAOAC **14,** 247(1931); **15,** 560(1932).

23.22   927.05—Moisture in Dried Milk
Final Action

Weigh 1–1.5 g sample into round, flat-bottom metal dish (≥5 cm diameter and provided with tight-fitting slip-in cover). Loosen cover and place dish on metal shelf (dish resting directly on shelf) in vacuum oven at 100°. Dry to constant weight (ca 5 h) under pressure ≤100 mm (4″) of Hg. During drying, admit slow current of air into oven (ca 2 bubbles/s), dried by passing through H_2SO_4. Stop vacuum pump and carefully admit dried air into oven. Press cover tightly into dish, remove from oven, cool, and weigh. Calculate % loss in weight as moisture.

References: JAOAC **10,** 308(1927); **11,** 289(1928).

23.23 934.01—Moisture in Animal Feed
Drying in Vacuo at 95–100°
Final Action

Dry amount sample containing ca 2 g dry material to constant weight at 95–100° under pressure ≤100 mm Hg (ca 5 h). For feeds with high molasses content, use temperature ≤70° and pressure ≤50 mm Hg. Use covered Al dish ≥50 mm diameter and ≤40 mm deep. Report loss in weight as moisture.

References: JAOAC **17**, 68(1934); **51**, 467(1968); **60**, 322(1977).

23.24 934.06—Moisture in Dried Fruits
Final Action

Spread 5–10 g prepared sample, **920.149(c)**, as evenly as possible over bottom of metal dish ca 8.5 cm diameter provided with tight-fit cover, weigh, and dry 6 h at 70 ± 1° under pressure ≤100 mm Hg (13.3 kPa). (Metal dish must be in direct contact with metal shelf of oven.) During drying, admit to oven slow current of air (ca 2 bubbles/s) dried by passing through H_2SO_4. Replace cover, cool dish in desiccator, and weigh. Disregard any temporary drop in oven temperature during early part of drying period owing to rapid evaporation of H_2O.

> **920.149** (Preparation of Fruit Sample)
>
> (c) *Fresh fruits, dried fruits, preserves, jams, and marmalades.*—Pulp by passing through food chopper, or by use of soil dispersion mixer, Hobart mixer, or other suitable mechanical mixing apparatus, or by grinding in large mortar, and mixing thoroughly, completing operation as quickly as possible to avoid loss of moisture. With dried fruits, pass sample through food chopper 3 times, mixing thoroughly after each grinding. Set burrs or blades of food chopper as close as possible without crushing seeds. Grind entire contents of No. 10 or smaller container. Mix contents of larger containers thoroughly by stirring and remove portion for grinding. With stone fruits, remove pits and determine their proportion in weighed sample.
>
> Prepare solution by weighing into 1.5–2 L beaker 300 g fresh fruit, or equivalent of dried fruit, preserves, jams, and marmalades, well-pulped and mixed in blender or other suitable type of mechanical grinder; add ca 800 mL H_2O; and boil 1 h replacing at intervals H_2O lost by evaporation. Transfer to 2 L volumetric flask, cool, dilute to volume, and filter. With unsweetened fruit, ashing is facilitated by addition of sugar before boiling; therefore weigh 150 g fruit, add 150 g sugar and 800 mL H_2O, and proceed as above.

With raisins, and other fruit rich in sugar, use ca 5 g sample and dry and weigh in dish with ca 2 g finely divided asbestos. Moisten with hot H_2O, mix sample and asbestos thoroughly, evaporate barely to dryness on steam bath, and complete drying as above.

Duplicate determinations should agree within 0.2%.

References: JAOAC **17**, 215(1934); **18**, 80(1935).

23.25 920.115—Sweetened Condensed Milk
Final Action

B. Preparation of Sample—Procedure

(a) Temper unopened can in H_2O bath at 30–35° until warm. Open, scrape out all milk adhering to interior of can, transfer to dish large enough to permit stirring thoroughly, and mix until whole mass is homogeneous.

(b) Weigh 100 g thoroughly mixed sample into 500 mL volumetric flask, dilute to volume with H_2O, and mix thoroughly. If sample will not emulsify uniformly, weigh out separate portion of (a) for each determination.

D. Total Solids

Transfer 10 mL prepared solution, **920.115B(b)**, to weighed flat-bottom dish, ≥5 cm diameter, containing 15–20 g previously dried sand or asbestos fiber. Heat on steam bath 30 min and then in vacuum oven at 100° to constant weight. Cool in desiccator and weigh quickly to avoid absorption of H_2O. Correct result for dilution.

23.26 925.30—Solids (Total) in Eggs
Vacuum Method
Final Action

A. Apparatus

Vacuum oven.—Connected with pump to maintain pressure ≤25 mm Hg (3.3 kPa) and provided with thermometer passing into oven with bulb near samples. Connect H_2SO_4 gas-drying bottle to oven for admitting dry air to release vacuum

B. Determination

(a) *Liquid eggs.*—Accurately weigh by difference, using weighing buret, ca 5 g samples, **925.29(a)** or (b), in covered dish previously dried at 98–100°, cooled in desiccator, and weighed soon after coming to room temperature. Remove cover and evaporate most of H_2O by heating on steam bath. Replace cover loosely and complete drying in vacuum oven as in (b).

(b) *Dried eggs.*—Weigh ca 2 g sample, **925.29(c)**, in covered dish previously dried at 98–100°, cooled in desiccator, and weighed soon after coming to room temperature. Loosen cover (do not remove) and heat at 98–100° to constant weight (ca 5 h) in vacuum oven. Admit dry air into oven to bring to atmospheric pressure. Immediately tighten cover of dish, transfer to desiccator containing fresh efficient desiccant, and weigh soon after coming to room temperature. Report as % total solids.

925.29 (Sampling of Eggs, Collection and Preparation of Sample)

No simple rules can be made for collection of sample representative of average of any particular lot of egg material, as conditions may differ widely. Experienced judgment must be used in each instance. For large lots, preferably draw several samples for separate analyses rather than attempt to get one composite representative sample.

302

Sampling for microbiological examination, if required, should be performed first; *see* **939.14A–B** [*Official Methods of Analysis* (1990) 15th Ed.].

(**a**) *Liquid eggs.*—Obtain representative container or containers. Mix contents of container thoroughly and draw ca 300 g. (Long-handle dipper or ladle serves well.) Keep sample in hermetically sealed jar in freezer or with solid CO_2. Report odor and appearance.

(**b**) *Frozen eggs.*—Obtain representative container or containers. Examine contents as to odor and appearance. (Condition of contents can be determined best by drilling to center of container with auger and noting odor as auger is withdrawn. If impossible to secure individual containers, samples may consist of composite of borings from contents of each container.) Take borings diagonally across can from ≥ 3 widely separated parts, starting 2–5 cm in from edge and extending to opposite side as near to bottom as possible. Pack shavings tightly into sample jar and fill it completely to prevent partial dehydration of sample. Seal jar tightly and store in freezer or with solid CO_2. Before analyzing, warm sample in bath held at $< 50°$, and mix well.

(**c**) *Dried eggs.*—Obtain representative container or containers. For small packages, take entire parcel or parcels for sample. For boxes and barrels, remove top layer to depth of ca 15 cm (6″) with scoop or other convenient instrument. Draw small amounts of sample totaling 300–500 g from accessible parts of container and place in hermetically sealed jar. Report odor and appearance. Prepare sample for analysis by mixing 3 times through domestic flour sifter to thoroughly break up lumps. (Grind flake albumen samples to pass entirely through No. 60 sieve. Mix well.) Keep in hermetically sealed jar in cool place.

References: JAOAC **8**, 599(1925); **53**, 439(1970); **58**, 314(1975).

References: JAOAC **8**, 600(1925); **9**, 354(1926); **14**, 395(1931).

23.27 925.09—Solids (Total) and Moisture in Flour
Vacuum Oven Method
Final Action

(Also applicable to flour mixes containing $NaHCO_3$ as ingredient)

A. Apparatus

(**a**) *Metal dish.*—Diameter ca 55 mm, height ca 15 mm, with inverted slip-in cover fitting tightly on inside.

(**b**) *Air-tight desiccator.*—Reignited CaO is satisfactory drying agent.

(**c**) *Vacuum oven.*—Connect with pump capable of maintaining partial vacuum in oven with pressure equivalent to ≤ 25 mm Hg (3.3 kPa) and provided with thermometer passing into oven in such way that bulb is near samples. Connect H_2SO_4 gas-drying bottle with oven to admit dry air when releasing vacuum.

B. Determination

Accurately weigh ca 2 g well-mixed sample in covered dish previously dried at 98–100°, cooled in desiccator, and weighed soon after reaching room temperature. Loosen cover (do not remove) and heat at 98–100° to constant weight (ca 5 h) in partial vacuum having pressure equivalent to ≤ 25 mm Hg (3.3 kPa). Admit dry air into oven to bring to atmospheric pressure. Immediately tighten cover on dish, transfer to desiccator, and weigh soon after reaching room temperature. Report flour residue as total solids and loss in weight as moisture (indirect method).

References: JAOAC **8,** 665(1925); **9,** 39, 88(1926); **34,** 278(1951).

23.28   945.43—Moisture in Fig Bars and Raisin-Filled Crackers
Gravimetric Method
Final Action

Place 25–30 g prepared sand and short stirring rod in dish ca 55 mm diameter and 40 mm deep, fitted with cover. Dry thoroughly, cover dish, cool in desiccator, and weigh immediately. Remove cover, place 3–5 g prepared sample, **926.04(b)**, in dish, and weigh accurately. Remove dish containing sand, stirring rod, and weighed sample from balance. Add 5–10 mL H_2O and mix with the sand. Heat carefully on H_2O bath, stirring at 2–3 min intervals, until excess H_2O is removed and contents of dish are consistency of heavy paste. Place uncovered dish in vacuum oven and dry ca 16 h at 70° under pressure ≤50 mm Hg (6.7 kPa). After drying, cover dish, transfer to desiccator, cool to room temperature, and weigh immediately.

> **926.04** (Bread, Preparation of Sample)
> (When total solids of original loaf are not desired)
> (**a**) *All types of bread not containing fruit.*—Cut loaf, or ½ loaf, of bread into slices 2–3 mm thick. Spread slices on paper and let dry in warm room until sufficiently crisp and brittle to grind well in mill. Grind entire sample to pass No. 20 sieve, mix well, and keep in air-tight container. References: JAOAC **9,** 42(1926); **15,** 72(1932); **17,** 65(1934).
> (**b**) *Raisin bread.*—Proceed as in (**a**), except comminute by passing twice through food chopper instead of grinder.

Notes: Quartz sand that passes No. 40 sieve but is retained on No. 60 sieve, has been digested with HCl, washed free of acid, and ignited, is recommended. Al dishes with fit-over covers are most convenient. Dish can be set in cover during heating on H_2O bath and during oven-drying period. After drying, cover can be easily and quickly refitted on dish as it is transferred to desiccator.

23.29   964.22—Solids (Total) in Canned Vegetables
Gravimetric Method
First Action 1964
Final Action 1965

To flat-bottom metal dish with tight-fitting cover, add ca 15 mg diatomaceous earth filter-aid/sq cm, dry ca 30 min at 110°, cool in desiccator, weigh, and to each dish add sample of such size that dry residue will be ≥9 but ≤30 mg/sq cm. Weigh as rapidly as possible to avoid moisture loss. Mix with filter-aid and distribute uniformly over bottom of dish, diluting with H_2O if necessary to facilitate distribution. Bring sample to apparent dryness (remaining moisture not more than ca 50% dry solids) by one of following methods:

(1) Place sample on boiling H_2O bath and remove when samples reach apparent dryness.

(2) Place sample in forced-draft oven at 70°. Oven must have rapid air circulation and enough interchange of outside air to remove moisture rapidly. Examine dishes at intervals of ≤30 min, and remove as soon as they reach apparent dryness.

(3) Place sample in vacuum oven at 70° with release cock left partly open to allow rapid flow of air through oven at ≥310 mm Hg (41.3 kPa) pressure. Examine dishes at 30 min intervals and remove any that reach apparent dryness.

Place partially dried samples in vacuum oven with bottoms of dishes in direct contact with shelf. Measure temperature of oven by thermometer in direct contact with shelf. Oven must be so constructed that temperature variations from one part of shelf to another do not exceed ca 2°. Admit dry air to oven at rate of 2–4 bubbles/s by bubbling through H_2SO_4. Dry samples 2 h at 69–71° (oven may be as low as 65° at start of drying, but must reach 69–71° before end of first h) at pressure ≤50 mm Hg (6.6 kPa). As dried sample will absorb appreciable amount of moisture on standing over most desiccating agents, cover quickly, and weigh as soon as possible after sample reaches room temperature.

Reference: JAOAC **47**, 492(1964).

23.30   925.45A,B,D—Moisture in Sugars

A. Vacuum Drying
—Final Action
(Applicable to cane and beet, raw and refined sugars)

Dry 2–5 g prepared sample, **920.175(a)**, in flat dish (Ni, Pt, or Al with tight-fit cover), 2 h at ≤70° (preferably 60°), under pressure ≤50 mm Hg (6.7 kPa). Bleed oven with current of air (dried by passing through anhydrous $CaSO_4$, P_2O_5, or other efficient desiccant) during drying to remove H_2O vapor. Remove dish from oven, cover, cool in desiccator, and weigh. Redry 1 h and repeat process until change in weight between successive dryings at 1 h intervals is ≤2 mg.

920.175 (Preparation of Sample)

(a) *Solids (sugars, etc.).*—Grind, if necessary, and mix to uniformity. Thoroughly mix raw sugars with spatula in minimum time. Break up any lumps either on glass plate with glass or iron rolling pin, or in large, clean, dry mortar, with pestle.

B. Drying at Atmospheric Pressure
—Procedure
(Applicable to cane and beet, raw and refined sugars)

Dry ca 5 g prepared sample, **920.175(a)**, in flat dish (Ni, Pt, or Al with tight-fit cover), 3 h at 100°. Remove dish, cover, cool in desiccator, and weigh. Redry 1 h and repeat process until change in weight between successive dryings at 1 h intervals is ≤2 mg. For large-grain sugars, increase temperature to 105–110° in final heating periods to expel last traces of occluded H_2O. Report loss in weight as H_2O.

305

D. Drying on Quartz Sand
—Final Action

(Applicable to massecuites, molasses, and other liquid and semiliquid products)

Digest pure quartz sand that passes No. 40 but not No. 60 sieve with HCl, wash acid-free, dry, and ignite. Preserve in stoppered bottle. Place 25–30 g prepared sand and short stirring rod in dish ca 55 mm diameter and 40 mm deep, fitted with cover. Dry thoroughly, cover dish, cool in desiccator, and weigh immediately. Add enough diluted sample of known weight to yield ca 1 g dry matter and mix thoroughly with sand. Heat on steam bath 15–20 min, stirring at 2–3 min intervals, or until mass becomes too stiff to manipulate readily. Dry at <70° (preferably 60°) under pressure ≤50 mm Hg (6.7 kPa), bleeding with dry air as in **925.45A**. Make trial weighings at 2 h intervals toward end of drying period (ca 18 h) until change in weight is ≤2 mg.

For materials containing no fructose or other readily decomposable substance, dry 8–10 h at atmospheric pressure in oven at 100°, cool in desiccator, and weigh, repeating heating and weighing until loss in 1 h heating is ≤2 mg. Report loss in weight as H_2O.

As dry sand, as well as dried sample, absorbs appreciable moisture on standing over most desiccating agents, make all weighings as quickly as possible after cooling in desiccator.

Reference: JAOAC **8**, 255(1925).

23.31   985.26—Solids (Total) in Processed Tomato Products
Microwave Oven Drying Method
First Action 1985

A. Principle

Tared sample on fiberglass pad is placed in microwave oven 4 min. Instrument automatically weighs sample before and after drying, and calculates % total solids.

B. Apparatus

(**a**) *Microwave oven.*—CEM Microwave Drying Moisture Solids Analyzer Model AVC-MP (replacement model AVC-80) (CEM Corp., PO Box 200, Matthews, NC 28106), or equivalent.

(**b**) *Fiberglass pads.*—CEM £20-20015, or equivalent. Dry in microwave oven before use.

(**c**) *Jumbo bulb pipet.*—6 in., Beral No. 028-795 (Curtin Matheson Scientific Inc.), or equivalent.

(**d**) *Spatula.*—Plastic or Teflon-coated.

(**e**) *Top loading balance.*—Accurate to 0.01 g.

C. Preparation of Sample

(**a**) *Tomato juice.*—Use 4 g, as is.

(**b**) *Puree.*—10–15% solids. Use 2 g, as is.

(**c**) *Paste.*—Up to 30% solids. Prepare 1 + 1 dilution (weight/volume) with H_2O by one of following techniques: (*1*) blending in mini-cup blender; (*2*) shaking in closed jar; (*3*) mixing with rubber spatula. Use 2 g of dilution.

(**d**) *Paste.*—Over 30% solids. Prepare thoroughly mixed dilution (1 + 3, weight/volume) as in (**c**) above. Use 2 g of dilution.

Use calibrated Beral pipet to deposit sample on fiberglass pad. To calibrate pipet, weigh 4 g sample (2 g puree or paste), draw completely into pipet, and mark level. Draw subsequent samples to this line.

D. Determination

Before starting each day's run, place 2 pads on oven balance ring, and run through complete cycle with oven set at 100% power. Then, place 2 pre-dried pads on balance ring. Press "weigh" button, then press "auto-tare" button until balance displays 0.0000 (±0.0002).

Remove both pads and deposit proper amount of sample on *rough* side of one pad. Use spatula to spread sample evenly over entire pad. Place second pre-dried pad on top of sample—rough side against sample. Work *rapidly* to minimize evaporation. Invert pads and place on balance ring. Drop cover over samples. Close door securely.

Closing door activates microprocessor. Display will indicate *increasing* weight for 4–5 s, then weight will begin to decrease. At exact point that weight starts to decrease, press "auto-time" button to begin drying cycle. At end of 4 min, record % solids. Determine % total solids on duplicate samples, and correct for sample dilution.

Reference: JAOAC **68**, 1081(1985).

23.32   972.16—Fat, Lactose, Protein, and Solids in Milk
Mid-Infrared Spectroscopic Method
First Action 1972

[*Note*: Methods for fat (*see* Chapter 18), lactose (*see* Chapter 32), and protein (*see* Chapter 28) are not included.]

A. Principle

Analysis of milk by IR is based on absorption of IR energy at specific wavelengths by CH groups in fatty acid chain of fat molecules (3.48 μm), by carbonyl groups in ester linkages of fat molecules (5.723 μm), by peptide linkages between amino acids of protein molecules (6.465 μm), and by OH groups in lactose molecules (9.610 μm). Total solids (TS) or solids-not-fat (SNF) are computed by assigning experimentally determined factor to percentage of all other solid milk components, and by adding this amount to appropriate % fat, protein, and lactose, or by direct multiple regression calculations using instrument signals at combinations of above-mentioned wavelengths. Latter method has been shown to be more accurate method of determining milk solids. Analysis by IR is dependent on calibration against suitable standard method. *See* "Definitions of Terms and Explanatory Notes" (1990) *Official Methods of Analysis*, 15th Ed., for calculation of regression lines.

B. Performance Specifications

Number of firms manufacture various model instruments based upon principle, **972.16A**. It is imperative that individual instrument utilized meets following performance specifications, based upon analysis of 8 samples:

Standard deviation of difference between duplicate instrument estimates:

Fat, protein, and lactose	≤0.02%	Total solids	≤0.04%

Mean difference between duplicate instrument estimates:

Fat, protein, and lactose	≤0.02%	Total solids	≤0.03%

Standard deviation of difference between instrument estimates and values by reference methods:

Fat (**905.02**), protein (**920.105**),	≤0.06%	Total solids [**925.23A** (*see* 23.8)]	≤0.12%

and lactose (**896.01B** or **930.28**)

Mean difference between instrument estimates and values by reference methods:

Fat, protein, and lactose	≤0.05%	Total solids	≤0.09%

Calculate standard deviation of difference as in **969.16D**, where S_D = algebraic difference either between duplicate instrument estimates or between instrument estimates and values by reference methods.

969.16D (Fat in Milk, Automated Turbidimetric Method I)

D. Calibration

Instruments should be operated in accordance with manufacturer's instructions.

Test in triplicate 20 representative milks, 3–6% fat for unhomogenized milks, by **905.02** or **924.05C** and instrument. If instrument is also to be used for testing homogenized milk, it is necessary to run 20 homogenized milks, 1–5% fat, by **905.02** and instrument. (Lower fat range for homogenized samples is to allow for testing homogenized low fat milks.) Calculate average for each sample by each method to nearest 0.01%. Calculate standard deviation of difference (S_D) as follows:

$$S_D = \sqrt{[\sum (D^2) - (\sum D)^2/N]/(N - 1)}$$

where D = average of results by **905.02** or **924.05C** on sample minus instrumental results on same sample, e.g.,

$$[(B_1 + B_2 + B_3)/3] - [(I_1 + I_2 + I_3)/3] = D$$

where B = reading by **905.02** or **924.05C**, I = reading by instrument, and N = number of samples tested.

Instrument is properly calibrated when S_D is <0.10 for individual cow sample or ≤0.06 for herd, composite, or homogenized samples. Should S_D exceed these values, see manufacturer's instructions on how to adjust calibration. After adjustments, rerun aliquots of ≥20 samples and recalculate. Instrument is properly calibrated when, after adjustments, S_D values do not exceed limits specified for milks tested.

During any calendar day of use, make performance check consisting of comparison of results obtained on 1 milk bulk sample, using both instrument and **905.02** or **924.05C**. If difference is >0.10% fat, repeat determination on 3 additional samples. If average differences of 3 additional samples is >0.10% fat, recalibrate instrument.

C. Precautions

Differences in fat readings for homogenized and unhomogenized samples of same milk should be <0.05% to assure accurate results at high fat levels. If larger differences occur and servicing homogenizer does not correct fault, consult manufacturer. Changes in moisture vapor content of instrument console will cause changes in optical 0 and shift in calibration level. Replace desiccant frequently, preferably at end of each day, as 3–4 h are required to restore equilibrium conditions. For best accuracy, calibrate with type of milk to be analyzed (herd, individual cow, homogenized, unhomogenized, market, etc.). Do not use mixtures of cream and milk for calibration. Avoid abnormal (low lactose) milks for calibration. Single pumping of milk through instrument sample cell should purge ≥99% of previous sample. To test purging efficiency, perform fat determinations on H_2O and single pasteurized, homogenized whole milk in sequence: H_2O, H_2O, milk, milk, H_2O, etc., until total of 20 determinations have been obtained. Calculate

$$\text{purging efficiency} = (\Sigma M_1 - \Sigma W_2) \times 100/(\Sigma M_2 - \Sigma W_2)$$

where M_1 and M_2 are first and second values for milk and W_2 second value for H_2O.

Instrument must be well maintained and functioning correctly. Malfunctions that influence calibration can cause large errors.

I. Fat

D. Calibration

Before first calibration, check linearity of output signals. Mix accurately measured volumes of H_2O and homogenized cream to prepare ca 8 mixtures of known relative fat contents covering required range. Prepare samples as in **925.21**, and pump each mixture into instrument twice, using second readings to prepare plot against relative concentrations. If plot is not linear, adjust as indicated in operating manual. Repeat measurements and adjustments until plot is linear.

If analyzing unhomogenized milks, check linearity again with ca 4 dilutions of unhomogenized cream or high fat milk. If these mixtures deviate significantly from linearity, *see* **972.16C** and check differences between readings for homogenized and unhomogenized milk samples.

Determine % fat for series of ≥8 preanalyzed (**905.02**) milk samples of type to be analyzed (*see* **972.16C**). Prepare samples as in **925.21** and analyze in triplicate. Compare averages of second and third instrument readings with standard values and follow instructions in operating manual for required changes to calibration.

Alternatively, for better accuracy, use simple linear regression equation that relates instrument estimates and standard reference values, using latter as dependent variable, to correct these tests. In earlier instruments, which do not have this capability in instrument software, this calculation must be performed ouside instrument. To perform this calculation on calibration data that are collected on successive days or weeks, it is necessary to record instrument estimates as well as final results. Purpose of this alternative, preferred procedure is to avoid adjusting instrument slope controls.

E. Determination

Prepare sample as in **925.21**. Operate instrument in accordance with manufacturer's instructions. Use A, B, or A + B filters for measurements.

II. Protein

F. Calibration

Proceed as in **972.16D**, first and third paragraphs, substituting Ca propionate solution (dissolve 15.0 g pure Ca propionate·H_2O in H_2O and dilute to 1 L with H_2O at 20°) for homogenized cream to prepare mixtures of known relative concentrations from 0 to required maximum for protein. Determine % protein for series of ≥8 preanalyzed (**920.105**) milk samples having range of protein content approximately that of population of milks to be analyzed. Prepare samples as in **925.21** and analyze in triplicate. Compare averages of second and third instrument readings with standard values and follow directions in operating manual for making required adjustments to calibration.

Alternatively, for better accuracy, use simple linear regression equation that relates instrument estimates and standard reference values, using latter as dependent variable, to correct these estimates. In earlier instruments, which do not have this capability in instrument software, this calculation must be performed outside instrument. To perform this calculation on calibration data that are collected on successive days or weeks, it is necessary to record instrument estimates as well as final results. Purpose of this alternative, preferred procedure is to avoid adjusting instrument slope controls.

G. Determination

Prepare sample as in **925.21**. Operate instrument according to manufacturer's instructions.

III. Lactose

H. Calibration

Proceed as in **972.16D**, paragraph 1, substituting lactose solution (dissolve 50.00 g lactose·H_2O and 0.25 g $HgCl_2$ in H_2O and dilute to 1 L with H_2O at 20°) for homogenized cream to prepare mixtures of known relative concentrations ranging from 0 to required maximum for lactose. Determine lactose for series of ≥8 preanalyzed (**896.01B** or **930.28**) milk samples having range of lactose content approximately that of population of milks to be analyzed.

Prepare samples as in **925.21** and analyze in triplicate. Use averages of second and third values for each sample in estimating calibration requirements. Adjust instrument controls, as directed in operating manual, to make $\Sigma L = \Sigma L'$, where L = instrument readings for lactose and L' = values from reference method.

Alternatively, for better accuracy, multiply instrument estimates by $\Sigma L'/\Sigma L$ to obtain final results. In earlier instruments, which do not have this capability in instrument software, this calculation must be performed outside instrument. To perform this calculation on calibration data that are collected on successive days or weeks, it is necessary to record instrument estimates as well as final results. Purpose of this alternative, preferred procedure is to avoid adjusting instrument slope controls.

I. Determination

Prepare sample as in **925.21**. Operate instrument according to manufacturer's instructions.

IV. Solids (Total)

J. Calibration

Use standard method **925.23A** to determine % total solids for series of ≥8 milks. Determine % fat, % protein, and % lactose. Calculate mean difference for total solids $(TS) - F - P - L = a$, where F, P, and L are estimates of fat, protein, and lactose, respectively. For routine control of calibration, analyze additional series of milks and adjust value for mean difference in accordance with accumulated data.

Calculate % total solids = $a + F + P + L$

Alternatively, calibrate by multiple regression to calculate equation for estimation of either TS or SNF as function of fat, protein, and lactose uncorrected signals. For recalibration, use simple linear regression equation which relates regression estimates and standard reference values, using latter as dependent variable, to correct these estimates and obtain final result. In earlier instruments, which do not have this capability in instrument software, this calculation must be performed outside instrument. To perform this calculation on calibration data that are collected on successive days or weeks, it is necessary to record regression estimates as well as final result. This alternative, preferred method has been demonstrated to be more accurate.

Note: For products that are fortified or diluted, both original multiple regression and simple regression calculations must be based on regression that forces calibration line through origin. First calculation procedure in this section, paragraph 1, cannot be used successfully with these products.

K. Computer-Based Calibration and Control

Program computer to:

(1) Calculate $S_2' = S_1 + [(S_2 - S_1)/PF]$, where S_2' is purge-corrected signal; S_2 is signal at any instrument channel; S_1 is same signal for previous sample; and PF is predicted purge fraction = purging efficiency/100 (see **972.16C**). Apply correction to all signals received from instrument.

(2) Calculate $(\Sigma CS_2')/10$, where CS_2' is purge-corrected control milk signal. Sum control milk signals at each channel for 10 control samples, and average. At time of calibration, store and designate as required control milk samples.

(3) Calculate $S = S_2' + CSE$, where S is purge- and drift-corrected signal; CSE is control signal error = (required control signal average) − (determined control signal average) for any check on control milk. Apply value to all except control milks.

(4) Calculate estimates from purge- and drift-corrected signals using calibration signals, and store. Equation type is Estimate = A + B (main equation). Initially, A = 0 and B = 1.

(5) Calculate calibration equations and store.

(6) Store random sample signals, estimates, and standard method reference results.

(7) Calculate and store mean difference, standard deviation of difference, limits for mean difference, and population standard deviation of difference for statistical quality control.

(8) Store results for checks on purging efficiency tests, homogenization efficiency tests, linearity tests, and repeatability tests.

L. Instrument Controls

For instrument with secondary slope controls, operate in uncorrected mode. For instruments without secondary slope controls, reduce interference correction coefficients to 0.

M. Control Milk

Prepare adequate supply of pasteurized, homogenized, preserved milks with % fat about that of population average. Transfer amounts for single tests to sample containers and keep refrigerated. Zero-adjust instrument channels. Heat 11 samples to 40°, and pump each through instrument, collecting signals. Average last 10 results for each signal to calculate required signal. Record required control milk signals to 4 decimals to prevent rounding errors in continuous control situation.

N. Setting Primary Slope Controls

Determine % fat, protein, and lactose on series of ≥8 preanalyzed (e.g., **905.02, 920.105, 896.01A, 984.15**) milks of type to be analyzed by instrument. Warm samples to 40°, mix thoroughly, and pump through instrument, collecting and correcting signals for purge and drift. For each signal, calculate regression equation of type $S = aF + bP + cL$, where S is signal and F, P, and L are results for standard. At fat channel, adjust slope amplification by 1/a. At protein and lactose channels, adjust by 1/b and 1/c, respectively. Check success of attempt to obtain coefficient of 1 for main components by repeating test.

Readjust slope amplifications if necessary. Lock slope controls and do not change settings thereafter. Warm 11 samples of control milk and redetermine required control milk values as indicated above.

O. First Calibration

Obtain 20 milk samples by random selection from population to be tested, and analyze by standard reference method for components to be estimated by IR method. Key standard results into computer. Warm and prepare 11 control milk samples and the calibration samples. Pump through instrument and collect and store signals. Computer applies purge correction, calculates control signal correction values, applies these to calculate milk signals, and stores these values in matrix with standard reference values. Select equation that is applicable to instrument from following main equation types.

Components	F_A	Signals F	L	F_B
1. F, P, L, TS, SNF	*	*	*	
2. F, P, L, TS, SNF		*	*	*
3. F	*	*	*	*
4. F		$[0.27 \times F(1)] + [0.73 \times F(2)]$		

Note: Except for TS and SNF, all main equation types force regression line through 0. With TS and SNF, either may be used, but equation with intercept is preferred and gives better results unless product being analyzed has been fortified or diluted.

Calculate by multiple linear regression main equations for components for which IR analysis is required. It is not necessary to calculate estimates for any component for which estimates are not required or to perform standard reference method analysis for that component except when slopes for initial calibration are adjusted. However, all signals must be controlled using required control milk signal values.

P. Production Analysis

At beginning of each production period and at definite intervals during production run, check control milk signals and recalculate drift corrections for application to product samples. Interval between checks can be shortened if drift for current interval is excessive. If instrument signals stability is acceptable, 1-h interval is satisfactory. Signals for product samples are corrected for purge and drift and then are used to calculate estimates.

Q. Quality Control

Select production samples at random at predetermined intervals and perform standard reference method analyses on these. Store signals, estimates, and reference values for these samples in matrix on accumulative basis. Check control milks and make adjustments to drift correction just prior to these selections. Interval between selection (days) and number selected may be varied to suit laboratory but ≥ 5 should be selected in 1 day and ≥ 20 in 1 week. Current population standard deviations of difference between estimate and reference methods may be calculated from last 50 differences in these accumulated data.

For quality control, calculate statistical limits for daily mean difference as $3 \times$ population standard deviation/$\sqrt{N}$ where, N is number of random samples tested that day. Action situations for changing A intercept in overall equations are:

(*1*) Daily mean difference is greater than limit.

(*2*) Six successive or 7 of 8 successive or 8 of 10 successive mean differences are on same side of 0. To correct this, adjust A in opposite direction to mean of differences. To correct for (*1*), adjust A in opposite direction by excess of difference over limit plus one-third of limit. Suggested additional statistical calculations are: (a) accumulated monthly mean difference standard deviation of difference, and limits for mean difference; and (b) accumulated annual mean difference, standard deviation of difference, and limits for mean difference. Overall objectives are to control current analyses as well as possible and to achieve annual mean difference very close to 0.

R. Recalibration

Use signals and standard reference values for last N samples in accumulated random sample data. Calculation may be made either to redetermine coefficients of main equation or by simple regression using estimates of main equation as independent variable and standard reference method values as dependent variable. Latter method would determine values for A and B in overall equation.

Whenever control milk is changed, whether at a time of recalibration or between calibrations, run 11 samples of both old and new control milks. Use drift errors of old control milk to adjust averages for new control milk signals in calculating required signals for it. Do not use control milk for longer than 1 week.

With random sample data accumulated over long periods of time, number of samples used for calibration and frequency of calibration can be optimized. Signals and standard reference values in data bank can be used to vary choices and determine net effect for different equations generated in this way.

For test population used first with this control method, optimum conditions were $N = 20$ and interval between calibrations = 1 week.

S. Precautions

See **972.16C** for normal precautions. This control method uses required control milk signals to control calibration level in preference to maintaining 0 settings at various channels with H_2O. Advantages are that drift errors identify signal subject to drift and that control of level is in range of test analysis. Water zeros may still be checked. Drift away from 0 indicates extraneous absorptions which could be due to excessive moisture in console, buildup of scale on cell windows, or other instrument faults. Continuous drifting in 1 direction for 0 signal should be investigated.

References: JAOAC **55,** 488(1972); **61,** 1015(1978); **62,** 1202, 1211(1979); **72,** 70, 184(1989).
CAS-63-42-3 (lactose)

Chapter 24
Niacin

24.1

960.46—Vitamin Assays
Microbiological Methods
Final Action

See Chapter 15.1.

24.2   ## 944.13—Niacin and Niacinamide (Nicotinic Acid and Nicotinamide) in Vitamin Preparations
Microbiological Methods
Final Action 1960

A. Basal Medium Stock Solution

Using ingredients in amounts prescribed for niacin, Table **960.46(c)** (*see* Chapter 15.1), proceed as below.

Using solutions prepared as in **960.46A**, add, with mixing, and in following order: acid-hydrolyzed casein solution, (**a**); cystine-tryptophan solution, (**e**); adenine-guanine-uracil solution, (**b**); vitamin solution IV, (**o**); vitamin solution V, (**p**); salt solution A, (**i**); and salt solution B, (**j**). Add ca 100 mL H_2O, and add, with mixing, anhydrous glucose and $NaOAc \cdot 3H_2O$. When solution is complete, adjust to pH 6.8 with NaOH solution, and dilute with H_2O to 250 mL.

Titrimetric Method

B. Niacin Standard Solutions

(**a**) *Stock solution.*—100 µg/mL. Accurately weigh, in closed system, 50–60 mg USP Niacin Reference Standard that has been dried to constant weight and stored in dark over P_2O_5 in desiccator. Dissolve in 25% alcohol, and dilute with additional 25% alcohol to make niacin concentration exactly 100 µg/mL. Store in dark at ca 10°.

(**b**) *Intermediate solution I.*—10 µg/mL. Dilute 100 mL stock solution, (**a**), with 25% alcohol to 1 L. Store in dark at ca 10°.

(**c**) *Working solution.*—Dilute suitable volume intermediate solution, (**b**), with H_2O to measured volume such that after incubation as in **960.46D** and **960.46E**, response at 5.0 mL level of this solution is equivalent to titration (as described in **960.46E**) of ca 8–12 mL. Designate this as standard solution. (This concentration is usually 0.1–0.4 µg niacin/mL standard solution.) Prepare fresh standard solution for each assay.

C. Inoculum

(a) *Liquid culture medium.*—Dilute measured volume basal medium stock solution, **944.13A**, with equal volume aqueous solution containing 0.2 μg niacin/mL. Add 10 mL portions diluted medium to test tubes, cover to prevent contamination, sterilize 15 min in autoclave at 121–123°, and cool tubes as rapidly as practicable to avoid color formation from overheating. Store in dark at ca 10°.

(b) *Inoculum.*—Make transfer of cells from stock culture of *Lactobacillus plantarum,* **960.46C(c)**, to sterile tube containing 10 mL liquid culture medium, (a). Incubate 6–24 h at any selected temperature between 30 and 40° held constant to within ±0.5°. Under aseptic conditions, centrifuge culture and decant supernate. Wash cells with 3 ca 10 mL portions sterile 0.9% NaCl solution or sterile suspension medium, **960.46B(c)**. Resuspend cells in 10 mL sterile 0.9% NaCl solution or sterile suspension medium. Cell suspension so obtained is inoculum.

D. Assay Solution

Place measured amount of sample in flask and proceed as below. Designate final measured volume so obtained as assay solution.

(a) *For dry or semidry materials containing no appreciable amount of basic substances.*—Add volume $1N$ H_2SO_4 equal in mL to ≥10 times dry weight sample in grams; resulting solution must contain ≤5.0 mg niacin/mL. If sample is not readily soluble, comminute to disperse it evenly in liquid; then agitate vigorously and wash down sides of flask with $1N$ H_2SO_4.

Autoclave mixture 30 min at 121–123° and cool. If lumping occurs, agitate mixture until particles are evenly dispersed. If dissolved protein is not present, adjust mixture to pH 6.8 with NaOH solution, dilute with H_2O to final measured volume containing, per mL, niacin ca equivalent to that of standard solution, **944.13B(c)**, and filter if solution is not clear.

If dissolved protein is present, adjust mixture, with vigorous agitation, to pH 6.0–6.5 with NaOH solution; then immediately add dilute HCl until no further precipitation occurs (usually ca pH 4.5, isoelectric point of many proteins). Dilute mixture to measured volume with H_2O, and filter. (In case of mixture difficult to filter, centrifuging and/or filtering through fritted glass, using suitable analytical filter-aid, may often be substituted for, or may precede, filtering through paper. Ash-free filter paper pulp and Celite Analytical Filter-Aid have been found satisfactory.) Take aliquot of clear filtrate and check for dissolved protein by adding dropwise, first dilute HCl, and if no precipitate forms, then, with vigorous agitation, NaOH solution, and proceed as follows with this aliquot:

(*1*) If no further precipitation occurs, add, with vigorous agitation, NaOH solution to pH 6.8, and dilute with H_2O to final measured volume containing, per mL, niacin ca equivalent to that of standard solution, **944.13B(c)**. If cloudiness occurs, refilter.

(*2*) If further precipitation occurs, adjust mixture again to point of maximum precipitation, dilute with H_2O to measured volume, and then filter. Take aliquot of clear filtrate and proceed as in (*1*).

(b) *For dry or semidry materials containing appreciable amounts of basic substances.*—Adjust mixture to pH 5.0–6.0 with dilute H_2SO_4. Add volume H_2O equal in mL to ≥10 times dry weight sample in g; resulting solution must contain ≤5.0 mg niacin/mL. Then add equivalent of 10 mL $10N$ H_2SO_4/100 mL liquid and proceed as in (a), beginning with second sentence, "If sample is not readily soluble . . . ."

(c) *For liquid materials.*—Adjust mixture to pH 5.0–6.0 with H_2SO_4 solution or NaOH solution and proceed as in (b), beginning with second sentence, "Add volume H_2O . . . ."

E. Assay

Using standard solution, **944.13B(c)**, assay solution, **944.13D**, basal medium stock solution, **944.13A**, and inoculum, **944.13C(b)**, proceed as in **960.46D**, **G**, and **H**. Value so obtained is potency of sample expressed as niacin. Multiply this value by 0.992 if potency is to be expressed as niacinamide.

Turbidimetric Method

F. Niacin Standard Solutions

(a) *Intermediate solution II.*—1.0 μg/mL. Dilute 10 mL niacin standard stock solution, **944.13B(a)**, with 25% alcohol to 1 L. Store in dark at ca 10°.

(b) *Working solution.*—Dilute suitable volume intermediate solution II, (a), with H_2O to measured volume such that after incubation as in **960.46D** and **960.46G**, with inoculated blank set at 100% T, % T at 5.0 mL level of this solution is equivalent to that for dried cell weight (as described in **960.46F**) of ≥1.25 mg. Designate this as standard solution. (This concentration is usually 0.01–0.04 μg niacin/mL standard solution.) Prepare fresh standard solution for each assay.

G. Inoculum

Proceed as in **944.13C(b)**.

H. Assay Solution

Proceed as in **944.13D**, except that where reference is made to niacin concentration ca equivalent to that of standard solution, **944.13B(c)**, replace by niacin concentration ca equivalent to that of standard solution, **944.13F(b)**. Designate solution so obtained as assay solution.

I. Assay

Using standard solution, **944.13F(b)**, assay solution, **944.13H**, basal medium stock solution, **944.13A**, and inoculum, **944.13G**, proceed as in **960.46D**, **G**, and **H**. Value so obtained is potency of sample expressed as niacin. Multiply this value by 0.992 if potency is to be expressed as niacinamide.

References: JAOAC **27,** 105(1944); **30,** 82(1947); **32,** 110, 479(1949); **39,** 172(1956); **40,** 856(1957); **41,** 61, 587(1958); **42,** 529(1959).
CAS-59-67-6 (niacin)
CAS-98-92-0 (niacinamide)

24.3   961.14—Niacin and Niacinamide in Drugs, Foods, and Feeds
Colorimetric Method
First Action 1961
Final Action 1962

A. Reagents

(a) *Niacin standard solutions.*—(*1*) *Stock solution.*—100 μg/mL. Dissolve 50 mg USP Niacin Reference Standard, previously dried and stored in dark in desiccator over P_2O_5, in 25% alcohol to make 500 mL. Store at ca 10°.

(*2*) *Working solution I.*—10 μg/mL. Remove small portion stock solution and let come to room temperature. Dilute 10 mL to 100 mL with H_2O. Use as standard solution in **961.14B(c)**.

(*3*) *Working solution II.*—4 μg/mL. Dilute 2 mL stock solution, allowed to come to room temperature as in (*2*), to 50 mL with H_2O. Use as standard solution in **961.14B(b)** and **961.14C(a)**.

(**b**) *Dilute ammonium hydroxide.*—Dilute 5 mL NH_4OH to 250 mL with H_2O.

(**c**) *Dilute hydrochloric acid.*—1 + 5.

(**d**) *Phosphate buffer solution.*—pH 8. Dissolve 60 g $Na_2HPO_4 \cdot 7H_2O$ and 10 g KH_2PO_4 in warm H_2O and dilute to 200 mL.

(**e**) *Cyanogen bromide solution.*—10%. Prepare under hood. Warm 370 mL H_2O to 40° in large flask and add 40 g CNBr. Shake until dissolved, cool, and dilute to 400 mL. Do not let CNBr or solution come in contact with skin. Store in refrigerator.

(**f**) *10% Sulfanilic acid solution.*—Add NH_4OH in 1 mL portions to mixture of 20 g sulfanilic acid and 170 mL H_2O until acid dissolves. Adjust to pH 4.5 with HCl (1 + 1), using bromocresol green indicator, **942.23A(b)**, and spot plate. Dilute to 200 mL. Solution should be almost colorless. Use in **961.14C(a)**.

> **942.23A(b)**
>
> *A. Reagents and Apparatus*
>
> (**b**) *Bromocresol green pH indicator.*—Dissolve 0.1 g indicator by triturating in agate mortar with 2.8 mL 0.05N NaOH, and dilute to 200 mL with H_2O. Transition range: 4.0 (green)–5.8 (blue).

(**g**) *55% Sulfanilic acid solution.*—Add 27 mL H_2O and 27 mL NH_4OH to 55 g sulfanilic acid and shake until dissolved, warming if necessary. Adjust to pH 7 with few drops NH_4OH or 5N HCl and dilute to 100 mL. Store in dark. Use in **961.14C(b)**.

B. Preparation of Sample and Standards

(**a**) *Pharmaceutical preparations.*—Disperse ≥5 tablets or capsules in small volume H_2O with heat. Tablets may be ground first. Cool, transfer to volumetric flask, and dilute to volume. Solution should contain 50–200 μg niacin/mL. Pipet 10 mL aliquot into 250 mL erlenmeyer and add 10 mL HCl. Evaporate on hot plate to ca 2 mL, cool, add ca 25–50 mL H_2O, and adjust to pH 2.5–4.5 with 40% NaOH or KOH solution. Transfer to volumetric flask of such size that solution contains ca 4 μg niacin/mL. Filter, if necessary, discarding first 10 mL filtrate. Proceed as in **961.14C(a)**.

(**b**) *Noncereal foods and feeds.*—Weigh 1 oz (28.35 g) sample into 1 L erlenmeyer, add 200 mL 1N H_2SO_4, mix, and heat 30 min in autoclave at 15 lb (104 kPa) pressure. Cool, adjust to pH 4.5 with 10N NaOH, using bromocresol green as outside indicator, dilute to 250 mL with H_2O, and filter. Weigh 17 g $(NH_4)_2SO_4$ into 50 mL volumetric flask, pipet in 40 mL sample solution, dilute to volume with H_2O, and shake vigorously. Filter, mix well, and use 1 mL for color development. In case of samples containing 16 mg niacin/lb, final solution contains 3.2 μg/mL.

Pipet 40 mL working solution II, **A(a)(3)**, into 17 g $(NH_4)_2SO_4$ in 50 mL volumetric flask, and dilute to volume with H_2O. This standard contains 3.2 μg/mL. Proceed as in **961.14C(a)**.

(**c**) *Cereal products.*—Run 1 reagent blank and 5 levels of working solution I, **A(a)(2)**, with samples throughout determination.

Place 1.5 g $Ca(OH)_2$ into each of six 250 mL erlenmeyers. From pipet add 0, 5, 10, 15, 20, and 25 mL working solution I, respectively. Accurately weigh ca 2.5 g sample containing ca 100 μg niacin into another flask containing ca 1.5 g $Ca(OH)_2$. To all flasks add H_2O to ca 90 mL, shake to mix, and autoclave 2 h at 15 lb (104 kPa) pressure. Mix thoroughly while still hot. Cool to ca 40°, transfer to 100 mL volumetric flasks, and dilute to volume. (When necessary, sample may be stored in refrigerator few days.)

Transfer ca 50 mL supernate from each volumetric flask to separate centrifuge tubes and place in ice bath 15 min or in refrigerator ≥ 2 h. Centrifuge 15 min and pipet 20 mL supernate from each tube into separate centrifuge tubes containing 8 g $(NH_4)_2SO_4$ and 2 mL phosphate buffer solution. Shake to dissolve and warm to 55–60°. Centrifuge 5 min and filter through Whatman No. 12 paper, or equivalent, refiltering if necessary to obtain clear solution. Proceed as in **961.14C(b)**.

C. Determination

(**a**) *For pharmaceutical preparations and noncereal foods and feeds.*—Add 10% sulfanilic acid solution, **A(f)**, and CNBr solution under hood from burets or pipets filled by mechanical suction. (*Caution: CNBr is toxic.*) Use working solution II, **A(a)(3)**. Prepare tubes as follows:

Standard Blank
1.0 mL standard solution
5.0 mL H$_2$O
0.5 mL dilute NH$_4$OH
2.0 mL 10% sulfanilic acid
0.5 mL dilute HCl

Sample Blank
1.0 mL sample solution
5.0 mL H$_2$O
0.5 mL dilute NH$_4$OH
2.0 mL 10% sulfanilic acid
0.5 mL dilute HCl

Standard Solution
1.0 mL standard solution
0.5 mL dilute NH$_4$OH
5.0 mL CNBr
2.0 mL 10% sulfanilic acid
0.5 mL H$_2$O

Sample Solution
1.0 mL sample solution
0.5 mL dilute NH$_4$OH
5.0 mL CNBr
2.0 mL 10% sulfanilic acid
0.5 mL H$_2$O

Prepare separate sample blank for each sample.

Pipet standard solution and sample solution into respective tubes; add 5 mL H$_2$O for standard blank and sample blank. Add all subsequent solutions to single tube and read color before proceeding with next tube. Starting with standard blank, swirl tube to impart rotary motion in liquid, immediately add dilute NH$_4$OH, swirl again, add sulfanilic acid, and swirl. Immediately add 0.5 mL dilute HCl, mix again, place in photoelectric colorimeter, and adjust instrument to 0 A at any specific wavelength between 430 and 450 nm within ca 30 s after addition of sulfanilic acid solution. Treat standard solution in same way as standard blank with respect to addition of dilute NH$_4$OH. Immediately swirl tube, add CNBr solution, and swirl again. At 30 s after addition of CNBr solution, swirl tube, add sulfanilic acid solution, and swirl again. Immediately add 0.5 mL H$_2$O, mix again, and stopper. With instrument set at 0 A for standard blank, as above, read A of standard solution at maximum. (Color reaches maximum in ca 1.5 min after addition of sulfanilic acid solution, remains at peak ca 2 min, and then fades slowly.)

With sample blank set at 0 A, determine A of sample solution similarly. Niacin content is proportional to A if standard and sample solutions are ca same concentration.

(**b**) *For cereal products.*—In each of 2 tubes place 5 mL standard and in each of 2 additional tubes place 5 mL sample solution. In additional tube to be used as reagent blank, place 5 mL H$_2$O. To one standard tube and one sample tube to be used as their respective blanks, add 10 mL H$_2$O. Let all tubes stand 30 min in bath of finely crushed ice, preferably in refrigerator. To remaining sample and standard tubes and to reagent blank, consecutively add 10 mL cold CNBr, followed in 30 s by 1.0 mL 55% sulfanilic acid solution, **A(g)**. Mix immediately after addition of each reagent (most conveniently done by swirling), and stopper tubes containing CNBr. Replace all tubes in ice bath. To standard and sample blank add 1.0 mL 55% sulfanilic acid solution.

Set colorimeter to 0 A at 470 nm with standard blank, and read A of other tubes 12–15 min after addition of sulfanilic acid. Tubes must be cooled uniformly and each tube must be wiped dry just before placing in colorimeter. If tubes fog, dip momentarily in hot H_2O and wipe before reading.

Plot standard curve of A of standard minus that of reagent blank against niacin concentration in $\mu g/mL$, drawing straight line of best fit. From this line read concentration, C, corresponding to A of sample corrected for sample blank and reagent blank.

$$mg\ Niacin/g\ sample = C/(10 \times g\ sample)$$

References: Anal. Chem. **23**, 983(1951). JAOAC **34**, 380(1951); **36**, 1018(1953); **42**, 625(1959); **44**, 431(1961); **45**, 449(1962); **51**, 506, 828(1968).
CAS-59-67-6 (niacin)
CAS-98-92-0 (niacinamide)

24.4   981.16—Niacin and Niacinamide in Foods, Drugs, and Feeds
Automated Method
First Action 1981
Final Action 1982
AACC-AOAC Method

(Applicable to products for which manual method, **961.14** (*see* 24.3),
is applicable and which contain $\geq 2\ \mu g/g$.)

A. Apparatus

(**a**) *Automatic analyzer.*—Technicon AutoAnalyzer II system with flow scheme as in Fig. **981.16**. (Technicon Instruments Corp., manifold No. 116-D137), or equivalent.

(**b**) *Collection funnels.*—Disposable funnels, 20 mL, are convenient.

(**c**) *Pipets.*—Rapid dispensing pipets are convenient in multiple analyses.

B. Reagents

(**a**) *Wetting agent.*—30% aqueous Brij 35 solution (Atlas Chemical Industries, Wilmington, DE 19899).

(**b**) *Phosphate buffer solutions.*—(*1*) *Stock solution.*—Dissolve 130 g Na_2HPO_4 and 71 g KH_2PO_4 in ca 900 mL warm H_2O. Cool to room temperature and dilute to 1 L with H_2O. (*2*) *Working solution.*—pH 6.7. Dilute 150 mL stock solution to 1 L with H_2O and add 1.5 mL wetting agent. Filter through Whatman 2V paper before use. (*3*) *Sample buffer solution.*—pH 7.6. Dissolve 272 g Na_2HPO_4 and 48 g KH_2PO_4 in ca 1.8 L warm H_2O. Cool to room temperature and dilute to 2 L with H_2O.

(**c**) *Sulfanilic acid solution.*—10%. Add 100 g sulfanilic acid to ca 500 mL H_2O. Add NH_4OH with mixing until dissolved (ca 40 mL). Adjust to pH 7.0 with HCl (1 + 3) and dilute to 1 L with H_2O. Filter, and store in cool, dark place. Prepare fresh every 2 weeks.

(**d**) *Cyanogen bromide solution.*—5%. Weigh ca 50 g CNBr into beaker containing 300 mL H_2O at ca 40°, and stir to dissolve. Cool, and dilute to 1 L with H_2O. Prepare fresh every 2 weeks. (*Caution:* CNBr is very poisonous. Weigh compound and prepare solution in hood.)

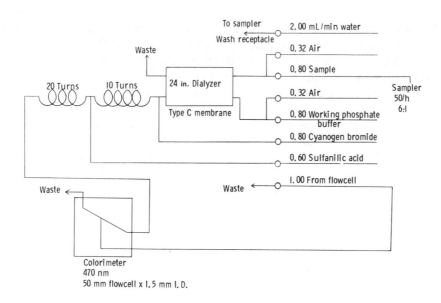

To sampler
Wash receptacle
Waste
2.00 mL/min water
0.32 Air
0.80 Sample
0.32 Air
0.80 Working phosphate buffer
0.80 Cyanogen bromide
0.60 Sulfanilic acid
1.00 From flowcell
Sampler 50/h 6:1
20 Turns
10 Turns
24 in. Dialyzer
Type C membrane
Waste
Waste
Colorimeter
470 nm
50 mm flowcell x 1.5 mm I.D.

Figure 981.16.—Flow diagram for automated determination of niacin and niacinamide.

(**e**) *Sample wash solution.*—Dilute 3.0 mL wetting agent to 2 L with H_2O and filter through Whatman 2V paper.

(**f**) *Calcium hydroxide slurry.*—Add 22 g $Ca(OH)_2$ to 200 mL volumetric flask and add ca 100 mL H_2O. Shake to disperse and dilute to volume with H_2O. To use, transfer to 250 mL beaker on magnetic stirrer and stir at rate to ensure homogeneity.

(**g**) *Basic solution for waste container.*—Dissolve 150 g NaOH in 300 mL H_2O in 4 L reagent bottle. Place bottle in hood and pump waste into this bottle.

(**h**) *Niacin standard solutions.*—(*1*) *Stock solution.*—10 μg/mL. Weigh 50.0 mg nicotinic acid (stored in desiccator) into 500 mL volumetric flask, dissolve and dilute to volume with H_2O. Daily, dilute 25.0 mL to 250 mL with H_2O. (*2*) *Working standard solutions.*—Pipet 30, 20, 10, and 5 mL stock solution into 100 mL volumetric flasks containing 5 mL $Ca(OH)_2$ slurry. Add H_2O to ca 55 mL, autoclave, and treat samples and standards alike. Final solutions will contain 3.0, 2.0, 1.0, and 0.5 μg niacin/mL.

C. Preparation of Sample

Grind representative portion to pass No. 40 sieve.

D. Determination

Transfer accurately weighed portion (1.5 g maximum) of ground sample containing ca 0.2 mg niacin to 100 mL volumetric flask. Add 5 mL $Ca(OH)_2$ slurry, using Rainin pipet, or weigh 0.55 g $Ca(OH)_2$ into flask. Add ca 50 mL H_2O, cover with foil, swirl, and autoclave 2 h at 121°. For products which spatter during hydrolysis (high oil content), use 125 mL erlenmeyer and transfer to 100 mL volumetric flask after autoclaving.

While solutions are still hot, add 10 mL 1.5N HCl (1 + 7) with auto pipettor, and swirl to dissolve remaining $Ca(OH)_2$. Be sure all $Ca(OH)_2$ is dissolved. Let cool to room temperature. (Solutions may be stored at this point.)

To sample and standard solutions, add 25 mL sample buffer solutions from pipettor, 2 drops wetting agent, and dilute to volume with H_2O. (Precipitate forms and final pH will be ca 6.7.) Shake, and filter through Whatman 2V paper (disposable collection funnels are convenient).

Pump high standard solution ($3\mu g/mL$) through system and set recorder pen at 100% with standard calibration adjustment. Aspirate and pump set of standards and sample filtrates through system. Use one standard with every series of 20 samples to correct for any drift. If sample is more concentrated than highest standard, dilute sample solution with sample buffer solution to bring peak height into range of standards. After all sample filtrates have been run, replace CNBr line with H_2O. Let pump ca 15 min and resample filtrates to obtain corresponding blank values. Alternatively, dual channel instrument may be used for simultaneous blank corrections. Determine concentration, C, ($\mu g/mL$) from standard curve:

$$\text{mg Niacin or Niacinamide/g} = C \times 10/W$$

where W = grams sample.

Reference: JAOAC **62,** 1027(1979).
CAS-59-67-6 (niacin)
CAS-98-92-0 (niacinamide)

24.5 975.41—Niacin and Niacinamide in Cereal Products
Automated Method
First Action 1975
Final Action 1976

A. Principle

Niacin and niacinamide are extracted from cereal products with $Ca(OH)_2$. Pyridine groups are cleaved by CNBr and reacted with sulfanilic acid to form yellow complex whose A is read at 470 nm.

B. Apparatus and Reagents

(**a**) *Automatic analyzer.*—AutoAnalyzer AAII with following modules (Technicon Instruments Corp.): Sampler IV, proportioning pump, colorimeter with 470 nm filters, recorder, and manifold No. 116-D137. *See* Fig. **975.41.**

(**b**) *Cyanogen bromide solution.*—10%. See **961.14A(e)** (*see* 24.3).

(**c**) *Phosphate buffer solution I.*—pH 8. See **961.14A(d)**.

(**d**) *Phosphate buffer solution II.*—pH 8. Dissolve 60 g $Na_2HPO_4 \cdot 7H_2O$ and 10 g KH_2PO_4 in warm H_2O and dilute to 2 L. Add 1 mL Brij-35 (Technicon Instruments Corp. No. T21-0110) and mix.

(**e**) *Sulfanilic acid solution.*—10%. Add 100 g sulfanilic acid to beaker containing 500 mL H_2O. Mix on magnetic stirrer and slowly add NH_4OH until acid dissolves (ca 40 mL). Adjust to pH 7 with HCl (1 + 3) and dilute to 1 L.

(**f**) *Niacin standard solutions.*—(*1*) *Stock solution.*—100 $\mu g/mL$. See **961.14A(a)(*1*)**. (*2*) *Working solution.*—25 $\mu g/mL$. Remove small portion stock solution and let come to room temperature. Dilute 25 mL to 100 mL with H_2O. (*3*) *Calibration solution.*—2.5 $\mu g/mL$. Dilute 10 mL working standard solution to 100 mL with H_2O.

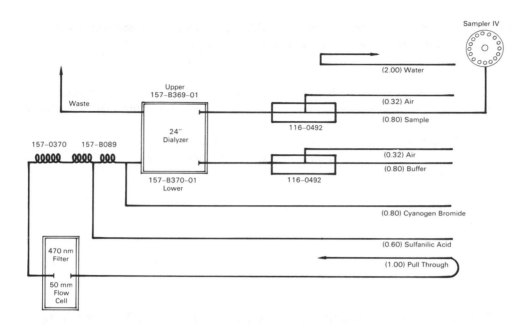

Figure 975.41.—Flow diagram for automated analysis for niacin and niacinamide.

C. Preparation of Samples and Standards

Run 4 levels of working standard solution with samples throughout determination.

Place 1.5 g $Ca(OH)_2$ into each of four 250 mL erlenmeyers. From pipet add 5, 10, 15, and 20 mL working standard solution, respectively. Accurately weigh ca 5 g sample containing ca 150–400 μg niacin into another flask containing 1.5 g $Ca(OH)_2$. To all flasks add H_2O to ca 90 mL, shake to mix, and autoclave 2 h at 15 lb (104 kPa) pressure. Mix thoroughly while still hot. Cool to ca 40°, transfer to 100 mL volumetric flasks, add 1 drop Brij-35, and dilute to volume. (When necessary, solution may be stored in refrigerator few days.)

Transfer ca 35 mL supernate from each volumetric flask to separate centrifuge tubes and place in ice bath 15 min or in refrigerator 2 h. Centrifuge 15 min, pipet 20 mL supernate from each tube into separate centrifuge tubes, add 2 mL phosphate buffer solution I, mix thoroughly, and filter through Whatman No. 2 paper, or equivalent.

D. Determination

(System should be operated under hood. If this is not possible, take following precautions to minimize CNBr fumes: Remove only portion of CNBr solution from refrigerator [usually 100 mL in 100 mL volumetric flask is sufficient]. Place tubing [polyethylene preferred] into flask and wrap opening with Al foil. Suspend waste lines from flowcell into 1 L erlenmeyer containing ca 100 mL 25% NaOH solution. Cover opening of flask with wet paper towel.)

Establish steady baseline with all reagents pumping through system. Adjust 2.5 μg/mL standard solution (250 μg/100 mL) to 50 scale units on recorder by using ''Standard Cal'' control on colorimeter. Fill sample cups in following order: standards, samples, and 2.5 μg/mL standard solution after every 10 samples. Dialyzer in system results in low blanks for most samples. Determine blank as follows: Place CNBr line into H_2O and flush system free of CNBr (ca 30 min). Keep all other tubing in respective reagents and "Standard Cal" setting locked in position as in analysis. Establish steady baseline and repeat determination on samples and standards in same order as in analysis.

E. Calculations

Plot standard curve of A (chart units) of standard minus blank against niacin concentration in μg/mL, drawing line of best fit. Read concentration, C, corresponding to A of sample corrected for blank and any shift in baseline during run.

For dilution to 100 mL for both samples and standards:

$$\text{mg Niacin/g} = C/(10 \times \text{g sample})$$

where $C = (\mu\text{g/mL}) \times 100$.

Reference: JAOAC **58,** 799(1975).
CAS-59-67-6 (niacin)
CAS-98-92-0 (niacinamide)

24.6   985.34—Niacin and Niacinamide (Nicotinic Acid and Nicotinamide) in Ready-to-Feed Milk-Based Infant Formula
Microbiological-Turbidimetric Method
First Action 1985
Final Action 1988

A. Basal Medium Stock Solution

Using solutions prepared as in **960.46A** (*see* Chapter 15.1), combine, with mixing, and in following order: 25 mL cystine-tryptophan solution, (**e**); 5 mL adenine-guanine-uracil solution, (**b**); 5 mL vitamin solution IV, (**o**); 5 mL vitamin solution V, (**p**); 5 mL salt solution A, (**i**); and 5 mL salt solution B, (**j**). Add ca 100 mL H_2O, and add, with mixing, 2.5 g vitamin-free casein, hydrolyzed, (**a**); 10 g anhydrous glucose; and 5 g NaOAc, anhydrous. When solution is complete, adjust to pH 6. with NaOH solution, and dilute with H_2O to 250 mL. (Some commercial sources of basal media have been found satisfactory, e.g., Difco niacin assay medium [0322-15].)

B. Niacin Standard Solutions

(**a**) *Stock solution.*—100 μg/mL. Accurately weigh, in closed system, 50–60 mg USP Niacin Reference Standard that has been dried to constant weight and stored in dark over P_2O_5 in desiccator. Dissolve in 25% alcohol, and dilute with additional 25% alcohol to make niacin concentration exactly 100 μg/mL. Store in dark at ca 10°.

(**b**) *Intermediate solution.*—1 μg/mL. Dilute 5 mL stock solution, (**a**), with 25% alcohol to 500 mL.

(**c**) *Working solution.*—0.014 μg/mL. Dilute 7 mL intermediate solution, (**b**), with H_2O to 500 mL. Also prepare secondary working solutions, one higher and one lower in niacin concentration (usually 0.01 and 0.02 μg/mL) than primary working solution. This is done in case sample niacin concentration is too high or too low for primary working solution to be used.

C. Inoculum

(a) *Liquid culture medium.*—Dilute measured volume basal medium stock solution, **985.34A**, with equal volume aqueous solution containing 0.2 µg niacin/mL. Add 10 mL portions diluted medium to test tubes, cover to prevent contamination, sterilize 15 min in autoclave at 121–123°, and cool tubes as rapidly as practicable to avoid color formation caused by overheating. Store in dark at ca 10°.

(b) *Inoculum.*—Make transfer of cells from stock culture of *Lactobacillus plantarum*, **960.46C(c)**, to sterile tube containing 10 mL liquid culture medium, (a). Incubate 6–24 h in constant temperature bath at 37°. Under aseptic conditions, centrifuge culture and decant supernate. Wash cells with 3 ca 10 mL portions sterile 0.9% NaCl solution. Resuspend cells in 10 mL sterile 0.9% NaCl solution. Cell suspension so obtained is inoculum.

D. Assay Solution

Place measured amount of composite containing 10–30 µg niacin in flask and add volume 1N H_2SO_4 equal in mL to ≥10 times dry weight sample in grams. Then agitate vigorously and wash down sides of flask with 1N H_2SO_4.

Autoclave mixture 30 min at 121–123° and cool. If lumping occurs, agitate mixture until particles are evenly dispersed.

If dissolved protein is present, adjust mixture, with vigorous agitation, to pH 6.0–6.5 with NaOH solution; then immediately add dilute HCl until no further precipitation occurs (usually ca pH 4.5, isoelectric point of many proteins). Dilute mixture to measured volume with H_2O, and filter. (In case of mixture difficult to filter, centrifuging and/or filtering through fritted glass, using suitable analytical filter-aid, may often be substituted for, or may precede, filtering through paper. Ash-free filter paper pulp and Celite Analytical Filter-Aid have been found satisfactory.) Take aliquot of clear filtrate and check for dissolved protein by adding dropwise, first dilute HCl, and if no precipitate forms, then with vigorous agitation, NaOH solution, and proceed as follows with this aliquot:

(1) If no further precipitation occurs, add, with vigorous agitation, NaOH solution to pH 6.8, and dilute with H_2O to final measured volume containing, per mL, niacin ca equivalent to that of standard solution, **985.34B(c)**. If cloudiness occurs, refilter.

(2) If further precipitation occurs, adjust mixture again to point of maximum precipitation, dilute with H_2O to measured volume, and then filter. Take aliquot of clear filtrate and proceed as in *(1)*.

Designate final measured volume obtained as assay solution.

E. Assay

Using standard solution, **985.34B(c)**, assay solution, **985.34D**, basal medium stock solution, **985.34A**, and inoculum, **985.34C(b)**, proceed as in **960.46D, G**, and **H**. Value so obtained is potency of sample expressed as niacin. Multiply this value by 0.992 if potency is to be expressed as niacinamide.

Reference: JAOAC **68,** 514(1985).
CAS-59-67-6 (niacin)
CAS-98-92-0 (niacinamide)

Chapter 25
Pantothenic Acid

25.1

960.46—Vitamin Assays
Microbiological Methods
Final Action

See Chapter 15.1.

25.2

945.74—Pantothenic Acid in Vitamin Preparations
Microbiological Methods
Final Action 1960

(Applicable only to materials containing Ca pantothenate or other free forms of pantothenic acid)

A. Basal Medium Stock Solution

Using ingredients in amounts prescribed for pantothenic acid, Table **960.46(d)** (*see* Chapter 15.1), proceed as below.

Using solutions prepared as in **960.46A**, add, with mixing, and in following order: acid-hydrolyzed casein solution, (**a**); cystine-tryptophan solution, (**e**); adenine-guanine-uracil solution, (**b**); vitamin solution IV, (**o**); vitamin solution VI, (**q**); salt solution A, (**i**); and salt solution B, (**j**). Add ca 100 mL H_2O and add, with mixing, anhydrous glucose and $NaOAc\cdot3H_2O$. When solution is complete, adjust to pH 6.8 with NaOH solution, add, with mixing, polysorbate 80 solution, (**h**), and dilute with H_2O to 250 mL.

Titrimetric Method
B. Pantothenic Acid Standard Solutions

(Do not shake standard solutions stored under toluene.)

(**a**) *Stock solution.*—40 µg/mL. Accurately weigh, in closed system, 45–55 mg USP Calcium Pantothenate Reference Standard that has been dried to constant weight and stored in dark over P_2O_5 in desiccator. Dissolve in ca 500 mL H_2O, add 10 mL 0.2*N* CH_3COOH and 100 mL 0.2*N* NaOAc, and dilute with additional H_2O to make Ca pantothenate concentration exactly 43.47 µg/mL (40 µg pantothenic acid/mL). Store under toluene in dark at ca 10°.

(**b**) *Intermediate solution.*—1.0 µg/mL. To 25 mL stock solution, (**a**), add ca 500 mL H_2O, 10 mL 0.2*N* CH_3COOH, and 100 mL 0.2*N* NaOAc, and dilute with additional H_2O to 1 L. Store under toluene in dark at ca 10°.

(c) *Working solution.*—Dilute suitable volume of intermediate solution, (b), with H_2O to measured volume such that after incubation as in **960.46D** and **960.46E**, response at 5.0 mL level of this solution is equivalent to titration (as described in **960.46E**) of ca 8–12 mL. Designate this as standard solution. (This concentration is usually 0.005–0.020 μg pantothenic acid/mL standard solution.) Prepare fresh standard solution for each assay.

C. Inoculum

(a) *Liquid culture medium.*—Dilute measured volume basal medium stock solution, **945.74A**, with equal volume aqueous solution containing 0.04 μg pantothenic acid/mL. Add 10 mL portions diluted medium to test tubes, cover to prevent contamination, sterilize 15 min in autoclave at 121– 123°, and cool tubes as rapidly as practicable to avoid color formation from overheating. Store in dark at ca 10°.

(b) Make transfer of cells from stock culture of *Lactobacillus plantarum,* **960.46C(c)**, to sterile tube containing 10 mL liquid culture medium, (a). Incubate 6–24 h at any selected temperature between 30 and 40° held constant to within ±0.5°. Under aseptic conditions, centrifuge culture and decant supernate. Wash cells with 3 ca 10 mL portions sterile 0.9% NaCl solution or sterile suspension medium, **960.46B(c)**. Resuspend cells in 10 mL sterile 0.9% NaCl solution or sterile suspension medium. Cell suspension so obtained is inoculum.

D. Assay Solution

(Throughout all stages, keep solution below pH 7.0 to prevent loss of pantothenic acid.)

Place measured amount of sample in flask and proceed as below. (Where directed to filter through paper, use paper known not to adsorb pantothenic acid. Ash-free papers have been found satisfactory.) Designate final measured volume so obtained as assay solution.

(a) *For dry or semidry materials containing no appreciable amount of basic substances.*—Add volume H_2O equal in mL to ≥10 times dry weight sample in g; resulting solution must contain ≤5 mg pantothenic acid/mL. Adjust mixture to pH 5.65 ± 0.05 with CH_3COOH solution or NaOAc solution. If sample is not readily soluble, comminute so that it may be evenly dispersed in liquid. Then agitate vigorously and wash down sides of flask with aqueous solution containing in each liter 10 mL 0.2N CH_3COOH and 100 mL 0.2N NaOAc.

Autoclave mixture 5–7 min at 121–123° and cool. Then proceed as in **944.13D(a)**, beginning with second sentence in second paragraph, ''If lumping occurs . . .'' except where reference is made to niacin concentration ca equivalent to that of standard solution, **944.13B(c)**, replace by pantothenic acid concentration ca equivalent to that of standard solution, **945.74B(c)**.

> I. **944.13B(c)**
>
> B. *Niacin Standard Solutions*
>
> (c) *Working solution.*—Dilute suitable volume intermediate solution, (b), with H_2O to measured volume such that after incubation as in **960.46D** and **960.46E**, response at 5.0 mL level of this solution is equivalent to titration (as described in **960.46E**) of ca 8–12 mL. Designate this as standard solution. (This concentration is usually 0.1–0.4 μg niacin/mL standard solution.) Prepare fresh standard solution for each assay.

> II. **944.13D(a)**
>
> D. *Assay Solution*
>
> Place measured amount of sample in flask and proceed as below. Designate final measured volume so obtained as assay solution.

(a) *For dry or semidry materials containing no appreciable amount of basic substances.*—Add volume $1N$ H_2SO_4 equal in mL to ≥ 10 times dry weight sample in grams; resulting solution must contain ≤ 5.0 mg niacin/mL. If sample is not readily soluble, comminute to disperse it evenly in liquid; then agitate vigorously and wash down sides of flask with $1N$ H_2SO_4.

Autoclave mixture 30 min at 121–123° and cool. If lumping occurs, agitate mixture until particles are evenly dispersed. If dissolved protein is not present, adjust mixture to pH 6.8 with NaOH solution, dilute with H_2O to final measured volume containing, per mL, niacin ca equivalent to that of standard solution, **944.13B(c)**, and filter if solution is not clear.

If dissolved protein is present, adjust mixture, with vigorous agitation, to pH 6.0–6.5 with NaOH solution; then immediately add dilute HCl until no further precipitation occurs (usually ca pH 4.5, isoelectric point of many proteins). Dilute mixture to measured volume with H_2O, and filter. (In case of mixture difficult to filter, centrifuging and/or filtering through fritted glass, using suitable analytical filter-aid, may often be substituted for, or may precede, filtering through paper. Ash-free filter paper pulp and Celite Analytical Filter-Aid have been found satisfactory.) Take aliquot of clear filtrate and check for dissolved protein by adding dropwise, first dilute HCl, and if no precipitate forms, then, with vigorous agitation, NaOH solution, and proceed as follows with this aliquot:

(*1*) If no further precipitation occurs, add, with vigorous agitation, NaOH solution to pH 6.8, and dilute with H_2O to final measured volume containing, per mL, niacin ca equivalent to that of standard solution, **944.13B(c)**. If cloudiness occurs, refilter.

(*2*) If further precipitation occurs, adjust mixture again to point of maximum precipitation, dilute with H_2O to measured volume, and then filter. Take aliquot of clear filtrate and proceed as in (*1*).

(b) *For dry or semidry materials containing appreciable amounts of basic substances.*—Adjust mixture to pH 5.0–6.0 with CH_3COOH solution. Add volume H_2O equal in mL to ≥ 10 times dry weight sample in g; resulting solution must contain ≤ 5 mg pantothenic acid/mL. Then proceed as in (a), beginning with second sentence: ''Adjust mixture to pH 5.65 $\pm$ 0.05 . . . .''

(c) *For liquid materials.*—Adjust mixture to pH 5.0–6.0 with CH_3COOH solution or NaOAc solution and proceed as in (b), beginning with second sentence: ''Add volume H_2O . . . .''

E. Assay

Using standard solution, **945.74B(c)**, assay solution, **945.74D**, basal medium stock solution, **945.74A**, and inoculum, **945.74C(b)**, proceed as in **960.46D**, **G**, and **H**. Value so obtained is potency of sample expressed as D-pantothenic acid. Multiply this value by 1.087 if potency is to be expressed as Ca D-pantothenate. Multiply this value by 1.100 if potency is to be expressed as Na pantothenate.

Turbidimetric Method

F. Pantothenic Acid Standard Solution

Dilute suitable amount of pantothenic acid intermediate solution, **945.74B(b)**, with H_2O to measured volume such that after incubation as in **960.46D** and **960.46G**, with inoculated blank set at 100% T, % T at 5.0 mL level of this solution is equivalent to that for dried cell weight (as described in **960.46F**) of

$\geq$1.25 mg. Designate this as standard solution. (This concentration is usually 0.003–0.012 μg pantothenic acid/mL standard solution.) Prepare fresh standard solution for each assay.

G. Inoculum

Proceed as in **945.74C(b)**.

H. Assay Solution

Proceed as in **945.74D**, except that where reference is made to pantothenic acid concentration ca equivalent to that of standard solution, **945.74B(c)**, replace by pantothenic acid concentration ca equivalent to that of standard solution, **945.74F**. Designate solution so obtained as assay solution.

I. Assay

Using standard solution, **945.74F**, assay solution, **945.74H**, basal medium stock solution, **945.74A**, and inoculum, **945.74G**, proceed as in **960.46D**, **G**, and **H**. Value so obtained is potency of sample expressed as D-pantothenic acid. Multiply this value by 1.087 if potency is to be expressed as Ca D-pantothenate.

References: JAOAC **28**, 567(1945); **35**, 103, 722(1952); **37**, 779(1954); **38**, 710(1955); **39**, 172(1956); **40**, 853, 856(1957); **41**, 61, 587, 739(1958); **42**, 525, 529(1959); J. Biol. Chem. **192**, 181(1951).
CAS-137-08-6 (calcium pantothenate)
CAS-79-83-4 (pantothenic acid)

Chapter 26
Phosphorus

26.1   **958.01—Phosphorus (Total) in Fertilizers**
Spectrophotometric Molybdovanadophosphate Method
Final Action

(Not applicable to materials yielding colored solutions or solutions containing ions other than orthophosphate which form colored complexes with molybdovanadate. Not recommended for basic slag.)

A. Apparatus

Photometer.—Beckman Instruments, Inc. Model DU (no longer available) spectrophotometer with stray light filter and matched 1 cm cells. With other photometers analyst must determine suitability for use and conditions for satisfactory performance. Means for dispelling heat from light source is desirable.

B. Reagents

(a) *Molybdovanadate reagent.*—Dissolve 40 g ammonium molybdate·4H$_2$O in 400 mL hot H$_2$O and cool. Dissolve 2 g ammonium metavanadate in 250 mL hot H$_2$O, cool, and add 450 mL 70% HClO$_4$. (*Caution: See Appendix* for safety notes on perchloric acid.) Gradually add molybdate solution to vanadate solution with stirring, and dilute to 2 L.

(b) *Phosphate standard solution.*—Dry pure KH$_2$PO$_4$ (52.15% P$_2$O$_5$) 2 h at 105°. Prepare solutions containing 0.4–1.0 mg P$_2$O$_5$/mL in 0.1 mg increments by weighing 0.0767, 0.0959, 0.1151, 0.1342, 0.1534, 0.1726, and 0.1918 g KH$_2$PO$_4$ and diluting each to 100 mL with H$_2$O. Prepare fresh solutions containing 0.4 and 0.7 mg P$_2$O$_5$/mL weekly.

C. Preparation of Standard Curve

Pipet 5 mL aliquots of 7 standard phosphate solutions (2–5 mg P$_2$O$_5$/aliquot) into 100 mL volumetric flasks and add 45 mL H$_2$O. Then, within 5 min for entire series, add 20 mL molybdovanadate reagent by buret or pipet, dilute to volume and mix. Let stand 10 min.

Select 2 absorption cells (standard and sample cells) and fill both with 2 mg standard. Set spectrophotometer to 400 nm and adjust to zero *A* with standard cell. Sample cell must check zero *A* within 0.001 unit; otherwise read *A* for sample cell and correct subsequent readings. (Choose cell showing positive *A* against other as sample cell so that this positive *A* is always subtracted.) Using sample cell, determine *A* of other standards with instrument adjusted to zero *A* for 2 mg standard. After each determination empty and refill cell containing 2 mg standard, and readjust zero to avoid error that might arise from temperature changes. Plot *A* against concentration in mg P$_2$O$_5$/mL standard solution.

D. Preparation of Solution

Treat 1 g sample as in **957.02B**, preferably (**e**), when these acids are suitable solvents. (Solution should be free of nitrogen oxides and NOCl.)

957.02 (Phosphorus [Total] in Fertilizers, Preparation of Sample Solution)

A. Reagent

Magnesium nitrate solution.—Dissolve 950 g P-free $Mg(NO_3)_2 \cdot 6H_2O$ in H_2O and dilute to 1 L.

B. Preparation of Solution

(*Caution: See Appendix* for safety notes on wet oxidation, nitric acid, perchloric acid, sulfuric acid, and oxidizers.)

Treat 1 g sample by (**a**), (**b**), (**c**), (**d**), or (**e**), as indicated. Cool solution, transfer to 200 or 250 mL volumetric flask, dilute to volume, mix, and filter through dry filter.

(**a**) *Materials containing small quantities of organic matter.*—Dissolve in 30 mL HNO_3 and 3–5 mL HCl, and boil until organic matter is destroyed (30 min for liquids and suspensions).

(**b**) *Fertilizers containing much Fe or Al phosphate, and basic slag.*—*See Official Methods of Analysis* (1965) 10th ed., **2.017**.

(**c**) *Organic material like cottonseed meal alone or in mixtures.*—Evaporate with 5 mL $Mg(NO_3)_2$ solution, **957.02A**, ignite, and dissolve in HCl.

(**d**) *Materials or mixtures containing large amounts of organic matter.*—*See Official Methods of Analysis* (1970) 11th ed., **2.017(d)**.

(**e**) *All fertilizers.*—Boil gently 30–45 min with 20–30 mL HNO_3 in suitable flask (preferably Kjeldahl for samples containing large amounts of organic matter) to oxidize all easily oxidizable matter. Cool. Add 10–20 mL 70–72% $HClO_4$. Boil very gently until solution is colorless or nearly so and dense white fumes appear in flask. Do not boil to dryness at any time (Danger!). (With samples containing large amounts of organic matter, raise temperature to fuming point, ca 170°, over period of ≥ 1 h.) Cool slightly, add 50 mL H_2O, and boil few minutes.

Reference: JAOAC **40,** 690(1957).

CAS-7723-14-0 (phosphorus)

(**a**) For P_2O_5 content $\leq 5\%$, dilute to 250 mL.

(**b**) For P_2O_5 content $> 5\%$, dilute to such volume that 5 or 10 mL aliquot contains 2–5 mg P_2O_5.

E. Determination

Pipet, into 100 mL volumetric flasks, 5 mL aliquots of standard phosphate solutions containing 2 and 3.5 mg P_2O_5/aliquot, respectively, and develop color as in **958.01C**. Adjust instrument to zero A for 2 mg standard, and determine A of 3.5 mg standard. (It is essential that A of latter standard be practically identical with corresponding value on standard curve.)

(**a**) *Samples containing up to 5% P_2O_5.*—Pipet, into 100 mL volumetric flask, 5 mL sample solution, **958.01D(a)**, and 5 mL standard phosphate solution containing 2 mg P_2O_5. Develop color and determine A concurrently with and in same manner as for standard phosphate solutions in preceding paragraph, with instrument adjusted to zero A for 2 mg standard. Read P_2O_5 concentration from standard curve. With series of sample solutions, empty and refill cell containing 2 mg standard after each determination.

$$\% \; P_2O_5 \text{ in sample} = 100 \times [(\text{mg } P_2O_5 \text{ from standard curve} - 2)/20]$$

(b) *Samples containing more than 5% P_2O_5.*—Pipet 5 or 10 mL sample solution, **958.01D(b)**, into 100 mL volumetric flask. Without adding standard phosphate solution, proceed as in (a).

% P_2O_5 in sample $= 100 \times$ (mg P_2O_5 from standard curve/mg sample in aliquot)

References: JAOAC **41,** 517(1958); **42,** 503(1959); **44,** 133(1961).
CAS-1314-56-3 (phosphorus pentoxide)

26.2   957.18—Microchemical Determination of Phosphorus
Kjeldahl Digestion Method
Final Action

A. Reagents

(a) *Nitric-sulfuric acid mixture.*—Slowly pour 420 mL HNO_3 into 580 mL H_2O; then slowly add 30 mL H_2SO_4.

(b) *Ammonium nitrate solution.*—2%. Prepare 2% solution of NH_4NO_3 in H_2O, add 2 drops HNO_3, and store in glass-stoppered bottle. Filter immediately before use.

(c) *Molybdate reagent.*—Dissolve 150 g powdered ammonium molybdate in 400 mL H_2O and cool under tap. Place 50 g $(NH_4)_2SO_4$ in 1 L volumetric flask, dissolve in mixture of 105 mL H_2O and 395 mL HNO_3, and cool under tap. Pour cooled molybdate solution slowly into $(NH_4)_2SO_4$ solution with constant stirring and cooling under tap. Dilute solution to 1 L, store in refrigerator 3 days, filter, and store in paraffin-lined, glass-stoppered, brown bottle in refrigerator. Filter reagent immediately before use and check by periodically analyzing standard sample.

B. Apparatus

(a) *Kjeldahl digestion flasks (30 mL), rack, and manifold.*—See **960.52B(a)** and **(c)**.

> **960.52B(a) and (c)** (Microchemical Determination of Nitrogen, Micro-Kjeldahl Method)
> *B. Apparatus*
> (a) *Digestion rack.*—With either gas or electric heaters which will supply enough heat to 30 mL flask to cause 15 mL H_2O at 25° to come to rolling boil in ≥ 2 but < 3 min.
> (c) *Digestion flasks.*—Use 30 mL regular Kjeldahl or Soltys-type flasks (Reference: Anal. Chem. **23,** 523(1951)). For small samples, 10 mL Kjeldahl flasks may be used.

(b) *Filter tubes and filtration assembly.*—See **952.24B(c)** and **(d)**.

> **952.24B (c)** and **(d)** (Microchemical Determination of Bromine, Chlorine, or Iodine, Carius Combustion Method)
> *B. Apparatus*
> (c) *Filter tubes.*—Micro 3 mL filter tube with medium-coarse porosity fritted disk (average pore diameter 15–25 μm).
> (d) *Siphon.*—Make from 3 mm od glass tubing, with parallel arms, one 50 and other 250 mm long, and with 110 mm connecting section rising with 13° slope to longer arm.

(c) *Rubber stoppers.*—Two or three small, solid rubber stoppers to loosen precipitate from walls of flask.

C. Determination

Weigh 3–20 mg sample, depending on P content and whether microchemical or semimicrochemical balance is used (maximum weight precipitate = 50 mg). Weigh in charging tube, if possible, and transfer to Kjeldahl flask. Use porcelain boat for sticky solids and viscous liquids, and glass capillary for volatile liquids.

Add 0.5 mL H_2SO_4 followed by 4–5 drops HNO_3. Heat on digestion rack to white SO_3 fumes and cool under tap. Add 4–5 drops HNO_3, repeat digestion, and cool under tap. Add 4–5 drops HNO_3 and again digest to SO_3 fumes. Cool to room temperature; add 2 mL acid mixture, A(a), and 12.5 mL H_2O, rinsing down neck of flask. (If porcelain boat was used to add sample, remove boat with Pt wire; if glass capillary was used, filter digestion mixture to remove capillary. Rinse filter and boat or capillary with 12.5 mL H_2O used to dilute sample.)

Place flask on steam bath 15 min to convert P to H_3PO_4. Remove from steam bath and pipet 15 mL molybdate reagent, A(c), into center of digest, not down walls of flask. Let stand 2–3 min; then gently swirl to mix contents, being careful to prevent reagents from splashing on neck of flask. Cover flask and set in dark place overnight.

Condition filter tube as described below and weigh empty tube. Connect tared filter tube to filtration assembly and transfer precipitate to filter through siphon tube. Wash flask alternately with 1–2 mL portions of the NH_4NO_3 solution and alcohol. Add 2–3 small rubber stoppers to digestion flask, shake to loosen any precipitate, and transfer with the NH_4NO_3 solution and alcohol. Disconnect siphon tube; rinse precipitate from tip and stopper into filter tube with the NH_4NO_3 solution and alcohol. Wash precipitate with more NH_4NO_3 solution, alcohol, and finally with acetone, and suck dry. Wipe filter tube with chamois skin, place in vertical position in vacuum desiccator containing no desiccant, and evacuate to 1 mm for 30 min with mechanical vacuum pump in continuous operation. Release vacuum and weigh *immediately* to nearest 0.1 mg. (Rapid weighing is essential because of hygroscopic nature of precipitate.)

$$\% \ P = \text{mg precipitate} \times 0.014524 \times 100/\text{mg sample}$$

Reference: JAOAC **40**, 386(1957).
CAS-7723-14-0 (phosphorus)

26.3   964.06—Phosphorus in Animal Feed
Alkalimetric Ammonium Molybdophosphate Method
Final Action

A. Reagents

(a) *Molybdate solution.*—Dissolve 100 g MoO_3 in mixture of 144 mL NH_4OH and 271 mL H_2O. Cool, and slowly pour solution, stirring constantly, into cool mixture of 489 mL HNO_3 and 1148 mL H_2O. Keep final mixture in warm place several days or until portion heated to 40° deposits no yellow precipitate. Decant solution from any sediment and keep in glass-stoppered vessels.

(b) *Acidified molybdate solution.*—To 100 mL molybdate solution, (a), add 5 mL HNO_3. Filter immediately before use.

(c) *Sodium hydroxide standard solution.*—Dilute 324.03 mL 1N alkali, carbonate-free, **936.16**, to 1 L. (100 mL of this solution should neutralize 32.40 mL 1N acid; 1 mL = 1 mg or 1% P_2O_5 on basis of 0.1 g sample.) (Since burets in constant use may become so corroded as to increase their capacity, test them at least annually.)

I. **936.16** (Standard Solution of Sodium Hydroxide)

Standard Potassium Hydrogen Phthalate Method

A. Apparatus

Use buret and pipet calibrated by NIST or by analyst. Protect exits to air of automatic burets from CO_2 contamination by suitable guard tubes containing soda-lime. Use containers of alkali-resistant glass.

B. Reagents

(**a**) *Carbon dioxide-free water.*—Prepare by one of following methods: (*1*) Boil H_2O 20 min and cool with soda-lime protection; (*2*) bubble air, freed from CO_2 by passing through tower of soda-lime, through H_2O 12 h.

(**b**) *Sodium hydroxide solution.*—(1 + 1). To 1 part NaOH (reagent quality containing <5% Na_2CO_3) in flask add 1 part H_2O and swirl until solution is complete. Close with rubber stopper. Set aside until Na_2CO_3 has settled, leaving perfectly clear liquid (ca 10 days).

(**c**) *Acid potassium phthalate.*—NIST SRM for Acidimetry 84. Crush to pass No. 100 sieve. Dry 2 h at 120°. Cool in desiccator containing H_2SO_4.

C. Preparation of Standard Solution

Following table gives approximate volumes of NaOH solution (1 + 1) necessary to make 10 L of standard solutions:

Approx. normality	*mL NaOH to be diluted to 10 L*
0.01	5.4
0.02	10.8
0.10	54.0
0.50	270.0
1.0	540.0

Add required volume of NaOH solution (1 + 1) to 10 L CO_2-free H_2O. Check normality, which should be slightly high, as in **936.16D**, and adjust to desired concentration by following formula:

$$V_1 = V_2 \times N_2/N_1$$

where N_2 and V_2 represent normality and volume stock solution, respectively, and V_1, volume to which stock solution should be diluted to obtain desired normality, N_1. Standardize final solution as in **936.16D** or **E**.

D. Standardization

Accurately weigh enough dried $KHC_8H_4O_4$ to titrate ca 40 mL and transfer to 300 mL flask that has been swept free from CO_2. Add 50 mL cool CO_2-free H_2O. Stopper flask and swirl gently until sample dissolves. Titrate to pH 8.6 with solution being standardized, taking precautions to exclude CO_2 and using as indicator either glass-electrode pH meter or 3 drops phenolphthalein. In latter case, determine end point by comparison with pH 8.6 buffer solution, **941.17C**, containing 3 drops phenolphthalein. Determine volume NaOH required to produce end point of blank by matching color in another flask containing 3 drops phenolphthalein and same volume CO_2-free H_2O. Subtract volume required from that used in first titration and calculate normality.

$$\text{Normality} = \text{g KHC}_8\text{H}_4\text{O}_4 \times 1000/\text{mL NaOH} \times 204.229$$

Refs.: JAOAC **19**, 107, 194(1936). NIST Certificate for Standard Reference Material 84.

Constant Boiling Hydrochloric Acid Method
E. Standardization
Accurately weigh from weighing buret enough constant boiling HCl, **936.15C**, to titrate ca 40 mL, into erlenmeyer previously swept free from CO_2. Add ca 40 mL CO_2-free H_2O, then 3–5 drops desired indicator, and titrate with solution being standardized.

$$\text{Normality} = \text{g HCl} \times 1000/\text{mL titer} \times G$$

where G has value given in **936.15C**.
Refs.: JAOAC **25**, 653(1942); **36**, 96, 354(1953); **37**, 122, 462(1954).

II. **941.17** (Standard Buffers and Indicators for Colorimetric pH Comparisons)
    A. Preparation of Sulfonphthalein Indicators

	X	pH
Bromocresol green	14.3	3.8—5.4
Chlorophenol red	23.6	4.8—6.4
Bromothymol blue	16.0	6.0—7.6
Phenol red	28.2	6.8—8.4

X = mL 0.01*N* NaOH/0.1 g indicator required to form mono-Na salt. Dilute to 250 mL for 0.04% reagent.

B. Preparation of Stock Solutions
Use recently boiled and cooled H_2O.
(**a**) *Acid potassium phthalate solution.*—0.2*M*. Dry to constant weight at 110–115°. Dissolve 40.836 g in H_2O and dilute to 1 L.
(**b**) *Monopotassium phosphate solution.*—0.2*M*. Dry KH_2PO_4 to constant weight at 110–115°. Dissolve 27.232 g in H_2O and dilute to 1 L. Solution should be distinctly red with methyl red, and distinctly blue with bromophenol blue.
(**c**) *Boric acid-potassium chloride solution.*—0.2*M*. Dry H_3BO_3 to constant weight in desiccator over $CaCl_2$. Dry KCl 2 days in oven at 115–120°. Dissolve 12.405 g H_3BO_3 and 14.912 g KCl in H_2O, and dilute to 1 L.
(**d**) *Sodium hydroxide standard solution.*—0.2*M*. Prepare and standardize as in **936.16**; 0.04084 g $KHC_8H_4O_4$ = 1 mL 0.2*M* NaOH. It is preferable to use factor with solution rather than try to adjust to exactly 0.2*M*.

C. Preparation of Buffer Solutions
Prepare standard buffer solutions from designated amounts stock solutions, **941.17**, and dilute to 200 mL. For use as colorimetric standard, mix 20 mL buffer solution with 0.5 mL indicator solution, **941.17A**.

Phthalate-NaOH Mixtures

pH	0.2M KH Phthalate (mL)	0.2M NaOH (mL)
5.0	50	23.65
5.2	50	29.75
5.4	50	35.25
5.6	50	39.70
5.8	50	43.10
6.0	50	45.40
6.2	50	47.00

KH_2PO_4-NaOH Mixtures

pH	0.2M KH_2PO_4 (mL)	0.2M NaOH (mL)
5.8	50	3.66
6.0	50	5.64
6.2	50	8.55
6.4	50	12.60
6.6	50	17.74
6.8	50	23.60
7.0	50	29.54
7.2	50	34.90
7.4	50	39.34
7.6	50	42.74
7.8	50	45.17
8.0	50	46.85

H_3BO_3-KCl-NaOH Mixtures

pH	0.2M H_3BO_3, KCl (mL)	0.2M NaOH (mL)
7.8	50	2.65
8.0	50	4.00
8.2	50	5.90
8.4	50	8.55
8.6	50	12.00

Refs.: JAOAC **24,** 583(1941). Clark, "Determination of Hydrogen-ions," 3rd Ed., pp. 91, 94, 192-202.

III. **936.15** (Standard Solution of Hydrochloric Acid)

  C. Constant Boiling Method

  Dilute 822 mL HCl (36.5–38% HCl) with 750 mL H_2O. Check specific gravity with spindle and adjust to 1.10. Place 1.5 L in 2 L flat-bottom distilling flask, add ca 10 SiC grains (ca "20 mesh"), and connect to long, straight inner-tube condenser. Heat on electric hot plate and distil at 5–10 mL/min, keeping end of condenser open to air. When 1125 mL has distilled, change receivers and catch next 225 mL, which is constant boiling HCl, in erlenmeyer with end of condenser inserted into flask, but above surface of liquid. Read barometer to nearest mm at beginning and end of collection of 225 mL portion and note barometer temperature. Average readings.

  Calculate air weight in grams (G) of this constant boiling HCl required to give one equivalent weight of HCl from one of following equations:

  For $P_0 = 540–669$ mm Hg:
  $$G = 162.255 + 0.02415\,P_0$$

  For $P_0 = 670–780$ mm Hg:
  $$G = 164.673 + 0.02039\,P_0$$

  where P_0 = barometric pressure in mm Hg corrected to 0°C for expansion of Hg and of barometer scale. For brass scale barometer, following correction is accurate enough:
  $$P_0 = P_t(1 - 0.000162t), \text{ where } t = \text{ barometer temperature in °C.}$$

  Weigh required amount of constant boiling HCl in tared, stoppered flask to at least 1 part in 10,000. Dilute immediately, and finally dilute to volume with CO_2-free H_2O at desired temperature.

  Refs.: JAOAC **25**, 653(1942); **36**, 96, 354(1953); **37**, 122, 462(1954).

  (d) *Standard acid solution.*—Prepare solution of HCl or of HNO_3, corresponding to concentration of **(c)** or to ½ this concentration, and standardize by titration against **(c)**, using phenolphthalein.

B. Determination

Prepare sample solution as in **935.13A(a)**. Pipet, into beaker or flask, aliquot corresponding to 0.4 g sample for P_2O_5 content of sample <5%; 0.2 g for 5–20%; 0.1 g for >20%. Add 5–10 mL HNO_3, depending on method of solution (or equivalent in NH_4NO_3); then add NH_4OH until precipitate that forms dissolves only slowly on vigorous stirring, dilute to 75–100 mL, and adjust to 25–30°. If sample does not give precipitate with NH_4OH as test of neutralization, make solution slightly alkaline to litmus paper with NH_4OH and then slightly acid with HNO_3 (1 + 3). Add 20–25 mL acidified molybdate solution for P_2O_5 content <5%; 30–35 mL for 5–20%; and enough acidified molybdate solution to ensure complete precipitation for >20%. Shake or stir mechanically 30 min at room temperature; decant *at once* through filter and wash precipitate twice by decanting with 25–30 mL portions H_2O, agitating thoroughly and allowing to settle. Transfer precipitate to filter and wash with cold H_2O until filtrate from 2 fillings of filter yields pink color on adding phenolphthalein and 1 drop of the standard alkali. Transfer precipitate and filter to beaker or precipitating vessel, dissolve precipitate in small excess of the standard alkali, add few drops of phenolphthalein, and titrate with standard acid. Report as % P.

935.13A(a) (Calcium in Animal Feed, Wet Ash Method)

  A. Preparation of Solution

  (*Caution: see Appendix* for safety notes on nitric acid and perchloric acid.)

(a) Weigh 2.5 g sample into 500 or 800 mL Kjeldahl flask. Add 20–30 mL HNO_3 and boil gently 30–45 min to oxidize all easily oxidizable matter. Cool solution somewhat and add 10 mL 70–72% $HClO_4$. Boil very gently, adjusting flame as necessary, until solution is colorless or nearly so and dense white fumes appear. Use particular care not to boil to dryness (Danger!) at any time. Cool slightly, add 50 mL H_2O, and boil to drive out any remaining NO_2 fumes. Cool, dilute, filter into 250 mL volumetric flask, dilute to volume, and mix thoroughly.

Reference: JAOAC **47,** 420(1964).
CAS-7723-14-0 (phosphorus)

26.4   965.17—Phosphorus in Animal Feed
Photometric Method
First Action 1965
Final Action 1966

(Not applicable to mineral-mix feeds. Dry ashing procedure is not applicable to feeds or mineral mixes containing monobasic calcium phosphate.)

A. Apparatus

Spectrophotometer.—Capable of isolating 400 nm band and accepting ≤15 mm diameter cells.

B. Reagents

(a) *Molybdovanadate reagent.*—Dissolve 40 g ammonium molybdate·$4H_2O$ in 400 mL hot H_2O and cool. Dissolve 2 g ammonium metavanadate in 250 mL hot H_2O and cool; add 250 mL 70% $HClO_4$. (*Caution: see Appendix* for safety notes on perchloric acid.) Gradually add molybdate solution to vanadate solution with stirring, and dilute to 2 L.
(b) *Phosphorus standard solutions.*—(*1*) *Stock solution.*—2 mg P/mL. Dissolve 8.788 g KH_2PO_4 in H_2O and dilute to 1 L. (*2*) *Working solution.*—0.1 mg P/mL. Dilute 50 mL stock solution to 1 L.

C. Preparation of Standard Curve

Transfer aliquots of working standard solution containing 0.5, 0.8, 1.0, and 1.5 mg P to 100 mL volumetric flasks. Treat as in **965.17D**, beginning ''Add 20 mL molybdovanadate reagent. . . .'' Prepare standard curve by plotting mg P against %T on semilog paper.

D. Determination

Ash 2 g sample, in 150 mL beaker, 4 h at 600°. Cool, add 40 mL HCl (1 + 3) and several drops HNO_3, and bring to bp. Cool, transfer to 200 mL volumetric flask, and dilute to volume with H_2O. Filter, and place aliquot containing 0.5–1.5 mg P in 100 mL volumetric flask. Add 20 mL molybdovanadate reagent, dilute to volume with H_2O, and mix well. Let stand 10 min; then read %T at 400 nm against 0.5 mg standard set at 100% T. (Use ≤15 mm diameter cells.) Determine mg P from standard curve.

$$\% \ P = mg \ P \ in \ aliquot/(g \ sample \ in \ aliquot \times 10)$$

References: JAOAC **48,** 654(1965); **59,** 937(1976).
CAS-7723-14-0 (phosphorus)

26.5   980.03—Metals in Plants
Direct Reading Spectrographic Method
Final Action 1988

See Chapter 12.3.

26.6   953.01—Metals in Plants
General Recommendations for Emission Spectrographic Methods
Final Action 1988

See Chapter 12.5.

26.7   985.01—Metals and Other Elements in Plants
Inductively Coupled Plasma Spectroscopic Method
First Action 1985
Final Action 1988

See Chapter 12.6.

26.8   966.01—Phosphorus in Plants
Gravimetric Quinolinium Molybdophosphate Method
Final Action 1974

A. Preparation of Solution

Accurately weigh ca 2 g plant sample in porcelain dish, and add 7.5 mL $Mg(NO_3)_2$ solution (dissolve 950 g P-free $Mg(NO_3)_2 \cdot 6H_2O$ in H_2O and dilute to 1 L). Dry in oven 2 h at 110–115° (or until dry). Ignite carefully over Fisher burner, or equivalent, until bubbling and smoking cease. Complete ashing in furnace 4 h at 550–600°. Dissolve ash in few mL HCl (2 + 1) and evaporate to dryness on steam bath. Take up residue in 10–15 mL HCl (1 + 9) and filter through coarse paper into 200 mL volumetric flask. Wash paper thoroughly with H_2O and let filtrate cool to room temperature. Dilute to volume with H_2O.

B. Determination

Pipet 40 mL aliquot into 300 or 500 mL Erlenmeyer and proceed as in **962.02C**.

962.02C (Phosphorus [Total] in Fertilizers, Gravimetric Quinolinium Molybdophosphate Method)

C. Determination

Pipet, into 500 mL Erlenmeyer, aliquot containing $\leq$25 mg P_2O_5 and dilute to ca 100 mL with H_2O. Continue by one of the following methods:

(**a**) Add 30 mL citric-molybdic acid reagent and boil gently 3 min. (Solution must be precipitate-free at this time.) Remove from heat and swirl carefully. Immediately add 10 mL quinoline solution from buret with continuous swirling. (Add first 3–4 mL dropwise and remainder in steady stream.) Or:

(**b**) Add 50 mL quimociac reagent, cover with watch glass, place on hot plate in well-ventilated hood, and boil 1 min.

After treatment by (**a**) or (**b**), cool to room temperature, swirl carefully 3–4 times during cooling, filter into gooch with glass fiber filter paper previously dried at 250° and weighed, and wash with five 25 mL portions of H_2O. Dry crucible and contents 30 min at 250°, cool in desiccator to room temperature, and weigh as $(C_9H_7N)_3H_3[PO_4 \cdot 12MoO_3]$. Subtract weight reagent blank. Multiply by 0.03207 to obtain weight P_2O_5 (or by 0.01400 for P). Report as % P_2O_5 (or % P).

References: Z. Anal. Chem. **189,** 243(1962). JAOAC **45,** 40, 201, 999(1962); **46,** 579(1963); **47,** 420(1964).

CAS-7723-14-0 (phosphorus)

CAS-1314-56-3 (phosphorus pentoxide)

Reference: JAOAC **49,** 284(1966).

26.9   931.01—Phosphorus in Plants
Micro Method
Final Action

A. Reagents

(**a**) *Phosphorus standard solution.*—0.025 mg P/mL. Dissolve 0.4394 g pure dry KH_2PO_4 in H_2O and dilute to 1 L. Dilute 50 mL of this solution to 200 mL.

(**b**) *Ammonium molybdate solution.*—Dissolve 25 g ammonium molybdate in 300 mL H_2O. Dilute 75 mL H_2SO_4 to 200 mL and add to ammonium molybdate solution.

(**c**) *Hydroquinone solution.*—Dissolve 0.5 g hydroquinone in 100 mL H_2O, and add 1 drop H_2SO_4 to retard oxidation.

(**d**) *Sodium sulfite solution.*—Dissolve 200 g Na_2SO_3 in H_2O, dilute to 1 L, and filter. Either keep this solution well stoppered or prepare fresh each time.

B. Preparation of Solution

To 1 or 2 g sample in small porcelain crucible add 1 mL $Mg(NO_3)_2$ solution (dissolve 950 g P-free $Mg(NO_3)_2 \cdot 6H_2O$ in H_2O and dilute to 1 L), and place on steam bath. After few minutes, cautiously add few drops HCl, taking care that gas evolution does not push portions of sample over edge of crucible. Make 2 or 3 further additions of few drops HCl while sample is on bath so that as it approaches dryness it tends to char. If contents become too viscous for further drying on bath, complete drying on hot plate. Cover crucible, transfer to cold furnace, and ignite 6 h at 500°, or until even gray ash is obtained. (If necessary, cool crucible, dissolve ash in little H_2O or alcohol-glycerol, evaporate to dryness, and return uncovered to furnace 4–5 h longer.) Cool, take up with HCl (1 + 4), and transfer to 100 mL beaker. Add 5 mL HCl and evaporate to dryness on steam bath to dehydrate SiO_2. Moisten residue with 2 mL HCl, add ca 50 mL H_2O, and heat few minutes on bath. Transfer to 100 mL volumetric flask, cool immediately, dilute to volume, mix, and filter, discarding first portion of filtrate.

C. Determination

To 5 mL aliquot filtrate in 10 mL volumetric flask add 1 mL ammonium molybdate solution, rotate flask to mix, and let stand few seconds. Add 1 mL hydroquinone solution, again rotate flask, and add 1 mL Na_2SO_3 solution. (Last 3 additions may be made with Mohr pipet.) Dilute to volume with H_2O, stopper flask with thumb or forefinger, and shake to mix thoroughly. Let stand 30 min, and measure A with spectrophotometer set at 650 nm. Report as % P.

References: JAOAC **14,** 216(1931). J. Biol. Chem. **59,** 255(1924).
CAS-7723-14-0 (phosphorus)

26.10   970.39—Phosphorus in Fruits and Fruit Products
Spectrophotometric Molybdovanadate Method
First Action 1970
Final Action 1980

(Do not clean glassware with P-containing detergents.)

A. Apparatus and Reagents

(**a**) *Spectrophotometer.*—Prism or grating, with matched 1 cm cells.

(**b**) *Molybdovanadate reagent.*—Dissolve 60 g NH_4 molybdate·$4H_2O$ in 900 mL hot H_2O, cool, and dilute to 1 L. Dissolve 1.5 g NH_4 metavanadate in 690 mL hot H_2O, add 300 mL HNO_3, cool, and dilute to 1 L. Gradually add molybdate solution to vanadate solution with stirring. Store at room temperature in polyethylene or glass-stoppered Pyrex bottle. (Reagent is stable indefinitely in polyethylene, but in Pyrex, precipitate gradually forms after several months. Discard reagent if precipitate forms.)

(**c**) *Phosphate standard solutions.*—(*1*) *Stock solution.*—0.5 mg P_2O_5/mL. Dissolve 0.2397 g pure (if assay <100% KH_2PO_4, 0.2397 g × 100/% KH_2PO_4 = correct weight) and dried (2 h at 105°) primary standard KH_2PO_4 in H_2O and dilute to 250 mL. (*2*) *Working solutions.*—Dilute 0, 5, 10, 15, 20, 25, 30, and 35 mL stock solution to 500 mL to obtain 0.00, 0.05, 0.10, 0.15, 0.20, 0.25, 0.30, and 0.35 mg P_2O_5/10 mL, respectively.

B. Preparation of Standard Curve

(*Caution: See Appendix* for safety notes on pipets and nitric acid.)

Pipet 10 mL of each working standard solution into 25 mL erlenmeyers and stopper immediately to prevent evaporation. As rapidly as possible for entire series, pipet 5 mL molybdovanadate reagent into each, stopper, and mix. Let stand 10 min for color development and read A of each solution within 1 h.

Fill 4 matched cells with 0.00 mg standard. Set spectrophotometer at 400 nm and adjust to 0 *A* with 1 cell. Read each cell *A* against this cell. Use cell with lowest *A* with 0.00 mg standard in future measurements. If *A* of 0.00 mg standard in other cells are >0.001 against this standard in reference cell, subtract these *A* from subsequent readings. Determine *A* of each standard with instrument adjusted to 0 *A* for 0.00 mg standard. After every 3 determinations, refill cell containing 0.00 mg standard to avoid error due to evaporation and temperature changes. Plot *A* against mg P_2O_5/10 mL (volume working standard solution).

(*Note:* Use Pyrex dropper to fill and empty cells. Do not remove cells from holder. Use dropper tube with greater capacity than cell to prevent liquid from entering bulb. Bulb should be just large enough that cell can be filled or emptied in one operation. Rinse cell with succeeding standard or sample solution. Use different dropper to fill and empty reference cell.)

C. Preparation of Sample

Proceed as in **940.26A** (*see* Chapter 10.1). (Add 1 teaspoon sucrose to samples low in sugar to speed ashing.) Dissolve ash in 10 mL HCl (1 + 3) and evaporate to dryness on steam bath. Dissolve residue in 10 mL HCl (1 + 9) on steam bath and transfer to 100 mL volumetric flask. Cool, dilute to volume, and mix. Filter through dry paper if any insoluble matter is present. If ash has >3.5 mg P_2O_5, dilute to >100 mL or make secondary dilutions so 10 mL aliquot contains <0.35 mg P_2O_5. (*See* Watt, B. K., and Merrill, A. L., *Composition of Foods,* USDA Handbook No. 8, p. 6–67, Superintendent of Documents, U.S. Government Printing Office, Washington, DC 20402, rev. Dec. 1963, for data on P content of fruit products and other foods.) If ash weight is not desired, use smaller sample aliquot to reduce drying and ashing time.

D. Determination

Into separate 25 mL erlenmeyers pipet 10 mL aliquots standard solutions containing 0.00 and 0.20 mg P_2O_5/10 mL. Develop color as for standard curve. Adjust instrument to 0 *A* for 0.00 mg standard and determine *A* of 0.20 mg standard. (*A* of this standard should be within ±1% of *A* of standard curve; if not, prepare new standard curve.) Develop color and determine *A* of sample ash solutions concurrently with and in same manner as for standard solutions. Calculate as follows:

(a) *From standard curve.*—mg P_2O_5/100 g sample = 100 × (mg P_2O_5/10 mL from standard curve)/g sample in 10 mL ash solution.

(b) *From formula.*—mg P_2O_5/100 g sample = $A \times S \times 100/W$, where *A* refers to sample solution at 400 nm, *S* = slope of standard curve = $(\Sigma r)/n$; Σr = sum of ratios of mg P_2O_5/10 mL to *A* of each standard, and *n* = number of standard solutions used in calculations; and *W* = g sample in 10 mL ash solution.

References: JAOAC **52,** 865(1969); **53,** 575(1970).
CAS-1314-56-3 (phosphorus pentoxide)

26.11   969.31—Phosphorus (Total) in Meat

A. Method I (Final Action)

Destroy organic matter as in **957.02B(c)** or (**d**) (*see* 26.1), and proceed as in **964.06B** (*see* 26.3) or **965.18C**.

965.18C (Phosphorus in Baking Powders, Gravimetric Method)

C. Determination

Pipet aliquot of prepared solution into 250 mL beaker; add NH_4OH in slight excess and barely dissolve precipitate formed with few drops HNO_3, stirring vigorously. If HCl or H_2SO_4 has been used as solvent, add ca 15 g crystalline NH_4NO_3 or solution containing that amount. To hot solution add 70 mL molybdate solution, **964.06A(a)**, for every 100 mg P_2O_5 present. Digest 1 h at ca 65° and test for complete precipitation of P_2O_5 by adding more molybdate solution to clear supernate. Filter, and wash with cold H_2O or preferably with the NH_4NO_3 solution. Dissolve precipitate on filter with NH_4OH (1 + 1) and hot H_2O, and wash into beaker to volume ≤100 mL. Neutralize with HCl, using litmus paper or *bromothymol blue* as indicator; cool, and from buret slowly add (ca 1 drop/sec), stirring vigorously, 15 mL magnesia mixture/100 mg P_2O_5 present. After 15 min add 12 mL NH_4OH and let stand until supernate is clear (usually 2 h); filter, wash precipitate with NH_4OH (1 + 9) until washings are practically Cl-free, dry, burn at low heat, and ignite to constant weight, preferably in furnace at 950–1000°; cool in desiccator, and weigh as $Mg_2P_2O_7$. Report as % P_2O_5.

B. Method II (First Action 1969)

Weigh, to nearest mg, 2.5 ± 0.1 g sample, prepared as in **983.18**, into ashing dish (Pt, Vycor, or other suitable material) and dry 30 min at 125° in forced-draft oven. Ash in furnace at 550° to whiteness or near whiteness. Cool, add 25 mL HNO_3 (1 + 4), and heat on steam bath ca 30 min. Quantitatively filter into 400 mL beaker, using H_2O in transfer. Adjust volume to ca 100 mL and proceed as in **962.02C(b)** (*see* 26.8).

983.18 (Meat and Meat Products, Preparation of Sample)

To prevent H_2O loss during preparation and subsequent handling, do not use small samples. Keep ground material in glass or similar containers with air- and H_2O-tight covers. Prepare samples for analysis as follows:

(**a**) *Fresh meats, dried meats, cured meats, smoked meats, etc.*—Separate as completely as possible from any bone; pass rapidly 3 times through food chopper with plate openings ≤⅛″ (3 mm), mixing thoroughly after each grinding; and begin all determinations promptly. If any delay occurs, chill sample to inhibit decomposition.

Alternatively, use a bowl cutter for sample preparation (benchtop model, ½ HP; 14 in. bowl, 22 rpm; two 3.5 in. knives, 1725 rpm; Model 84145, Hobart Corp., 711 Pennsylvania Ave, Troy, OH, 45374, or equivalent). Chill all cutter parts before preparation of each sample.

(**b**) *Canned meats.*—Pass entire contents of can through food chopper, as in (**a**).

(**c**) *Sausages.*—Remove from casings and pass through food chopper, as in (**a**).

Dry portions of samples of (**a**), (**b**), and (**c**) not needed for immediate analysis, either *in vacuo* <60° or by evaporating on steam bath 2 or 3 times with alcohol. Extract fat from dried product with petroleum ether (bp <60°) and let petroleum ether evaporate spontaneously, finally expelling last traces by heating short time on steam bath. Do not heat sample or separated fat longer than necessary because of tendency to decompose.

Reserve fat in cool place for examination as in chapter on oils and fats and complete examination before it becomes rancid.
Reference: JAOAC **66**, 579(1983).

Reference: JAOAC **52**, 634(1969).
CAS-7723-14-0 (phosphorus)

26.12   972.22—Phosphorus in Meat
Automated Method
First Action 1972

A. Principle

Phosphate and Mo^{+6} react in acid solution to produce 12-molybdophosphoric acid, which is reduced with 1-amino-2-naphthol-4-sulfonic acid to phosphomolybdenum blue. Maximum A at 660 nm is proportional to amount P present. Method is applicable to 0.05–0.4% P.

B. Apparatus

(**a**) *Automatic analyzer.*—AutoAnalyzer with following modules (Techniqueon Instruments Corp.): Sampler II; proportioning pump I; continuous digestor; proportioning pump II; current stabilizer; constant temperature bath equipped with variable temperature regulator (set at 70°); colorimeter with 15 mm tubular flowcell, 660 nm filters, and No. 9 aperture; voltage stabilizer; recorder with transmittance paper; vacuum pump; 2 manifolds (Figs. **972.22A** and **972.22B**); and 8.5 mL sample cups.

(**b**) *Pipet.*—Automatic zeroing, 50 mL (Kontes Glass Co., K-763280).

(**c**) *Tubing.*—Fluran F-5000, 0.125″ id, or Teflon, 0.133″ id.

(**d**) *Pipetting machine.*—Automatic Model 60453, with Model 60480 valve syringe (Scientific Equipment Products [SEPCO]).

C. Reagents

(**a**) *Vanadium pentoxide solution.*—Weigh 40.0 g NaOH pellets and transfer to 1 L volumetric flask. Add 500 mL H_2O, dissolve, and cool. Add 12.5 g V_2O_5 to flask, dissolve, dilute to volume, and mix.

(**b**) *Digestion mixture.*—Mix in order: 150 mL V_2O_5 solution, 90 mL 60–62% $HClO_4$, and 3460 mL H_2SO_4. (*Caution: See Appendix for safety notes on perchloric acid and sulfuric acid.*) Rate of consumption is 495 mL/h.

(**c**) *Wash solution.*—H_2SO_4 (1 + 1). To 1 L H_2O in 2 L volumetric flask, add 1 L H_2SO_4 slowly with swirling. Cool to room temperature, dilute to volume with H_2O, and mix. Rate of consumption is 234 mL/h.

(**d**) *1-Amino-2-naphthol-4-sulfonic acid (ANSA).*— (*1*) *Solution A.*—Add 2.0 g Na_2SO_3 and 60 g $NaHSO_3$ to 320 mL H_2O in 500 mL volumetric flask. Heat to 50° and add 1 g ANSA. Dissolve, cool, dilute to volume, and mix. Store in amber bottle; discard when precipitate forms. (*2*) *Solution B.*— Dilute 100 mL Solution *A* to 1 L with H_2O. Add 0.5 mL Levor IV wetting agent (slurry containing 40% Na nonylbenzene sulfonate, Techniqueon Instruments Corp.). Store in amber bottle. Refrigerate when not in use. Rate of consumption is 36 mL/h.

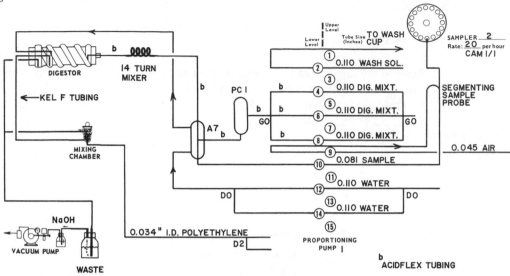

Figure 972.22A.—Helix inlet manifold.

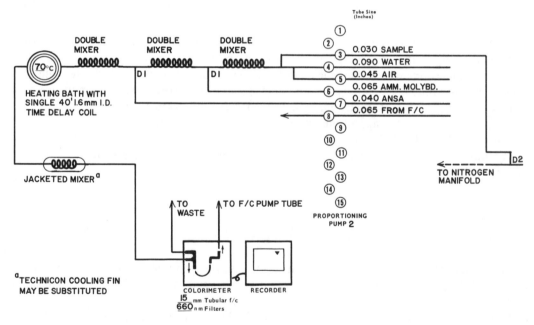

Figure 972.22B.—Phosphorus analytical manifold.

(e) *Ammonium molybdate solution.*—Dissolve 30 g $(NH_4)_6Mo_7O_{24}\cdot4H_2O$ in ca 1 L H_2O. Dilute to 2 L and mix. Rate of consumption is 96 mL/h.

(f) *Dilution water.*—(*1*) Pumped through A7 fitting (Fig. **972.22A**). Rate of consumption is 468 mL/h. (*2*) Pumped through P analytical manifold (Fig. **972.22B**). Rate of consumption is 174 mL/h.

D. Preparation of Standards

Weigh 10.9839 g KH_2PO_4 into 250 mL volumetric flask, add H_2O to dissolve, and dilute to volume. Transfer 5.0, 7.5, 10.0, 15.0, 20.0, 25.0, 30.0, and 40.0 mL to 8 separate 1 L volumetric flasks. Add H_2O to 500 mL. Place flasks in ice bath and slowly add 500 mL H_2SO_4 to each. Cool, dilute to volume with H_2O, and store in 1 L polyethylene bottles. Based on 10 g sample, as prepared in **972.22E**, % P = 0.050, 0.075, 0.100, 0.150, 0.200, 0.250, 0.300, and 0.400.

E. Preparation of Sample

Accurately weigh 10.00 g sample into 200 mL tall-form beaker. Pipet 53 mL H_2O into beaker with pipetting machine, **B(d)**. Add 1″ (2.5 cm) Teflon-coated stirring bar, cover with 60 mm watch glass, and disperse sample, using magnetic stirrer. With stirring, add 50 mL H_2SO_4, using automatic pipet, **B(b)**, and continue stirring until sample is dissolved. Cool to room temperature in cooling bath.

F. Analytical System

Use standard 0.0625″ id transmission tubing throughout system unless otherwise specified. Pump sample at 2.5 mL/min and segment with air pumped at 0.8 mL/min. Pump digestion mixture at 8.28 mL/min through PC1 fitting and add to sample at A7 fitting. Pass sample stream through 14-turn mixing coil into inlet of digestor helix. Pump dilution H_2O at 7.80 mL/min through A7 fitting to outlet end of digestor helix. Aspirate diluted sample into bubble chamber and remove aliquot for analysis at 0.35 mL/min. Dilute aliquot with H_2O pumped at 2.90 mL/min and segment with air at 0.80 mL/min. Pass stream through 28-turn mixer, and add NH_4 molybdate at 1.60 mL/min. Pass stream through second 28-turn mixer followed by addition of ANSA Solution *B* pumped at 0.60 mL/min. After final 28-turn mixer, pass stream into 70° heating bath for color development, cool in jacketed mixer, and pass into colorimeter equipped with 660 nm filters and 15 mm tubular flowcell. Measure *A* at 660 nm. Pump stream from flowcell at 1.60 mL/min.

G. Start-Up Procedure

Place all reagent lines, except Acidflex, in water; turn on both proportioning pumps and digestor power. Turn on vacuum pump, setting gage at 12–15 psi. Pump digestion mixture and all analytical reagents through their respective lines after determining that system is operating properly. After 5 min, turn on heat switch and adjust amperage to proper settings. Amperage should be adjusted to give temperature readout in range of 280–400° in first stage and 250–380° in second and third stages. Warm-up time is ca 20 min (older digestor units may require longer). Set recorder baseline at 99% *T* or 0.01 *A*.

H. Shut-Down Procedure

Turn off heat switch and let first stage temperature reach 200°. Remove helix cover and place all reagent lines except digestion mixture in H_2O after first stage temperature is <150°. Place digestion mixture line in empty erlenmeyer and let Acidflex pump tubes "air-wash." Rinse entire system for 15 min. Shut off proportioning pumps and break vacuum in liquid waste bottle. Turn off digestor power switch and replace helix cover.

I. Determination

Pour standard and prepared samples into 8.5 mL cups and place in Sampler II turntable. Adjust sampling rate to 20/h with 1:1 sample-to-wash ratio to provide 1.5 min sampling and 1.5 min wash. Press reset button and activate sampler turntable, thus passing standards and samples into analytical system. Place stop bar in turntable. (Formation of excessive fat deposits in sample line between segmenting sample probe and input manifold can be retarded by passing wash solution through double mixer wrapped with heating tape and covered with layer of Al foil and layer of asbestos; adjust temperature to 60° with variable transformer connected to heating tape.)

Read % T of samples from recorder strip chart and compare with standard curves of % T against % P on 1 cycle, 70 division semilog paper. A strip chart paper may also be used. Include standard curve with every 30 samples. (% P can be converted to % Na tripolyphosphate, using gravimetric factor 3.96, after % P naturally occurring in meat is deducted.) Dilution error caused by variation in moisture content of samples does not significantly affect P determination. Standard curve is linear through range of standards.

Reference: JAOAC **53**, 911(1970); **55**, 123(1972).
CAS-7723-14-0 (phosphorus)

26.13   991.27—Phosphorus in Meat and Meat Products
Spectrophotometric Method
First Action 1991

(Applicable to smoked ham, water-added ham, canned ham, pork sausage, cooked sausage, and hamburger)

Method Performance:

Smoked ham, 0.22–0.30% P
s_r = 0.005–0.010; s_R = 0.009–0.010; RSD_r = 1.70–4.66%; RSD_R = 3.50–4.66%
Water-added ham, 0.23–0.26% P
s_r = 0.007–0.012; s_R = 0.012–0.013; RSD_r = 2.87–4.48%; RSD_R = 4.75–5.51%
Pork sausage, 0.10–0.13% P
s_r = 0.004–0.005; s_R = 0.009–0.011; RSD_r = 3.75–3.98%; RSD_R = 6.88–9.87%
Cooked sausage, 0.12–0.13% P
s_r = 0.004–0.008; s_R = 0.007–0.011; RSD_r = 3.72–6.16%; RSD_R = 5.64–8.65%
Canned ham, 0.23–0.24% P
s_r = 0.004–0.009; s_R = 0.012–0.013; RSD_r = 1.82–4.06%; RSD_R = 5.20–5.59%
Hamburger (70–90% lean), 0.14–0.18% P
s_r = 0.003–0.010; s_R = 0.010–0.014; RSD_r = 2.22–7.28%; RSD_R = 7.27–8.05%

A. Principle

Sample is dispersed in water and digested in H_2SO_4 and H_2O_2. Digestion is complete in ca 10 min. Phosphorus is determined in dilute aliquot of digest in 2 steps using 2 solutions. In first step, orthophosphate reacts with molybdate in acid solution to form yellow phosphomolybdate complex. Then, yellow complex is reduced by ascorbic acid to form characteristic molybdenum blue species, which can be measured spectrophotometrically vs standards.

B. Apparatus

(a) *Spectrophotometer.*—For operation at 890 ± 1 nm; wavelength repeatability ±0.2 nm. With pour-through cell of ca 1 in. path length. (Hach Model DR 3000 Spectrophotometer with Pour Thru Cell [Hach Co., PO Box 389, Loveland, CO 80539] meets these requirements.)

(b) *Digestion equipment.*—For operation at 470°. Temperature control within ±15° of setting at idling temperature. Calibrate temperature setting according to manufacturer's instructions. Capable of delivering H_2O_2 at controlled rate of ca 3.5 mL/min. Digestion fumes removed by mechanical or water aspiration. (Hach Model 23130 Digesdahl apparatus meets these requirements.)

C. Reagents

Prepared reagents are available from Hach Co. as indicated.

(a) *Phosphorus standard solutions.*—Use ACS grade monobasic potassium phosphate to prepare 0.0, 5.0, 10.0, 15.0, 20.0, and 25.0 mg/L phosphate-phosphorus (PO_4-P) in 3% H_2SO_4 solution (Hach Cat. No. 22204-05).

(b) *Hydrogen peroxide.*—50% (w/w). Food grade.

(c) *Phosphorus 1 solution.*—Contains H_2SO_4, cyclohexanediaminetetraacetic acid, ammonium molybdate tetrahydrate, and potassium antimoryl tartrate (Hach Cat. No. 22605-11).

(d) *Phosphorus 2 solution.*—Contains ascorbic acid and dimethyl sulfoxide (Hach Cat. No. 22606-11).

D. Sample Preparation and Digestion

Caution: Sulfuric acid and hydrogen peroxide can cause burns. Wear gloves and eye protection when handling.

Place 1 in. Teflon-coated stirring bar in 200 mL Berzelius beaker and record combined weight as (A). Tare balance. Add ca 10 g sample prepared as in **983.18** (*see* 26.11) to beaker and record exact weight as (B). Add 50 mL H_2O to sample and disperse using magnetic stirrer. With stirring, add 50 mL H_2SO_4 and cover beaker with 65 mm watch glass. Continue stirring until sample is dissolved (ca 1 min). Remove watch glass and record weight of beaker and contents as (C). Tare a digestion flask. Let any molten fat rise to surface, then, avoiding fat layer, withdraw 5 mL of sample and transfer to tared flask. Record exact weight of 5 mL sample as (D). Add 1 boiling chip to flask.

Place flask on digestion unit preheated to 470°. Place fractionating head on flask, turn on water aspirator for fume removal, and heat 4 min. Add 10 mL 50% H_2O_2 to capillary funnel. Heat sample for 1 min after flow of H_2O_2 has ended. Remove flask from heat and disconnect fractionating head. Cool sample digest and dilute to 100 mL with water and mix.

E. Preparation of Standard Curve

Adjust wavelength of spectrophotometer to 890 nm. Zero (100% T) spectrophotometer on deionized water. Construct best-fit linear calibration using phosphorus standard solutions. Pipet 0.5 mL of each phosphorus standard solution into separate 25 mL tall-form graduated mixing cylinders. Dilute each solution to 23 mL with deionized water. Add 1.0 mL phosphorus 1 solution, and then add 1.0 mL phosphorus 2 solution to each standard. Invert cylinders several times to mix contents. (Hach Model 42800-03 Diluter/Dispenser may be used for sample dilution and reagent additions.) Let solutions stand ≥3 min, but ≤10 min before measurement. Based on 10 g sample, this series of standards represents 0.0, 0.2, 0.4, 0.6, 0.8, and 1.0% P, respectively.

Record % T readings for standards and construct calibration curve of % T vs % P on 1 cycle, 70 division semilog paper. (If Hach DR/3000 Spectrophotometer is used, enter calibration line directly into instrument according to manufacturer's instructions.) Standard curve is linear through range of standards specified. Calibrate with each new lot of reagents.

F. Determination

Develop color in sample digest as for standards. Read % T of samples and compare with standard curve. (For Hach Spectrophotometer, read apparent % P directly from instrument display.)

Perform calculation as follows:

Actual phosphorus, % = [0.25 x apparent % P x (C - A)]/(B x D)

Ref.: JAOAC **74**, 22(1991).
CAS-7723-14-0 (phosphorus)

26.14   948.09—Phosphorus in Flour
Final Action

A. Reagent

(a) *Magnesium nitrate solution.*—Dissolve 8 g MgO in HNO_3 (1 + 1), avoiding excess acid; add little MgO in excess, boil, filter from excess MgO, Fe_2O_3, etc., and dilute to 100 mL.

(b) *Molybdate solution.*—Dissolve 100 g MoO_3 in mixture of 144 mL NH_4OH and 271 mL H_2O. Cool, and slowly pour solution, stirring constantly, into cool mixture or 489 mL HNO_3 and 1148 mL H_2O. Keep final mixture in warm place several days or until portion heated to 40° deposits no yellow precipitate. Decant solution from any sediment and keep in glass-stoppered vessels.

B. Determination

(a) Transfer 1.00 g sample to ca 140 mL porcelain casserole, add 3 mL $Mg(NO_3)_2$ solution, and mix well, using small glass rod. Clean rod with small piece filter paper and place in casserole. Dry in oven at 100° ca 2 h, transfer to cold furnace, and ignite at 550° to white or gray ash (6-8 h). Cool, cover with watch glass, take up with 10 mL HCl (1 + 4), and add 5 mL HCl. Rinse watch glass and evaporate to dryness on steam bath. Add 5 mL HCl and 50 mL H_2O, heat 15 min on steam bath, filter into 100 mL volumetric flask, cool, and dilute to volume. Pipet 50 mL into 300 mL erlenmeyer, neutralize to litmus paper with NH_4OH, make just faintly acid with HNO_3, dilute to 75–100 mL, add ca 15 g NH_4NO_3, and add 20–25 mL acidified molybdate solution for P_2O_5 content <5%; 30–35 mL for 5–20%; and enough acidified molybdate solution to ensure complete precipitation for >20%. Shake or stir mechanically 30 min at room temperature; decant *at once* through filter and wash precipitate twice by decanting with 25–30 mL portions H_2O, agitating thoroughly and allowing to settle. Transfer precipitate to filter and wash with cold H_2O until filtrate from 2 fillings of filter yields pink color on adding phenolphthalein and 1 drop of the standard alkali. Transfer precipitate and filter to beaker or precipitate vessel, dissolve precipitate in small excess of the standard acid. Report as % P. Or:

(b) Transfer 5.00 g sample to 35 mL porcelain evaporating dish, mix well with 0.5 g Na_2CO_3, and ignite at 550° to gray ash. Cool, cover with watch glass, take up with 2 mL HCl (1 + 4), and add 5 mL HCl. Rinse watch glass, evaporate to dryness, add 5 mL HCl and 10 mL H_2O, heat ca 10 min on steam bath, filter into 100 mL volumetric flask, cool, and dilute to volume. Pipet 10 mL aliquot into 300 mL erlenmeyer and proceed as in (a), beginning ". . . neutralize to litmus paper with NH_4OH. . . ." Report results as % P.

Reference: JAOAC **31,** 269(1948).
CAS-7723-14-0 (phosphorus)

26.15   990.24—Phosphorus (Total) in Cheese and Processed Cheese Products
Photometric Method
First Action 1990
IDF-ISO-AOAC Method

(Applicable to all cheeses and processed cheese products)

Method Performance:

Low level, 0.75% P

$s_r = 0.010$; $s_R = 0.017$; $RSD_r = 1.23\%$; $RSD_R = 2.28\%$

Medium level, 1.0–1.5% P

$s_r = 0.011–0.035$; $s_R = 0.025–0.043$; $RSD_r = 0.89–2.37\%$; $RSD_R = 2.14–2.94\%$

High level, 1.75% P

$s_r = 0.012–0.021$; $s_R = 0.038–0.068$; $RSD_r = 0.69–1.16\%$; $RSD_R = 2.24–3.81\%$

A. Principle

Cheese is digested by H_2SO_4 and H_2O_2. Molybdenum blue complex formed by addition of molybdate-ascorbic acid solution is measured by photometer at 820 nm.

B. Apparatus

Thoroughly clean all glassware with phosphorus-free detergent and rise with water.

(a) *Digestion flasks (Kjeldahl) or digestion tubes.*—25 mL.

(b) *Graduated cylinders.*—5 and 25 mL.

(c) *Volumetric flasks.*—50 and 100 mL.

(d) *Pipets.*—To deliver 1, 2, 3, 5, and 10 mL.

(e) *Spectrophotometer.*—Suitable for measurements at 820 nm, with cells of 10 mm optical path length.

(f) *Grinder.*—Capable of being easily cleaned. Retain cheese in covered container so that it does not change weight.

(g) *Other apparatus.*—Boiling water bath. Micro gas burners (electric heaters may also be used). Glass beads.

C. Reagents

Use analytical grade reagents and distilled or deionized water that is free of phosphorus compounds.

(a) *Concentrated sulfuric acid.*—Density at 20° = 1.84 g/mL.

(b) *Hydrogen peroxide solution.*—About 30 g H_2O_2/100 mL.

(c) *Sodium molybdate solution.*—Dissolve 12.5 g sodium molybdate dihydrate ($Na_2MoO_4 \cdot 2H_2O$) in 5 mol/L H_2SO_4 solution, dilute to 500 mL with same H_2SO_4 solution and mix.

(d) *Ascorbic acid solution.*—Dissolve 10 g ascorbic acid ($C_6H_8O_6$) in water, dilute to 200 mL, and mix. *Note:* This solution cannot be stored.

(e) *Molybdate-ascorbic acid solution.*—Immediately before use, add 25 mL sodium molybdate solution, (c), to 10 mL ascorbic acid solution, (d), dilute to 100 mL with water, and mix.

(f) *Phosphorus standard solution.*—100 μg P/mL. Dry ca 1 g potassium dihydrogen orthophosphate (KH_2PO_4) for ≥48 h in desiccator over efficient drying agent (e.g., concentrated H_2SO_4). Dissolve 0.4394 g dried phosphate in water, dilute to 1L, and mix.

D. Sampling

See **920.122**, **968.12**, and **970.30**. Store sample in manner that prevents deterioration and change in composition.

I. **920.122** (Cheese, Collection of Samples, Procedure)
(*See also* **968.12** and **970.30**.)
When cheese can be cut, take narrow wedge reaching from outer edge to center. When not permissible to cut cheese, take sample with cheese trier. If only one plug can be obtained, take it perpendicular to surface of cheese at point ⅓ distance from edge to center and extending either entirely or half-way through. When >1 plug can be taken, draw 3 plugs, 1 from center, 1 near outer edge, and 1 midway between other two. Use ca 2 cm (¾ ″) of rind portion of core to reseal hole.

Sample bulk containers of cottage and similar cheeses by stirring can thoroughly for ≥5 min with dairy stirrer (ca 14 cm [5.5″] perforated concave metal disk attached to ca 70 cm [27″] metal rod as handle) so that all portions of container are reached. Remove portions from top surface with small spoon to fill 0.5 L (1 pt) jar, and cover.

II. **968.12** (Sampling of Dairy Products, General Instructions)
A. Instructions of Administrative Character
(This section is usually prescribed by specific regulatory agency. It is included for completeness.) Sampling should be performed by authorized or sworn independent agent, properly trained in appropriate technique. Agent should be free from any infectious disease. If possible, representatives of parties concerned should be given opportunity to be present when sampling is performed.

Samples should be accompanied by report, signed by sworn or authorized sampling agent and countersigned by any witnesses present. Report should give particulars of place, date, and time of sampling; name and designation of agent and of any witnesses; precise method of sampling which is followed if this deviates from prescribed standard method; nature and number of units constituting consignment together with their batch code markings, where available; number of samples duly identified as to batches from which they are drawn; and place to which the samples will be sent.

When appropriate, report should also include any relevant conditions or circumstances, e.g., condition of packages and their surroundings, temperature and humidity of atmosphere, method of sterilization of sampling equipment, whether preservative has been added to samples, and any other special information relating to material being sampled.

Each sample should be sealed and labeled to give nature of product, identification number, and any code markings of batch from which sample has been taken, date of sampling, and name and signature of sampling agent. When necessary, additional information may be required, for example, weight of sample and unit from which it was taken.

All samples should be taken at least in duplicate, one set being held, if necessary, in cold storage and put at disposal of second party as soon as possible. Precise method of sampling and weight or volume of product to be taken as sample vary with nature of product and purpose for which sampling is required and are defined for each particular case.

When previously agreed between parties, take additional sets of samples and retain for independent arbitration, if necessary. Send samples to testing laboratory immediately after sampling.

B. Technical Instructions

(*See* sampling equipment specifications laid down for each product to be sampled.)

(**a**) *Sampling for chemical purposes.*—Clean and dry all equipment.

(**b**) *Sampling for bacteriological purposes.*—Clean and treat equipment by one of following methods: (*1*) Expose to hot air 2 h at 170° (may be stored if kept under sterile conditions). (*2*) Autoclave 15–20 min at 120° (may be stored if kept under sterile conditions). (*3*) Expose to steam 1 h at 100° (use equipment same day). (*4*) Immerse in H_2O 1 min at 100° (use equipment immediately). (*5*) Immerse in 70% alcohol and flame to burn off alcohol immediately before use. (*6*) Expose to hydrocarbon (propane, butane) torch flame so that all working surfaces contact flame immediately before use.

Choice of treatment depends on nature, shape, and size of equipment and on conditions of sampling. Sterilize wherever possible by method (*1*) or (*2*).

Methods (*3*), (*4*), (*5*), and (*6*) are regarded as secondary methods only.

(**c**) *Sampling for organoleptic purposes.*—Use equipment as in (**a**) or (**b**), or as specified for specific product. Equipment should not impart any flavor or odor to product.

C. Sample Containers

(**a**) *For liquids.*—Use clean and dry containers of suitable waterproof, greaseproof material (glass, stainless metal, suitable plastic material) of quality suitable for sterilization by **968.12B(b)**, if necessary, and of suitable shape and capacity for material to be sampled (as defined in each particular case).

Securely close containers either with suitable rubber or plastic stopper or by screw cap of metal or plastic having, if necessary, liquid-tight plastic liner which is insoluble, nonabsorbent, and greaseproof, and which will not influence odor, flavor, or composition of milk products.

If rubber stoppers are used, cover with nonabsorbent, flavorless material (such as suitable plastic) before pressing into sample container. Suitable plastic bags may also be used.

(**b**) *For solids or semisolids.*—Use clean and dry wide-mouth, cylindrical receptacles of suitable waterproof, greaseproof material (glass, stainless metal, suitable plastic material) of quality suitable for sterilization by **968.12B(b)**, if necessary, and of capacity suited to size of sample to be taken (as defined in each particular case). Make air-tight as in (**a**). Suitable plastic bags may also be used.

(**c**) *Small retail containers.*—Contents of intact and unopened containers constitute samples.

D. Preservation of Samples

To samples of liquid products or cheese intended for chemical analysis, suitable preservative may be added. Such preservative should not interfere with subsequent analysis. Indicate nature and amount of addition on label and in any reports.

Do not add preservatives to samples of semisolid, solid (except cheese), or dried products intended for chemical analysis. Rapidly cool and store samples in refrigerator at 0–5°. Dried milks may be kept at room temperature.

Do not add preservatives to samples intended for bacteriological or organoleptic examination. Hold at 0–5°, except for condensed (conserved) milk products when sample comprises unopened hermetically sealed containers in which products are sold. Keep liquid products and butter cold. Start bacteriological examination of liquid products as soon as possible and never >24 h after sampling.

E. Transport of Samples

Transport samples to laboratory as quickly as possible after sampling. Take precautions to prevent, during transit, exposure to direct sunlight, or to temps $<0°$ or $>10°$ in case of perishable products. For samples intended for bacteriological examination, use insulated transport container capable of maintaining temperature at $0-5°$, except for samples of condensed (conserved) milk products in unopened containers, or in case of very short journeys.

Maintain samples of cheese under such conditions as to avoid separation of fat or moisture. Maintain soft cheese at $0-5°$.

References: JAOAC **49,** 58(1966); **50,** 531(1967).

III. **970.30** (Sampling of Cheese)

A. Sampling Equipment

(**a**) *Cheese triers of shape and size suited to cheese to be sampled.*

(**b**) *Stainless steel knife with pointed blade.*

(**c**) *Sealing compounds.*—(*1*) Mix by heating paraffin, beeswax, and white petrolatum (1 + 1 + 2); or (*2*) mix by heating white petrolatum and paraffin (1 + 1).

B. Sampling Technique

Draw enough subsamples to give total sample of ≥ 50 g. Use one of following techniques, depending on shape, weight, type, and maturity of cheese (when choice is necessary between (**a**) and (**b**), method (**a**) is preferable but (**b**) is acceptable, especially with hard cheese of large size).

(**a**) *Sampling by cutting.*—Using knife with pointed blade, make 2 cuts radiating from center of cheese, if cheese has circular base, or parallel to sides if base is rectangular. Size of piece thus obtained should be such that, after removal of inedible surface layer, remaining edible portion weighs ≥ 50 g.

(**b**) *Sampling by means of trier.*—According to shape, weight, and type of cheese, use one of following sampling techniques: (*1*) Insert trier obliquely towards center of cheese once or several times into one of flat surfaces at point ≥ 10 cm from edge. (*2*) Insert trier perpendicularly into one face and pass through center of cheese to reach opposite face. (*3*) Insert trier horizontally into vertical face of cheese, midway between 2 plane faces, toward center of cheese. (*4*) In case of cheese transported in barrels, boxes, or other bulk containers, or cheese which is formed into large compact blocks, perform sampling by passing trier obliquely through contents of container from top to base. (*5*) For large cheeses, use outer 2 cm or more of plug containing rind for closing hole made in cheese. Remainder of plug constitutes sample. Close plug holes with great care and, if possible, seal over with sealing compound, **970.30A(c)**.

(**c**) *Sampling by taking entire cheese.*—Normally use for small cheese and for wrapped portions of cheese packaged in small containers. Take enough packages to have ≥ 50 g.

Weigh, at time of sampling, cheese sold by piece for which minimum weight dry matter in unit is specified by national legislation, and state weight on label.

(**d**) *Sampling of cheese in brine.*—Take fragments of ≥ 200 g each and enough brine to cover cheese in sample container. Before analysis, place sample on filter paper 1–2 h.

(For additional instructions, *see* **920.122.**)

C. Sampling Technique for Barrels

Sampling by means of trier.—Insert 30.5 cm (12 in.) blade length trier 7 cm (2.75 in.) from edge of cheese and toward nearest outside edge of barrel at 11° from vertical. Center of plug hole shall be 7 cm from edge of cheese. Trier guide fixed at 11° angle may be used as aid.

If cheese barrel is full, i.e., not >2–3 cm headspace, it is possible to draw reliable sample through bung or sample port in cover which permits insertion of trier at 7 cm point. If headspace is >3 cm, remove cover; otherwise, point of trier insertion will be distorted. In no instance should barrel containing cheese from more than 1 vat be selected as sample for moisture analysis.

For reliable sample, insert trier to draw full 27.9–30.5 cm (11–12 in.) plug from full container. If plug breaks short of 25.4 cm (10 in.), draw another plug from different location 7 cm from edge. For plug between 25.5 and 30.5 cm, remove top 11.4 cm (4.5 in.) for sealing plug hole. Transfer next 10.2 cm (4 in.) portion to sample container. Discard remaining bottom portion of plug.

Reference: JAOAC **68,** 718(1985).

D. Sample Containers

Use sample containers with air-tight closures. Immediately after sampling, place samples (plugs, sectors, entire small cheese, fragments of brine cheese) in container of suitable size and shape. Sample may be cut into pieces for insertion into container but do not compress or grind.

E. Treatment of Samples

In preparation of sample, whatever method of sampling is used, carefully remove only inedible surface layer of cheese, if any, such as moldy and horny portions, unless prescribed otherwise. Do not remove outer rind or crust from soft cheese sold by piece, and for which minimum weight of dry matter in unit is specified by national legislation.

(For additional instructions, *see* **955.30.**)

IV. 955.30 (Cheese, Preparation of Samples, Procedure)

Cut wedge sample into strips and pass 3 times through food chopper. Grind plugs in food chopper (preferable method), or cut or shred very finely and mix thoroughly.

With creamed cottage and similar cheeses, place 300–600 g sample at <15° in 1 L (1 qt) cup of high-speed blender and blend for minimum time (2–5 min) required to obtain homogeneous mixture. Final temperature should be ≤25°. This may require stopping blender frequently after channeling and spooning cheese back into blades until blending action starts. (Use of variable transformer in line to permit slow speed at first minimizes channeling when speed is increased later.)

E. Sample Preparation

Remove rind or moldy surface layer of cheese so that sample represents cheese as it is usually consumed. Use appropriate device, **B(f),** to grind sample. Pulse grinder on and off for best grinding. Do not grind too long or heat developed will oil off sample. Mix ground mass quickly and, if possible, grind sample a second time and again mix thoroughly. If the sample cannot be ground, mix it thoroughly by intensive stirring and kneading. Place test sample in air-tight container so that it will not lose moisture on standing. Analyze sample as soon as possible after grinding. If delay is unavoidable, take precautions to ensure proper preservation of sample and to prevent condensation of moisture on inside surface of container. Clean grinder after use.

F. Determination

Note: Sample may be dry-ashed provided results are same as for wet digestion.

Weigh, to nearest 1 mg, 0.5–1.0 g test portion of prepared test sample into digestion flask, **B(a)**. If water content of cheese is <50% (w/w), ca 0.5 g test portion is sufficient. For fresh cheese, take ca 1.0 g test portion. For processed cheese, take 0.2–0.5 g test portion. Add 3 glass beads and 4 mL H_2SO_4, **C(a)**, to flask.

Working under well-ventilated fume hood, place flask in inclined position and heat with micro burner. Control height of flame to limit production of foam in flask. Foam may be allowed to enter neck of flask, but do not let foam escape. Keep mixture at gentle boil. Avoid local overheating and do not heat flask above surface of liquid contents.

As soon as foaming stops, cool flask to room temperature. Carefully add ca 2 mL H_2O_2 solution, **C(b)**, and reheat. Repeat this procedure until contents are clear and colorless. During heating, mix contents from time to time by careful swirling. Avoid local overheating.

Rinse neck of flask with ca 2 mL H_2O. Heat contents again until water has evaporated. Let liquid boil 30 min to destroy traces of H_2O_2. Avoid local overheating.

Cool flask to room temperature. Quantitatively transfer liquid contents to 100 mL volumetric flask. Dilute to volume with water and mix well. Pipet 1 mL diluted digestate into 50 mL volumetric flask and add ca 25 mL H_2O. Add 20 mL molybdate-ascorbic acid solution, **C(e)**. Dilute to volume with water and mix well. Heat flask in boiling water bath for 15 min.

Cool flask to room temperature in cold water. Within 1 h, measure absorbance of solution vs that of blank test solution at 820 nm. (*Note:* Prepare blank test solution by performing above steps without test portion.)

G. Calibration Curve

Pipet 10 mL phosphorus standard solution, **C(f)**, into 200 mL volumetric flask. Dilute to volume with water and mix well. Into series of five 50 mL volumetric flasks, pipet 0 (reagent blank), 1, 2, 3, and 5 mL, respectively, of diluted standard solution, i.e., equivalent to 0, 10, 20, 30, and 50 μg P, respectively. Dilute contents of each flask to ca 25 mL with water.

Add to contents of each volumetric flask 20 mL molybdate-ascorbic acid solution, **C(e)**. Dilute each solution to volume with water and mix well. Heat flasks in boiling water bath for 15 min.

Cool flasks to room temperature in cold water or in air. Within 1 h, measure absorbance of each standard colorimetric solution vs that of reagent blank at 820 nm. Plot these absorbances vs amounts of phosphorus added.

H. Calculations

Calculate total phosphorus content as follows:
$$P, \text{wt } \% = w_1/(100 \text{ x } w_0)$$
where w_0 = weight, g, of test portion; and w_1 = weight, μg, of phosphorus read from calibration curve (or calculated from regression line obtained by method of least squares).

Report result to second decimal place.

I. Repeatability and Reproducibility

(a) *Repeatability.*—In normal and correct operation of method, difference between 2 single results obtained on identical test material by one analyst using same apparatus within short time interval will exceed 0.05 g P/100 g product on average not more than once in 20 cases.

(b) *Reproducibility.*—In normal and correct operation of method, difference between 2 single and independent results obtained by 2 operators working in different laboratories on identical test material will exceed 0.10 g P/100 g product on average not more once in 20 cases.

Ref.: International Dairy Federation Bulletin, No. 207, 94(1986).
CAS-7723-24-0 (phosphorus)

26.16   991.25—Calcium, Magnesium, and Phosphorus in Cheese
Atomic Absorption Spectrophotometric
and Colorimetric Methods
First Action 1991

(*Caution*: *See Appendix* for safety note on magnesium.)

(Applicable to determination of calcium, magnesium, and phosphorus in processed American, mozzarella, cheddar, Romano, and Parmesan cheeses at levels studied.)

Method Performance:

Calcium, 608–1107 mg/100 g
s_r = 9.9–17.8; s_R = 15.1–32.6; av. RSD_r = 1.5%; av. RSD_R = 2.6%
Magnesium, 23.9–25.1 mg/100 g
s_r = 0.91–1.06; s_R = 1.08–1.27; av. RSD_r = 4.0%; av. RSD_R = 4.8%
Magnesium, 40.0–50.6 mg/100 g
s_r = 0.29–0.56; s_R = 1.01–1.17; av. RSD_r = 0.9%; av. RSD_R = 2.4%
Phosphorus, 444–695 mg/100 g
s_r = 5.9–7.6; s_R = 7.6–9.6; av. RSD_r = 1.2%; av. RSD_R = 1.6%

A. Principle

Sample is dried and ashed. Residue is dissolved and diluted in acidified aqueous solution. Portions are diluted for colorimetric (P) and AAS (Ca and Mg) determinations.

B. Apparatus

Note: Before use, rinse all glassware (volumetric flasks, stoppers, and pipets) and crucibles with HCl (1 + 1) and then with water.

(a) *Atomic absorption spectrophotometer.*—Capable of determining absorbance response to 3 decimal places and of integrating response for 9 s. Determine Ca at 422.7 nm and Mg at 285.2 nm using an air–acetylene flame. Allow 5 min warm-up with flame and source lamp lit.

Several commercial models are available, which have varying requirements of light source, burner flow rate, and detector sensitivity. Operators must become familiar with settings and procedures for their apparatus. Linear range and detector response must be comparable with manufacturer's specifications.

(b) *Spectrophotometer.*—With 1 cm glass cuvets. Capable of measuring absorbance response to 3 decimal places. Determine P at 400 nm. Allow 5 min warm-up with source lit.

C. Reagents

Note: Reagents for Ca, P, and Mg standards must be ultra-pure (99.95%). Opened reagents should be resealed and stored in desiccator in inert atmosphere.

(a) *Calcium carbonate.*—$CaCO_3$, 99.95% pure. Dry overnight at 200°.

(b) *Ammonium dihydrogen phosphate.*—$(NH_4)H_2PO_4$, 99.99% pure. Dry overnight at 110°.

(c) *Magnesium metal.*—99.95% pure.

(d) *Magnesium stock solution.*—1000 mg Mg/L. Place 1.0000 g pure Mg metal, (c), in 50 mL H_2O and slowly add 10 mL HCl. Dilute solution to 1 L.

(e) *Concentrated stock solution.*—500 mg Ca/L, 300 mg P/L, and 25 mg Mg/L. To 1 L volumetric flask, add 1.249 g $CaCO_3$, (a), 1.114 g $(NH_4)H_2PO_4$, (b), and 25 mL Mg stock solution, (d). Add 30 mL HCl (1 + 3), mix until dissolved, and dilute to volume. Store solution in clean Nalgene or poly(ethylene) bottle.

(f) *Dilute stock solution.*—20 mg Ca/L, 12 mg P/L, and 1 mg Mg/L. Dilute 20 mL concentrated stock solution, (e), to 500 mL with water.

(g) *Molybdovanadate reagent.*—Dissolve 60 g ammonium molybdate tetrahydrate in 900 mL hot H_2O, cool to 20°, and dilute to 1 L. Dissolve 1.5 g ammonium metavanadate in 690 mL hot H_2O, add 300 mL HNO_3, cool to 20°, and dilute to 1 L. While stirring, gradually add molybdate solution to vanadate solution. Store at room temperature in poly(ethylene) or glass-stoppered Pyrex bottle. (*Note:* Reagent is stable indefinitely in poly(ethylene) bottle; in Pyrex bottle, precipitate gradually forms after several months. Discard reagent if precipitate forms.)

(h) *Lanthanum stock solution.*—1% La. Dissolve 11.73 g La_2O_3 in 25 mL HNO_3, adding acid slowly. Dilute solution to 1 L.

D. Sample Preparation

Thoroughly mix cheese as in **955.30** (*see* 26.15). Weigh ca 1 g cheese to nearest mg in 100 mL Vycor® dish or Pt crucible and dry 1 h in 100° forced-air oven. Char dried cheese on hot plate. Ash in furnace overnight (16 h) at 525°, and cool in desiccator.

Dissolve ash in 1 mL HNO_3. Transfer to 250 mL volumetric flask and dilute to volume (Solution A).

E. Determination of Phosphorus

(a) *Standard curve.*—Pipet 0, 5, 10, 15, 20, 25, 30, and 35 mL portions of dilute stock solution, C(f), into series of 50 mL volumetric flasks. Add 10 mL molybdovanadate reagent, C(g), to each flask. Mix each solution and dilute each to volume to obtain 0, 1.2, 2.4,...8.4 ppm P standards. Read absorbance of each solution within 1 h. Set spectrophotometer at 400 nm and adjust instrument to 0 A with 0 ppm standard. Plot A vs ppm P.

Linear regression analysis of this curve should yield coefficient of variation of ≥0.99980, with intercept 0 ± 0.004 AU.

(b) *Samples.*—Pipet 10 mL Solution A into 50 mL volumetric flask. Develop color and read absorbance as for standard curve. Determine ppm P from standard curve. (*Note:* Although standards and molybdovanadate reagent are stable for several months, periodically check reproducibility of curve by concurrently running 4.8 ppm standard with assay. Prepare new curve if absorbance of this standard differs from curve by ±1%.)

Calculate mg P/100 g cheese as follows:

Phosphorus, mg/100 g $= (Y \times 125)/W$

where Y = ppm P in assay solution as extrapolated from standard curve and W = weight of cheese taken, g. Report results to nearest mg.

F. Determination of Calcium and Magnesium

(a) *Standard curve.*—Pipet 0, 5, 10, 15, 20, 25, and 30 mL portions of dilute stock solution, **C(f)**, into series of 100 mL volumetric flasks. To each flask, add 10 mL La stock solution, **C(h)**, and dilute to volume to obtain 0–6 ppm Ca and 0–0.3 ppm Mg in 0.1% La. Use 4 or 5 standards in range that approximates anticipated assay level. Adjust instrument to 0 A with 0 ppm standard and run samples along with standards under conditions in **B(a)**. Plot A vs ppm Ca and ppm Mg.

Linear regression analysis of these curves should yield correlation coefficient of ≥ 0.99960 with intercept 0 ± 0.002 AU.

(b) *Samples.*—Pipet 10 mL Solution A into 100 mL volumetric flask. Add 10 mL La stock solution and dilute to volume. With AAS system set for optimum response, determine ppm Ca and Mg in Solution A vs 4 or 5 standards of respective material. Periodically check absorbance of 4.0 ppm Ca (0.2 ppm Mg) standard. Response should not differ by more than 1%. If absorbance of sample is beyond range of curve (above 6.0 ppm Ca [0.3 ppm Mg]), use smaller portion of Solution A for assay.

Calculate mg Ca/100 g and mg Mg/100 g cheese as follows:

Calcium or magnesium, mg/100 g $= (Z \times 2500)/(W\!/V)$

where Z = ppm Ca or Mg in assay solution as extrapolated from standard curve; W = weight of cheese taken, g; and V = volume of Solution A taken for assay, mL. Report Ca results to nearest mg and Mg results to nearest 0.1 mg.

Ref.: JAOAC **74**, 27(1991).
CAS-7440-70-2 (calcium)
CAS-7439-95-4 (magnesium)
CAS-7723-14-0 (phosphorus)

26.17

984.27—Calcium, Copper, Iron, Magnesium, Manganese, Phosphorus, Potassium, Sodium, and Zinc in Infant Formula
Inductively Coupled Plasma Emission Spectroscopic Method
First Action 1984
Final Action 1986

See Chapter 12.13.

26.18　　　　　**986.24—Phosphorus in Milk-Based Infant Formula**
Spectrophotometric Method
First Action 1986
Final Action 1988

A. Principle

P is determined by spectrophotometry on ashed sample by complexing with molybdovanadate reagent.

B. Apparatus

(a) *Spectrophotometer.*—Capable of operation at 400 nm.

(b) *Muffle furnace.*—Equipped with pyrometer and controller.

(c) *Ashing dishes.*—Silica or porcelain.

C. Solutions

(a) *Dilute hydrochloric acid.*—(1 + 3). Add 250 mL HCl to 750 mL H_2O.

(b) *Molybdovanadate reagent.*—Dissolve 20 g ammonium molybdate in 200 mL hot H_2O and cool. Dissolve 1.0 g ammonium metavanadate in 125 mL hot H_2O, cool, and add 160 mL HCl. Gradually add, with stirring, molybdate solution to vanadate solution and dilute with H_2O to 1.0 L.

(c) *Phosphorus standard solution.*—*(1) Stock standard solution.*—2 mg P/mL. Weigh 8.7874 g KH_2PO_4, dried 2 h at 105°. Quantitatively transfer to 1 L volumetric flask and add ca 750 mL H_2O to dissolve. Dilute to volume with H_2O. Store in refrigerator. *(2) Working standard solution.*—0.1 mg P/mL. Dilute 50 mL stock standard solution with H_2O to 1 L. Store in refrigerator. Prepare fresh on day of analysis.

D. Preparation of Sample

Accurately weigh 10.0 g sample (ca 4.0 mg P) into ashing dish and evaporate to dryness on hot plate or steam bath. Ignite sample in muffle furnace at maximum temperature of 600° until free of C (3–4 h). Cool and add 40 mL HCl (1 + 3) and several drops of HNO_3 and bring to boil on hot plate. Cool, transfer quantitatively to 100 mL volumetric flask, and dilute to volume with H_2O.

E. Determination

Transfer aliquots of working standard solution of 0.0, 5.0, 8.0, 10.0, and 15.0 mL to respective 100 mL volumetric flasks. These represent 0.0, 0.5, 0.8, 1.0, and 1.5 mg P. Pipet 20.0 mL sample solution into 100 mL volumetric flask. To each standard and sample flask, add 20.0 mL molybdovanadate reagent, dilute to volume with H_2O, and mix well. Let flasks stand 10 min for complete color development.

Determine *A* of standards and samples in 1 cm cells at maximum near 400 nm, using 0.0 mg standard to zero spectrophotometer. Use linear regression of standard *A* vs mg P of standards to determine mg P for each sample.

F. Calculations

P, mg/L = mg P × 5000 × sample density/g sample

Sample density should be ca 1.03 g/mL for ready-to-feed formula.

Reference: JAOAC **69,** 777(1986).

26.19   **935.59—Phosphorus (Total) in Food Dressings**
Final Action

Use 10 g sample and proceed as in **931.06A(a)** and **931.06B**, except use Pt dish in place of beaker and burn off oil before ashing in furnace.

    I. **931.06** (Phosphorus [Total] [P_2O_5] in Eggs)

        A. Preparation of Solution

        (a) *Liquid eggs.*—From well-mixed sample, **925.29(a)** or **(b)**, accurately weigh, by difference, into 250 mL Pyrex beaker, ca 2 g yolks, 4 g whole eggs, or 10 g whites. Add 20 mL 10% Na_2CO_3 solution and evaporate to dryness on hot plate or in oven overnight at 100–105°. Transfer beaker while hot to furnace at 500° (faint red), and keep at this temperature 1 h. Cool, add few drops H_2O, break up residue with flat-end glass rod, and cover beaker with watch glass; slowly add 10 mL HNO_3 (1 + 3) while stirring, mix, wash watch glass, and filter, collecting filtrate in 300 or 500 mL erlenmeyer. Thoroughly wash charred material and filter with H_2O.

        (b) *Dried eggs.*—Transfer 1 g well-mixed sample, **925.29(c)**, to 150 mL Pyrex beaker, add 20 mL 10% Na_2CO_3 solution, and proceed as in **(a)**.

        B. Determination

        Determine P_2O_5 in prepared filtrate as in **964.06B** (*see* 26.3), using 40–50 mL molybdate solution. Report as total P_2O_5.

        References: JAOAC **14**, 416(1931); **16,** 298(1933).

    II. **925.29** (Sampling of Eggs, Collection and Preparation of Sample, Procedure)

        No simple rules can be made for collection of sample representative of average of any particular lot of egg material, as conditions may differ widely. Experienced judgment must be used in each instance. For large lots, preferably draw several samples for separate analyses rather than attempt to get one composite representative sample. Sampling for microbiological examination, if required, should be performed first; *see* **939.14A–B**.

        939.14 (Sampling of Eggs and Egg Products, Microbiological Methods)

            ("Compendium of Methods for the Microbiological Examination of Foods." Prepared by the APHA Intersociety/Agency Committee on Microbiological Methods for Foods. 1984. Marvin L. Speck, Ed., should be used as guide for further study of microorganisms obtained in culturing techniques described.)

            A. Equipment

            (a) *Liquid eggs.*—Sampling tube or dipper, sterile sample containers with tight closures (pint [500 mL] Mason jars or friction top cans are most practical), alcohol, alcohol lamp or other burner, absorbent cotton, clean cloth or towel, and H_2O pail.

            (b) *Frozen eggs.*—Electric (high-speed) or hand drill with 1 × 16″ auger, hammer and steel strip (12 × 2 × 0.25″), or other tool for opening cans; tablespoon, hatchet or chisel, precooled sterile containers, etc., as in **(a)**.

(c) *Dried eggs.*—Grain trier long enough to reach to bottom of containers to be sampled. Clean sample containers with tight closures (pint [500 mL] Mason jars or paperboard cartons), clean cloth or towel, and tablespoon.

B. Methods

Take samples from representative number of containers in lot, **925.29**. Sterilize sampling tube or dipper, auger, spoon, and hatchet by wiping with alcohol-soaked cotton and flaming over alcohol lamp or other burner. Between samplings, thoroughly wash instruments, dry, and resterilize. Open and sample all containers under as nearly aseptic conditions as possible.

(a) *Liquid eggs.*—Thoroughly mix contents of container with sterile sample tube or dipper, and transfer ca 400 mL (0.75 pint) to sterile sample container. Keep samples at <5° but avoid freezing. Observe and record odor of each container sampled as normal, abnormal, reject, or musty.

(b) *Frozen eggs.*—Remove top layer of egg with sterilized hatchet or chisel. Drill 3 cores from top to bottom of container: first core in center, second core midway between center and periphery, and third core near edge of container. Transfer drillings from container to sample container with sterile spoon. Examine product organoleptically by smelling at opening of fourth drill-hole made after removal of bacteriological sample. (Heat produced by electric drill intensifies odor of egg material, thus facilitating organoleptic examination.) Record odors as normal, abnormal, reject, or musty. Refrigerate samples with solid CO_2 or other suitable refrigerant if analysis is to be delayed or sampling point is at some distance from laboratory.

(c) *Dried eggs.*—For small packages, take entire parcel or parcels for sample. For boxes and barrels, remove top layer with sterile spoon or other sterile instrument, and with sterile trier remove ≥3 cores as in (**b**). (Samples should consist of ca 400 mL [0.75 pint].) Aseptically transfer core to sample container with sterile spoon or other suitable instrument. Store samples under refrigeration or in cool place.

Reference: JAOAC **22**, 625(1939).

(a) *Liquid eggs.*—Obtain representative container or containers. Mix contents of container thoroughly and draw ca 300 g. (Long-handle dipper or ladle serves well.) Keep sample in hermetically sealed jar in freezer or with solid CO_2. Report odor and appearance.

(b) *Frozen eggs.*—Obtain representative container or containers. Examine contents as to odor and appearance. (Condition of contents can be determined best by drilling to center of container with auger and noting odor as auger is withdrawn. If impossible to secure individual containers, samples may consist of composite of borings from contents of each container.) Take borings diagonally across can from ≥3 widely separated parts, starting 2–5 cm in from edge and extending to opposite side as near to bottom as possible. Pack shavings tightly into sample jar and fill it completely to prevent partial dehydration of sample. Seal jar tightly and store in freezer or with solid CO_2. Before analyzing, warm sample in bath held at <50°, and mix well.

(c) *Dried eggs.*—Obtain representative container or containers. For small packages, take entire parcel or parcels for sample. For boxes and barrels, remove top layer to depth of ca 15 cm (6″) with scoop or other convenient instrument. Draw small amounts of sample totaling

300–500 g from accessible parts of container and place in hermetically sealed jar. Report odor and appearance. Prepare sample for analysis by mixing 3 times through domestic flour sifter to thoroughly break up lumps. (Grind flake albumen samples to pass entirely through No. 60 sieve. Mix well.) Keep in hermetically sealed jar in cool place.
References: JAOAC **8,** 599(1925); **53,** 439(1970); **58,** 314(1975).

26.20   930.35—Vinegars (*1*)

(Unless otherwise directed, express results as g/100 mL.)

D. Ash—Final Action

Measure 25 mL sample into weighed Pt dish, evaporate to dryness on H_2O or steam bath, and heat in furnace 30 min at 500–550°. Break up charred mass in Pt dish, add hot H_2O, filter through ashless paper, and wash *thoroughly* with H_2O. Return paper and contents to dish, dry, and heat 30 min at ca 525°, or until all C is burned off. Add filtrate, evaporate to dryness, and heat 15 min at ca 525°. Cool in desiccator and weigh (weight *x*). Reheat 5 min at ca 525°, and cool ≤1 h in desiccator containing efficient desiccant. Put 1 or 2 dishes (preferably only 1) in desiccator at a time. Place weight *x* on balance pan before removing dish from desiccator, and weigh rapidly to nearest mg. Calculate total ash from last weight.

E. Soluble and Insoluble Ash—Final Action

Treat ash, **930.35D,** as in **900.02D** (*see* Chapter 10.5).

F. Alkalinity of Soluble Ash—Final Action

Proceed as in **900.02E,** using soluble ash obtained in **930.35E.** Express result as number mL 1*N* acid required to neutralize soluble ash from 100 mL vinegar. If relationship of ash to alkalinity of soluble ash is abnormal, study composition of ash, especially content of chlorides, sulfates, phosphates, and alkalies (J. Amer. Chem. Soc. **22,** 218[1900]).

> **900.02E** (Surplus 1989. From **31.016,** 14th ed.)
> Cool filtrate from **900.02D** and titrate with 0.1N HCl, using 0.05% methyl orange indicator. Express alkalinity in terms of mL 1N acid/100 g sample.

G. Soluble Phosphorus (2)—Final Action 1965

Proceed as in **964.06B** (*see* 26.3); **965.18C**; or **935.45** [*see Official Methods of Analysis* (1970) 11th ed., **22.037–22.039**], using solution obtained in **930.35F.** If either volumetric or colorimetric method is used, standardize with sample of known phosphate content. Express results as mg P_2O_5/100 mL vinegar.

965.18 (Phosphorus in Baking Powders, Gravimetric Method)

A. Reagents

(**a**) *Ammonium nitrate solution.*—Dissolve 100 g P-free NH_4NO_3 in H_2O and dilute to 1 L.

(**b**) *Magnesia mixture.*—*(1)* Dissolve 55 g crystallized $MgCl_2 \cdot 6H_2O$ in H_2O, add 140 g NH_4Cl and 130.5 mL NH_4OH, and dilute to 1 L. Or: *(2)* Dissolve 55 g crystallized $MgCl_2 \cdot 6H_2O$ in H_2O, add 140 g NH_4Cl, dilute to 870 mL, and add NH_4OH to each required portion of solution just before using, at rate of 15 mL/100 mL solution.

(**c**) *Ammonium hydroxide solution for washing.*—(1 + 9). Should contain $\geq 2.5\%$ NH_3 by weight.

B. Preparation of Solution

Mix 5 g sample with little $Mg(NO_3)_2$ solution, (dissolve 950 g P-free $Mg(NO_3)_2 \cdot 6H_2O$ and H_2O and dilute to 1 L), dry, ignite, dissolve in HCl (1 + 2.5), and dilute to definite volume. In aliquot of solution determine P as in **965.18C** or as in **964.06B**, beginning with 2nd sentence.

C. Determination

Pipet aliquot of prepared solution into 250 mL beaker; add NH_4OH in slight excess and barely dissolve precipitate formed with few drops HNO_3, stirring vigorously. If HCl or H_2SO_4 has been used as solvent, add ca 15 g crystalline NH_4NO_3 or solution containing that amount. To hot solution add 70 mL molybdate solution, **964.06A(a)**, for every 100 mg P_2O_5 present. Digest 1 h at ca 65° and test for complete precipitation of P_2O_5 by adding more molybdate solution to clear supernate. Filter, and wash with cold H_2O or preferably with the NH_4NO_3 solution. Dissolve precipitate on filter with NH_4OH (1 + 1) and hot H_2O, and wash into beaker to volume ≤ 100 mL. Neutralize with HCl, using litmus paper or *bromothymol blue* as indicator; cool, and from buret slowly add (ca 1 drop/s), stirring vigorously, 15 mL magnesia mixture/100 mg P_2O_5 present. After 15 min add 12 mL NH_4OH and let stand until supernate is clear (usually 2 h); filter, wash precipitate with NH_4OH (1 + 9) until washings are practically Cl-free, dry, burn at low heat, and ignite to constant weight, preferably in furnace at 950–1000°; cool in desiccator, and weigh as $Mg_2P_2O_7$. Report as % P_2O_5.

D. Qualitative Test

Add 10 mL H_2O to 1–2 g sample in 150 mL beaker. Make just acid with HNO_3, filter, take equal volumes filtrate and molybdate solution, **964.06A(a)**, and warm at 40–50°. Yellow precipitate indicates presence of phosphate.

CAS-7723-14-0 (phosphorus)

H. Insoluble Phosphorus (2)—Final Action 1965

Dissolve H_2O-insoluble ash, **930.35E**, in ca 50 mL boiling HNO_3 (1 + 8) (use 25 mL H_2SO_4 [1 + 9] for colorimetric method) and proceed as in **964.06B**, or **965.18C**, or **935.45**. If either volumetric or colorimetric method is used, standardize with sample of known phosphate content. Express result as mg P_2O_5/100 mL vinegar.

I. Total Phosphorus (2)—Final Action

Dissolve ash, **930.35D**, or both soluble and insoluble ash, **930.35E**, in ca 50 mL boiling HNO$_3$ (1 + 8) (use 25 mL H$_2$SO$_4$ [1 + 9] for colorimetric method) and proceed as in **964.06B**, or **965.18C**, or **935.45**. If either volumetric or colorimetric method is used, standardize with sample of known phosphate content. Express result as mg P$_2$O$_5$/100 mL vinegar. If desired, digest vinegar as in **935.45**, instead of using ash from **930.35D**.

Chapter 27
Potassium

27.1   **985.35—Minerals in Ready-to-Feed Milk-Based Infant Formula**
Atomic Absorption Spectrophotometric Method
First Action 1985
Final Action 1988

See Chapter 12.14

27.2   **956.01—Potassium and/or Sodium in Plants**
Flame Photometric Method
Final Action 1965

A. Reagents

(**a**) *Potassium stock solution.*—1000 ppm K. Dissolve 1.907 g dry KCl in H_2O and dilute to 1 L.

(**b**) *Sodium stock solution.*—1000 ppm Na. Dissolve 2.542 g dry NaCl in H_2O and dilute to 1 L.

(**c**) *Lithium stock solution.*—1000 ppm Li. Dissolve 6.108 g LiCl in H_2O and dilute to 1 L. (Needed only if internal standard method of evaluation is to be used.)

(**d**) *Ammonium oxalate stock solution.*—0.24N. Dissolve 17.0 g $(NH_4)_2C_2O_4 \cdot H_2O$ in H_2O and dilute to 1 L.

(**e**) *Extracting solutions.*—(*1*) *For potassium.*—For internal standard method, dilute required volume LiCl stock solution to 1 L; otherwise use H_2O. (*2*) *For sodium.*—To 250 mL ammonium oxalate stock solution add required volume LiCl stock solution (if internal standard method is used) and dilute to 1 L. If internal standard requirements are same for both Na and K determinations, this reagent may be used as common extracting solution.

B. Preparation of Standard Solutions

Dilute appropriate aliquots of stock solutions to prepare series of standards containing K and/or Na in stepped amounts (including 0) to cover instrument range, and Li and ammonium oxalate (if required) in same concentrations as in corresponding extracting solutions. (If common extracting solution is used, 1 set of standards containing both K and Na suffices.)

C. Sample Extraction

Transfer weighed portion of finely ground and well-mixed sample to Erlenmeyer of at least twice capacity of volume of extracting solution to be used. Add measured volume extracting solution, stopper flask, and shake vigorously at frequent intervals during ≥ 15 min. Filter through dry, fast paper. If paper clogs, pour contents onto additional fresh paper and combine filtrates. Use filtrate for determination.

Note: Do not make extracts more concentrated than required for instrument because there is tendency toward incomplete extraction as ratio of sample weight to volume extracting solution increases. Prepare separate extracts for K and Na when their concentrations in sample differ greatly. For K, use weight sample ≤ 0.1 g/50 mL extracting solution; for low Na concentrations use ≥ 1.0 g/50 mL extracting solution; and for higher concentrations, prepare weaker extracts by reducing ratio of sample to extracting solution rather than by diluting stronger extracts.

D. Determination

(*Caution: See Appendix* for safety notes on flame photometer.)

Rinse all glassware used in Na determination with dilute HNO_3, followed by several portions H_2O. Protect solutions from air-borne Na contamination.

Operate instrument according to manufacturer's instructions. Permit instrument to reach operating equilibrium before use. Aspirate portions of standard solutions toward end of warm-up period until reproducible readings for series are obtained.

Run standards, covering concentration range of samples involved, at frequent intervals within series of sample solution determinations. Repeat this operation with both standard and sample solutions enough times to result in reliable average reading for each solution. Plot curves from readings of standards, and calculate % K and/or Na in samples.

Reference: JAOAC **39**, 419(1956).
CAS-7440-09-7 (potassium)
CAS-7440-23-5 (sodium)

27.3   953.01—Metals in Plants
General Recommendations for Emission Spectrographic Methods
First Action 1988

See Chapter 12.5.

27.4   985.01—Metals and Other Elements in Plants
Inductively Coupled Plasma Spectroscopic Method
First Action 1985
Final Action 1988

See Chapter 12.6.

27.5

975.03—Metals in Plants
Atomic Absorption Spectrophotometric Method
First Action 1975
Final Action 1988

See Chapter 12.2.

27.6

980.03—Metals in Plants
Direct Reading Spectrographic Method
Final Action 1988

See Chapter 12.3.

27.7

965.30—Potassium in Fruits and Fruit Products
Rapid Flame Photometric Method
First Action 1965
Final Action 1968

(*Caution: See Appendix* for safety notes on flame photometers.)

Prepare sample solution as in **920.149**. Dilute, if necessary, to reduce K concentration to range covered by flame photometer (preferably 40–80 ppm). Aspirate sample solution (diluted or undiluted) directly into flame.

I. **920.149** (Preparation of Fruit Sample)

Transfer samples received in open packages (i.e., not sterile) without delay to glass-stoppered containers and keep in cool place. To avoid effects of fermentation, make prompt determinations of alcohol, total and volatile acids, solids, and sugars, particularly in case of fruit juices and fresh fruits. (Portions for determination of sucrose and reducing sugars may be weighed and kept several days without fermenting if the slight excess of neutral $Pb(OAc)_2$ solution required in determination is added. *Note:* $Pb(OAc)_2$ is toxic. Label samples to show its addition.) Prepare various products for analysis as follows:

(**a**) *Juices.*—Mix thoroughly by shaking to ensure uniform sample, and filter through absorbent cotton or rapid paper. Prepare fresh juices by pressing well-pulped fruit and filtering. Express juice of citrus fruits by commercial device, and filter.

(**b**) *Jellies and sirups.*—Mix thoroughly to ensure uniform sample. Prepare solution by weighing 300 g thoroughly mixed sample into 2 L flask and dissolve in H_2O, heating on steam bath if necessary. Apply as little heat as possible to minimize inversion of sucrose. Cool, dilute to volume, mix thoroughly by shaking, and use aliquots for the various determinations. If insoluble material is present, mix thoroughly and filter first.

369

(c) *Fresh fruits, dried fruits, preserves, jams, and marmalades.*—Pulp by passing through food chopper, or by use of soil dispersion mixer, Hobart mixer, or other suitable mechanical mixing apparatus, or by grinding in large mortar, and mixing thoroughly, completing operation as quickly as possible to avoid loss of moisture. With dried fruits, pass sample through food chopper 3 times, mixing thoroughly after each grinding. Set burrs or blades of food chopper as close as possible without crushing seeds. Grind entire contents of No. 10 or smaller container. Mix contents of larger containers thoroughly by stirring and remove portion for grinding. With stone fruits, remove pits and determine their proportion in weighed sample.

Prepare solution by weighing into 1.5–2 L beaker 300 g fresh fruit, or equivalent of dried fruit, preserves, jams, and marmalades, well-pulped and mixed in blender or other suitable type of mechanical grinder; add ca 800 mL H_2O; and boil 1 h replacing at intervals H_2O lost by evaporation. Transfer to 2 L volumetric flask, cool, dilute to volume, and filter. With unsweetened fruit, ashing is facilitated by addition of sugar before boiling; therefore weigh 150 g fruit, add 150 g sugar and 800 mL H_2O, and proceed as above.

(d) *Canned fruits.*—*See* **968.30**. Carefully invert by hand all fruits having cups or cavities if they fall on sieve with cups or cavities up. Cups or cavities in soft products may be drained by tilting sieve, but no other handling of these products while draining is permissible. Examination of sirup in which fruits are preserved is often enough. Separate liquor by draining, **968.30B**, and treat as in (a).

II. **968.30** (Canned Vegetables, Drained Weight)

A. Sieves

See Definition of Terms and Explanatory Notes, Official Methods of Analysis, 15th ed. Use 8″ (20 cm) diameter for containers ≤3 lb (1.36 kg) or 12″ (30 cm) diameter for containers >3 lb.

B. Determination

Weigh full can, open, and pour entire contents on No. 8 sieve (use 7/16″ sieve for canned tomatoes). Without shifting product, incline sieve at ca 17–20° angle to facilitate drainage. Drain 2 min, directly weigh either drained solids or free liquid, and weigh dry empty can. From weights obtained, determine % liquid and % drained solid contents.

Prepare standards as in **963.13A(a)** except cover range 10–100 ppm K in 10 ppm steps. Determine %*T* for standards or follow instructions of manufacturer, making check determinations as necessary. If internal standard instrument is used, add appropriate amount of LiCl to both standard and sample solutions.

963.13A(a) (Potassium and Sodium in Wines, Flame Photometric Method)

A. Reagents and Apparatus

(a) *Potassium and sodium standard solution.*—Dry reagent grade KCl and NaCl at 100° overnight. Dilute 1.716 g KCl and 2.288 g NaCl to 1 L with H_2O. This solution contains 900 mg K/L and 900 mg Na/L.

From %*T* of sample and standard curve, determine ppm K. Report as mg K_2O/100 g sample. K × 1.2046 = K_2O.

Reference: JAOAC **48,** 521(1965).
CAS-7440-09-7 (potassium)

27.8   990.23—Sodium and Potassium in Dried Milk
Flame Emission Spectrometric Method
First Action 1990
IDF-ISO-AOAC Method

(Applicable to all types of dried milk)

Method Performance:
    Sodium
    $s_r = 0.008$; $s_R = 0.012$; $RSD_r = 1.93\%$; $RSD_R = 2.90\%$
    Potassium
    $s_r = 0.028$; $s_R = 0.035$; $RSD_r = 1.88\%$; $RSD_R = 2.36\%$

A. Principle

Dried milk is dissolved in warm water. Test solution and reference solutions are atomized directly into flame of flame emission spectrometer and intensity of emitted light is measured.

B. Apparatus

Thoroughly clean and rinse all glassware with distilled water to be sure that it is free from extractable Na and K under test conditions.

(a) *Volumetric flasks.*—100, 500, and 1000 mL.

(b) *Graduated cylinder.*—50 mL.

(c) *Pipets.*—To deliver 10, 15, 20, 25, 30, 40, 45, 50, and 60 mL. (*Note:* Where appropriate, burets may be used instead of pipets.)

(d) *Flame emission spectrometer.*—With burner fed with mixture of either acetylene and air or propane and air, and with filters with maximum transmittance at ca 589 and 768 nm for Na and K, respectively, or fitted with a monochromator.

C. Reagents

(a) *Hydrochloric acid.*—About 4M. Dilute 300 mL 37% (w/w) HCl to 1 L with water, and mix.

(b) *Standard solutions.*—(*Note:* Store standard solutions in hard poly(ethylene) containers or in others of at least equivalent quality.)

    Dry NaCl and KCl to constant weight at 110–120°.

(*1*) *Sodium standard solution.*—0.4 mg Na/mL. Dissolve 1.0168 g dried NaCl in water, dilute to 1 L, and mix. (*2*) *Potassium standard solution.* 1 mg K/mL. Dissolve 1.9068 g dried KCl in water, dilute in 1 L, and mix. (*3*) *Phosphorus standard solution.*—2.5 mg P/mL. Dissolve 10.660 g diammonium hydrogen phosphate [$(NH_4)_2HPO_4$] in water, dilute to 1 L, and mix.

D. Sampling

Proceed as in **935.41A**, **968.12**, and **970.28A**. Store sample in manner that prevents deterioration and change in composition.

    I. **935.41** (Sampling of Dried Milk)
        A. Sampling
        (*See also* **968.12** and **970.28**.)

Avoid sampling on rainy day or when humidity is high, so as to reduce moisture absorption from air to minimum.

On surface of milk at top of barrel locate point on each end of a diameter and on radius perpendicular to this diameter, 2.5–5 cm (1–2″) in from edge of barrel. Midway on each side of triangle between these points locate one point. At 6 points so located, using tubular trier long enough to extend full length of barrel, draw core parallel to vertical axis of barrel. Transfer cores to clean, dry, air-tight container and seal immediately.

Before opening sample for analysis, make homogeneous either by shaking or by alternately rolling and inverting container. Avoid excessive temperature and humidity when opening sample container.
Reference: JAOAC **18,** 402(1935).

B. Preparation of Sample
Avoid absorption of moisture during preparation of sample. Mix sample by transferring to dry, air-tight container with capacity ca twice volume of sample. Carefully mix by shaking and inverting repeatedly. When sampling, operate as rapidly as possible. If lumps are present, sift sample through No. 20 sieve, rubbing material through sieve and tapping vigorously, if necessary.

II. **968.12** (Sampling of Dairy Products)
A. Instructions of Administrative Character
(This section is usually prescribed by specific regulatory agency. It is included for completeness.)

Sampling should be performed by authorized or sworn independent agent, properly trained in appropriate technique. Agent should be free from any infectious disease. If possible, representatives of parties concerned should be given opportunity to be present when sampling is performed.

Samples should be accompanied by report, signed by sworn or authorized sampling agent and countersigned by any witnesses present. Report should give particulars of place, date, and time of sampling; name and designation of agent and of any witnesses; precise method of sampling which is followed if this deviates from prescribed standard method; nature and number of units constituting consignment together with their batch code markings, where available; number of samples duly identified as to batches from which they are drawn; and place to which the samples will be sent.

When appropriate, report should also include any relevant conditions or circumstances, e.g., condition of packages and their surroundings, temperature and humidity of atmosphere, method of sterilization of sampling equipment, whether preservative has been added to samples, and any other special information relating to material being sampled.

Each sample should be sealed and labeled to give nature of product, identification number, and any code markings of batch from which sample has been taken, date of sampling, and name and signature of sampling agent. When necessary, additional information may be required, for example, weight of sample and unit from which it was taken.

All samples should be taken at least in duplicate, one set being held, if necessary, in cold storage and put at disposal of second party as soon as possible. Precise method of sampling and weight or volume of product to be taken as sample vary with nature of product and purpose for which sampling is required and are defined for each particular case.

When previously agreed between parties, take additional sets of samples and retain for independent arbitration, if necessary. Send samples to testing laboratory immediately after sampling.

B. Technical Instructions

(*See* sampling equipment specifications laid down for each product to be sampled.)

(**a**) *Sampling for chemical purposes.*—Clean and dry all equipment.

(**b**) *Sampling for bacteriological purposes.*—Clean and treat equipment by one of following methods: (*1*) Expose to hot air 2 h at 170° (may be stored if kept under sterile conditions). (*2*) Autoclave 15–20 min at 120° (may be stored if kept under sterile conditions). (*3*) Expose to steam 1 h at 100° (use equipment same day). (*4*) Immerse in H_2O 1 min at 100° (use equipment immediately). (*5*) Immerse in 70% alcohol and flame to burn off alcohol immediately before use. (*6*) Expose to hydrocarbon (propane, butane) torch flame so that all working surfaces contact flame immediately before use.

Choice of treatment depends on nature, shape, and size of equipment and on conditions of sampling. Sterilize wherever possible by method (*1*) or (*2*).

Methods (*3*), (*4*), (*5*), and (*6*) are regarded as secondary methods only.

(**c**) *Sampling for organoleptic purposes.*—Use equipment as in (**a**) or (**b**), or as specified for specific product. Equipment should not impart any flavor or odor to product.

C. Sample Containers

(**a**) *For liquids.*—Use clean and dry containers of suitable waterproof, greaseproof material (glass, stainless metal, suitable plastic material) of quality suitable for sterilization by **968.12B(b)**, if necessary, and of suitable shape and capacity for material to be sampled (as defined in each particular case).

Securely close containers either with suitable rubber or plastic stopper or by screw cap of metal or plastic having, if necessary, liquid-tight plastic liner which is insoluble, nonabsorbent, and greaseproof, and which will not influence odor, flavor, or composition of milk products.

If rubber stoppers are used, cover with nonabsorbent, flavorless material (such as suitable plastic) before pressing into sample container. Suitable plastic bags may also be used.

(**b**) *For solids or semisolids.*—Use clean and dry wide-mouth, cylindrical receptacles of suitable waterproof, greaseproof material (glass, stainless metal, suitable plastic material) of quality suitable for sterilization by **968.12B(b)**, if necessary, and of capacity suited to size of sample to be taken (as defined in each particular case). Make air-tight as in (**a**). Suitable plastic bags may also be used.

(**c**) *Small retail containers.*—Contents of intact and unopened containers constitute samples.

D. Preservation of Samples

To samples of liquid products or cheese intended for chemical analysis, suitable preservative may be added. Such preservative should not interfere with subsequent analysis. Indicate nature and amount of addition on label and in any reports.

Do not add preservatives to samples of semisolid, solid (except cheese), or dried products intended for chemical analysis. Rapidly cool and store samples in refrigerator at 0–5°. Dried milks may be kept at room temperature.

Do not add preservatives to samples intended for bacteriological or organoleptic examination. Hold at 0–5°, except for condensed (conserved) milk products when sample comprises unopened hermetically sealed containers in which products are sold. Keep liquid products and butter cold. Start bacteriological examination of liquid products as soon as possible and never >24 h after sampling.

E. Transport of Samples

Transport samples to laboratory as quickly as possible after sampling. Take precautions to prevent, during transit, exposure to direct sunlight, or to temperatures <0° or >10° in case of perishable products. For samples intended for bacteriological examination, use insulated transport container capable of maintaining temperature at 0–5°, except for samples of condensed (conserved) milk products in unopened containers, or in case of very short journeys.

Maintain samples of cheese under such conditions as to avoid separation of fat or moisture. Maintain soft cheese at 0–5°.

References: JAOAC **49,** 58(1966); **50,** 531(1967).

III. **970.28** (Sampling of Dried Milk and Its Products)

(Perform sampling for bacteriological examination first, independent of other sampling, from same bulk container, whenever possible.)

A. Sampling for Chemical Analysis and Organoleptic Examination

(**a**) *Sampling equipment.*—Use suitable clean, dry borer tube or trier of stainless steel, Al, or Al alloy.

(**b**) *Sampling technique.*—Pass tube steadily through powder at even rate of penetration. When tube reaches bottom of container withdraw contents and discharge immediately into sample container. Do not touch powder with fingers. Take ≥1 bores to make up 300–500 g samples.

(**c**) *Sample containers.*—Place samples in clean, dry containers, air-tight and, if required for examination, opaque. Use sample container large enough to allow mixing by shaking.

(**d**) Submit unopened original container of gas-packed dried milk if gas analysis is required.

B. Sampling for Bacteriological Examination

Take samples for bacteriological examination, whenever possible, from same package as for chemical and organoleptic examination. Take sample for bacteriological examination first.

(**a**) *Sampling equipment.*—Sterilize suitable stainless steel or Al spoon or trier as in **968.12B(b)**(*1*), (*2*), (*5*), or (*6*).

(**b**) *Sampling technic.*—Using sterile metal implement (e.g., broad-bladed knife or spoon), remove surface layer of powder from sampling area. With another sterile spoon or trier, take sample of 50–200 g, if possible, from point near center of container. Place sample as quickly as possible into sample container, and close immediately, using aseptic precautions. In case of dispute concerning bacteriological conditions of top layer of powder in packing, take special sample from this top layer.

(**c**) *Sample containers.*—Place samples in clean, dry, sterile containers, preferably brown if transparent, capable of air-tight closure.

(For additional instructions, *see* **935.41A.**)

E. Sample Preparation

Note: Avoid contamination, especially with perspiration.

(**a**) *Test sample.*—Transfer sample to container of capacity about twice sample volume. Immediately close container with airtight lid and mix sample thoroughly by repeatedly shaking and inverting container. During preparation, avoid exposing sample to atmosphere as far as possible in order to minimize absorption of atmospheric moisture.

(**b**) *Test portion.*—Weigh, to nearest 1 mg, 1.25 g portion of test sample into 50 mL glass beaker.

(**c**) *Test solution.*—Dissolve test portion in ca 20 mL warm water (40–50°) while stirring with glass rod. Quantitatively transfer contents of beaker by rinsing with water into 500 mL volumetric flask, cool to about 20°, and dilute to volume. Mix contents of flask thoroughly.

Notes: (*1*) Using dried normal whole milk, this solution contains ca 10 mg Na and 40 mg K per liter.

(*2*) Results will not be reliable if this solution contains insoluble particles.

F. Preparation of Reference Solutions

Into seven 1000 mL volumetric flasks, successively pipet volumes of Na and K standard solutions, **C(b)**, listed in Table **990.23**, and dilute to 900 mL with water. To each flask, add 10 mL P standard solution, dilute to volume with water, and mix.

G. Determination

(**a**) *Sodium.*—Alternately atomize reference solutions, starting with solution with lowest Na concentration, and test solution, into flame of flame emission spectrometer, following manufacturer's instructions and using Na filter, or monochromator, adjusted to 589 nm. Note readings.

(**b**) *Potassium.*—Proceed as in (**a**), using reference solutions starting with solution with lowest K content, and K filter, or monochromator, adjusted to 768 nm. Note readings.

Note: If reading for test solution exceeds that of reference solution with highest concentration, repeat spectrometric measurements using appropriate dilution of test solution and appropriate reference solutions. For this purpose, prepare reference solutions that have concentrations of Na, K, and P as close as possible to expected concentrations in diluted test solution.

H. Calculations

Calculation Na and K contents of sample as follows:

$$\text{Na or K, wt \%} = \{[(I_x - I_1)/I_2 - I_1)]$$
$$\times [(C_2 - C_1) + C_1]\} \times (f/w)$$

where I_x = spectrometer reading for test solution; I_1 = nearest lower spectrometer reading for reference solution of concentration C_1; I_2 = nearest higher spectrometer reading for reference solution with concentration C_2; C_1 = concentration, mg/L, of reference solution that gives reading I_1; C_2 = concentration, mg/L, of reference solution that gives reading I_2; f = conversion factor to express results at % by weight (for Na and K, f = 0.04); w = weight, g, of test portion. (*Note:* Take into account any dilution of test solution.)

Report Na and K contents to nearest 0.01% (w/w).

I. Repeatability and Reproducibility

(**a**) *Repeatability.*—Difference between results of 2 determinations, carried out simultaneously or in rapid succession by same analyst using same apparatus, shall not exceed 6% relative of arithmetic mean of results for both Na and K.

(**b**) *Reproducibility.*—Difference between 2 single and independent results, obtained by 2 different analysts working in different laboratories on identical test material, shall not exceed 8% relative of arithmetic mean of results for both Na and K.

Table 990.23 Preparation and Composition of Sodium and Potassium Reference Solutions[a]

Ref. Soln	Na Std Soln, Vol. Taken, mL	Na Ref. Soln, Concn, mg Na/L	K Std Soln, Vol. Taken, mL	K Ref. Soln, concn, mg K/L
1	15	6	50	50
2	20	8	45	45
3	25	10	40	40
4	30	12	40	40
5	40	16	35	35
6	50	20	30	30
7[b]	60	24	25	25

[a]10 mL P standard solution is added to each reference solution to provide 25 mg P/L in reference solutions at all Na and K levels. Reference solutions are stable at least 1 month stored in containers of hard polyethylene or of other material of at least equivalent quality.
[b]Use of reference solution 7 is optional.

Ref.: International Dairy Federation Bulletin, No 207, 143(1986).
CAS-7440-23-5 (sodium)
CAS-7440-09-7 (potassium)

27.9　　　　969.23—Sodium and Potassium in Seafood
Flame Photometric Method
First Action 1969
Final Action 1971

A. Apparatus and Reagents

(a) *Glassware.*—Borosilicate glassware and intact Vycor, Pt, or Si crucible precleaned with dilute HNO_3 and rinsed in distilled H_2O immediately before use.

(b) *Distilled water.*—H_2O, free from Na and K; either double-distilled or deionized. Use for preparing standards and dilutions.

(c) *Sodium standard solutions.*—(*1*) *Stock solution.*—1 mg Na/mL. Dry reagent grade NaCl 2 h at 110°; cool in desiccator. Weigh 2.5421 g into 1 L volumetric flask and dilute to volume with H_2O. (*2*) *Working solutions for flame emission.*—0.01, 0.03, and 0.05 mg Na/mL. Pipet 1, 3, and 5 mL Na stock solution into separate 100 mL volumetric flasks; add 7 mL K stock solution and 2 mL HNO_3 to each flask; dilute to volume with H_2O. (*3*) *Working solutions for flame absorption.*—0.00003, 0.0001, 0.0003, and 0.0005 mg Na/mL. Pipet 1 mL Na stock solution into 100 mL volumetric flask and dilute to volume with H_2O. Pipet 0.3, 1.0, 3.0, and 5.0 mL diluted stock solution into separate 100 mL volumetric flasks and dilute to volume with H_2O.

(**d**) *Potassium standard solutions.*—(*1*) *Stock solution.*—1 mg K/mL. Dry and cool reagent grade KCl as in (**c**). Weigh 1.9068 g into 1 L volumetric flask and dilute to volume with H_2O. (*2*) *Working solutions for flame emission.*—0.04, 0.07, and 0.10 mg K/mL. Pipet 4, 7, and 10 mL stock solution into separate 100 mL volumetric flasks; add 3 mL Na stock solution to each flask; dilute to volume with H_2O. (*3*) *Working solutions for flame absorption.*—0.0001, 0.0005, 0.0007, and 0.0010 mg K/mL. Pipet 1 mL K stock solution into 100 mL volumetric flask and dilute to volume with H_2O. Pipet 1, 5, 7, and 10 mL diluted stock solution into separate 100 mL volumetric flasks and dilute to volume with H_2O.

B. Wet Ashing

(*Caution: See Appendix* for safety notes on distillation, wet oxidation, and nitric acid.)
Prepare sample as in **937.07**.

937.07 (Fish and Marine Products, Treatment and Preparation of Sample)

Procedure

To prevent loss of H_2O during preparation and subsequent handling, use samples as large as practicable. Keep ground material in container with air-tight cover. Begin all determinations as soon as practicable. If any delay occurs, chill sample to inhibit decomposition. In general, prepare sample of fish as it is usually prepared by consumer, by including skin and discarding bones, but subject to overall rule of edibility, e.g., inedible catfish skin is discarded; softened canned salmon bones are included; sardines are examined whole. Instructions may be modified in accordance with purpose of specific examination. Prepare samples for analysis as follows:

(**a**) *Fresh fish.*—Clean, scale, and eviscerate fish. In case of small fish ≤15 cm (6″), use 5–10 fish. In case of large fish, from each of ≥3 fish cut 3 cross-sectional slices 2.5 cm (1″) thick, 1 slice from just back of pectoral fins, 1 slice halfway between first slice and vent, and 1 slice just back of vent. Remove bone. For intermediate-size fish, remove and discard heads, scales, tails, fins, guts, and inedible bones; fillet fish to obtain all flesh and skin from head to tail and from top of back to belly on both sides. For determination of fat and fat-soluble components, skin must be included, since many fish store large amounts of fat directly beneath skin.

Pass sample rapidly through meat chopper 3 times. Remove unground material from chopper after each grinding and mix thoroughly with ground material. Meat chopper should have holes as small as practicable (1.5–3 mm (1/16–⅛″) diameter) and should not leak around handle end. As alternative for soft fish, high-speed blender may be used. Blend several minutes, stopping blender frequently to scrape down sides of cup.

(**b**) *Canned fish, shellfish, and other canned marine products.*—Place entire contents of can (meat and liquid) in blender and blend until homogeneous or grind 3 times through meat chopper. For large cans, drain meat 2 min on No. 8–12 sieve and collect all liquid. Determine weight of meat and volume of liquid. Recombine portion of each in proportionate amounts. Blend recombined portions in blender (or grind) until homogeneous.

(**c**) *Canned marine products packed in oil, sauce, broth, or water.*—Drain 2 min on No. 8 sieve. Prepare solid portion as in (**b**). Liquid may be analyzed separately, if desired, or reincorporated with solids. H_2O is usually discarded.

(**d**) *Fish packed in salt or brine.*—Drain and discard brine and rinse off adhering salt crystals with saturated NaCl solution. Drain again 2 min and proceed as in (**a**).

(**e**) *Dried smoked or dried salt fish.*—Proceed as in (**a**).

(**f**) *Frozen fish.*—Let thaw at room temperature, and discard draining. (*1*) *Fillet.*—Use entire piece. (*2*) *Whole fish.*—Proceed as in (**a**).

(g) *Shellfish other than oysters, clams, and scallops.*—If sample is received in shell, wash as in (h) and separate edible portions in usual way. Prepare edible portion for analysis as in (a).

(h) *Shell oysters, shell clams, and scallops.*—Wash shells in potable H_2O to remove all loose silt and dirt, and drain well. Shuck enough oysters or clams into clean dry container to yield ≥500 mL (1 pint) drained meats. Transfer shellfish meats to skimmer, **953.11A**, pick out pieces of shell, drain 2 min on skimmer, and proceed as in (i) or (j).

953.11A (Drained Liquid from Shucked Oysters)

A. Apparatus

Skimmer or strainer.—Flat-bottom metal pan or tray with ca 5 cm (2″) sides, with area of ≥1900 cm^2 (300 square inches) for each gallon of oysters to be poured on tray, and with perforations 0.6 cm (0.25″) diameter and 3.2 cm (1.25″) apart in square pattern, or perforations of equivalent area and distribution. Support skimmer over slightly larger solid tray so that liquid drains into solid tray.

(i) *Shucked clams or scallops.*—Prepare as in (b).

(j) *Shucked oysters.*—Blend meats, including liquid, 1–2 min in high-speed blender.

(k) *Breaded fish, raw or cooked.*—Do not remove breading or skin. Proceed as in (a).

References: JAOAC **20**, 70(1937); **21**, 85(1938); **35**, 218(1952); **36**, 608(1953); **38**, 194(1955); **59**, 312(1976).

Weigh 1 g sample into 50 mL Pyrex beaker. Dry 2.5 h at 110°, cool, and weigh if % solids is to be determined.

(a) *Samples with unknown or known high oil content.*—Add ca 10 mL petroleum ether, and warm on steam bath or low temperature hot plate until oil is extracted. Decant and repeat until sample is defatted. Proceed as in (b).

(b) *Samples with low oil content.*—Add 5 mL HNO_3 (if total Cl content is desired, add enough 0.1N $AgNO_3$ to precipitate chlorides (3.0 mL)) to each beaker. Digest on steam bath or low temperature hot plate until sample dissolves; evaporate to dryness. Add 5 mL HNO_3 and take to dryness. Repeat. Add 2 mL HNO_3 and warm to dissolve. Proceed as in (c) or (d).

(c) *For flame emission.*—Transfer digest to 25 mL volumetric flask with hot H_2O, wash down sides of beaker 3 times with hot H_2O, and add washings to flask. Cool, and dilute to volume with H_2O. If particles are too finely dispersed to settle, centrifuge aliquot at 2000 rpm.

(d) *For flame absorption.*—Transfer digest to 100 mL volumetric flask and proceed as above. Dilute for direct readout as follows: Place 1 mL aliquot in 25 mL volumetric flask and dilute to volume with H_2O for Na; place 2 mL aliquot in 10 mL volumetric flask and dilute to volume with H_2O for K.

Prepare blank solution by diluting 2 mL HNO_3 to 100 mL with H_2O.

C. Dry Ashing

Prepare sample as in **937.07**.

Weigh 4 g sample into crucible, and char on electric hot plate or over low flame. Place in cold furnace and bring to 525°. Ash 2 h to white ash. Cool, and weigh if total ash is desired.

Add 15 mL dilute HNO_3 (1 + 4) to crucible, breaking up ash with stirring rod if necessary. Filter through acid-washed quantitative paper into 100 mL volumetric flask. Wash residue and paper 3 times with H_2O. Dilute to volume. Proceed as in (a) or (b).

(a) *For flame emission.*—Read directly.

(b) *For flame absorption.*—Dilute for direct readout as follows: Place 1 mL aliquot in 100 mL volumetric flask and dilute to volume with H_2O for Na; place 1 mL aliquot in 25 mL volumetric flask and dilute to volume with H_2O for K.

Prepare blank solution by diluting 2 mL HNO_3 to 100 mL with H_2O.

D. Determination

(*Caution: See Appendix* for safety notes on AAS and flame photometers.)

Follow manufacturer's directions for type of instrument available. Dilute samples if necessary to bring T readings within range of working standards. Read blank, standards, and samples at 589 nm for Na and 767 nm for K until results are reproducible; record % T or % absorption for each.

E. Calculations

For flame emission photometers not equipped with direct readout:

mg Na or K/100 g

$$= 100 \times F \times \left\{ \left[\frac{(E_x + E_1)}{(E_2 - E_1)} \times (C_2 - C_1) \right] + C_1 \right\} / g \ sample$$

where E_x = (% T of unknown) − (% T of blank); E_1 = (% T of standard of lower concentration than sample) − (% T of blank); E_2 = (% T of standard of higher concentration than sample) − (% T of blank); C_1 = mg Na or K/mL in standard of lower concentration than sample; C_2 = mg Na or K/mL in standard of higher concentration than sample; F = dilution factor.

For flame absorption photometers: Convert % absorption to absorbance (*A*). Plot standard curve of *A* against concentration. Read unknown concentrations.

mg Na or K/100 g = (concentration unknown $\times F \times 100$)/g sample

Reference: JAOAC **52**, 55(1969).
CAS-7440-09-7 (potassium)
CAS-7440-23-5 (sodium)

27.10   **984.27—Calcium, Copper, Iron, Magnesium,
Manganese, Phosphorus, Potassium, Sodium,
and Zinc in Infant Formula**
Inductively Coupled Plasma Emission Spectroscopic Method
First Action 1984
Final Action 1986

See Chapter 12.13.

Chapter 28
Protein

28.1

981.10—Crude Protein in Meat
Block Digestion Method
First Action 1981
Final Action 1983

A. Reagents

(a) *Catalyst tablets.*—Containing 3.5 g K_2SO_4 and 0.175 g HgO (Kjeltabs "MT" available from Tecator, Inc., 2875C Towerview Rd, Herndon, VA 22071, or equivalent).

(b) *Boric acid solution.*—4%. Dissolve 4 g H_3BO_3 in H_2O containing 0.7 mL 0.1% alcoholic solution of methyl red and 1.0 mL 0.1% alcoholic solution of bromocresol green, and dilute to 100 mL with H_2O.

(c) *Sodium hydroxide-sodium thiosulfate solution.*—Dissolve 2000 g NaOH and 125 g $Na_2S_2O_3$ in H_2O and dilute to 5 L (ca 50 mL is used per analysis).

(d) *Hydrochloric acid standard solution.*—0.2N (**936.15**).

936.15 (Standard Solution of Hydrochloric Acid)

A. Preparation of Standard Solutions

Following table gives approximate volumes of 36.5–38% HCl required to make 10 L standard solutions:

Approx. normality	mL HCl to be diluted to 10 L
0.01	8.6
0.02	17.2
0.10	86.0
0.50	430.1
1.0	860.1

B. Standard Sodium Hydroxide Method

Titrate 40 mL against standard alkali solution, **936.16C-E** (*see* 28.2), of ca same concentration as acid being standardized in 300 mL flask that has been swept free from CO_2, using CO_2-free H_2O and 3 drops phenolphthalein.

Normality = (mL standard alkali × normality of alkali)/mL HCl

If more concentrated than desired, dilute solution to required normality value by following formula:

$$V_1 = V_2 \times N_2/N_1$$

where N_2 and V_2 represent normality and volume of stock solution, respectively, and V_1 = volume to which stock solution should be diluted to obtain desired normality, N_1.

Check exact concentration of final solution by titration as above. Normality will be exact only if same indicator is used in determination as in standardization. Restandardize if indicators other than phenolphthalein are used.

Refs.: JAOAC **19**, 107, 194(1936). **49**, 250(1966). Kolthoff & Stenger, "Volumetric Analysis," **II**, 52(1947).

C. Constant Boiling Method

Dilute 822 mL HCl (36.5–38% HCl) with 750 mL H_2O. Check specific gravity with spindle and adjust to 1.10. Place 1.5 L in 2 L flat-bottom distilling flask, add ca 10 SiC grains (ca "20 mesh"), and connect to long, straight inner-tube condenser. Heat on electric hot plate and distil at 5–10 mL/min, keeping end of condenser open to air. When 1125 mL has distilled, change receivers and catch next 225 mL, which is constant boiling HCl, in erlenmeyer with end of condenser inserted into flask, but above surface of liquid. Read barometer to nearest mm at beginning and end of collection of 225 mL portion and note barometer temperature. Average readings.

Calculate air weight in grams (G) of this constant boiling HCl required to give one equivalent weight of HCl from one of following equations:

For $P_0 = 540$–669 mm Hg:
$$G = 162.255 + 0.02415\, P_0$$

For $P_0 = 670$–780 mm Hg:
$$G = 164.673 + 0.02039\, P_0$$

where P_0 = barometric pressure in mm Hg corrected to 0°C for expansion of Hg and of barometer scale. For brass scale barometer, following correction is accurate enough:
$$P_0 = P_t(1 - 0.000162t),\ \text{where } t = \text{barometer temperature in °C.}$$

Weigh required amount of constant boiling HCl in tared, stoppered flask to at least 1 part in 10,000. Dilute immediately, and finally dilute to volume with CO_2-free H_2O at desired temperature.

Refs.: JAOAC **25**, 653(1942); **36**, 96, 354(1953); **37**, 122, 462(1954).

Standard Borax Method

D. Reagents

(**a**) *Methyl red indicator.*—Dissolve 100 mg methyl red in 60 mL alcohol and dilute with H_2O to 100 mL.

(**b**) *Reference solution.*—Prepare reference solution of H_3BO_3, NaCl, and indicator corresponding to composition and volume of solution at equivalence point. For use in determination of end point of titration with $0.1N$ HCl, reference solution should be $0.1M$ in H_3BO_3 and $0.05M$ in NaCl.

(**c**) *Standard borax.*—Saturate 300 mL H_2O at 55° (not higher) with $Na_2B_4O_7 \cdot 10H_2O$ (ACS) (ca 45 g). Filter at this temperature through folded paper into 500 mL erlenmeyer. Cool filtrate to ca 10°, with continuous agitation during crystallization. Decant supernate, rinse precipitate once with 25 mL cold H_2O, and dissolve crystals in just enough H_2O at 55° to ensure complete solution (ca 200 mL). Recrystallize by cooling to ca 10°, agitating flask during crystallization.

Filter crystals onto small buchner with suction, wash precipitate once with 25 mL ice-cold H_2O, and dry crystals by washing with two 20 mL portions alcohol, drying after each washing with suction. Follow with two 20 mL portions ether. (Just before use, free alcohol and ether from any possible reacting acids by vigorously shaking each with 2–3 g of the pure, dry $Na_2B_4O_7 \cdot 10H_2O$ and then filtering.) Spread crystals on watch glass, immediately place dried $Na_2B_4O_7 \cdot 10H_2O$ in closed container over solution saturated with respect to both sucrose and NaCl, and let it remain ≥ 24 h before using. Then transfer the pure $Na_2B_4O_7 \cdot 10H_2O$ to glass-stoppered container and store in closed container over solution saturated with respect to both sucrose and NaCl (stable under these conditions 1 year).

E. Standardization

Accurately weigh enough standard $Na_2B_4O_7 \cdot 10H_2O$ to titrate ca 40 mL and transfer to 300 mL flask. Add 40 mL CO_2-free H_2O, **936.16B(a)** (see 28.2), and stopper flask. Swirl gently until sample dissolves. Add 4 drops methyl red and titrate with solution that is being standardized to equivalence point as indicated by reference solution.

$$\text{Normality} = \text{g } Na_2B_4O_7 \cdot 10H_2O \times 1000/\text{mL acid} \times 190.69$$

Standard Sodium Carbonate Method

F. Reagents

(a) *Methyl orange indicator.*—0.1% in H_2O.

(b) *Reference solution.*—80 mL CO_2-free H_2O containing 3 or 4 drops methyl orange.

(c) *Anhydrous sodium carbonate.*—Heat 250 mL H_2O to 80° and add $NaHCO_3$ (ACS), stirring until no more dissolves. Filter solution through folded paper (use of hot H_2O funnel is desirable) into erlenmeyer. Cool filtrate to ca 10°, swirling constantly during crystallization. Fine crystals of trona that separate out have approximate composition: $Na_2CO_3 \cdot NaHCO_3 \cdot 2H_2O$. Decant supernate, drain crystals by suction, and wash once with cold H_2O.

Transfer precipitate, being careful not to include any paper fibers, to large flat-bottom Pt dish. Heat 1 h at 290° in electric oven or furnace with pyrometer control. Stir contents occasionally with Pt wire. Cool in desiccator. Place the anhydrous Na_2CO_3 in glass-stoppered container and store in desiccator containing efficient desiccant. Dry at 120° and cool just before weighing.

Refs.: Kolthoff & Stenger, "Volumetric Analysis," **II**, 80(1947). Ind. Eng. Chem., Anal. Ed. **9**, 141(1937). JAOAC **22**, 563(1939).

G. Standardization

Accurately weigh enough anhydrous Na_2CO_3, (c), to titrate ca 40 mL, transfer to 300 mL erlenmeyer, and dissolve in 40 mL H_2O. Add 3 drops methyl orange and titrate until color begins to deviate from H_2O tint (reference solution). (Equivalence point has not been reached.) Boil solution gently 2 min, and cool. Titrate until color is barely different from H_2O tint of indicator.

$$\text{Normality} = \text{g } Na_2CO_3 \times 1000/\text{mL acid} \times 52.994$$

Ref.: JAOAC **22**, 102, 563(1939).

B. Apparatus

(a) *Digestion block and associated glassware.*—Tecator DS-6 or DS-20 (Tecator), or equivalent.

(b) *Distillation unit and associated glassware.*—Kjeltec 1003 (Tecator), or equivalent.

C. Determination

Accurately weigh ca 2 g well-ground and mixed sample of 7 cm N-free filter paper (e.g., Whatman 541), fold, and transfer to 250 mL digestion tube. Place tubes in fume hood and add 2 or 3 boiling stones, 2 catalyst tablets, 15 mL H_2SO_4, and *slowly* 3 mL 30–35% H_2O_2. Let reaction subside and place tubes in block digestor preheated at 410°. (Digestor must be placed in perchloric acid fume hood or be equipped with exhaust system.) Digest at 410° until mixture is clear, ca 45 min. Remove tubes and let cool ca 10 min. Do not let precipitate form; if precipitate forms, reheat. Carefully add 50–75 mL H_2O.

Place $NaOH$-$Na_2S_2O_3$ solution in alkali tank of steam distillation unit. Make sure that 50–75 mL is dispensed from unit before conducting distillation. Attach digestion tube containing diluted digest to distillation unit. Place 250 mL receiving flask containing 25 mL H_3BO_3 solution with mixed indicator on receiving platform, with tube from condenser extending below surface of absorbing solution. Steam distil until 100–125 mL collects (absorbing solution turns green from liberated NH_3). Remove digestion tube and receiving flask from unit.

Titrate absorbing solution with 0.2N HCl to neutral gray end point and record volume acid required to 0.01 mL. Titrate reagent blank similarly.

$$\% \text{ N} = (V_A - V_B) \times 1.4007 \times N/\text{g sample}$$
$$\% \text{ Protein} = (V_A - V_B) \times 1.4007 \times N \times 6.25/\text{g sample}$$

where V_A and V_B = volume standard acid required for sample and blank, respectively; 1.4007 = milliequivalent weight N $\times$ 100(%); N = normality of standard acid; and 6.25 = protein factor for meat products (16% N).

Reference: JAOAC **65**, 1339(1982).

28.2   955.04—Nitrogen (Total) in Fertilizers
Kjeldahl Method
Final Action

(Provide adequate ventilation in laboratory and do not permit accumulation of exposed Hg. *See Appendix* for safety notes on Hg.)

A. Reagents

(a) *Sulfuric acid.*—93–98% H_2SO_4, N-free.

(b) *Mercuric oxide or metallic mercury.*—HgO or Hg, reagent grade, N-free.

(c) *Potassium sulfate (or anhydrous sodium sulfate).*—Reagent grade, N-free.

(d) *Salicylic acid.*—Reagent grade, N-free.

(e) *Sulfide or thiosulfate solution.*—Dissolve 40 g commercial K_2S in 1 L H_2O. (Solution of 40 g Na_2S or 80 g $Na_2S_2O_3 \cdot 5H_2O$ in 1 L may be used.)

(f) *Sodium hydroxide.*—(*Caution: See Appendix* for safety notes on sodium and potassium hydroxide.) Pellets or solution, nitrate-free. For solution, dissolve ca 450 g solid NaOH in H_2O, cool, and dilute to 1 L. (Specific gravity of solution should be ≥ 1.36.)

(g) *Zinc granules.*—Reagent grade.

(h) *Zinc dust.*—Impalpable powder.

(i) *Methyl red indicator.*—Dissolve 1 g methyl red in 200 mL alcohol.

(j) *Hydrochloric or sulfuric acid standard solution.*—$0.5N$, or $0.1N$ when amount of N is small. Prepare as in **936.15** (*see* 28.1) or **890.01A**.

890.01A (Standard Solutions of Sulfuric Acid)

A. Preparation of Standard Solution

Following table gives approximate volumes of 95–98% H_2SO_4 necessary to make 10 L standatrd solutions:

Approx. normality	mL H_2SO_4 to be diluted to 10 L
0.01	2.8
0.02	5.6
0.10	27.7
0.50	138.1
1.0	276.1

(k) *Sodium hydroxide standard solution.*—$0.1N$ (or other specified concentration). Prepare as in **936.16**.

I. **936.16** (Standard Solution of Sodium Hydroxide)

Standard Potassium Hydrogen Phthalate Method

A. Apparatus

Use buret and pipet calibrated by NIST or by analyst. Protect exits to air of automatic burets from CO_2 contamination by suitable guard tubes containing soda-lime. Use containers of alkali-resistant glass.

B. Reagents

(a) *Carbon dioxide-free water.*—Prepare by one of following methods: (*1*) Boil H_2O 20 min and cool with soda-lime protection; (*2*) bubble air, freed from CO_2 by passing through tower of soda-lime, through H_2O 12 h.

(b) *Sodium hydroxide solution.*—$(1 + 1)$. To 1 part NaOH (reagent quality containing $<5\%$ Na_2CO_3) in flask add 1 part H_2O and swirl until solution is complete. Close with rubber stopper. Set aside until Na_2CO_3 has settled, leaving perfectly clear liquid (ca 10 days).

(c) *Acid potassium phthalate.*—NIST SRM for Acidimetry 84. Crush to pass No. 100 sieve. Dry 2 h at 120°. Cool in desiccator containing H_2SO_4.

C. Preparation of Standard Solution

Following table gives approximate volumes of NaOH solution $(1 + 1)$ necessary to make 10 L of standard solutions:

Approx. normality	mL NaOH to be diluted to 10 L
0.01	5.4
0.02	10.8
0.10	54.0
0.50	270.0
1.0	540.0

Add required volume of NaOH solution (1 + 1) to 10 L CO_2-free H_2O. Check normality, which should be slightly high, as in **936.16D**, and adjust to desired concentration by following formula:

$$V_1 = V_2 \times N_2/N_1$$

where N_2 and V_2 represent normality and volume stock solution, respectively, and V_1, volume to which stock solution should be diluted to obtain desired normality, N_1. Standardize final solution as in **936.16D** or **E**.

D. Standardization

Accurately weigh enough dried $KHC_8H_4O_4$ to titrate ca 40 mL and transfer to 300 mL flask that has been swept free from CO_2. Add 50 mL cool CO_2-free H_2O. Stopper flask and swirl gently until sample dissolves. Titrate to pH 8.6 with solution being standardized, taking precautions to exclude CO_2 and using as indicator either glass-electrode pH meter or 3 drops phenolphthalein. In latter case, determine end point by comparison with pH 8.6 buffer solution, **941.17C**, containing 3 drops phenolphthalein. Determine volume NaOH required to produce end point of blank by matching color in another flask containing 3 drops phenolphthalein and same volume CO_2-free H_2O. Subtract volume required from that used in first titration and calculate normality.

$$Normality = g\ KHC_8H_4O_4 \times 1000/mL\ NaOH \times 204.229$$

Refs.: JAOAC **19,** 107, 194(1936). NIST Certificate for Standard Reference Material 84.

Constant Boiling Hydrochloric Acid Method
E. Standardization

Accurately weigh from weighing buret enough constant boiling HCl, **936.15C** (*see* 28.1), to titrate ca 40 mL, into erlenmeyer previously swept free from CO_2. Add ca 40 mL CO_2-free H_2O, then 3–5 drops desired indicator, and titrate with solution being standardized.

$$Normality = g\ HCl \times 1000/mL\ titer \times G$$

where G has value given in **936.15C**.

Refs.: JAOAC **25,** 653(1942); **36,** 96, 354(1953); **37,** 122, 462(1954).

II. **941.17** (Standard Buffers and Indicators for Colorimetric pH Comparisons)
A. Preparation of Sulfonphthalein Indicators

	X	pH
Bromocresol green	14.3	3.8—5.4
Chlorophenol red	23.6	4.8—6.4
Bromothymol blue	16.0	6.0—7.6
Phenol red	28.2	6.8—8.4

X = mL 0.01*N* NaOH/0.1 g indicator required to form mono-Na salt. Dilute to 250 mL for 0.04% reagent.

B. Preparation of Stock Solutions
Use recently boiled and cooled H_2O.

(**a**) *Acid potassium phthalate solution.*—*0.2M.* Dry to constant weight at 110–115°. Dissolve 40.836 g in H_2O and dilute to 1 L.

(**b**) *Monopotassium phosphate solution.*—*0.2M.* Dry KH_2PO_4 to constant weight at 110–115°. Dissolve 27.232 g in H_2O and dilute to 1 L. Solution should be distinctly red with methyl red, and distinctly blue with bromophenol blue.

(**c**) *Boric acid-potassium chloride solution.*—*0.2M.* Dry H_3BO_3 to constant weight in desiccator over $CaCl_2$. Dry KCl 2 days in oven at 115–120°. Dissolve 12.405 g H_3BO_3 and 14.912 g KCl in H_2O, and dilute to 1 L.

(**d**) *Sodium hydroxide standard solution.*—*0.2M.* Prepare and standardize as in **936.16**; 0.04084 g $KHC_8H_4O_4$ = 1 mL 0.2*M* NaOH. It is preferable to use factor with solution rather than try to adjust to exactly 0.2*M*.

C. Preparation of Buffer Solutions
Prepare standard buffer solutions from designated amounts stock solutions, **941.17**, and dilute to 200 mL. For use as colorimetric standard, mix 20 mL buffer solution with 0.5 mL indicator solution, **941.17A**.

Phthalate-NaOH Mixtures

pH	0.2M KH Phthalate (mL)	0.2M NaOH (mL)
5.0	50	23.65
5.2	50	29.75
5.4	50	35.25
5.6	50	39.70
5.8	50	43.10
6.0	50	45.40
6.2	50	47.00

KH_2PO_4-NaOH Mixtures

pH	0.2M KH_2PO_4 (mL)	0.2M NaOH (mL)
5.8	50	3.66
6.0	50	5.64
6.2	50	8.55
6.4	50	12.60
6.6	50	17.74
6.8	50	23.60
7.0	50	29.54

pH	50	34.90
7.2	50	34.90
7.4	50	39.34
7.6	50	42.74
7.8	50	45.17
8.0	50	46.85

H_3BO_3-KCl-NaOH Mixtures

pH	0.2M H_3BO_3, KCl (mL)	0.2M NaOH (mL)
7.8	50	2.65
8.0	50	4.00
8.2	50	5.90
8.4	50	8.55
8.6	50	12.00

Refs.: JAOAC **24**, 583(1941). Clark, "Determination of Hydrogen-ions," 3rd Ed., pp. 91, 94, 192-202.

Standardize each standard solution with primary standard and check one against the other. Test reagents before use by blank determination with 2 g sugar, which ensures partial reduction of any nitrates present.

Caution: Use freshly opened H_2SO_4 or add dry P_2O_5 to avoid hydrolysis of nitriles and cyanates. Ratio of salt to acid (weight:volume) should be ca 1:1 at end of digestion for proper temperature control. Digestion may be incomplete at lower ratio; N may be lost at higher ratio. Each g fat consumes 10 mL H_2SO_4, and each g carbohydrate 4 mL H_2SO_4 during digestion.

B. Apparatus

(**a**) *For digestion.*—Use Kjeldahl flasks of hard, moderately thick, well-annealed glass with total capacity ca 500–800 mL. Conduct digestion over heating device adjusted to bring 250 mL H_2O at 25° to rolling boil in ca 5 min or other time as specified in method. To test heaters, preheat 10 min if gas or 30 min if electric. Add 3–4 boiling chips to prevent superheating.

(**b**) *For distillation.*—Use 500–800 mL Kjeldahl or other suitable flask, fitted with rubber stopper through which passes lower end of efficient scrubber bulb or trap to prevent mechanical carryover of NaOH during distillation. Connect upper end of bulb tube to condenser tube by rubber tubing. Trap outlet of condenser in such way as to ensure complete absorption of NH_3 distilling over into acid in receiver.

C. Improved Method for Nitrate-Free Samples

(*Caution: See Appendix* for safety notes on sulfuric acid, sodium hydroxides, and mercury.)

Place weighed sample (0.7–2.2 g) in digestion flask. Add 0.7 g HgO or 0.65 g metallic Hg, 15 g powdered K_2SO_4 or anhydrous Na_2SO_4, and 25 mL H_2SO_4. If sample >2.2 g is used, increase H_2SO_4 by 10 mL for each g sample. Place flask in inclined position and heat gently until frothing ceases (if necessary, add small amount of paraffin to reduce frothing); boil briskly until solution clears and then ≥30 min longer (2 h for samples containing organic material).

Cool, add ca 200 mL H_2O, cool $<25°$, add 25 mL of the sulfide or thiosulfate solution, and mix to precipitate Hg. Add few Zn granules to prevent bumping, tilt flask, and add layer of NaOH without agitation. (For each 10 mL H_2SO_4 used, or its equivalent in diluted H_2SO_4, add 15 g solid NaOH or enough solution to make contents strongly alkaline.) (Thiosulfate or sulfide solution may be mixed with the NaOH solution before addition to flask.) Immediately connect flask to distilling bulb on condenser, and, with tip of condenser immersed in standard acid and 5–7 drops indicator in receiver, rotate flask to mix contents thoroughly; then heat until all NH_3 has distilled (≥ 150 mL distillate). Remove receiver, wash tip of condenser, and titrate excess standard acid in distillate with standard NaOH solution. Correct for blank determination on reagents.

$$\% \text{ N} = [(\text{mL standard acid} \times \text{normality acid}) - (\text{mL standard NaOH} \\ \times \text{ normality NaOH})] \times 1.4007/\text{g sample}$$

Reference: JAOAC **38,** 56(1955).

D. Improved Kjeldahl Method for Nitrate-Containing Samples

(Not applicable to liquids or to materials with high Cl:NO_3 ratio. *Caution: See Appendix* for safety notes on sulfuric acid and mercury.)

Place weighed sample (0.7–2.2 g) in digestion flask. Add 40 mL H_2SO_4 containing 2 g salicylic acid. Shake until thoroughly mixed and let stand, with occasional shaking, ≥ 30 min; then add (*1*) 5 g $Na_2S_2O_3 \cdot 5H_2O$ or (*2*) 2 g Zn dust (as impalpable powder, not granulated Zn or filings). Shake and let stand 5 min; then heat over low flame until frothing ceases. Turn off heat, add 0.7 g HgO (or 0.65 g metallic Hg) and 15 g powdered K_2SO_4 (or anhydrous Na_2SO_4), and boil briskly until solution clears, then ≥ 30 min longer (2 h for samples containing organic material).

Proceed as in second paragraph of **955.04C**.

Reference: JAOAC **51,** 446(1968).
CAS-7727-37-9 (nitrogen)

28.3   977.02—Nitrogen (Total) (Crude Protein) in Plants
First Action 1977

A. Automated Method
Proceed as in **976.05**.

976.05 (Protein [Crude] in Animal Feed, Automated Kjeldahl Method)
A. Principle
Automation of macro Kjeldahl method is in 6 steps: sample and reagent addition, initial and final digestion, cooling and dilution, NaOH addition, steam distillation and titration, and automatic pumping of flask contents to waste. Chemistry is carried out in macro Kjeldahl flasks equipped with side arms which are rotated at 3 min intervals through each successive step.

B. Apparatus

(**a**) *Kjeldahl (protein/nitrogen) analyzer.*—Kjel-Foss Automatic, Model 16210 (Foss Food Technology Corp.), or equivalent.

(**b**) *Weighing papers.*—120 × 120 mm N-free tissues, Foss Food Technology Corp., or equivalent.

C. Reagents

(**a**) *Kjel-tabs.*—Containing 5 g K_2SO_4 and 0.25 g HgO (Foss Food Technology Corp.).

(**b**) *Kjeldahl (protein/nitrogen) analyzer reagents.*—Prepare following according to manufacturer's instructions: (*1*) *Sulfuric acid.*—96–98%. (*2*) *Hydrogen peroxide.*—30–35%. (*3*) *Ammonium sulfate standard solutions.*—(*a*) *Standard solution I.*—Dissolve 30.000 ± 0.030 g $(NH_4)_2SO_4$ in H_2O and dilute to 1 L with H_2O. (*b*) *Standard solution II.*—Dissolve 0.750 ± 0.001 g $(NH_4)_2SO_4$ in H_2O and dilute to 1 L with H_2O. (*4*) *Mixed indicator solution.*—Dissolve 1.000 g methyl red and 0.250 g methylene blue in alcohol and dilute to 1 L with alcohol. Dilute 10 mL this solution to 1 L with H_2O. (*5*) *Sodium hydroxide-sodium thiosulfate solution.*—40% NaOH-8% $Na_2S_2O_3 \cdot 5H_2O$. (*6*) *Dilute sulfuric acid solution.*—0.6%. Dilute 30 mL 96–98% H_2SO_4 to 5 L with H_2O.

D. Determination

(*Caution: See Appendix* for safety notes on wet oxidation, sulfuric acid, mercury, and peroxides.)

Place 3 Kjel-tabs in special flask (500 mL of design compatible to Foss instrument) in position 1. Shift dispenser arm over flask and depress H_2SO_4 lever, initiating simultaneous addition of 10 mL 30–35% H_2O_2 and 12–15 mL 96–98% H_2SO_4 (depending on fat content of sample). To flask, add accurately weighed sample (ca 1.0 g if <45% protein, and ca 0.5 g if >45% protein) wrapped in weighing paper and close lid. Flask automatically rotates to position 2 where sample digests 3 min, and then to position 3 for 3 min additional digestion. In position 4, flask is cooled by centrifugal blower, lid opens automatically, and 140 mL H_2O is added automatically. Flask rotates to position 5, where NaOH-$Na_2S_2O_3$ solution is automatically introduced in excess. Released NH_3 is steam distilled quantitatively into 200 mL tall-form titration beaker containing 50 mL mixed indicator solution, and is simultaneously titrated automatically with dilute H_2SO_4 solution delivered by photometrically regulated syringe. Final position of syringe is measured by potentiometer, output of which feeds electronic circuitry for conversion to visual display and/or printout in % N or % protein with appropriate conversion factors. In position 6, flask is emptied. Calibrate instrument initially each day with aliquots of $(NH_4)_2SO_4$ standard solutions and check periodically as stated in operating manual.

Reference: JAOAC **59**, 141(1976).

B. Semiautomated Method

Proceed as in **976.06**

976.06 (Protein [Crude] in Animal Feed, Semiautomated Method)

A. Principle

Samples are digested in 250 mL calibrated tubes, using block digestor. *A* of NH_3-salicylate complex is read in flowcell at 660 nm, or NH_3, is distilled into standard acid and back-titrated with standard alkali.

B. Apparatus

(a) *Block digestor.*—Model BD-20 (Technicon Instruments Corp., instrument now available from Bran and Luebbe, Inc., 1025 Bush Parkway, Buffalo Grove, IL 60089). Capable of maintaining 410° and digesting 20 samples at a time in 250 mL calibrated volumetric tubes constricted at top. Block must be equipped with removable shields to enclose exposed area of tubes completely at or above height of constriction.

(b) *Automatic analyzer.*—AutoAnalyzer with following modules (Technicon Instruments Corp., instrument now available from Bran and Luebbe, Inc., 1025 Bush Parkway, Buffalo Grove, IL 60089), or equivalent: Sampler II or IV with 40/h (2:1) cam (higher ratio cams result in carry-over and poorer peak separation); proportioning pump III; NH_3 analysis cartridge No. 116-D531-01 (or construct equivalent manifold from flow diagram); AAII single channel colorimeter with 15 × 1.5–2.0 mm id tubular flowcell, matched 660 nm interference filters, and voltage stabilizer; and recorder of appropriate span. (*See* Fig. **976.06**.)

C. Reagents

(a) *Phosphate-tartrate buffer solution.*—pH 14.0. Dissolve 50 g sodium potassium tartrate and 26.8 g $Na_2HPO_4 \cdot 7H_2O$ in 600 mL H_2O. Add 54 g NaOH and dissolve. Add 1 mL Brij-35 (Technicon Instruments Corp.), dilute to 1 L with H_2O, and mix.

(b) *Sodium chloride-sulfuric acid solution.*—Dissolve 200 g NaCl in H_2O in 2 L volumetric flask. Add 15 mL H_2SO_4 and 2 mL Brij-35. Dilute to volume with H_2O and mix.

(c) *Sodium hypochlorite solution.*—Dilute 6 mL commercial bleach solution containing 5.25% available Cl to 100 mL with H_2O and mix. Prepare fresh daily.

(d) *Sodium nitroprusside-sodium salicylate solution.*— Dissolve 150 g $NaC_7H_5O_3$ and 0.3 g $Na_2Fe(CN)_5 \cdot NO \cdot 2H_2O$ in 600 mL H_2O. Add 1 mL Brij-35, dilute to 1 L with H_2O, and mix.

(e) *Nitrogen standard solutions.*—Prepare 6 standards by accurately weighing (±10 mg) 59, 118, 177, 236, 295, and 354 mg $(NH_4)_2SO_4$ primary standard (Fisher Scientific Co. No. A-938, or equivalent; dry 2 h at 105° before use and assume theoretical value of 21.20% N after drying) into individual 250 mL digestion tubes. Proceed as in **976.06G**, beginning "Add 9 g K_2SO_4, 0.42 g HgO, and 15 mL H_2SO_4 . . . ." Standards may be stored and reused until exhausted.

(f) *Sodium hydroxide-potassium sulfide solution.*—Dissolve 400 g NaOH in H_2O. While still warm, dissolve 30 g K_2S in solution, and dilute to 1 L.

D. Analytical System

If manifold is to be constructed, use clear standard pump tubes for all air and solution flows. All fittings, coils, and glass transmission lines are AAII type and size. Use glass transmission tubing for all connections after pump to colorimeter. Construct modified AO fitting on sample dilution loop using AO fitting, N13 stainless steel nipple connector, and ½″ length of 0.035″ id Tygon tubing. Insert N13 nipple approximately halfway into 0.035″ Tygon tubing. Insert tubing into side arm of AO fitting far enough so resample line will not pump any air. Space pump tubes equally across pump rollers. Cut 0.16 mL/min resample pump tube ≤1″ at entrance before connecting to side arm of AO fitting. In operation, add buffer and hypochlorite solutions through metal side arms of A10 type fittings; add salicylate solution, (**d**), through metal insert to 20T coil. Air, reagents, and sample are combined immediately after pump through injection fittings.

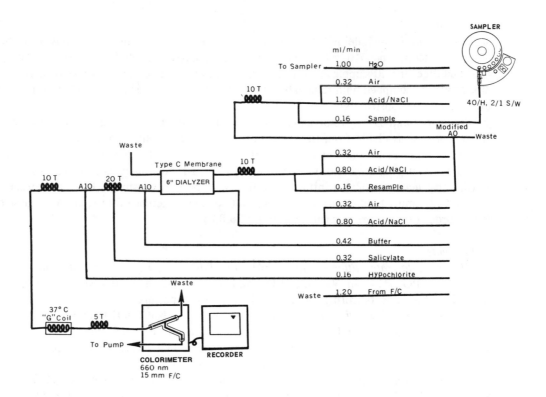

Figure 976.06.—Flow diagram for semiautomatic analysis of crude protein.

E. Start-Up

Start automatic system and place all lines except salicylate line in respective solutions. After ≥ 5 min, place salicylate line in respective solution and let system equilibrate. If precipitate forms after addition of salicylate, pH is too low. Immediately stop proportioning pump and flush coils with H_2O, using syringe. Before restarting system, check concentrations of $NaCl$-H_2SO_4 solution and phosphate-tartrate buffer solution.

Pump lowest concentration N standard solution continuously through system ≥ 5 min and adjust baseline control on colorimeter to read 10% full scale. Pump highest concentration N standard solution continuously through system until no drift exists (usually ≥ 10 min) and adjust "std. cal." control to read 85% full scale. Recorder tracings must be stable and show <0.3 division noise. If noisy conditions exist, replace dialyzer membrane. When recorder tracing indicates stable condition, immediately start sampling.

F. Shut-Down

Place reagent lines in H_2O, removing salicylate line first. Let system wash out ≥ 20 min.

G. Colorimetric Determination
(*Caution: See Appendix* for safety notes on mercury.)

Weigh samples (*See* Table **976.06**) into dry digestion tubes. Add 9 g K_2SO_4, 0.42 g HgO, and 15 mL H_2SO_4 to each tube. (Calibrated metal scoops may be used for solids.) Insert tubes into digestor block preheated to 410°, place shields around tubes, and digest 45 min.

After digestion, remove rack of tubes from block, place in hood, and let cool 8–10 min. (Time depends upon air flow around tubes.) Direct rapid spray of H_2O (kitchen sink dish rinsing sprayer works well) to bottom of each tube to dissolve acid digest completely. If precipitate forms, place tube in ultrasonic bath to aid in redissolving salt. Let cool, dilute to volume, and mix thoroughly. Transfer portion of each sample solution to AutoAnalyzer beaker.

Place standards in tray in increasing order of concentration, followed by group of samples. Analyze lowest concentration standard in duplicate, discarding first peak. Precede and follow each group of samples with standard reference curve to correct for possible drift. Analyze standards and samples at rate of 40/h, 2/1 sample-to-wash ratio. Prepare standard curve by averaging peak heights of first and second set of standards. Plot average peak height standards against N concentration contained in each 250 mL tube.

$$\% \text{ Protein} = [(\text{mg N}/250 \text{ mL from graph}) \times 6.25 \times 100]/\text{mg sample}$$

Table 976.06. Sample weight

Protein, %	Sample, g
6-24	1.5 ± 0.1
25-40	1.0 ± 0.1
41-50	0.8 ± 0.1
51-60	0.7 ± 0.1
61-90	0.5 ± 0.01
>90	Weigh sample equiv. to 50 mg N

H. Titrimetric Determination
Digest as in **976.06G**. Cool 5 min and add only enough H_2O to dissolve salts (70–75 mL). Cool and attach digestion tube to distillation head according to manufacturer's directions. Place receiver flask containing 25 mL standard acid, **936.15A** (*see* 28.1) or **890.01A** (*see* 28.2) and 5–7 drops methyl red indicator on platform. Condenser tip must be below surface of standard acid solution. Add 50 mL NaOH-K_2S solution to tube and steam distil vigorously until 125 mL distillate collects. Titrate excess acid with standard 0.1N NaOH solution, **936.16**. Correct for reagent blank.

$$\%N = [(\text{mL standard acid} \times \text{normality acid}) - (\text{mL standard NaOH} \times \text{normality NaOH})] \times 1.4007/\text{g sample}$$

$$\% \text{ crude protein} = \% \text{ N} \times 6.25$$

References: JAOAC **59**, 134(1976); **62**, 290(1979).

28.4   978.04—Nitrogen (Total) (Crude Protein) in Plants
Kjeldahl Methods
First Action 1976
Final Action 1978

A. Kjeldahl Method for Nitrate-free Samples

Proceed as in **955.04** (*see* 28.2).

B. Kjeldahl Method for Nitrate-Containing Samples

Poceed as in **955.04D**.

28.5   920.152—Protein in Fruit Products
Kjeldahl Method
Final Action

Proceed as in **955.04C** (*see* 28.2), using 5 g jelly or other fruit product containing large amount of sugar, or 10 g juice or fresh fruit, and larger amount of H_2SO_4 if necessary for complete digestion. % N $\times$ 6.25 = % protein.

28.6   992.15—Crude Protein in Meat and Meat Products
Combustion Method
First Action 1992

(Applicable to meat and meat products with 10–20% crude protein)

Method Performance:

s_r = 0.12–0.41; s_R = 0.18–0.46; RSD_r = 0.60–2.23%; RSD_R = 1.32–3.35%

A. Principle

Combustion method determines nitrogen released at high temperature into pure oxygen and measured by thermal conductivity. Nitrogen is converted to protein equivalent by using appropriate factor, 6.25 for meat and meat products.

B. Apparatus

Note: Manufacturer's recommendations must be followed for safe and accurate operation of instruments. For proper laboratory precautions in handling compressed gases required for instruments, *see* "Compressed Gas Cylinders" in *Appendix*.

(a) *Combustion instrument.*—Suitable for detecting 1–5% nitrogen (ca 5–30% protein) in meat and meat products, to within ±0.15% of theoretical nitrogen content of standard, and be repeatable with standard deviation of ≤0.15 for 10 successive determinations on same standard. Instrument capable of analyzing single sample of at least 200 mg (to reduce impact of nonhomogeniety of meat and meat products). Instrument to provide oven to operate at ≥850° in pure oxygen (for complete release of nitrogen from samples), to isolate nitrogen from other combustion products (i.e., CO_2, H_2O) for subsequent quantitation, and capable of thermal conductivity measurement of nitrogen (Leco FP428, Leco Corp., 3000 Lakeview Ave, St Joseph, MI 49085, USA; Macro-N Analyzer, Foss Hereaus Analysensysteme GmbH, Hanau 1, Germany; and PE2410, Perkin-Elmer Corp., Norwalk, CT 06859, USA are suitable). Calibrations, required by most instruments, must be conducted by using theoretical % nitrogen in pure primary standard organic compounds, such as EDTA.

(b) *Food chopper.*—With 1/8" (or less) plate, capable of grinding meat samples.

C. Reagents

The following reagents are typical but may vary depending on instrument. Consult manufacture's instructions for specific instruments.

(a) *Compressed oxygen gas.*—99.99%.

(b) *Compressed helium gas.*—99.99%.

(c) *Compressed inert gas.*—Nitrogen, or equivalent, oil and water free.

(d) *Nitrogen standard.*—Ethylenediaminetetraacetic acid (EDTA), 9.59% nitrogen, or other suitable organic material of high purity and known nitrogen content (e.g.: nicotinic acid, lysine hydrochloride).

(e) *Quartz wool.*

(f) *Glass wool.*

(g) *Alumina oxide pellets.*

(h) *Anhydrous magnesium perchlorate (MgClO$_4$).*

(i) *Sodium hydroxide on silicate carrier.*

(j) *Cu sticks.*

(k) *Cu metal turnings.*

(l) *Al foil combustion cups.*

Reagents available from several commercial manufacturers of combustion analyzer instruments [*See* **B(a)**].

D. Preparation of Sample

Pass samples through grinder 2× in succession for emulsified meat products, mixing thoroughly after each grinding; 3× in succession for non-emulsified (coarse or whole muscle) products.

E. Determination

Set instrument operating parameters (oven temperature, oxygen flow, calibration values, etc.) according to manufacturer's instructions. Allow furnace and instrument to reach operating temperature and to stabilize. Warmup time may be ca 6 h from cold start. Establish system blanks as appropriate for analysis and calibrate to blanks if necessary. At least 5 blank analyses are recommended. Calibrate instrument by using 3–5 analyses of nitrogen standard as follows:

(1) Accurately weigh 110–150 mg EDTA to nearest 0.1 mg, or equivalent amount of nitrogen if using other nitrogen standard, into tared combustion cup or foil and transfer cup/foil to open loading port on instrument. Enter or record protein conversion factor required, if appropriate for instrument used.

(2) Close port, move sample into furnace, and begin analysis.

(3) When analysis is complete (3–5 min), repeat sequence for next sample.

(4) Adjust instrument as necessary based on results from nitrogen standard.

(5) Analyze samples by repeating steps *(1)* to *(3)*.

(6) Read nitrogen results directly from instrument.

F. Calculation

$$\text{Crude protein, \%} = \text{\% nitrogen} \times 6.25$$

(*Note*: Results using this method average $1.01 \times$ results using **928.08**.)

Ref.: J. AOAC Int., in press.

28.7   939.02—Protein (Milk) in Milk Chocolate
Kjeldahl Method
Final Action

(Not applicable to chocolate products containing milk protein which has been subjected to high heat treatment)
Weigh 10.0 g finely divided milk chocolate into 250 mL or larger centrifuge bottle and extract twice with ca 100 mL ether by shaking until uniform, centrifuging, and decanting ether layer each time. Place in bottle 2-hole stopper carrying bent glass tube, and straight glass tube that extends into bottle ca ⅓ of way to bottom. Expel ether by applying suction to bent tube and drawing moderate air current through bottle while it is in moderately warm (not hot) place. When ether is expelled, pipet 100 mL H_2O into bottle. Stopper, and shake vigorously 4 min. Pipet in 100 mL *1% $Na_2C_2O_4$ solution*. Stopper, and shake vigorously 3 min. Let stand ca 10 min and again shake 1–2 min. centrifuge ca 15 min at high speed (ca 1800 rpm).

Decant supernate into beaker. Pipet 100 mL into dry 250 mL beaker and add 1 mL CH_3COOH while stirring gently. Let stand few minutes so precipitate can partly separate, and add, with stirring, 4 mL *10% tannic acid solution* (solution should be ≤ 1 week old). Let precipitate settle few minutes; then filter on 7 cm buchner with moderate suction. Filtrate should be clear. Use as filter S&S 589 white ribbon paper, or equivalent, overlaid with medium layer of paper pulp, prepared by shaking one 15 cm No. 1 Whatman paper, torn to bits, with H_2O. Using *wash solution* (add 1 mL CH_3COOH and 2 mL 10% tannic acid solution to 100 mL 1% $Na_2C_2O_4$ solution), transfer all precipitate to funnel with aid of policeman. Wash on filter 1 or 2 times. Loosen filter around edge with spatula. Carefully roll up and remove filter and precipitate to Kjeldahl flask. Transfer to flask any particles of precipitate clinging to funnel or spatula with small pieces of damp filter paper. Determine N as in **955.04C** (*see* 28.2). N $\times$ 2×6.38 = total casein and albumin in the 10 g taken for analysis. Casein and albumin $\times 1.07$ = total milk protein.

References: JAOAC **22**, 603(1939); **24**, 715(1941); **25**, 716(1942). Analyst **93**, 116(1968).

28.8   990.03—Protein (Crude) in Animal Feed
Combustion Method
First Action 1990

(Applicable to solid feeds containing 0.2–20% N)

Method Performance:

$s_r = 0.28$; $s_R = 0.52$; $RSD_r = 0.59\%$; $RSD_R = 1.10\%$

A. Principle

Nitrogen freed by combustion at high temperature in pure oxygen is measured by thermal conductivity detection and converted to equivalent protein by appropriate numerical factor.

B. Apparatus

Any instrument or device designed to measure nitrogen by combustion may be used, which is equipped to provide following conditions. Caution: Follow manufacturer's recommendation for safe operation of instrument.

(a) *Furnace.*—To maintain minimum operating temperature of 950° for pyrolysis of sample in pure (99.9%) oxygen. Some systems may require higher temperature.

(b) *Isolation system.*—To isolate liberated nitrogen gas from other combustion products for subsequent measurement by thermal conductivity detector. Device for converting NO_x products to N_2 or measuring N as NO_2 may be required and included in the design.

(c) *Detection system.*—To interpret detection response as % nitrogen w/w. May include features such as calibration on standard material, blank determination, and barometric pressure compensation. Any required calibration must be based on theoretical % nitrogen in pure primary standard organic material such as EDTA.

C. Performance Requirements

System equipped as in (**B**) must meet or exceed following minimum performance specifications.

(*1*) System must be capable of measuring nitrogen in feed materials containing 0.2–20% nitrogen.

(*2*) Accuracy of system is demonstrated by making 10 successive determinations of nitrogen in nicotinic acid and 10 successive determinations in lysine·HCl. Means of determinations must be within ±0.15 of the respective theoretic values, with standard deviations ≤0.15. Standard tryptophan may be substituted for lysine·HCl.

(*3*) Suitable fineness of grind is that which gives relative standard deviation (RSD) ≤2.0% for 10 successive determinations of nitrogen in mixture of corn grain and soybeans (2 + 1) that has been ground for analysis. RSD, % = (SD/mean %N) x 100.

    Fineness (ca 0.5 mm) required to achieve this precision must be used for all mixed feeds and other nonhomogeneous materials.

D. Calculation

Crude protein, % = %N x 6.25, or %N x 5.70 in case of wheat grains.

Ref.: JAOAC **72**, 770(1989)

28.9   990.02—Protein (Crude) in Animal Feed
Semiautomated Method—Alternative System
First Action 1990

A. *Principle*

See **976.06A** (*see* 28.3).

B. *Apparatus*

(**a**) *Block digestor.*—Capable of maintaining temperature of 410°.

(**b**) *Autoanalyzer.*—Traacs 800 continuous flow autoanalyzer with protein manifold No. 165-D004-03, as illustrated in Fig. **990.02** (Bran & Luebbe, Technicon Industrial Systems). Sample probe should be either Kel-F- or Teflon-coated.

C. *Reagents*

(**a**) *Sodium hypochlorite solution.*—Dilute 6 mL concentrated bleach solution containing 5.25% available Cl (Clorox, or equivalent) to 100 mL with water, and mix. Prepare fresh daily.

(**b**) *Wetting agent.*—Add 50 mL methanol to 50 mL Triton X-100® (Sigma Chemical Co.), and mix.

(**c**) *System wash solution.*—Add 1 mL wetting agent, (**b**), to 1 L H_2O, and mix.

(**d**) *Sodium chloride–sulfuric acid solution.*—Dissolve 10 g NaCl in water, add 7.5 mL H_2SO_4 and 1 mL wetting agent, (**b**), dilute to 1 L with water, and mix.

(**e**) *Sodium salicylate–sodium nitroprusside solution.*—Dissolve 150 g $NaC_7H_5O_3$ and 0.3 g $Na_2[Fe(NO)(CN)_5] \cdot 2H_2O$ in 600 mL H_2O, dilute to 1 L with water, and mix. Vacuum filter through 0.45 μm porosity filter and transfer to light-resistent container.

(**f**) *Phosphate–tartrate buffer solution.*—pH 14.0. Dissolve 50

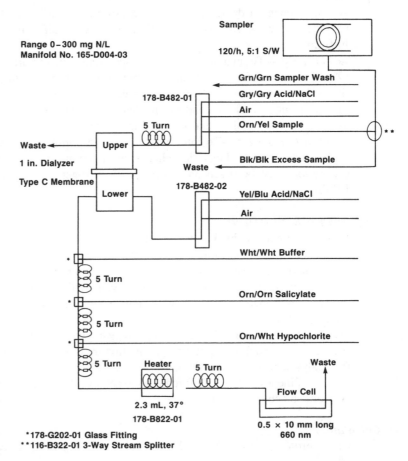

Figure 990.02.—Flow diagram for crude protein determination on alternative system.

g NaK tartrate and 26.8 g $Na_2HPO_4 \cdot 7H_2O$ in 600 mL H_2O. Add 54 g NaOH and dissolve. Cool, dilute to 1 L with water, and mix.

(**g**) *Sampler wash solution.*—6% H_2SO_4. Dissolve 60 mL H_2SO_4 in 800 mL H_2O, cool, dilute to 1 L, and mix.

(**h**) *Nitrogen standard solutions.*—Prepare 6 standards by accurately weighing to 4 decimal places primary standard $(NH_4)_2SO_4$ (Fisher Scientific Co. No. A-938, or equivalent; dry 2 h at 105° before use) to following target amounts, ± 10 mg: 0, 60, 120, 180, 240, and 300 mg. Transfer to individual 250 mL digestion tubes and proceed as in **976.06G**, beginning "Add 9 g K_2SO_4, 0.42 g HgO, and 15 mL H_2SO_4. . . ." Determine nitrogen content as [wt $(NH_4)_2SO_4$] x (%N actually certified). Standards may be stored and used up to 45 days.

D. Determination

Prepare samples as in **976.06G**, paragraphs 1 and 2.

When starting instrument, begin pumping salicylate reagent only after other reagents have been pumping 3–4 min. Follow reverse procedure to shut down instrument.

Use the following parameters to analyze samples: 120 samples/h; 5.0 sample:wash ratio; no pecking; use base correction; cubic standard curve fit; base not in calibration curve. Use protocol P,2N,6C,H,2L (10S,I) times m, H,2L,2N,G,4N,E, where m can be any number from 1 to 4.

Enter standard concentrations as mg N/250 mL. Arrange standards in descending order, with gain peak referenced to initial high standard. Null and internal standard peaks are to be high standard solution.

Exercise caution when using repeated sampling from same cup, other than for null peaks, because probe will gradually contaminate solution.

$$\text{Protein, \%} = [(C/W) \times 6.25] \times 100$$

where C = calculated sample concentration, mg N/250 mL; W = sample weight, mg; and 6.25 = nitrogen-to-protein conversion factor.

Ref.: JAOAC **73**, 31(1990)

28.10 920.87—Protein (Total) in Flour
Final Action

Place weighed sample (0.7–2.2 g) in digestion flask. Add 0.7 g HgO or 0.65 g metallic Hg, 15 g powdered K_2SO_4 or anhydrous Na_2SO_4, and 25 mL H_2SO_4. If sample >2.2 g is used, increase H_2SO_4 by 10 mL for each g sample. Place flask in inclined position and heat gently until frothing ceases (If necessary, add small amount of paraffin to reduce frothing.); boil briskly until solution clears and then ≥30 min longer (2 h for samples containing organic material).

Cool, add ca 200 mL H_2O, cool <25°, add 25 mL of the sulfide or thiosulfate solution, and mix to precipitate Hg. Add few Zn granules to prevent bumping, tilt flask, and add layer of NaOH without agitation. (For each 10 mL H_2SO_4 used, or its equivalent in diluted H_2SO_4, add 15 g solid NaOH or enough solution to make contents strongly alkaline.) (Thiosulfate or sulfide solution may be mixed with the NaOH solution before addition to flask.) Immediately connect flask to distilling bulb on condenser, and, with tip of condenser immersed in standard acid and 5–7 drops indicator in receiver, rotate flask to mix contents thoroughly; then heat until all NH_3 had distilled

(≥ 150 mL distillate). Remove receiver, wash tip of condenser, and titrate excess standard acid in distillate with standard NaOH solution. Correct for blank determination on reagents.

$$\% \text{ N} = [(\text{mL standard acid} \times \text{normality acid}) - (\text{mL standard NaOH} \times \text{normality NaOH})] \times 1.4007/\text{g sample}$$

Multiply % N by 5.7 to obtain % protein.

28.11 945.18B—Cereal Adjuncts
Final Action

B. Protein
Proceed as in **920.49** and **920.53**. Multiply results by 6.25.

I. 920.49 (Beer, Preparation of Sample)
Remove CO_2 by transferring sample to large flask and shaking, gently at first and then vigorously, keeping temperature of beer at 20–25°. If necessary, remove suspended material by passing the CO_2-free beer through dry filter paper.

II. 920.53 (Protein in Beer, Kjeldahl Method)
To 25 mL prepared sample, **920.49**, at 20° in Kjeldahl flask, add 2–3 mL H_2SO_4 and concentrate to sirupy consistency. Determine N as follows: Place weighed sample (0.7–2.2 g) in digestion flask. Add 0.7 g HgO or 0.65 g metallic Hg, 15 g powdered K_2SO_4 or anhydrous Na_2SO_4, and 25 mL H_2SO_4. If sample >2.2 g is used, increase H_2SO_4 by 10 mL for each g sample. Place flask in inclined position and heat gently until frothing ceases (if necessary, add small amount of paraffin to reduce frothing); boil briskly until solution clears and then ≥ 30 min longer (2 h for samples containing organic material).

Cool, add ca 200 mL H_2O cool, to <25°, add 25 mL of the sulfide or thiosulfate solution, and mix to precipitate Hg. Add few Zn granules to prevent bumping, tilt flask, and add layer of NaOH without agitation.

(For each 10 mL H_2SO_4 used, or its equivalent in diluted H_2SO_4, add 15 g solid NaOH or enough solution to make contents strongly alkaline.) (Thiosulfate or sulfide solution may be mixed with the NaOH solution before addition to flask.) Immediately connect flask to distilling bulb on condenser, and, with tip of condenser immersed in standard acid and 5–7 drops indicator in receiver, rotate flask to mix contents thoroughly; then heat until all NH_3 has distilled (≥ 150 mL distillate). Remove receiver, wash tip of condenser, and titrate excess standard acid in distillate with standard NaOH solution. Correct for blank determination on reagents.

$$\% \text{ N} = [(\text{mL standard acid} \times \text{normality acid}) - (\text{mL standard NaOH} \times \text{normality NaOH})] \times 1.4007/\text{g sample}$$

$$\% \text{ N} \times 6.25 = \% \text{ protein}$$

$$\text{\% Protein} = [(\text{mL } 0.1N \text{ acid} - \text{mL } 0.1N \text{ base}) \times 1.4 \times 6.25 \times 100]/(\text{specific gravity} \times \text{mL sample} \times 1000)$$

28.12   930.25—Protein in Macaroni Products
Final Action

Determine N as in **920.87** (*see* 28.10), using 1 g prepared sample, **926.06**. Percent protein = % N × 5.7 × for wheat, % N × 6.25 for all other grains.

> **926.06** (Macaroni Products, Preparation of Samples)
> Select from lot to be analyzed enough strips or pieces to assure representative sample, break these into small fragments with hands or in mill, and mix well. Grind 300–500 g in mill until all material passes through No. 20 sieve. Keep ground sample in sealed container to prevent moisture changes.
> Reference: JAOAC **9**, 43, 396(1926).

Reference: JAOAC **9**, 43(1926).

28.13   950.36—Protein in Bread
Final Action

Determine N as in **920.87** (*see* 28.10), using 2 g prepared air-dried ground sample, **926.04**. Multiply % N by factor 5.7 to obtain % protein.

> **926.04** (Bread, Preparation of Sample)
> (a) *All types of bread not containing fruit.*—Cut loaf, or ½ loaf, of bread into slices 2–3 mm thick. Spread slices on paper and let dry in warm room until sufficiently crisp and brittle to grind well in mill. Grind entire sample to pass No. 20 sieve, mix well, and keep in air-tight container.
> References: JAOAC **9**, 42(1926); **15**, 72(1932); **17**, 65(1934).
> (b) *Raisin bread.*—Proceed as in (a), except comminute by passing twice through food chopper instead of grinder.

28.14   991.20—Nitrogen (Total) in Milk
Kjeldahl Methods
First Action 1991

(*Caution*: *See Appendix* for safety notes on H_2SO_4, HCl, fuming acids, NaOH, ethanol,
and use of electrical equipment.)

Method Performance:
$s_r = 0.014$; $s_R = 0.017$; $RSD_r = 0.385\%$; $RSD_R = 0.504\%$

A. Principle

Milk is digested in H_2SO_4, using $CuSO_4 \cdot 5H_2O$ as catalyst with K_2SO_4 as boiling point elevator, to release nitrogen from protein and retain nitrogen as ammonium salt. Concentrated NaOH is added to release NH_3, which is distilled, collected in H_3BO_3 solution, and titrated.

Traditional Method

B. Apparatus

(a) *Digestion flasks.*—Kjeldahl. Hard, moderately thick, well-annealed glass. Total capacity ca 500 or 800 mL.

(b) *Distillation flasks.*—Same Kjeldahl flask as in (a), fitted with rubber stopper through which passes lower end of efficient rubber bulb or trap to prevent mechanical carryover of NaOH during distillation. Connect upper end of bulb to condenser tube by rubber tubing. Use graduated 500 mL Erlenmeyer titration flask to collect distillate. Trap outlet of condenser in manner to ensure complete absorption of NH_3 distilled into boric acid solution.

(c) *Digestion/distillation system.*—Traditional apparatus with adjustable controls for individual flasks.

(d) *Titration buret.*—50 mL. Class A or equivalent.

C. Reagents

(a) *Sulfuric acid.*—95–98% H_2SO_4. Nitrogen free.

(b) *Copper catalyst solution.*—$CuSO_4 \cdot 5H_2O$. Nitrogen free. Prepare solution 0.05 g/mL H_2O.

(c) *Potassium sulfate.*—K_2SO_4. Nitrogen free.

(d) *Sodium hydroxide solution.*—50% w/w nitrate-free NaOH.

(e) *Boiling chips.*—Mesh size 10 suggested. High purity, amphoteric alundum granules, plain.

(f) *Methyl red/bromocresol green indicator solution.*—Dissolve 0.2 g methyl red and dilute to 100 mL in 95% ethanol. Dissolve 1.0 g bromocresol green and dilute to 500 mL in 95% ethanol. Mix 1 part methyl red solution with 5 parts bromocresol green solution (combine all of both solutions).

(g) *Boric acid solution.*—4%, with indicator. Dissolve 40 g H_3BO_3 and dilute to 1 L in water and add 3 mL methyl red/bromocresol green indicator solution, (f). Solution will be light orange color.

(h) *Hydrochloric acid standard solution.*—0.1000N. Prepare as in **936.15** (*see* 28.1) or use premade solution of certified specification range 0.0995–0.1005N and use 0.1000N for calculation.

(i) *Ammonium sulfate.*—99.9% $(NH_4)_2SO_4$.

(j) *Tryptophan or lysine hydrochloride.*—99% $C_{11}H_{12}N_2O_2$ or $C_6H_{15}ClN_2O_2$.

(k) *Sucrose.*—Nitrogen free.

D. Sample Preparation

Add 15.00 g K_2SO_4, 1 mL $CuSO_4 \cdot 5H_2O$ catalyst solution, and 8–10 boiling chips to digestion flask. Warm milk to 38 ± 1°. Mix milk as in **925.21**. Weigh warm sample (5 ± 0.1 mL) and immediately place in digestion flask. (*Note*: Weights must be recorded to nearest 0.0001 g.) Add 25 mL H_2SO_4, rinsing any milk on neck of flask down into bulb. Flask may be stoppered and held for digestion at later time. Digest and distill a blank (all reagents and no sample) each day.

> **925.21** (Preparation of Milk Sample, Procedure)
> Bring sample to ca 20°, mix until homogeneous by pouring into clean receptacle and back repeatedly, and promptly weigh or measure test portion. If lumps of cream do not disperse, warm sample in H_2O bath to ca 38° and keep mixing until homogeneous, using policeman, if necessary, to reincorporate any cream adhering to container or stopper. Where practical and fat remains dispersed, cool warmed samples to ca 20° before transferring test portion.
>
> When Babcock method, **989.04C** (*see* Chapter 18.12), is used, adjust both fresh and composite samples to ca 38°, mix until homogeneous as above, and immediately pipet portions into test bottles.

E. Determination

(**a**) *Digestion burner setting*.—Conduct digestion over heating device that can be adjusted to bring 250 mL H_2O at 25° to rolling boil in ca 5–6 min. To determine maximum heater setting to be used during digestion, preheat 10 min (gas) or 30 min (electric) at burner setting to be evaluated. Add 3 or 4 boiling chips to 250 mL H_2O at 25° and place flask on preheated burner. Determine heater setting that brings water from 25° to rolling boil in 5–6 min on each burner. This is maximum burner setting to be used during digestion.

(**b**) *Digestion*.—Place flask in inclined position with fume ejection system on. Start on setting low enough so that sample does not foam up neck of Kjeldahl flask. Digest at least 20 min or until white fumes appear in flask. Next, increase burner setting half way to maximum burner setting determined in (**a**) and heat for 15 min. At end of another 15 min, increase heat to maximum setting determined in (**a**). When digest clears (clear with light blue–green color), continue to *boil* 1–1.5 h at maximum setting (total time ca 1.8–2.25 h).

To determine specific boil time needed for analysis conditions in your laboratory, select a high protein, high fat milk sample and determine protein content using different boil times (1–1.5 h) after clearing. Mean protein test increases with increasing (0–1.5 h) boil time, becomes constant, and then decreases when boil time is too long. Select boil time that yields maximum protein test.

At end of digestion, digest should be clear and free of undigested material. Cool acid digest to room temperature (ca 25 min). Cooled digest should be liquid or liquid with few small crystals. (Large amount of crystallization before addition of water indicates too little residual H_2SO_4 at end of digestion and can result in low test values.) After digest is cooled to room temperature, add 300 mL H_2O to flask and swirl to mix (for 800 mL flasks add 400 mL H_2O). When room temperature water is added some crystals may form and then go into solution; this is normal. Let mixture cool to room temperature before distillation. Flasks can be stoppered for distillation at later time.

(**c**) *Distillation*.—Turn on condenser water. Add 50 mL H_3BO_3 solution with indicator to graduated 500 mL Erlenmeyer titration flask and place flask under condenser tip so that tip is well below H_3BO_3 solution surface. To room temperature diluted digest, carefully add 75 mL 50% NaOH down sidewall of Kjeldahl flask with no agitation. NaOH forms clear layer under the diluted digest. Immediately connect flask to distillation bulb on condenser. Vigorously swirl flask to mix contents thoroughly; heat until all NH_3 has been distilled ($\geq$ 150 mL distillate; $\geq$ 200 mL total volume). Do not leave distillation unattended. Flasks (500 mL) may bump at this point (ca 150 mL distillate; 200 mL total volume). Lower receiving flask and let liquid drain from condenser tip. Turn off distillation heater. Titrate H_3BO_3 receiving solution with standard 0.1000N HCl solution to first trace of pink. Lighted stir plate may aid visualization of end point. Record mL HCl to at least nearest 0.05 mL.

F. Nitrogen Recovery Verification

Run nitrogen recoveries to check accuracy of procedure and equipment.

(a) *Nitrogen loss.*—Use 0.12 g ammonium sulfate and 0.85 g sucrose per flask. Add all other reagents as stated in *Sample Preparation*, **D**. Digest and distill under same conditions as for a milk sample. Recoveries shall be at least 99%.

(b) *Digestion efficiency.*—Use 0.16 g lysine hydrochloride or 0.18 g tryptophan, with 0.67 g sucrose per flask. Add all other reagents as stated in *Sample Preparation*, **D**. Digest and distill under same conditions as for a milk sample. Recoveries shall be at least 98%.

G. Calculations

Calculate results as follows:

$$\text{Nitrogen, \%} = [1.4007 \times (V_s - V_b) \times N]/W$$

where V_s and V_b = mL HCl titrant used for sample and blank, respectively; N = normality of HCl solution; and W = sample weight, g.

Multiply percent nitrogen by factor 6.38, to calculate percent "protein." This is "protein" on a total nitrogen basis.

Maximum recommended difference between duplicates is 0.03% "protein."

H. Repeatability and Reproducibility Values

For method performance parameters obtained in collaborative study of this method, r value = 0.038 and R value = 0.049.

Block Digestor/Steam Distillation Method

I. Apparatus

(a) *Digestion block.*—Aluminum alloy block or equivalent apparatus, with adjustable temperature control and device for measuring block temperature.

(b) *Digestion block tubes.*—250 mL capacity.

(c) *Distillation unit.*—For steam distillation. To accept 250 mL digestion tubes and 500 mL titration flasks.

(d) *Distillation titration flask.*—500 mL graduated Erlenmeyer titration flask.

(e) *Titration buret.*—50 mL. Class A or equivalent.

J. Reagents

See **C(a)–(k)**.

Note: 40% w/w NaOH may be used instead of 50% w/w. Boiling chips should not be used if equipment manufacturer does not recommend such use.

K. Sample Preparation

Add 12 g K_2SO_4 and 1 mL $CuSO_4 \cdot 5H_2O$ catalyst solution to digestion tube. Warm milk to 38 $\pm$ 1°. Mix milk as in **925.21**. Weigh warm sample (5 $\pm$ 0.1 mL) and immediately place in digestion tube. (*Note*:

Weights must be recorded to nearest 0.0001 g.) Add 20 mL H_2SO_4. Tube may be stoppered and held for digestion at later time. Digest and distill a blank (all reagents and no sample) each day.

L. Determination

(a) *Digestion*.—Set block at low initial temperature to control foaming (ca 180–230°). Place tubes with aspirator connected in block digestor; suction should be just enough to remove fumes. Digest 30 min or until white fumes develop. Increase temperature to 410–430° and digest until clear. It may be necessary to increase temperature gradually over ca 20 min to control foaming. Do not let foam within tube rise higher than ca 4–5 cm below surface of fume collection device inserted into top of tube. After digest clears (clear with light blue–green color), continue to *boil* (H_2SO_4 must be boiling) for at least 1 h, total digestion time ca 1.75–2.5 h.

To determine specific length of boil time needed for analysis conditions in your laboratory, select high protein, high fat milk sample and determine protein content using different boil times (1–1.5 h) after clearing. Mean protein test increases with increasing (0–1.5 h) boil time, becomes constant, and then decreases when boil time is too long. Select boil time that yields maximum protein test. (*Note*: Before removing hot tubes from block, make sure there is no condensate layer in aspirator manifold. If there is a liquid layer, increase aspiration to remove liquid.)

At end of digestion, digest should be clear and free of undigested material. Cool digest to room temperature (ca 25 min). Cooled digest should be liquid or liquid with few small crystals at bottom of tube. (Excessive crystallization indicates too little residual H_2SO_4 at end of digestion and may cause low results. To reduce acid loss during digestion, reduce fume aspiration rate.) After digest has cooled to room temperature, add 85 mL H_2O (blanks may require 100 mL) to each tube, swirl to mix, and let cool to room temperature. When room temperature water is added some crystals may form and then go into solution; this is normal. Tubes can be stoppered for distillation at later time.

(b) *Distillation*.—Place 50% (or 40%) NaOH in alkali tank of distillation unit. Adjust volume dispensed to 55 mL (65 mL for 40% NaOH). Attach digestion tube containing diluted digest to distillation unit. Place graduated 500 mL Erlenmeyer titration flask containing 50 mL H_3BO_3 solution with indicator on receiving platform, with tube from condenser extending below surface of H_3BO_3 solution. Steam-distill until ≥150 mL distillate is collected (≥200 mL total volume). Remove receiving flask. Titrate H_3BO_3 receiving solution with standard 0.1000N HCl to first trace of pink. Lighted stir plate may aid visualization of end point. Record mL HCl to at least nearest 0.05 mL.

M. Nitrogen Recovery Verification

Run nitrogen recoveries to check accuracy of procedure and equipment.

(a) *Nitrogen loss*.—Use 0.12 g ammonium sulfate and 0.85 g sucrose per flask. Add all other reagents as stated in *Sample Preparation*, **K**. Digest and distill under same conditions as for a milk sample. Recoveries shall be at least 99%.

(b) *Digestion efficiency*.—Use 0.16 g lysine hydrochloride or 0.18 g tryptophan, with 0.67 g sucrose per flask. Add all other reagents as stated in *Sample Preparation*, **K**. Digest and distill under same conditions as for a milk sample. Recoveries shall be at least 98%.

N. Calculations

See **G**.

O. Repeatability and Reproducibility Values

For method performance parameters obtained in collaborative study of this method, r value = 0.038 and R value = 0.049.

Ref.: JAOAC **73**, 849(1990).

28.15   991.22—Protein Nitrogen Content of Milk
Kjeldahl Method
First Action 1991

Direct Method

Method Performance:

$s_r = 0.008$; $s_R = 0.021$; $RSD_r = 0.285\%$; $RSD_R = 0.702\%$

A. Principle

Protein is precipitated from milk by trichloroacetic acid (TCA) solution. Precipitation *must be* done in Kjeldahl flask or tube. Final concentration of TCA in mixture is ca 12%. The 12% TCA solution, which contains nonprotein nitrogen components of sample, is separated from protein precipitate by filtration. Nitrogen content of protein precipitate is determined as in **991.20** (*see* 28.14).

B. Apparatus

See **991.20B** or **991.20I**.

C. Reagents

See **991.20C** or **991.20J** and in addition:

(a) *Trichloroacetic acid solution.*—15% w/v analytical grade CCl_3COOH. (*Caution: See Appendix* for safety note on trichloroacetic acid.) TCA is soft, white, deliquescent crystal, which should be stored in container protected from light and moisture.

D. Preparation of Sample

Warm milk to 38 ± 1°. Mix milk as in **925.21** (*see* 28.14). Immediately place weighed sample (5 ± 0.1 mL) in Kjeldahl digestion flask. Record all weights to nearest 0.0001 g. Add 5 ± 0.1 mL H_2O, rinsing any milk on neck of flask into bulb. Add 40 ± 0.5 mL 15% TCA solution to flask. Swirl mixture. Let precipitate settle (ca 5 min). Pour mixture from Kjeldahl flask through filter paper (Whatman No. 1, 15 cm, N-free; or equivalent) and collect filtrate. (Some protein precipitate will remain in Kjeldahl flask and some will be collected on paper. It is not necessary to remove precipitate from flask.)

Immediately after pouring mixture (do not let precipitate dry on neck of Kjeldahl flask), use pump dispenser to add 10 ± 0.5 mL 15% TCA to Kjeldahl flask and rinse any precipitate on neck of flask down into bulb. Swirl to mix. Pour mixture from Kjeldahl flask through same filter paper, and add filtrate to that previously collected. Immediately rinse neck of Kjeldahl flask with another 10 ± 0.5 mL rinse of 15% TCA solution. Swirl to mix and pour mixture from flask through same filter paper used earlier. Collect entire filtrate. Filtrate should be clear and free of particulate matter. At this point, filtrate is no longer needed and may be discarded in an appropriate manner.

Wearing TCA-resistant gloves, pick up filter paper; take care not to lose any precipitate. Pinch paper at top and twist sides and bottom to form oblong shape. If any precipitate remains on either inner or outer lip of Kjeldahl flask, wipe with filter paper so precipitate adheres to paper. Drop filter paper into Kjeldahl flask. Add boiling chips, K_2SO_4, $CuSO_4 \cdot 5H_2O$ catalyst solution, and H_2SO_4 as in **991.20D** or **991.20K**. Flask may be stoppered and held for digestion at later time. Digest and distill a blank solution (filter paper plus all reagents) each day that samples are analyzed. Keep record of blank values. If blank values change, identify cause.

E. Determination

Proceed as in **991.20E** or **991.20L**.

F. Calculation

Calculate protein nitrogen in milk as in **991.20G**.

G. Repeatability and Reproducibility

For method performance parameters obtained in collaborative study of this method, r value = 0.024 and R value = 0.059.

Ref.: JAOAC **74**, March/April issue (1991).

28.16   991.23—Protein Nitrogen Content of Milk
Kjeldahl Method
First Action 1991

Indirect Method

Method Performance:

$s_r = 0.014$; $s_R = 0.031$; $RSD_r = 0.483\%$; $RSD_R = 1.051\%$

A. Principle

Total nitrogen and nonprotein nitrogen contents of milk sample are determined separately. Difference between results of these 2 determinations is protein nitrogen content of milk.

B. Determination

(**a**) *Total nitrogen.*—Determine as in **991.20** (*see* 28.14).

(**b**) *Nonprotein nitrogen.*—Determine as in **991.21** (*see* 28.17).

C. Calculation

Subtract nonprotein nitrogen content from total nitrogen content of milk sample and multiply result by 6.38.

D. Repeatability and Reproducibility

For method performance parameters obtained in collaborative study of this method, r value = 0.040 and R value = 0.088.

Ref.: JAOAC **74**, March/April issue (1991).

28.17   991.21—Nonprotein Nitrogen in Whole Milk
Kjeldahl Method
First Action 1991

Method Performance:

$s_r = 0.006$; $s_R = 0.012$; $RSD_r = 2.817\%$; $RSD_R = 5.707\%$

A. Principle

Protein is precipitated from milk by addition of trichloroacetic acid (TCA) solution. Final concentration of TCA in the mixture is about 12%. Precipitated milk protein is removed by filtration. Filtrate contains nonprotein nitrogen components of milk. Nitrogen content of filtrate is determined as in **991.20** (*see* 28.14).

B. Apparatus

See **991.20B** or **991.20I**.

C. Reagents

See **991.20C** or **991.20J** and in addition:

(**a**) *Trichloroacetic acid solution.*—15% w/v analytical grade CCl_3COOH. (*Caution: See Appendix* for safety note on trichloroacetic acid.) TCA is soft, white, deliquescent crystal, which should be stored in container protected from light and moisture.

(**b**) *Hydrochloric acid standard solution.*—0.010N HCl. Prepare as in **936.15** (*see* 28.1). Alternatively, use premade solution of certified specification range 0.0101–0.0099N and use 0.010 for calculation.

D. Preparation of Sample

Warm milk to 38 ± 1°. Mix milk as in **925.21** (*see* 28.14). Immediately pipet milk (10 ± 0.1 mL) into preweighed 125 mL Erlenmeyer flask and weigh. Record all weights to nearest 0.0001 g. Add 40 ± 0.5 mL 15% TCA solution to flask. Weigh flask and contents. Swirl to mix. Let precipitate settle (ca 5 min). Filter (Whatman No. 1 paper, 15 cm, N-free; or equivalent) and collect entire filtrate. Filtrate should be clear and free of particulate matter; if it is not, repeat sample preparation. Swirl filtrate to mix. Pipet 20 ± 0.2 mL filtrate into a 50 mL beaker and weigh. Pour filtrate from beaker into Kjeldahl digestion flask that contains boiling chips, K_2SO_4, and $CuSO_4 \cdot 5H_2O$ catalyst solution as in **991.20D** or **991.20K**. Immediately reweigh empty beaker. Add H_2SO_4 as in **991.20D** or **991.20K**. Flask may be stoppered and held for digestion at later time. Digest and distill a blank solution (16 ± 0.5 mL 15% TCA and no sample) each day samples are analyzed. Keep record of blank values. If blank values change, identify cause.

E. Determination

Proceed as in **991.20E** or **991.20L**, substituting 0.010N HCl solution for 0.100N HCl solution as titrant in **991.20E(c)** or **991.20L(b)**.

F. Calculation

Calculate results as follows:

$$\text{Nitrogen, \%} = [1.4007 \times (V_s - V_b) \times N]/\{(W_f \times W_m)/[W_t - (W_m \times 0.065)]\}$$

where V_s and V_b = mL titrant used for sample and blank, respectively; N = normality of HCl solution; W_f = weight, g, of 20 mL filtrate; W_m = weight, g, of milk; and W_t = weight, g, of milk plus 40 mL 15% TCA solution. *Note:* Factor 0.065 in denominator assumes that milk contains about 3.5% fat and 3.0% true protein (i.e., 0.035 + 0.030). Factor may need to be adjusted if liquid dairy products of different composition are analyzed (i.e., concentrated or fractionated skim or whole milk products, etc.).

$$\text{"Protein equivalent," \%} = \text{\% nitrogen} \times 6.38$$

which is nonprotein nitrogen expressed as protein equivalent.

G. Repeatability and Reproducibility

For method performance parameters obtained in collaborative study of this method, r value = 0.016 and R value = 0.033.

Ref.: JAOAC **74**, March/April issue (1991).

28.18   930.33—Protein in Ice Cream and Frozen Desserts
Final Action

A. Kjeldahl Method

Proceed as in **920.105**, using 4–5 g sample.

920.105 (Nitrogen [Total] in Milk, Kjeldahl Method, *IDF-ISO-AOAC Method*)

Transfer 5 g sample to Kjeldahl digestion flask. Add 0.7 g HgO or 0.65 g metallic Hg, 15 g powdered K_2SO_4 or anhydrous Na_2SO_4, and 25 mL H_2SO_4. If sample >2.2 g is used, increase H_2SO_4 by 10 mL for each g sample. Place flask in inclined position and heat gently until frothing ceases (if necessary, add small amount of paraffin to reduce frothing); boil briskly until solution clears and then ≥30 min longer (2 h for samples containing organic material).

Cool, add ca 200 mL H_2O, cool <25°, add 25 mL of the sulfide or thiosulfate solution, and mix to precipitate Hg. Add few Zn granules to prevent bumping, tilt flask, and add layer of NaOH without agitation. (For each 10 mL H_2SO_4 used, or its equivalent in diluted H_2SO_4, add 15 g solid NaOH or enough solution to make contents strongly alkaline.) (Thiosulfate or sulfide solution may be mixed with the NaOH solution before addition to flask.) Immediately connect flask to distilling bulb on condenser, and, with tip of condenser immersed in standard acid and 5–7 drops indicator in receiver, rotate flask to mix contents thoroughly; then heat until all NH_3 has distilled (≥150 mL distillate). Remove receiver, wash tip of condenser, and titrate excess standard acid in distillate with standard NaOH solution. Correct for blank determination on reagents.

$$\% \text{ N} = [(\text{mL standard acid} \times \text{normality acid}) - (\text{mL standard NaOH} \times \text{normality NaOH})] \times 1.4007/\text{g sample}$$
$$\% \text{ N} \times 6.38 = \% \text{ "protein"}$$

B. Dye Binding Method

Proceed as in **967.12** (*see* 28.20).

28.19   930.29—Protein in Dried Milk
Final Action

A. Kjeldahl Method

Weigh 1 g sample into Kjeldahl digestion flask and determine N as in **920.105** (*see* 28.18).
$$\% \text{ N} \times 6.38 = \% \text{ "protein"}$$

B. Dye Binding Method

Proceed as in **967.12** (*see* 28.20).

28.20   967.12—Protein in Milk
Dye Binding Method I
First Action 1967
Final Action 1970

A. Reagents

(**a**) *Purified Acid Orange 12.*—Dissolve 100 g dye in 400 mL boiling H_2O and stir in 400 mL boiling denatured alcohol. Let cool at 0–5° ca 15 h. Filter through buchner, wash once with cold alcohol, and continue suction until alcohol is removed. Dry at 125°. Repeat recrystallization and dry in vacuum oven at 100°.

(**b**) *Reagent dye solution.*—(*1*) *Formulation I.*—Dissolve 1.300 g (corrected for assay) twice recrystallized Acid Orange 12 in 1 L 0.05M phosphate buffer, (**d**). (*2*) *Formulation II.*[1]—Dissolve 1.320 g (corrected for assay) twice recrystallized Acid Orange 12 in 1 L solution containing 60 mL CH_3COOH and 10 g oxalic acid.

Make assay correction by calculating dye concentration, c, in solution from A, using equation $c = A/(5.90 \times b)$, where b is mm path length of cell. Check solution further against either milk of known protein content or previous valid dye solution. (Same dye formulation must be used for assay and calibration.)

---

[1]Official First Action as an alternative for, but not interchangeable with, Formulation I.

(c) *Reference dye solution.*—Dissolve 0.600 g twice recrystallized Acid Orange 12 and 1 mL propionic acid in ca 900 mL H_2O. Dilute to 1 L with H_2O. Correct for assay as in (b) above.

(Recrystallized dye and solutions available from Udy Corporation, 201 Rome Ct, Fort Collins, CO 80524.)

(d) *0.05M Phosphate buffer.*—pH 1.8–1.9. Dissolve 3.4 g KH_2PO_4, 3.4 mL H_3PO_4 (1 (85%) + 1), 60 mL CH_3COOH, 1 mL propionic acid, and 2 g oxalic acid in ca 800 mL H_2O. Dilute to 1 L with H_2O.

B. Apparatus

(a) *Spectrophotometer.*—Photoelectric colorimeter or spectrophotometer set at 480 nm. Use buffer dilutions of reagent dye solution representing 0.350, 0.600, 0.750, and 0.850 g/L to calibrate spectrophotometer. Plot A against concentration to use as calibration chart.

(b) *Short-path cell.*—Cell with path length ca 0.3 mm; flow-through type is convenient. Measure A_s at 370 nm of 0.0400 g/L K_2CrO_4 in 0.05N KOH. Calculate path length in mm, b, from $b = A_s/0.09914$. Arrange drain tube, and supply tube if any, according to manufacturer's instructions to ensure proper flow and liquid levels.

Suitable colorimeter with short-path, flow-through cell, and calibration curve are available from Udy Corporation.

(c) *Automatic pipet.*—Adjust to deliver 40.44 g reagent dye solution at 20° (equivalent to 39.887 g H_2O; 40 mL). Adjust so that 10 successive deliveries are all within 40.44 ± 0.02 g by weight.

(d) *Syringe.*—Standardize sampling syringe to deliver 2.24 mL at 20° (equivalent to 2.2337 g H_2O).

(e) *Poly(ethylene) plastic bag.*—6 oz, Whirlpak (available from Fisher Scientific Co.), or equivalent.

C. Preparation of Samples

(a) *Fluid milk, ice cream mix.*—Use as received.

(b) *Buttermilk, half-and-half, chocolate drink.*— Warm to 35–38° and agitate thoroughly.

(c) *Nonfat dry milk (NFDM).*—Use as powder or reconstitute as follows: Weigh plastic bag to nearest 0.5 mg. Add 1 level tablespoon NFDM (ca 7.5 g) and reweigh. Add ca 75 mL (ca 60°) H_2O. Seal bag and shake vigorously 3 min. Let cool to room temperature. Do not use H_2O bath. Reweigh. Refrigerate overnight. Reconstitute new portion of NFDM sample for each replicate.

D. Determination

Zero spectrophotometer. Adjust gain so that reference dye solution, (c), reads 42%T at 480 nm. Place 2.24 mL milk, buttermilk, or half-and-half, 2.5–2.8 mL chocolate drink or reconstituted NFDM, from syringe, or 2.0–2.3 g ice cream mix or 0.22–0.24 g NFDM powder in 2 oz squeeze-type polyethylene dispenser bottle with fitted spun glass paper inside cap. Determine sample weight to 0.5 mg. Add 40.44 g reagent dye solution, (b), to bottle by automatic pipet. Shake vigorously 30 s, except shake bottle containing NFDM powder 3 min. Reset reference dye solution reading at 42%T, if necessary. Drop filtrate from dispenser bottle into cell funnel and draw into cell. When reading is constant, record to nearest 0.1%, avoiding parallax. Check spectrophotometer gain. If reading is not 42% with reference dye solution, adjust instrument, and reread sample.

All solutions must be 25 ± 1° when placed in cell. Measure temperature before reading; solution warms while in instrument.

E. Calculations

(a) *For formulation I.*—Using calibration chart prepared for instrument, determine dye concentration (mg/mL) in sample filtrate from observed reading. Volume = (1/1.012) × (g sample + 40.44); mg dye not bound = volume × dye concentration; mg bound dye = 52 mg dye available − mg dye not bound. Protein in mg = mg bound dye/0.312.

$$\% \text{ Protein} = \text{mg protein}/(\text{g sample} \times 10)$$
$$\% \text{ Protein in NFDM} = \% \text{ protein in reconstituted NFDM}$$
$$\times \text{ g reconstituted NFDM prepared}/\text{g NFDM sample used}$$

(b) *For formulation II.*—Using calibration chart prepared for instrument, determine dye concentration (mg/mL) in sample filtrate from observed reading.

$$\% \text{ Protein} = (1.250 - \text{sample dye concentration})/0.1824$$

References: JAOAC **50**, 542, 557(1967); **51**, 811(1968); **52**, 138(1969); **58**, 773(1975).

28.21   975.17—Protein in Milk
Dye Binding Method II
First Action 1975
IDF-ISO-AOAC Method

A. *Reagents and Apparatus*

(a) *Reagent dye solutions.*—(*1*) *Working solution.*—Dissolve 9.0–9.5 g Amido Black 10B (available from Merck and Co., Inc.) in ca 3 L H_2O by heating to ca 70°. Separately dissolve 158.40 g citric acid·H_2O, 19.80 g Na_2HPO_4·$2H_2O$, and 3 g thymol in ca 2 L H_2O. Add resulting buffer solution to dye solution. Add exactly 10 kg H_2O. Let dye solution stand overnight before use. (*2*) *Reference standard solution.*—Dilute 1 part working solution with 2.5 parts (w/w) H_2O.

(b) *Spectrophotometer.*—Photoelectric colorimeter or spectrophotometer set at 620 nm with 0–100 scale and nonlinear protein scale from 2.5 to 5.5% (such as ProMilk Mark II apparatus or automatic Pro-Milk PMA manufactured by Foss Food Technology Corp.); protein extremes correspond to ca 18 and 84, respectively, on 0–100 scale.

(c) *Short path cell.*—Flow-through, with ca 0.2 mm path length.

(d) *Automatic pipet.*—Adjustable to deliver ca 20 g reagent working solution at 20°. Adjust to maintain agreement of results with Kjeldahl method, **920.105** (*see* 28.18).

(e) *Syringe.*—Adjust to deliver 1.00 g H_2O at 20°.

(f) *Pneumatic pressure filter.*—Apparatus for using slight air pressure to force sample-reagent mixture through Fiberglass filter and filtrate into cell.

(Suitable equipment ((**b**)–(**f**)) is available from Foss Food Technology Corp.)

B. *Start-Up*

Zero spectrophotometer using 0–100 scale. Dispense reagent working solution through filter into cell according to manufacturer's directions. If reading is not 0 ± 0.25 scale division, adjust zero control. Dispense standard reference solution through filter into cell according to manufacturer's instructions. Adjust gain control to obtain reading of 45 on 0–100 scale. Repeat every 50 samples.

(If either gain or zero control is adjusted, repeat above steps until both readings are correct without further adjustment. This constitutes double-scale expansion.)

C. Determination

Install clean filter in mixing tube on filtration apparatus. Place 1 mL prepared sample, **967.12C** (*see* 28.20), in tube, using syringe. Dispense 20 mL reference dye solution into mixing tube. Mix according to manufacturer's directions. Apply air pressure (e.g., from squeeze bulb) to force filtrate through filter and into cell. Release pressure and read protein content from 2.5–5.5 scale. Remove and clean mixing tube, and renew filter according to manufacturer's directions.

D. Calibration

Determine protein content, **920.105**, of ca 10 milk samples of type to be analyzed containing as wide a range of protein contents as possible. Perform each determination in triplicate.

Analyze known milk samples by **975.17**. If mean difference between methods is >0.02% protein, adjust volume of reference dye solution delivered by dispenser. Increase dye volume if values from **975.17C** are high relative to **920.105** and decrease volume if low. Test known milk daily as check on validity of calibration.

Complete recalibration is necessary in event of disassembly, replacement, or repair of either sample syringe or dye-dispensing syringe; adjustments or repair to any part of photometric system, other than zero and gain adjustments referred to in **975.17B**; or use of new batch of reagent or reference dye solutions.

References: JAOAC **57**, 1338(1974); **58**, 770(1975).

28.22   975.18—Protein in Milk
Mid-Infrared Spectroscopic Method
First Action

See **972.16G** and **F** (*see* 28.23).

28.23   972.16—Fat, Lactose, Protein, and Solids in Milk
Mid-Infrared Spectroscopic Method
First Action 1972

(*Note*: Methods for fat [**905.02**, **924.05**: *see* Chapter 18], lactose [**896.01**, **930.28**, **984.15**: *see* Chapter 33] and solids [**925.23**: *see* Chapter 23] are not included.)

A. Principle

Analysis of milk by IR is based on absorption of IR energy at specific wavelengths by CH groups in fatty acid chain of fat molecules (3.48 μm), by carbonyl groups in ester linkages of fat molecules (5.723 μm), by peptide linkages between amino acids of protein molecules (6.465 μm), and by OH groups in lactose molecules (9.610 μm). Total solids (TS) or solids-not-fat (SNF) are computed by assigning experimentally determined factor to percentage of all other solid milk components, and by adding this amount to appropriate % fat, protein, and lactose, or by direct mulitple regression calculations using instrument signals at combinations of above-mentioned wavelengths. Latter method has been shown to be more accurate method of determining milk solids. Analysis by IR is dependent on calibration against suitable standard method. *See* "Definitions of Terms and Explanatory Notes," (1990) *Official Methods of Analysis*, 15th ed., for calculation of regression lines.

B. Performance Specifications

Number of firms manufacture various model instruments based upon principle, **972.16A**. It is imperative that individual instrument utilized meet following performance specifications, based upon analysis of 8 samples:

Standard deviation of difference between duplicate instrument estimates:

Fat, protein, and lactose	$\leq 0.02\%$	Total solids	$\leq 0.04\%$

Mean difference between duplicate instrument estimates:

Fat, protein, and lactose	$\leq 0.02\%$	Total solids	$\leq 0.03\%$

Standard deviation of difference between instrument estimates and values by reference methods:

Fat (**905.02**), protein [**920.105** (*see* 28.18)], and lactose(**896.01B** or **930.28**)	$\leq 0.06\%$	Total solids (**925.23A**)	$\leq 0.12\%$

Mean difference between instrument estimates and values by reference methods:

Fat, protein, and lactose	$\leq 0.05\%$	Total solids	$\leq 0.09\%$

Calculate standard deviation of difference as in **969.16D**, where S_D = algebraic difference either between duplicate instrument estimates or between instrument estimates and values by reference methods.

969.16D (Fat in Milk, Automated Turbidimetric Method I)

D. Calibration

Instruments should be operated in accordance with manufacturer's instructions.

Test in triplicate 20 representative milks, 3–6% fat for unhomogenized milks, by **905.02** or **924.05C** and instrument. If instrument is also to be used for testing homogenized milk, it is necessary to run 20 homogenized milks, 1–5% fat, by **905.02** and instrument. (Lower fat range for homogenized samples is to allow for testing homogenized low fat milks.) Calculate average for each sample by each method to nearest 0.01%. Calculate standard deviation of difference (S_D) as follows:

$$S_D = \sqrt{[\sum (D^2) - (\sum D)^2/N]/(N - 1)}$$

where D = average of results by **905.02** or **924.05C** on sample minus instrumental results on same sample, e.g.,

$$[(B_1 + B_2 + B_3)/3] - [(I_1 + I_2 + I_3)/3] = D$$

where B = reading by **905.02** or **924.05C**, I = reading by instrument, and N = number of samples tested.

Instrument is properly calibrated when S_D is <0.10 for individual cow sample or ≤0.06 for herd, composite, or homogenized samples. Should S_D exceed these values, see manufacturer's instructions on how to adjust calibration. After adjustments, rerun aliquots of ≥20 samples and recalculate. Instrument is properly calibrated when, after adjustments, S_D values do not exceed limits specified for milks tested.

During any calendar day of use, make performance check consisting of comparison of results obtained on 1 milk bulk sample, using both instrument and **905.02** or **924.05C**. If difference is >0.10% fat, repeat determination on 3 additional samples. If average differences of 3 additional samples is >0.10% fat, recalibrate instrument.

C. Precautions

Differences in fat readings for homogenized and unhomogenized samples of same milk should be <0.05% to assure accurate results at high fat levels. If larger differences occur and servicing homogenizer does not correct fault, consult manufacturer. Changes in moisture vapor content of instrument console will cause changes in optical 0 and shift in calibration level. Replace desiccant frequently, preferably at end of each day, as 3–4 h are required to restore equilibrium conditions. For best accuracy, calibrate with type of milk to be analyzed (herd, individual cow, homogenized, unhomogenized, market, etc.). Do not use mixtures of cream and milk for calibration. Avoid abnormal (low lactose) milks for calibration. Single pumping of milk through instrument sample cell should purge ≥99% of previous sample. To test purging efficiency, perform fat determinations on H_2O and single pasteurized, homogenized whole milk in sequence: H_2O, H_2O, milk, milk, H_2O, etc., until total of 20 determinations have been obtained. Calculate purging efficiency = $(\Sigma M_1 - \Sigma W_2) \times 100/(\Sigma M_2 - \Sigma W_2)$ where M_1 and M_2 are first and second values for milk and W_2 second value for H_2O.

Instrument must be well maintained and functioning correctly. Malfunctions that influence calibration can cause large errors.

I. Fat

D. Calibration

Before first calibration, check linearity of output signals. Mix accurately measured volumes of H_2O and homogenized cream to prepare ca 8 mixtures of known relative fat contents covering required range. Prepare samples as in **925.21** (*see* 28.14), and pump each mixture into instrument twice, using second readings to prepare plot against relative concentrations. If plot is not linear, adjust as indicated in operating manual. Repeat measurements and adjustments until plot is linear.

If analyzing unhomogenized milks, check linearity again with ca 4 dilutions of unhomogenized cream or high fat milk. If these mixtures deviate significantly from linearity, *see* **972.16C** and check differences between readings for homogenized and unhomogenized milk samples.

Determine % fat for series of ≥8 preanalyzed (**905.02**) milk samples of type to be analyzed (*see* **972.16C**). Prepare samples as in **925.21** and analyze in triplicate. Compare averages of second and third instrument readings with standard values and follow instructions in operating manual for required changes to calibration.

Alternatively, for better accuracy, use simple linear regression equation that relates instrument estimates and standard reference values, using latter as dependent variable, to correct these tests. In earlier instruments, which do not have this capability in instrument software, this calculation must be performed ouside instrument. To perform this calculation on calibration data that are collected on successive days or weeks, it is necessary to record instrument estimates as well as final results. Purpose of this alternative, preferred procedure is to avoid adjusting instrument slope controls.

E. Determination

Prepare sample as in **925.21**. Operate instrument in accordance with manufacturer's instructions. Use A, B, or A + B filters for measurements.

II. Protein

F. Calibration

Proceed as in **972.16D**, first and third paragraph, substituting Ca propionate solution (dissolve 15.0 g pure Ca propionate·H_2O in H_2O and dilute to 1 L with H_2O at 20°) for homogenized cream to prepare mixtures of known relative concentrations from 0 to required maximum for protein. Determine % protein for series of ≥8 preanalyzed (**920.105**) milk samples having range of protein content approximately that of population of milks to be analyzed. Prepare samples as in **925.21** (*see* 28.14) and analyze in triplicate. Compare averages of second and third instrument readings with standard values and follow directions in operating manual for making required adjustments to calibration.

Alternatively, for better accuracy, use simple linear regression equation that relates instrument estimates and standard reference values, using latter as dependent variable, to correct these estimates. In earlier instruments, which do not have this capability in instrument software, this calculation must be performed outside instrument. To perform this calculation on calibration data that are collected on successive days or weeks, it is necessary to record instrument estimates as well as final results. Purpose of this alternative, preferred procedure is to avoid adjusting instrument slope controls.

G. Determination

Prepare sample as in **925.21**. Operate instrument according to manufacturer's instructions.

III. Lactose

H. Calibration

Proceed as in **972.16D**, paragraph 1, substituting lactose solution (dissolve 50.00 g lactose·H_2O and 0.25 g $HgCl_2$ in H_2O and dilute to 1 L with H_2O at 20°) for homogenized cream to prepare mixtures of known relative concentrations ranging from 0 to required maximum for lactose. Determine lactose for series of ≥8 preanalyzed (**896.01B** or **930.28**) milk samples having range of lactose content approximately that of population of milks to be analyzed.

Prepare samples as in **925.21** and analyze in triplicate. Use averages of second and third values for each sample in estimating calibration requirements. Adjust instrument controls, as directed in operating manual, to make $\Sigma L = \Sigma L'$, where L = instrument readings for lactose and L' = values from reference method.

Alternatively, for better accuracy, multiply instrument estimates by $\Sigma L'/\Sigma L$ to obtain final results. In earlier instruments, which do not have this capability in instrument software, this calculation must be performed outside instrument. To perform this calculation on calibration data that are collected on successive days or weeks, it is necessary to record instrument estimates as well as final results. Purpose of this alternative, preferred procedure is to avoid adjusting instrument slope controls.

I. Determination

Prepare sample as in **925.21**. Operate instrument according to manufacturer's instructions.

IV. Solids (Total)

J. Calibration

Use standard method **925.23A** to determine % total solids for series of ≥ 8 milks. Determine % fat, % protein, and % lactose. Calculate mean difference for total solids $(TS) - F - P - L = a$, where F, P, and L are estimates of fat, protein, and lactose, respectively. For routine control of calibration, analyze additional series of milks and adjust value for mean difference in accordance with accumulated data.

Calculate % total solids $= a + F + P + L$

Alternatively, calibrate by multiple regression to calculate equation for estimation of either TS or SNF as function of fat, protein, and lactose uncorrected signals. For recalibration, use simple linear regression equation which relates regression estimates and standard reference values, using latter as dependent variable, to correct these estimates and obtain final result. In earlier instruments, which do not have this capability in instrument software, this calculation must be performed outside instrument. To perform this calculation on calibration data that are collected on successive days or weeks, it is necessary to record regression estimates as well as final results. This alternative, preferred method has been demonstrated to be more accurate.

Note: For products that are fortified or diluted, both original multiple regression and simple regression calculations must be based on regression that forces calibration line through origin. First calculation procedure in this section, paragraph 1, cannot be used successfully with these products.

K. Computer-Based Calibration and Control

Program computer to:

(*1*) Calculate $S_2' = S_1 + [(S_2 - S_1)/PF]$, where S_2' is purge-corrected signal; S_2 is signal at any instrument channel; S_1 is same signal for previous sample; and PF is predicted purge fraction $=$ purging efficiency/100 (*see* **972.16C**). Apply correction to all signals received from instrument.

(*2*) Calculate $(\Sigma CS_2')/10$, where CS_2' is purge-corrected control milk signal. Sum control milk signals at each channel for 10 control samples, and average. At time of calibration, store and designate as required control milk samples.

(*3*) Calculate $S = S_2' + CSE$, where S is purge- and drift-corrected signal; CSE is control signal error $=$ (required control signal average) $-$ (determined control signal average) for any check on control milk. Apply value to all except control milks.

(*4*) Calculate estimates from purge- and drift-corrected signals using calibration signals, and store. Equation type is Estimate $=$ A $+$ B (main equation). Initially, A $= 0$ and B $=1$.

(*5*) Calculate calibration equations and store.

(*6*) Store random sample signals, estimates, and standard method reference results.

(*7*) Calculate and store mean difference, standard deviation of difference, limits for mean difference, and population standard deviation of difference for statistical quality control.

(*8*) Store results for checks on purging efficiency tests, homogenization efficiency tests, linearity tests, and repeatability tests.

L. Instrument Controls

For instrument with secondary slope controls, operate in uncorrected mode. For instruments without secondary slope controls, reduce interference correction coefficients to 0.

M. Control Milk

Prepare adequate supply of pasteurized, homogenized, preserved milks with % fat about that of population average. Transfer amounts for single tests to sample containers and keep refrigerated. Zero-adjust instrument channels. Heat 11 samples to 40°, and pump each through instrument, collecting signals. Average last 10 results for each signal to calculate required signal. Record required control milk signals to 4 decimals to prevent rounding errors in continuous control situation.

N. Setting Primary Slope Controls

Determine % fat, protein, and lactose on series of ≥ 8 preanalyzed (e.g., **905.02**, **920.105**, **896.01A**, or **984.15**) milks of type to be analyzed by instrument. Warm samples to 40°, mix thoroughly, and pump through instrument, collecting and correcting signals for purge and drift. For each signal calculate regression equation of type $S = aF + bP + cL$, where S is signal and F, P, and L are results for standard. At fat channel, adjust slope amplification by $1/a$. At protein and lactose channels, adjust by $1/b$ and $1/c$, respectively. Check success of attempt to obtain coefficient of 1 for main components by repeating test. Readjust slope amplifications if necessary. Lock slope controls and do not change settings thereafter. Warm 11 samples of control milk and redetermine required control milk values as indicated above.

O. First Calibration

Obtain 20 milk samples by random selection from population to be tested, and analyze by standard reference method for components to be estimated by IR method. Key standard results into computer. Warm and prepare 11 control milk samples and the calibration samples. Pump through instrument and collect and store signals. Computer applies purge correction, calculates control signal correction values, applies these to calculate milk signals, and stores these values in matrix with standard reference values. Select equation that is applicable to instrument from following main equation types.

Components	Signals			
	F_A	F	L	F_B
1. F, P, L, TS, SNF	*	*	*	
2. F, P, L, TS, SNF		*	*	*
3. F	*	*	*	*
4. F	$[0.27 \times F(1)] + [0.73 \times F(2)]$			

Note: Except for TS and SNF, all main equation types force regression line through 0. With TS and SNF, either may be used, but equation with intercept is preferred and gives better results unless product being analyzed has been fortified or diluted.

Calculate by multiple linear regression main equations for components for which IR analysis is required. It is not necessary to calculate estimates for any component for which estimates are not required or to perform standard reference method analysis for that component except when slopes for initial calibration are adjusted. However, all signals must be controlled using required control milk signal values.

P. Production Analysis

At beginning of each production period and at definite intervals during production run, check control milk signals and recalculate drift corrections for application to product samples. Interval between checks can be shortened if drift for current interval is excessive. If instrument signals stability is acceptable, 1-h interval is satisfactory. Signals for product samples are corrected for purge and drift and then are used to calculate estimates.

Q. Quality Control

Select production samples at random at predetermined intervals and perform standard reference method analyses on these. Store signals, estimates, and reference values for these samples in matrix on accumulative basis. Check control milks and make adjustments to drift correction just prior to these selections. Interval between selection (days) and number selected may be varied to suit laboratory but ≥ 5 should be selected in 1 day and ≥ 20 in 1 week. Current population standard deviations of difference between estimate and reference methods may be calculated from last 50 differences in these accumulated data.

For quality control, calculate statistical limits for daily mean difference as $3 \times$ population standard deviation/$\sqrt{N}$ where, N is number of random samples tested that day. Action situations for changing A intercept in overall equations are:

(*1*) Daily mean difference is greater than limit.

(*2*) Six successive or 7 of 8 successive or 8 of 10 successive mean differences are on same side of 0. To correct this, adjust A in opposite direction to mean of differences. To correct for (*1*), adjust A in opposite direction by excess of difference over limit plus one-third of limit. Suggested additional statistical calculations are: (a) accumulated monthly mean difference, standard deviation of difference, and limits for mean difference; and (b) accumulated annual mean difference, standard deviation of difference, and limits for mean difference. Overall objectives are to control current analyses as well as possible and to achieve annual mean difference very close to 0.

R. Recalibration

Use signals and standard reference values for last N samples in accumulated random sample data. Calculation may be made either to redetermine coefficients of main equation or by simple regression using estimates of main equation as independent variable and standard reference method values as dependent variable. Latter method would determine values for A and B in overall equation.

Whenever control milk is changed, whether at a time of recalibration or between calibrations, run 11 samples of both old and new control milks. Use drift errors of old control milk to adjust averages for new control milk signals in calculating required signals for it. Do not use control milk for longer than 1 week.

With random sample data accumulated over long periods of time, number of samples used for calibration and frequency of calibration can be optimized. Signals and standard reference values in data bank can be used to vary choices and determine net effect for different equations generated in this way.

For test population used first with this control method, optimum conditions were $N = 20$ and interval between calibrations $= 1$ week.

S. Precautions

See **972.16C** for normal precautions. This control method uses required control milk signals to control calibration level in preference to maintaining 0 settings at various channels with H_2O. Advantages are that drift errors identify signal subject to drift and that control of level is in range of test analysis. Water zeros may still be checked. Drift away from 0 indicates extraneous absorptions which could be due to excessive moisture in console, buildup of scale on cell windows, or other instrument faults. Continuous drifting in 1 direction for 0 signal should be investigated.

References: JAOAC **55**, 488(1972); **61**, 1015(1978); **62**, 1202, 1211(1979); **72**, 70, 184(1989).
CAS-63-42-3 (lactose)

28.24   986.25C—Proximate Analysis of Milk-Based Infant Formula
First Action 1986
Final Action 1988

C. Protein

Proceed as in **920.105** (*see* 28.18) and **955.04** (*see* 28.2), except use 12 g sample and do not increase amount H_2SO_4 for each g sample.

28.25   928.08—Nitrogen in Meat
Kjeldahl Method
Final Action 1974

A. Reagents

    (**a**) *Kjeldahl catalyst.*—15 g K_2SO_4 + 0.7 g HgO (commercially prepared catalysts are available containing pumice, if desired).

    (**b**) *Sulfuric acid.*—ACS.

    (**c**) *NaOH solution.*—Prepare 1200 mL NaOH (1 + 1). Let stand until clear (ca 10 days).

    (**d**) *Metallic zinc.*—Powder, ACS, to be used if catalyst does not contain pumice.

    (**e**) *Indicator solution.*—Fleisher Methyl Purple, or equivalent.

    (**f**) *Acid potassium phthalate.*—NIST Standard.

    (**g**) *Standard NaOH solution.*—0.2000 ± 0.0004N. Add 108 mL NaOH (1 + 1) to CO_2-free H_2O and dilute to 10 L. Standardize against potassium acid phthalate, using phenolphthalein indicator.

    (**h**) *Standard acid solution.*—0.2000 ± 0.0004N. Prepare either HCl or H_2SO_4 solution.

    (**i**) *Hydrochloric acid.*—Dilute 178 mL 35–37% HCl to 10 L. Standardize against standard NaOH solution, and adjust strength accordingly.

    (**j**) *Sulfuric acid.*—Dilute 55 mL 98% H_2SO_4 to 10 L. Standardize against standard NaOH solution, and adjust strength accordingly.

    (**k**) *Sodium hydroxide.—sodium thiosulfate solution.*—Dissolve 460 g $Na_2S_2O_3 \cdot 5H_2O$ in H_2O; dilute to 1 L with H_2O, and add this solution to 15,250 g NaOH dissolved in 14,250 mL H_2O. This will yield 20 L 50% (weight/volume) NaOH solution. If other volumes are desired, adjust weights of NaOH and $Na_2S_2O_3 \cdot 5H_2O$ accordingly. Specific gravity of final solution should be 1.45.

B. Determination

Place weighed sample (2.0–2.2 g) in digestion flask. Add 0.7 g HgO or 0.65 g metallic Hg, 15 g powdered K_2SO_4 or anhydrous Na_2SO_4, and 40 mL H_2SO_4. If sample >2.2 g is used, increase H_2SO_4 by 10 mL for each g sample. Place flask in inclined position and heat gently until frothing ceases (if necessary, add small amount of paraffin to reduce frothing); boil briskly until solution clears and then ≥30 min longer (2 h for samples containing organic material).

    Cool, add ca 200 mL H_2O, cool <25°, add 25 mL of the sulfide or thiosulfate solution, and mix to precipitate Hg. Add few Zn granules to prevent bumping, tilt flask, and add layer of NaOH without agitation. (For each 10 mL H_2SO_4 used, or its equivalent in diluted H_2SO_4, add 15 g solid NaOH or enough solution to make contents strongly alkaline.) (Thiosulfate or sulfide solution may be mixed with the NaOH solution before addition to flask.) Immediately connect flask to distilling bulb on condenser, and, with tip of condenser immersed in standard acid and 5–7 drops indicator in receiver, rotate flask to mix contents thoroughly; then heat until all NH_3 has distilled (≥ 150 mL distillate). Remove receiver, wash tip of condenser, and titrate excess standard acid in distillate with standard NaOH solution. Correct for blank determination on reagents.

$$\% \text{ N} = [(\text{mL standard acid} \times \text{normality acid})$$
$$- (\text{mL standard NaOH} \times \text{normality NaOH})] \times 1.4007/\text{g sample}$$

Reference: JAOAC **11**, 408(1928).

28.26   977.14—Nitrogen in Meat
Automated Method II
First Action 1977
Final Action 1981

Proceed as in **976.05** (*see* 28.3).

28.27   950.48—Protein (Crude) in Nuts and Nut Products
Improved Kjeldahl Method
First Action

Determine N as in **955.04C** (*see* 28.2), and multiply result by 5.46 for peanuts and brazil nuts, 5.18 for almonds, and 5.30 for other tree nuts and coconut. (It may be desirable to defat with petroleum ether.)

References: JAOAC **33**, 753(1950); **34**, 357(1951); **37**, 845(1954); **58**, 316(1975).

28.28   935.39C—Baked Products
Final Action

(Other than bread; not containing fruit)

C. Protein
Proceed as in **950.36** (*see* 28.13).

Chapter 29
Protein Quality

29.1 **991.29—True Protein Digestibility of Foods and Food Ingredients**
Rat Bioassay
First Action 1991

Method Performance:
$s_r = 1.0$; $s_R = 2.2$; $RSD_r = 0.9\%$; $RSD_R = 2.4\%$

A. Principle

Before protein can be absorbed, it must first undergo hydrolysis, which is initiated in the stomach and continues in the small intestine, catalyzed by proteases and peptidases. Indigestible food passes to the colon and is excreted in the feces, along with small amounts of nondietary nitrogen from bacterial cells and sloughed intestinal mucosal cells. Thus, to determine true digestibility, corrections must be made for nondietary (metabolic) nitrogen, which can be estimated as the amount of fecal nitrogen excreted when the animal is consuming protein-free diet.

B. Reagents

(a) *Mineral mixture.*—AIN-76 (Nutritional Biochemicals, Cleveland, OH) or mixture of same proportions (g/kg): calcium phosphate, dibasic, 500; sodium chloride, 74; potassium citrate, monohydrate, 220; potassium sulfate, 52; magnesium oxide, 24; manganous carbonate, 3.5; ferric citrate, 6.0; zinc carbonate, 1.6; cupric carbonate, 0.3; potassium iodate, 0.01; sodium selenite, 0.01; chromium potassium sulfate, 0.55; sucrose, finely powdered, 118.

(b) *Corn oil.*

(c) *Cellulose.*

(d) *Vitamin mixture.*—Rat Fortification Vitamin Mix (Cat. No. 904654, Nutritional Biochemicals), or equivalent that provides optimum growth of rats.

(e) *Butylated hydroxyanisole.*—BHA (Cat. No. 1253, Sigma Chemical Co.; or equivalent). Add 0.005% BHA as antioxidant if diets are stored >1 week.

(f) *Cornstarch.*

C. Preparation of Diets

Standardize diets and perform proximate analysis to adjust diet so that comparisons between samples are made with diets that have same contents of N, moisture, and fat. Freeze-dry wet samples or, alternatively, dry overnight in 100° vacuum oven. Fat content of high-fat food samples, which when added to diet mix to give 10% protein would result in >10% fat in final diet, must be lowered by extraction with ether or methanol. Grind all food samples to pass 20-mesh screen before use. Final composition of mixed diets (dry weight basis) should be 10% protein, 10% fat (allowance must be made for fat provided by test food), 2%

vitamin mix, 3.5% mineral mix, 5% cellulose (need not be added if total dietary fiber content of test food is high enough to provide ≥5% dietary fiber in final diet mix), and cornstarch to equal 100%.

Mix all dry ingredients in single batch for 5 min with mechanical mixer, add corn oil when necessary and continue mixing additional 10 min or more.

D. Proximate Analysis of Diets

Determine N by **955.04C**, **976.05**, or other appropriate Kjeldahl method (*see* Chapter 28); moisture by **927.05** or **934.01** (*see* Chapters 23.22 and 23.23, respectively); fat by **920.38A**, **983.23**, or an equivalent method (*see* Chapter 18); and dietary fiber by **985.29** (*see* Chapter 16.1).

E. Test Animals

Male weanling laboratory rats of 50–70 g from same colony. After transport from breeding colony to test laboratory, feed standard laboratory chow during acclimation for ≥2 days but ≤7 days before using.

F. Assay Groups

After acclimation, assemble groups of ≥4 rats according to weight so that total number of rats in each group is equal and all groups are within 5 g mean weight. Feed one group protein-free diet concurrently with test group(s).

G. Assay

Throughout assay period, keep each rat in individual cage of metabolic or standard type suitable for collecting spilled food and feces. Use highly absorbent paper to avoid excessive wetting of spilled feed by urine. Maintain environmental conditions as uniform as possible within 18–26° and 40–70% relative humidity. Provide water *ad libitum*, but restrict diets to 15 g/day.

Weigh diets into glass or stainless steel cups. Feed protein-free diet concurrently with test diets, in duplicate, for 4-day preliminary period and 5-day balance period (total 9 days). On each day of 5-day balance period, weigh feed consumed and collect spilled food and feces, and carefully separate and composite into open containers (one for feces and one for food). At end of 5-day balance period, air-dry spilled food for 3 days and weigh. Dry feces overnight in 100° vacuum oven, weigh, grind (micro mill or mechanical equivalent), and determine N by Kjeldahl method.

H. Calculations

Calculate true protein digestibility (*TD*) as follows:

$$TD, \% = \{[Ni - (Fn - Mn)]/Ni\} \times 100$$

where Ni = N intake, Fn = fecal N, and Mn = fecal metabolic N loss. Find N intake and fecal N by multiplying food intake and fecal weights by their respective N values. Metabolic N is value obtained from feces of rats fed protein-free diet. Use metabolic value, expressed as mg N/g diet consumed, for test diets, corrected for weight consumed, i.e., if metabolic N is 1.5 mg/g protein-free diet consumed, and 50 g of test diet is consumed, then 1.5×50 gives metabolic N for test diet.

Ref.: JAOAC **73**, 801(1990).

29.2 982.30—Protein Efficiency Ratio
Calculation Method
First Action

A. Principle

Protein efficiency ratio is calculated from the essential amino acid composition of sample protein (DC-PER) or from both essential amino acid composition and enzymatic digestibility of sample protein (C-PER). Used together, C-PER and DC-PER models are capable of providing reliable estimates of protein quality for majority of foods and food ingredients currently in use. Rat bioassay, **936.14** (*See* Chapter **38.2**), remains official method for determining protein quality; C-PER and DC-PER assays are alternative methods for routine quality control screening of foods and food ingredients. Use of both assays is recommended when estimating protein quality to provide internal check. Experience indicates that, in rare cases, the 2 models will report quite different estimates of protein quality. When this occurs, it should be regarded as a warning that the sample under analysis is probably:

(*1*) single-cell protein or protein surrounded by heavy cell walls (e.g., yeast or wheat bran), where DC-PER will overestimate protein quality, or

(*2*) partially or completely predigested proteins (e.g., liquid protein supplements), where C-PER will underestimate protein quality or

(*3*) protein sources known to possess significant quantities of proteolytic inhibitors (e.g., improperly heat-treated soy protein), where DC-PER will overestimate protein quality.

For major discrepancies in PER predictions of the 2 models, use rat assay as assay of choice to estimate protein quality.

Computational procedures for obtaining C-PER and DC-PER estimates are too lengthy for repetitive hand calculation. For routine use of assay, it is recommended that algorithm be placed on computer.

B. Apparatus

(**a**) *Amino acid analyzer.*—Able to accurately measure individual amino acids at concentrates as low as 20 nmolar. Must be standardized using known amino acid standards at least once every 24 h.

(**b**) *Hydrolysis tubes.*—Any standard Kimax/Pyrex test tube or ampule ≥15 mL capacity.

(**c**) *Water-jacketed chamber.*—To fit on stir plate and connected to 37° circulating H_2O bath.

(**d**) *Water bath.*—55°.

(**e**) *pH meter.*—Having combination pH electrode and capable of reading to 0.01 pH unit.

C. Reagents

(**a**) *ANRC reference casein.*—Available from New Zealand Milk Products, 1269 N McDowell, PO Box 80816, Petaluma, CA 94975-8016; or Teklad, a Harlan Sprague Dawley, Inc., Co., PO Box 4220, Madison, WI 53711.

(**b**) *Amino acid standards.*—ASP, TH SER, GLU, PRO, GLY, ALA, VAL, MET, ILE, LEU, TRY, PHE, LYS, HIS, AMM, ARG, CYS, and TRP. Available from any amino acid analyzer supply house (e.g., Beckman Instruments, Inc., No. 338088; Pierce Chemical Co., Amino Acid Standard Kit 22, No 20065.

(**c**) *Performic acid.*—Add 1 mL 30% H_2O_2 to 9 mL formic acid (88%). Let stand 1 h and cool to 0°.

(**d**) *Buffer solution.*—Use buffer recommended for sample dilution for amino acid analyzer.

(**e**) *Enzyme solutions.*—Use the following enzymes (Sigma Chemical Co.) or their equivalent: porcine pancreatic trypsin (Type IX), porcine intestinal peptidase (Grade I), bovine pancreatic α-chymotrypsin (Type II), bacterial protease (Pronase P or E). *Solution A.*—Dissolve 227 040 BAEE units of trypsin +

1860 BAEE units of α-chymotrypsin + 0.520 L-leucine β-naphthylamide units of peptidase in 10 mL H_2O. *Solution B.*—Dissolve 65 casein units of bacterial protease in 10 mL H_2O. Store both solutions on ice.
(**f**) *Control protein.*—Suspend 10 g ANRC Na caseinate (**a**) in 200 mL H_2O and adjust to pH 8 with NaOH. Maintain at pH 8 ≥ 1 h. Freeze-dry and determine N content by Kjeldahl method.

D. Nitrogen Determination
Determine N by **955.04C**, **930.29A**, **976.05A**, or other appropriate Kjeldahl method (*See* Chapter 28).

E. Sample Hydrolysis
(**a**) *Acid hydrolysis.*—Place ca 0.1 g (weigh to 0.1 mg accuracy) sample in hydrolysis tube, add 10 mL 6N HCl, and mix. Freeze in dry ice-alcohol bath. Draw and hold vacuum of $\leq 50\ \mu$ for 1 min; seal tube under vacuum. Hydrolyze 24 h at 110 $\pm$ 1°. Cool, open tube, and filter hydrolysate through Whatman No. 1 paper; rinse tube 3 times with H_2O and filter each rinse. Dry filtrate at 65° under vacuum. Dissolve dry hydrolysate in volume of buffer appropriate for amino acid analyzer. Store hydrolysate not > 1 week before analysis. Use this hydrolysate to determine all amino acids except methionine, cystine and/or cysteine, and tryptophan.
(**b**) *Performic acid oxidation followed by acid hydrolysis.*—Place ca 0.1 g (0.1 mg accuracy) sample in hydrolysis tube, add 2 mL cold performic acid, and let sit overnight at 0–5°. Add 3 mL cold HBr + 0.04 mL 1-octanol (antifoam); immediately mix contents 30 s in ice-H_2O bath and evaporate to dryness at 40° under vacuum. Add 10 mL 6N HCl to tube and perform acid hydrolysis as described above. This treatment will quantitatively convert methionine to methionine sulfone and cystine and/or cysteine to cysteic acid. Use this hydrolysate to determine methionine (MET) and cystine/cysteine (CYS).
(**c**) *Alkaline hydrolysis.*—Place ca 0.1 g (0.1 mg accuracy) sample into glass hydrolysis tube having Nalgene polypropylene centrifuge tube as internal liner. Add 25 mg hydrolyzed potato starch (omit if sample is high in starch). Add 0.6 mL fresh 4.2N NaOH + 0.04 mL 1-octanol. Mix contents 2 min under partial vacuum. Freeze tube contents in dry ice-alcohol bath. Draw and hold vacuum $\leq 50\ \mu$ 1 min; seal tube while under vacuum. Hydrolyze 22 h at 110 $\pm$ 1°. Cool, open tube, and transfer contents to 5 mL volumetric flask containing sufficient cold 6N HCl to neutralize hydrolysate; dilute to volume using buffer appropriate for amino acid analyzer. Centrifuge or filter hydrolysate and store frozen. Use this hydrolysate to determine tryptophan (TRP).

F. Amino Acid Analysis
Analyze each of the 3 hydrolysates using parameters optimal for amino acid analyzer being used. Use standard amino acid solutions to calibrate analyzer at least every 24 h. Each amino acid peak should have $\geq 85\%$ resolution. When alkaline hydrolysate is analyzed, tryptophan must be separated from lysinoalanine. Compute for each of the following amino acids, the uncorrected g/16 g N: ASP, TH SER, GLU, PRO, GLY, ALA, VAL, MET, ILE, LEU, TRY, PHE, LYS, HIS, AMM, ARG, CYS, and TRP according to:
g amino acid (uncorrected)/16 g sample N = (η moles aa $\times$ initial sample volume (mL) $\times$ MW aa)/
(volume sample injected (mL) $\times$ sample weight (g) $\times$ %N for sample $\times$ 6.25 $\times$ 10^5)
Compute percentage recovery by determining N content for each amino acid:
g N contributed by each aa/16 g sample N
= (14 $\times$ No. of N atoms in aa/mW aa)$\times$ (uncorrected g aa/16 g sample N)
% Recovery = Σ(g aa N for each aa/16 g sample N) $\times$ 100
Note: If percent recovery is <86 or >105, error was made in hydrolysis procedure (weighing errors, dilution, instrument calibration) or in computational process of percent recovery. Hydrolysis, analysis,

and/or computation of percent recovery must be repeated until percent recovery falls within 86–105 tolerance *before* proceeding further. Adjust amino acid profile to normalize to 95% hydrolysis:

Correction factor = 95%/% recovery

Note: For each amino acid, compute the corrected g/100 g protein by:

g amino acid/16 g N (corrected) = correction factor × g aa/16 g N

G. *In Vitro Protein Digestion—For C-PER*

Use sample or control weight containing 10 mg N.

Place appropriate quantity of control protein, ANRC Na caseinate, (**f**), or sample, in labeled vial containing magnetic stirring bar. Add 10 mL H_2O and let soak 1 h. Using pH meter, 37° bath, and stirrer, equilibrate sample and control to pH 8 ± 0.03 at 37° by additions of dilute HCl and NaOH. At this time also equilibrate enzyme solutions to pH 8 ± 0.03 at 37°. Replace enzymes on ice; hold sample and control at 37°.

To equilibrated control vial, add 1 mL enzyme solution A while stirring. Exactly 10 min after addition of solution A, add 1 mL enzyme solution B, and then transfer vial to 55° H_2O bath. Exactly 19 min after adding solution A, transfer vial back to 37° bath, insert pH electrode, and read pH at 20 min. pH of casein control should read 6.42 ± 0.05 at 20 min. After proper pH reading is obtained for control, carry each sample through identical procedure and read 20 min pH (*X*) for each. Calculate % protein digestibility as

$$\% \text{ Digestibility} = 234.84 - 22.56(X)$$

H. *Computing the C-PER*

Compute C-PER using % digestibility and g amino acid/16 g N of: LYS, MET + CYS, THR ILE, LEU, VAL, PHE + TRY, and TRP. When combining ME + CYS and PHE + TYR, the CYS and TYR can be no >50% of MET + CYS and PHE + TYR totals, respectively. For example, if g amino acid/16 g N were: MET = 2 and CYS = 3, use 4 for MET + CYS total, because maximum CYS can only be 50% of MET + CYS total.

Step 1: Express each essential amino acid as percentage of FAO/WHO standard:

$$\% \text{ FAO} = [(\text{g aa}/16 \text{ g N})/\text{FAO/WHO standard}] \times \% \text{ digestibility}$$

where FAO/WHO standard is assumed to be: LYS = 5.44, MET + CYS = 3.52, THR = 4.00, ILE = 4.00, LEU = 7.04, VAL = 4.96, PHE + TYR = 6.08, TRP = 0.96.

Step 2: Examine each percentage of FAO/WHO standard and adjust as follows: (a) If *all* percentages are >90% (before rounding to nearest integer) of FAO/WHO standard, *and* LEU is <135% (before rounding to nearest integer) proceed to Step 3; otherwise, (b) if any percentage is >100, *reduce* to 100 and proceed to Step 3.

Step 3: Compute the following for sample protein and reference casein:

$$X = \Sigma[(1/\% \text{ FAO/WHO for each aa})(\text{weight})]$$

$$Y = \Sigma \text{ weights used}$$

Weights to be used in Step 3 computations:

% FAO/WHO[a]	Wt
≥100	1
91-99	2
81-90	2.83
71-80	4

% FAO/WHO[a]	Wt
61-70	5.66
51-60	8
41-50	11.31
31-40	16
21-30	22.63
11-20	32
0-10	45.25

[a] Round to nearest integer.

Step 4: Divide the sum of weights (Y) by sum of reciprocols (X) for both sample protein and reference casein. Results will be termed essential amino acid scores for sample and casein.

Step 5: Divide score of sample by score of reference casein. Result expresses sample as the ratio of reference casein, and is termed RATIO. If RATIO is >0.99 and <1.01, then PER of sample is 2.5 and program should terminate at this point, i.e., the sample is casein or its equivalent.

Step 6: Compute the following: $Z = \text{RATIO} \times 2.5$.

Step 7: Compute 4 discriminant values to determine group into which sample is to be classified. Discriminant equations are:

Group 1 = −671.8418 − 6.57689(LYS) + 3.56696(MET + CYS) + 13.10145(THR) + 2.54503(ILE) + 16.9981(LEU) − 0.43395(VAL) − 11.5244(PHE + TYR) + 31.55321(TRP) + 14.59278(Digestibility)

Group 2 = −666.4492 − 2.78584(LYS) + 5.17441(MET + CYS) + 13.08564(THR) + 4.61808(ILE) + 16.22603(LEU) − 1.63223(VAL) − 10.13673(PHE + TYR) + 32.60196(TRP) + 14.11668(Digestibility)

Group 3 = −619.0813 − 3.13909(LYS) + 4.26918(MET + CYS) + 10.00988(THR) − 1.42144(ILE) + 15.7547(LEU) + 5.6604(VAL) − 11.28705(PHE + TYR) + 30.49168(TRP) + 13.79953(Digestibility)

Group 4 = −744.7122 − 0.37674(LYS) + 6.03697(MET + CYS) + 11.51527(THR) + 1.63251(ILE) + 17.29687(LEU) + 3.0294(VAL) − 11.5033(PHE + TYR) + 37.88725(TRP) + 14.68169(Digestibility)

Step 8: Compute C-PER by examining the 4 group values computed in Step 7. Choose group number that has largest value and use that number to pick correct C-PER equation. For PER predictions, use following group equations when digestibility was estimated by the 4 enzyme procedure:

Group 1: C-PER = $1.12683 - 1.61426(Z) + 0.99306(Z^2)$

Group 2: C-PER = $-7.25391 + 8.14063(Z) - 1.79517(Z^2)$

Group 3: C-PER = $4.30469 - 1.99609(Z) + 0.45996(Z^2)$

Group 4: C-PER = $12.75 - 8.21484(Z) + 1.66016(Z^2)$

I. Computing the DC-PER

DC-PER is computed using steps just described in computing C-PER, with one additional step—percent protein digestibility is computed from amino acid profile instead of being determined via in vitro procedure. Coefficients for discriminant equations (Step 7) and PER predictive equations (Step 8) are also changed.

Compute digestibility from amino acid profile as follows:

Step 1: Compute the 3 group discriminant values for sample *and* reference casein.

Group 1 = −203.7537 − 2.59402(LYS) + 9.27153(LEU) + 19.36964(ASP) + 4.19676(PRO) + 12.46035(CYS) + 34.3075(AMM)

Group 2 = −150.3707 − 0.78115(LYS) + 7.6239(LEU) + 15.46558(ASP) + 3.8947(PRO) + 12.79949(CYS) + 29.74493 (AMM)

Group 3 = −155.9532 + 4.61135(LYS) + 7.85429(LEU) + 13.25949(ASP)
+ 4.68431(PRO) + 13.2907(CYS) + 19.89403(AMM)

Examine resulting discriminant values for sample protein and reference casein, and choose group number associated with highest discriminant value. Use group number to determine which digestibility equation to use. If for sample, group equation No. 3 has highest value, then use digestibility equation No. 3 below to compute sample digestibility. If reference casein had highest value from group No. 2 equation, then use digestibility equation No. 2 below to compute digestibility for casein.

Group 1 Digestibility = 67.8263 + 0.60144(LYS) − 1.73309(LEU) + 2.48377(ASP)
+ 2.03523(PRO) − 0.97312(CYS) − 6.44299(AMM)

Group 2 Digestibility = 160.5607 + 5.7998(LYS) − 2.20744(LEU) − 7.35627(ASP)
− 0.85275(PRO) + 6.11058(CYS) − 14.54944(AMM)

Group 3 Digestibility = 116.5451 + 0.99537(LYS) − 4.37473(LEU) − 0.10243(ASP)
− 0.06304(PRO) − 0.14005(CYS) + 3.48679(AMM)

Previous Step 1 (C-PER procedure) now becomes 1-A. Steps 2–6 remain as before.

Step 7: Substitute following discriminant group equations:

Group 1 = −350.9675 + 2.34642(LYS) − 8.60862(MET + CYS) − 13.80721(THR) + 11.71013(ILE) + 11.7984(LEU) − 12.10787(VAL) + 9.68089(PHE + TYR) + 46.88927(TRP) + 7.291(Digestibility)

Group 2 = −454.6516 + 7.83575(LYS) − 14.3054(MET + CYS) − 15.64592(THR) + 13.32306(ILE) + 14.1817(LEU) − 17.40405(VAL) + 12.36894(PHE + TYR) + 64.39914(TRP) + 8.00712(Digestibility)

Group 3 = −405.9275 + 5.01252(LYS) − 8.46439(MET + CYS) − 15.014(THR) + 10.1986(ILE) + 11.91023(LEU) − 9.50181(VAL) + 9.46879(PHE + TYR) + 49.43095(TRP) + 7.78124(Digestibility)

Group 4 = −488.5569 + 9.3207(LYS) − 11.36379(MET + CYS) − 15.24675(THR) + 10.60119(ILE) + 13.93578(LEU) − 12.14625(VAL) + 10.15707(PHE + TYR) + 63.1489(TRP) + 8.22588(Digestibility)

Step 8: Substitute the following predictive equations:

Group 1: DC-PER = 1.254 − 2.04932(Z) + 1.30629(Z^2)
Group 2: DC-PER = −4.08594 + 5.125(Z) − 1.08398(Z^2)
Group 3: DC-PER = 4.66406 − 2.29297(Z) + 0.50586(Z^2)
Group 4: DC-PER = 10.44141 − 5.93359(Z) + 1.13281(Z^2)

Reference: JAOAC **65**, 798(1982).

29.3   960.48—Protein Efficiency Ratio
Rat Bioassay
First Action 1960
Final Action 1962

(Applicable to materials containing >1.80% N)

A. Reagents

(a) *ANRC reference casein.*—Available from New Zealand Milk Products, 1269 N McDowell, PO Box 80816, Petaluma, CA 9475–8016.

(b) *Salt mixture USP.*—Either USP salt mixture or salt mixture having essentially same proportions of the elements. Prepare *U.S. Pharmacopeia* XIX (p. 612) salt mixture (or corresponding USP XX item) as follows: Grind in mortar portion of 139.3 g NaCl with 0.79 g KI. Similarly grind together remainder of the NaCl with 389.0 g KH_2PO_4, 57.3 g $MgSO_4$ anhydrous, 381.4 g $CaCO_3$, 27.0 g $FeSO_4 \cdot 7H_2O$, 4.01 g $MnSO_4 \cdot H_2O$, 0.548 g $ZnSO_4 \cdot 7H_2O$, 0.477 g $CuSO_4 \cdot 5H_2O$, and 0.023 g $CoCl_2 \cdot 6H_2O$, finally adding the NaCl-KI mixture. Reduce entire mixture to fine powder.

(c) *Vitamin mixture.—*

Ingredient	mg/100 g ration
Vitamin A (dry, stabilized)	2000(IU)
Vitamin D (dry, stabilized)	200(IU)
Vitamin E (dry, stabilized)	10(IU)
Menadione	0.5
Choline	200
p-Aminobenzoic acid	10
Inositol	10
Niacin	4
Ca D-pantothenate	4
Riboflavin	0.8
Thiamine·HCl	0.5
Pyridoxine·HCl	0.5
Folic acid	0.2
Biotin	0.04
Vitamin B_{12}	0.003
Glucose, to make	1000

(d) *Cottonseed oil.*

(e) *Cellulose.*—Cellu Flour, Solka Floc, or equivalent.

(f) *Protein evaluation basal diet.—*

Sample	X^*
Cottonseed oil	$8 - (X \times \% \text{ ether extract})/100$
Salt mixture USP	$5 - (X \times \% \text{ ash})/100$
Vitamin mixture	1
Cellulose	$1 - (X \times \% \text{ crude fiber})/100$
Water	$5 - (X \times \% \text{ moisture})100$
Sucrose or corn starch, to make 100	$^*X = 1.60 \times 100/\% \text{ N of sample}$

All % figures refer to sample. Proximate analysis is needed to adjust diet so that all comparisons between samples and reference material shall be made with diets having same content of N, fat, ash, moisture, and crude fiber. These suggested levels of fat, ash, moisture, and crude fiber are desirable whenever proximate analysis of sample permits.

B. Experimental Animals

Laboratory rats, males, shall be from same colony, and maintained during period before weaning upon diet and under environmental conditions that will provide for normal development in all respects; weaned; ≥ 21 days of age but ≤ 28 days of age; range of individual rat weights among animals used shall be ≤ 10 g.

When animals are transported from breeding colony to test laboratory, acclimation period of ≥ 3 days but < 7 should precede test.

C. Assay Groups

Assemble groups of ≥ 10 rats. In assay of each material provide 1 group that will receive ANRC reference casein. One reference casein group may be used for concurrent assay of > 1 assay material. When assembling of all groups is complete, total number of rats in each group must be the same, and average weight of rats in any 1 group on day beginning assay period must not exceed by > 5 g average weight of rats in any other group.

D. Assay Period

Throughout assay period keep each rat in individual cage and provide with appropriate assay diet and H_2O *ad libitum*. During assay period maintain all conditions of environment as uniform as possible with respect to each of groups being compared to ANRC reference casein. Record body weight of each rat on beginning day of assay period and body weight and food intake of each rat at regular intervals, not > 7 days, and on 28th day after beginning of assay period.

E. Calculation and Tabulation of Results

Calculate average 28-day weight gain and protein (N $\times$ 6.25) intake per rat for each group. Calculate Protein Efficiency Ratio (PER) (weight gain/protein intake) for each group. Determine ratio $\times$ 100 of PER for each assay group to PER for ANRC casein reference group. Tabulate 28-day weight gains, protein intake, PER, and ratio $\times$ 100 of sample PER to ANRC Reference Casein PER for each assay group. Report protein quality of sample as ratio $\times$ 100 of sample PER to ANRC Reference Casein PER.

References: JAOAC **43,** 38(1960); **48,** 847(1965).

Chapter 30
Pyridoxine

30.1   **960.46—Vitamin Assays**
                                            Microbiological Methods
                                            Final Action

See Chapter 15.1.

30.2   **961.15—Vitamin B$_6$ (Pyridoxine, Pyridoxal, Pyridoxamine)**
                              in Food Extracts
                            Microbiological Method
                            Final Action 1975

A. Reagents

(Work in subdued light with all solutions containing vitamin B$_6$.)

(**a**) *Potassium acetate buffers.*—(*1*) *0.01M, pH 4.5.*—Dissolve 0.981 g KOAc in H$_2$O and dilute to 1 L. Adjust pH with CH$_3$COOH. (*2*) *0.02M, pH 5.5.*—Dissolve 1.96 g KOAc in H$_2$O and dilute to 1 L. Adjust pH with CH$_3$COOH. (*3*) *0.04M, pH 6.0.*—Dissolve 3.92 g KOAc in H$_2$O and dilute to 1 L. Adjust pH with CH$_3$COOH. (*4*) *0.1M, pH 7.0.*—Dissolve 9.815 g KOAc in H$_2$O and dilute to 1 L. Adjust pH with CH$_3$COOH or KOH solution.

(**b**) *Potassium chloride-phosphate buffer.*—pH 8.0. Dissolve 74.6 g KCl and 17.4 g K$_2$HPO$_4$ in 800 mL H$_2$O and adjust pH with CH$_3$COOH. Dilute to 1 L.

(**c**) *Ion exchange resin.*—Dowex AG 50W-X8, 100–200 mesh.

(**d**) *Acid-hydrolyzed casein solution.*—100 mg/mL. (*Caution: See Appendix* for safety notes on distillation and vacuum.) Mix 100 g vitamin-free casein with 500 mL constant-boiling HCl (ca 5*N* HCl, 208 mL HCl diluted to 500 mL with H$_2$O) and reflux 8 h. Remove HCl from mixture by distillation under vacuum until very thick sirup remains, keeping H$_2$O bath temperature <80°. Dissolve sirup in H$_2$O and concentrate again in same manner. Redissolve sirup in H$_2$O.

Adjust to pH 4 with 40% NaOH, add H$_2$O to ca 600 mL, add 40 g activated C, stir 4 h and filter with vacuum through buchner with thin pad of HCl-washed Filter-Cel. Continue following activated C treatments only if solution is not clear and colorless: Add 20 g activated C to filtrate, stir 1 h and refilter. Repeat with fresh 10 g portion activated C and filter. When solution is clear and colorless, dilute to 1 L with H$_2$O. (Before solution is diluted to volume, 2–3 mL 6*N* HCl may be added to extend time before microbial growth occurs.) Store in refrigerator.

(e) *Vitamin solution I.*—Dissolve 10 mg thiamine and 1 g inositol in ca 200 mL H_2O and dilute to 1 L. Store in refrigerator. (1 mL = 10 μg thiamine and 1 mg inositol.)

(f) *Vitamin solution II.*—Dissolve 10 mg biotin in 100 mL 50% alcohol. Store in refrigerator. (1 mL = 100 μg biotin.) Dissolve 200 mg Ca pantothenate and 200 mg niacin in ca 200 mL H_2O; add 8 mL biotin solution and dilute to 1 L with H_2O. Store in refrigerator. (1 mL = 200 μg each Ca pantothenate and niacin and 0.8 μg biotin.)

(g) *Salt solution I.*—Dissolve 17 g KCl, 10.3 g $MgSO_4 \cdot 7H_2O$, 100 mg $FeCl_3 \cdot 6H_2O$, and 100 mg $MnSO_4 \cdot H_2O$ in ca 800 mL H_2O. Add 2 mL HCl. Dissolve 5 g $CaCl_2 \cdot 2H_2O$ in ca 100 mL H_2O, add to first solution, and dilute to 1 L with H_2O. Store in refrigerator. (1 mL = 17 mg KCl, 10.3 mg $MgSO_4 \cdot 7H_2O$, 100 μg $FeCl_3 \cdot 6H_2O$, 100 μg $MnSO_4 \cdot H_2O$, and 5 mg $CaCl_2 \cdot 2H_2O$.)

(h) *Salt solution II.*—Dissolve 22 g KH_2PO_4 and 40 g $(NH_4)_2HPO_4$ in H_2O and dilute to 1 L. Store in refrigerator. (1 mL = 22 mg KH_2PO_4 and 40 mg $(NH_4)_2HPO_4$.)

(i) *Polysorbate 80 solution.*—Weigh 2.5 g polysorbate 80 (Tween 80) in small beaker. Transfer with warm (45°) H_2O and dilute to 500 mL. Store in refrigerator. (1 mL = 5 mg polysorbate 80.)

(j) *Citric acid solution.*—(1 + 1). Dissolve 50 g citric acid in 50 mL H_2O. Store at room temperature in bottle with plastic stopper.

(k) *Ammonium phosphate solution.*—(1 + 2). Dissolve 25 g $(NH_4)_2HPO_4$ in 50 mL H_2O. Store at room temperature in bottle with plastic stopper.

(l) *Pyridoxine, pyridoxal, and pyridoxamine standard solutions.*—Prepare separate solutions for each as follows: (*1*) *Stock solution.*—10.0 μg/mL. Dissolve 12.16 mg pyridoxine·HCl, 12.18 mg pyridoxal·HCl, and 14.34 mg pyridoxamine·HCl, respectively, in 1N HCl and dilute to 1 L with 1N HCl. Store in glass-stoppered bottles in refrigerator.

(*2*) *Intermediate solution.*—1.0 μg/mL. Dilute 10 mL stock solution to 100 mL with H_2O.

(*3*) *Working solution.*—1.0 ng/mL. Dilute 5 mL intermediate solution to 500 mL with H_2O and mix. Dilute 10 mL to 100 mL with H_2O. Prepare fresh for each assay.

(m) *Mixed pyridoxine, pyridoxal, pyridoxamine solutions (for liquid broth culture).*—Pipet 2 mL of each intermediate solution (1.0 μg/mL) into 1 L volumetric flask and dilute to volume with H_2O.

(n) *Citrate buffer solution.*—Dissolve 100 g K citrate and 20 g citric acid in H_2O and dilute to 1 L. Store in refrigerator. (1 mL = 100 mg K citrate and 20 mg citric acid.)

(o) *Basal medium stock solution (for 200 tubes).*—To make 1 L medium, add to ca 400 mL H_2O: 100 mL citrate buffer, 100 mL hydrolyzed casein solution, 50 mL vitamin solution I, 25 mL vitamin solution II, 50 mL salt solution I, and 50 mL salt solution II. Dissolve 100 g glucose in this solution. Dissolve 22 mg DL-tryptophan, 27 mg L-histidine·HCl, 100 mg DL-methionine, 216 mg DL-isoleucine, and 256 mg DL-valine in 10 mL HCl (1 + 9) in small beaker and add to above. Add 20 mL polysorbate 80 solution. Adjust to pH 4.5 with citric acid (1 + 1) or $(NH_4)_2HPO_4$ (1 + 2) solutions. Dilute to 1 L with H_2O. Store in Pyrex bottle plugged with cotton in refrigerator. Prepare ≤24 h before use. When ready, steam 10 min and cool.

(p) *Test organism.*—*Saccharomyces uvarum* (ATCC No. 9080). Maintain by weekly transfers on wort agar slants (**q**). Incubate these freshly seeded agar slants 24 h at 30° and refrigerate.

(q) *Agar culture medium.*—Suspend 25 g Bactowort agar in ca 400 mL H_2O in marked 500 mL wide-mouth erlenmeyer. Cover to prevent contamination, steam ca 10 min to dissolve agar, and adjust volume to 500 mL. Pipet hot agar in ca 10 mL portions into 20 × 150 mm test tubes, plug with absorbent cotton, and autoclave 15 min at 121°. Since this medium has acid reaction, avoid overheating, which results in softer medium. Tilt hot agar tubes to form slants and cool in this position.

(r) *Liquid culture medium.*—Pipet 5 mL mixed solution, (m), into 16 × 150 mm test tubes containing two 4 mm glass beads, cover to prevent contamination, and autoclave 10 min at 121°. Add 5 mL steamed vitamin B_6-free basal medium, (o), under aseptic conditions. Store tubes in refrigerator.

(s) *Inoculum rinse.*—Pipet 5 mL H_2O into test tubes, cover to prevent contamination, and autoclave 10 min at 121°. Add 5 mL steamed vitamin B_6-free basal medium, (o), under aseptic conditions. Store tubes in refrigerator.

B. Assay Inoculum

(*Caution: See Appendix* for safety notes on centrifuges.)

Incubate cells for inoculum on agar 24 h at 30° before use. Transfer these cells under aseptic conditions to liquid broth culture tubes. Plug with absorbent cotton held on with masking tape (or other cover to prevent contamination) and place tubes on shaker 20 h in 30° room. Replace cotton plugs aseptically with sterile rubber stoppers; centrifuge 1.5 min at 2500 rpm. Decant liquid and resuspend in 10 mL inoculum rinse. Separate by centrifuging 1.5 min at 2500 rpm. Decant liquid, resuspend in second 10 mL sterile inoculum rinse, centrifuge 1.5 min, and decant. Cells suspended in third 10 mL inoculum rinse are assay inoculum.

C. Preparation of Exchange Resin and Column

To 250 g Dowex AG 50W-X8 (100–200 mesh) in H form, add excess 6N KOH until supernate is blue to litmus. Let settle, decant, and rinse resin with H_2O until supernate is clear. Add ca 600 mL 3N HCl, stir, and heat 0.5 h in boiling H_2O bath. Decant and repeat treatment with 3N HCl twice. Rinse resin until rinse H_2O is neutral. Add 6N KOH until pH is strongly basic and stir 1 h. Rinse with H_2O until rinse H_2O is neutral. Suspend in 2M KOAc and store in refrigerator until needed. Just before use, wash resin with H_2O until H_2O is green to bromothymol blue. Resin can be regenerated, beginning with 3N HCl treatment.

Prepare tubes by sealing capillary stopcock, 1.5 mm bore and 50 mm side arms, to 22 mm od × ≥400 mm tube. Pour 5–10 mL H_2O into tube. Place glass wool plug in bottom of tube and remove bubbles from capillary and glass wool. Rinse measured 30 mL prepared resin, settled out of H_2O suspension, into tube with H_2O. After resin settles in tube, place glass wool plug on top of resin. Rinse column with 50 mL hot H_2O followed by two 50 mL portions hot 0.01M KOAc (pH 4.5). pH of last buffer rinse from column should be 4.5; otherwise, more rinsing with buffer is required. Do not permit liquid level on column to fall below top glass wool plug at any time.

D. Preparation of Sample

Weigh 1–2 g dry product into 500 mL erlenmeyer. For plant products, add 200 mL 0.44N HCl and for animal products, add 200 mL 0.055N HCl. Autoclave plant solution 2 h at 121°, and animal solution 5 h at 121°. Cool to room temperature, adjust to pH 4.5 with 6N or saturated KOH, and dilute to 250 mL with H_2O in volumetric flask. Filter through Whatman No. 40 paper. Take 40–200 mL filtered aliquot for chromatography.

E. Chromatography

Place desired amount of filtered extract on ion exchange column in ca 50 mL portions and let pass completely through with no flow regulation. Wash beaker and column 3 times with ca 5 mL portions hot 0.02M KOAc (pH 5.5), followed by similar washing to column sides. Wash column with same solution until total of 100 mL 0.02M KOAc (pH 5.5) solution is used. Elute pyridoxal with two 50 mL portions boiling 0.04M KOAc (pH 6.0), using 100 mL volumetric flask as receiver. Elute pyridoxine with two 50 mL portions boiling 0.1M KOAc (pH 7.0), using 100 mL volumetric flask as receiver. Elute pyridoxamine with two 50 mL portions boiling KCl-K$_2$HPO$_4$ (pH 8.0) solution, using 250 mL beaker as receiver. Adjust pH to 4.5. Dilute pyridoxine and pyridoxal eluates to 100 mL and pyridoxamine eluate to 200 mL with H$_2$O unless otherwise desired.

For standard pyridoxine, pyridoxal, and pyridoxamine, mix 10 mL each intermediate solution, neutralize with KOH, and adjust to pH 4.5 with CH$_3$COOH. Put this solution on column, wash, and elute fractions as above. Dilute eluted pyridoxine and pyridoxal standards to 100 mL and dilute eluted pyridoxamine, after pH is adjusted to 4.5, to 200 mL with H$_2$O. Dilute eluted standards to 1.0 ng/mL with H$_2$O.

F. Assay

Heat clean tubes and glass beads 2 h at 260°. Place two 4 mm glass beads in each 16 × 150 mm screw-cap glass culture tube. For standard curve, pipet into triplicate tubes appropriate freshly prepared standard working solutions to give 0.0, 0.0, 1.0, 2.0, 3.0, 4.0, and 5.0 ng pyridoxine, pyridoxal, or pyridoxamine/tube. Similarly prepare set of tubes for eluted standards, omitting blanks. Dilute sample eluates from chromatographic column to contain ca 1 ng vitamin B$_6$ component/mL. Pipet 1, 2, 3, 4, and 5 mL diluted eluates into triplicate tubes. Pipet H$_2$O into all tubes to bring volume to 5 mL/tube. Cap tubes with plastic caps with 3 mm (1/8″) hole through top. Autoclave entire set 10 min at 121°. Cool tubes to room temperature. Using automatic pipet with sterilized delivery attachments, pipet 5 mL steamed medium, A(o), through hole in cap. Cover tubes with sterile cheesecloth and place in refrigerator. Remove from refrigerator 1 h before inoculation. Aseptically inoculate through cap of each tube, except first set of 0.0 level for standard curves, with 1 drop assay inoculum of *S. uvarum* suspended cells. Take care to maintain uniform cell suspension, since cells may settle out during inoculation step. Incubate tubes on constant rotary shaker 22 h in temperature-regulated room (30°). Steam tubes in autoclave 5 min, cool, and remove caps. Read % *T* at 550 nm on spectrophotometer. Set 100% *T* with H$_2$O to read uninoculated blank. Set 100% *T* with uninoculated blank to read inoculated blank. Mix 9 inoculated blank tubes, and with this mixture set at 100% *T* on instrument, read all other tubes.

Average readings of triplicate tubes and plot % *T* against ng eluted standard pyridoxine, pyridoxal, or pyridoxamine/tube on semilog paper. Determine amount of pyridoxine, pyridoxal, or pyridoxamine/sample tube by interpolation. Report μg pyridoxine, pyridoxal, and pyridoxamine/g sample.

References: JAOAC **44**, 426(1961); **47**, 750(1964); **53**, 546(1970).
CAS-66-72-8 (pyridoxal)
CAS-85-87-0 (pyridoxamine)
CAS-65-23-6 (pyridoxine)

30.3 **985.32—Vitamin B₆ (Pyridoxine, Pyridoxal, Pyridoxamine) in Ready-to-Feed Milk-Based Infant Formula**
Microbiological Method
First Action 1985
Final Action 1988

(*Caution:* Loosen caps or stoppers on tubes when liquids are being autoclaved.)

A. Reagents

(Work in subdued light with all solutions containing vitamin B_6.)

(a) *Vitamin solution I.*—Dissolve 10 mg thiamine and 1 g inositol in ca 200 mL H_2O and dilute to 1 L. Store in refrigerator. (1 mL = 10 µg thiamine and 1 mg inositol.)

(b) *Vitamin solution II.*—Dissolve 10 mg biotin in 100 mL 50% alcohol. Store in refrigerator. (1 mL = 100 µg biotin.) Dissolve 200 mg Ca pantothenate and 200 mg niacin in ca 200 mL H_2O; add 8 mL biotin solution and dilute to 1 L with H_2O. Store in refrigerator. (1 mL = 200 µg each Ca pantothenate and niacin and 0.8 µg biotin.)

(c) *Salt solution I.*—Dissolve 17 g KCl, 10.3 g $MgSO_4 \cdot 7H_2O$, 100 mg $FeCl_3 \cdot 6H_2O$, and 100 mg $MnSO_4 \cdot H_2O$ in ca 800 mL H_2O. Add 2 mL HCl. Dissolve 5 g $CaCl_2 \cdot 2H_2O$ in ca 100 mL H_2O, add to first solution, and dilute to 1 L with H_2O. Store in refrigerator. (1 mL = 17 mg KCl, 10.3 mg $MgSO_4 \cdot 7H_2O$, 100 µg $FeCl_3 \cdot 6H_2O$, 100 µg $MnSO_4 \cdot H_2O$, and 5 mg $CaCl_2 \cdot 2H_2O$.)

(d) *Salt solution II.*—Dissolve 22 g KH_2PO_4 and 40 g $(NH_4)_2HPO_4$ in H_2O and dilute to 1 L. Store in refrigerator. (1 mL = 22 mg KH_2PO_4 and 40 mg $(NH_4)_2HPO_4$.)

(e) *Polysorbate 80 solution.*—Weigh 2.5 g polysorbate 80 (Tween 80) in small beaker. Transfer with warm (45°) H_2O and dilute to 500 mL. Store in refrigerator. (1 mL = 5 mg polysorbate 80.)

(f) *Citric acid solution.*—(1 + 1). Dissolve 50 g citric acid in 50 mL H_2O. Store at room temperature in bottle with plastic stopper.

(g) *Ammonium phosphate solution.*—(1 + 2). Dissolve 25 g $(NH_4)_2HPO_4$ in 50 mL H_2O. Store at room temperature in bottle with plastic stopper.

(h) *Pyridoxine standard solution.*—(*1*) *Stock solution.*–10.0 µg/mL. Dissolve 12.16 mg pyridoxine·HCl in 1N HCl and dilute to 1 L with 1N HCl. Store in glass-stoppered bottle in refrigerator. *(2) Intermediate solution.*—100 ng/mL. Dilute 5 mL stock solution to 500 mL with H_2O. Prepare fresh for each assay. *(3) Working solution.*—1.0 ng/mL. Dilute 5 mL intermediate solution to 500 mL with H_2O and mix. Prepare fresh for each assay.

(i) *Citrate buffer solution.*—Dissolve 65 g KOH and 82 g citric acid in H_2O and dilute to 1 L with H_2O.

(j) *Basal medium stock solution (for 200 tubes).*—To make 1 L medium, add to ca 400 mL H_2O: 100 mL citrate buffer, 2 g asparagine, 50 mL vitamin solution I, 50 mL vitamin solution II, 50 mL salt solution I, and 50 mL salt solution II. Dissove 100 g glucose in this solution. Dissolve 22 mg DL-tryptophan, 27 mg L-histidine·HCl, 100 mg DL-methionine, 216 mg DL-isoleucine, and 256 mg DL-valine in 10 mL (1 + 9) in small beaker and add to above. Add 20 mL polysorbate 80 solution. Adjust to pH 4.5 with citric acid (1 + 1) or $(NH_4)_2HPO_4$ (1 + 2) solutions. Dilute to 1 L with H_2O. Store in refrigerator in Pyrex bottle plugged with cotton. Prepare ≤24 h before use.

(k) *Test organism.*—*Saccharomyces uvarum* (ATCC No. 9080). Maintain by weekly transfers on wort agar slants (**l**). Incubate these freshly seeded agar slants 24 h at 30° and refrigerate.

(l) *Agar culture medium.*—Suspend 25 g Bactowort agar in ca 400 mL H_2O in marked 500 mL wide-mouth erlenmeyer. Cover to prevent contamination, steam ca 10 min to dissolve agar, and adjust volume to 500 mL. Pipet hot agar in ca 7 mL portions into 20 × 150 mm test tubes, plug with absorbent cotton, and autoclave 15 min at 121°. Since this medium has acid reaction, avoid overheating, which results in softer medium. Tilt hot agar tubes to form slants and cool in this position.

(**m**) *Liquid culture medium.*—Dilute 20 mL intermediate solution, (**h**)*(2)*, to 1 L with H_2O in volumetric flask. Pipet 5 mL of this solution and 5 mL basal medium stock solution, (**j**), into 16 × 150 mm screw-cap tubes containing two 4 mm glass beads. Autoclave 10 min at 121°. Cap, and store tubes in refrigerator.

(**n**) *Inoculum rinse.*—Pipet 5 mL H_2O and 5 mL basal medium stock solution, (**j**), into stainless steel-cap or screw-cap 16 × 150 mm test tubes. Autoclave 10 min at 121°.

B. Assay Inoculum

(*Caution: See Appendix* for safety notes on centrifuges.)

Incubate cells for inoculum on agar 24 h at 30° before use. Transfer these cells under aseptic conditions to liquid broth culture tubes. Place tubes on shaker 20 h in 30° room or in mechanical shaker H_2O bath 20 h at 30°. Centrifuge 1.5 min at 2500 rpm. Decant liquid and resuspend in 10 mL inoculum rinse. Separate by centrifuging 1.5 min at 2500 rpm. Decant liquid, resuspend in second 10 mL sterile inoculum rinse, centrifuge 1.5 min, and decant. Resuspend in third 10 mL sterile inoculum rinse. Add 1 mL of third suspension to 10 mL inoculum rinse. This is assay inoculum.

C. Preparation of Sample

Weigh 10.0 g composite into 500 mL erlenmeyer. Add 200 mL 0.05N HCl. Autoclave 5 h at 121°. Cool to room temperature, and adjust to pH 4.5 with 6N KOH. Quantitatively transfer solution to 250 mL volumetric flask, and dilute to volume with H_2O. Filter through Whatman No. 40 paper. Dilute 1 mL of this solution to 20 mL with H_2O. This is assay solution.

D. Assay

Heat 16 ×150 mm screw-cap tubes containing two 4 mm glass beads 2 h at 260°. For standard curve, pipet into triplicate tubes, 0.0, 0.0, 1.0, 2.0, 3.0, 4.0, and 5.0 mL pyridoxine working solution, (**h**)*(3)*. Similarly pipet 1.0, 2.0, 3.0, and 4.0, mL assay solution into duplicate tubes. Pipet H_2O into all tubes to bring volume to 5 mL/tube. Add 5 mL basal medium stock solution, (**j**), to all tubes for total volume of 10 mL/tube. Cap all tubes and autoclave 10 min at 121°. Cool to room temperature using H_2O bath or refrigerator. Aseptically inoculate, except first set of 0.0 level for standard curve, with 1 drop assay inoculum. Incubate tubes on constant reciprocal shaker 22 h in temperature-regulated room (30°) or in mechanical shaker H_2O bath 22 h at 30°. Steam tubes in autoclave 5 min. Cool and read $\%T$ at 550 nm on spectrophotometer. Set $100\% \ T$ with H_2O to read uninoculated blanks. Set $100\% \ T$ with uninoculated blank to read inoculated blank. Mix the 3 inoculated blank tubes, and with this mixture set at $100\% \ T$, read all remaining tubes.

Average readings for standard curve triplicate tubes and plot $\%T$ against ng pyridoxine for each level of standard solution on semilog paper. Determine amount of pyridoxine/sample tube by interpolation. Calculate μg pyridoxine/g sample. (Calculation may be performed using computer program as in JAOAC **56,** 754(1973).)

Reference: JAOAC **68,** 514(1985).
CAS-65-23-6 (pyridoxine)

Chapter 31
Riboflavin

31.1

960.46—Vitamin Assays
Microbiological Methods
Final Action

See Chapter 15.1.

31.2

940.33—Riboflavin (Vitamin B₂) in Vitamin Preparations
Microbiological Methods
Final Action 1960

(Not applicable in presence of materials which adsorb riboflavin)

A. Basal Medium Stock Solution

Using ingredients in amounts prescribed for riboflavin, Table **960.46(e)** (*see* Chapter 15.1), proceed as below.

Using solutions prepared as in **960.46A**, add, with mixing, and in following order: photolyzed peptone solution, (**g**); cystine solution, (**d**); yeast supplement solution, (**s**); salt solution A, (**i**); and salt solution B, (**j**). Add ca 100 mL H_2O, and add anhydrous glucose with mixing. When solution is complete, adjust to pH 6.8 with NaOH solution, and dilute with H_2O to 250 mL.

Titrimetric Method

B. Riboflavin Standard Solutions

(Do not shake standard solutions stored under toluene.)

(**a**) *Stock solution.*—100 µg/mL. Accurately weigh, in closed system, 50–60 mg USP Riboflavin Reference Standard that has been dried to constant weight and stored in dark over P_2O_5 in desiccator. Suspend in ca 300 mL 0.02N CH_3COOH and warm on steam bath, with stirring, until solid dissolves. Cool, and dilute with 0.02N CH_3COOH to make riboflavin concentration exactly 100 µg/mL. Store under toluene in dark at ca 10°.

(**b**) *Intermediate solution I.*—10 µg/mL. Dilute 100 mL stock solution, (**a**), with 0.02N CH_3COOH to 1 L. Store under toluene in dark at ca 10°.

(**c**) *Working solution.*—Dilute suitable volume intermediate solution, (**b**), with H_2O to measured volume such that after incubation as in **960.46D** and **960.46E**, response at 5.0 mL level of this solution is equivalent to titration (as described in **960.46E**) of ca 8–12 mL. Designate this as standard solution. (This concentration is usually 0.05–0.20 μg riboflavin/mL standard solution.) Prepare fresh standard solution for each assay.

C. Inoculum

(a) *Liquid culture medium.*—Dilute measured volume basal medium stock solution, **940.33A**, with equal volume aqueous solution containing 0.1 μg riboflavin/mL. Add 10 mL portions diluted medium to test tubes, cover to prevent contamination, sterilize 15 min in autoclave at 121–123°, and cool tubes as rapidly as practicable to avoid color formation from overheating. Store in dark at ca 10°.

(b) Make transfer of cells from stock culture of *Lactobacillus casei,* **960.46C(d)**, to sterile tube containing 10 mL liquid culture medium, (a). Incubate 6–24 h at any selected temperature between 30 and 40° held constant to within ±0.5°. Under aseptic conditions, centrifuge culture and decant supernate. Wash cells with 3 ca 10 mL portions sterile 0.9% NaCl solution or sterile suspension medium, **960.46B(c)**. Resuspend cells in 10 mL sterile 0.9% NaCl solution or sterile suspension medium. Cell suspension so obtained is inoculum.

D. Assay Solution

(Throughout all stages, keep solution below pH 7.0 to prevent loss of riboflavin.)

Place measured amount of sample in flask and proceed as below. (Where directed to filter through paper, use paper known not to adsorb riboflavin. Ash-free papers have been found satisfactory.) Designate final measured volume so obtained as assay solution.

(a) *For dry or semidry materials containing no appreciable amount of basic substances.*—Add volume 0.1N HCl equal in mL to ≥10 times dry weight sample in grams; resulting solution must contain ≤0.1 mg riboflavin/mL. If sample is not readily soluble, comminute so that it may be evenly dispersed in liquid. Then agitate vigorously and wash down sides of flask with 0.1N HCl.

Then proceed as in **944.13D(a)**, beginning with second paragraph, ''Autoclave mixture 30 min … '' except that where reference is made to niacin concentration ca equivalent to that of standard solution, **944.13B(c)**, replace by riboflavin concentration ca equivalent to that of standard solution, **940.33B(c)**.

944.13 (Niacin and Niacinamide [Nicotinic Acid and Nicotinamide] in Vitamin Preparations, Microbiological Methods)

D. Assay Solution

Place measured amount of sample in flask and proceed as below. Designate final measured volume so obtained as assay solution.

(a) *For dry or semidry materials containing no appreciable amount of basic substances.*—Add volume 1N H₂SO₄ equal in mL to ≥10 times dry weight sample in grams; resulting solution must contain ≤5.0 mg niacin/mL. If sample is not readily soluble, comminute to disperse it evenly in liquid; then agitate vigorously and wash down sides of flask with 1N H₂SO₄.

Autoclave mixture 30 min at 121–123° and cool. If lumping occurs, agitate mixture until particles are evenly dispersed. If dissolved protein is not present, adjust mixture to pH 6.8 with NaOH solution, dilute with H₂O to final measured volume containing, per mL, niacin ca equivalent to that of standard solution, **944.13B(c)**, and filter if solution is not clear.

If dissolved protein is present, adjust mixture, with vigorous agitation, to pH 6.0–6.5 with NaOH solution; then immediately add dilute HCl until no further precipitation occurs (usually ca pH 4.5, isoelectric point of many proteins). Dilute mixture to measured volume with H₂O, and filter. (In case of mixture difficult to filter, centrifuging and/or filtering through fritted glass, using suitable analytical filter-aid, may often be substituted for, or may precede, filtering through paper. Ash-free filter paper pulp and Celite Analytical Filter-Aid have been found satisfactory.) Take aliquot of clear filtrate and check for dissolved protein by adding dropwise, first dilute HCl, and if no precipitate forms, then, with vigorous agitation, NaOH solution, and proceed as follows with this aliquot:

(*1*) If no further precipitation occurs, add, with vigorous agitation, NaOH solution to pH 6.8, and dilute with H_2O to final measured volume containing, per mL, niacin ca equivalent to that of standard solution, **944.13B(c)**. If cloudiness occurs, refilter.

(*2*) If further precipitation occurs, adjust mixture again to point of maximum precipitation, dilute with H_2O to measured volume, and then filter. Take aliquot of clear filtrate and proceed as in (*1*).

If riboflavin content of sample is so low that these requirements cannot be met, concentrate clear filtrate obtained at ca pH 4.5 to suitable volume with heat under reduced pressure. Filter if necessary, and proceed as in **944.13D(a)(*1*)**.

(**b**) *For dry or semidry materials containing appreciable amounts of basic substances.*—Adjust mixture to pH 5.0–6.0 with dilute HCl. Add volume H_2O equal in mL to ≥ 10 times dry weight sample in grams; resulting solution must contain ≤ 0.1 mg riboflavin/mL. Then add equivalent of 1.0 mL 10*N* HCl/100 mL liquid and proceed as in (**a**), beginning with second sentence, "If sample is not readily soluble. . . ."

(**c**) *For liquid materials.*—Adjust mixture to pH 5.0– 6.0 with dilute HCl, or with vigorous agitation, NaOH solution, and proceed as in (**b**), beginning with second sentence, "Add volume H_2O. . . ."

E. Assay

Using standard solution, **940.33B(c)**, assay solution, **940.33D**, basal medium stock solution, **940.33A**, and inoculum, **940.33C(b)**, proceed as in **960.46D**, **G**, and **H**.

Turbidimetric Method

F. Riboflavin Standard Solutions

(Do not shake standard solutions stored under toluene.)

(**a**) *Intermediate solution II.*—1.0 µg/mL. Dilute 10 mL riboflavin stock solution, **940.33B(a)**, with 0.02*N* CH_3COOH to 1 L. Store under toluene in dark at ca 10°.

(**b**) *Standard solution.*—Dilute suitable volume intermediate solution II, (**a**), with H_2O to measured volume such that after incubation as in **960.46D** and **960.46G**, with inoculated blank set at 100% *T*, % *T* at 5.0 mL level of this solution is equivalent to that for dried cell weight (as described in **960.46F**) of ≥ 1.25 mg. Designate this as standard solution. (This concentration is usually 0.01–0.04 µg riboflavin/mL standard solution.) Prepare fresh standard solution for each assay.

G. Inoculum

Proceed as in **940.33C(b)**.

H. Assay Solution

Proceed as in **940.33D**, except that where reference is made to riboflavin concentration ca equivalent to that of standard solution, **940.33B(c)**, replace by riboflavin concentration ca equivalent to that of standard solution, **940.33F(b)**. Designate solution so obtained as assay solution.

I. Assay

Using standard solution, **940.33F(b)**, assay solution, **940.33H**, basal medium stock solution, **940.33A**, and inoculum, **940.33G**, proceed as in **960.46D**, **G**, and **H**.

References: JAOAC **23**, 346(1940); **24**, 413(1941); **25**, 459(1942); **26**, 81(1943); **27**, 540(1944); **28**, 560(1945); **29**, 25(1946); **30**, 79, 391(1947); **31**, 701(1948); **32**, 105, 461(1949); **33**, 88, 631(1950); **37**, 770(1954); **39**, 172(1956); **40**, 856(1957); **41**, 61, 587(1958); **42**, 529(1959).
CAS-83-88-5 (riboflavin)

31.3   970.65—Riboflavin (Vitamin B₂) in Foods and Vitamin Preparations

Fluorometric Method
First Action 1970
Final Action 1971

A. Apparatus

Photofluorometer.—Use fluorometer suitable for accurately measuring fluorescence of solutions containing riboflavin in concentrations of 0.05–0.2 μg/mL. Input filter of narrow T range with maximum ca 440 nm and output filter of narrow T range with maximum ca 565 nm have been found satisfactory.

B. Reagents

(Do not shake standard solutions stored under toluene.)

(a) *Riboflavin standard solutions.*—(*1*) *Stock solution.*—100 μg/mL. Dissolve 50 mg USP Riboflavin Reference Standard, previously dried and stored in dark in desiccator over P_2O_5, in 0.02N CH_3COOH to make 500 mL. (To facilitate solution, warm with ca 300 mL 0.02N CH_3COOH on steam bath with constant stirring until dissolved, cool, and add 0.02N CH_3COOH to make 500 mL.) Store under toluene at ca 10°.

(*2*) *Intermediate solution.*—10 μg/mL. Dilute 100 mL stock solution to 1 L with 0.02N CH_3COOH. Store under toluene at ca 10°.

(*3*) *Working solution I.*—1 μg/mL. Dilute 10 mL intermediate solution to 100 mL with H_2O. Prepare fresh for each assay. Use as standard solution in **970.65D**.

(*4*) *Working solution II.*—0.1 μg/mL. Dilute 10 mL intermediate solution to 1 L with H_2O. Prepare fresh for each assay. Use as standard solution in **970.65E**.

(b) *Sodium hydrosulfite.*—High purity and stored to avoid undue exposure to light and air. Check suitability as follows: To each of ≥2 tubes add 10 mL H_2O and 1 mL standard riboflavin solution containing 20 μg/mL, and proceed as in **970.65D** with respect to addition of CH_3COOH, $KMnO_4$ solution, and H_2O_2 solution. Then when 8 mg $Na_2S_2O_4$ is added with mixing, riboflavin should be completely reduced in ≤5 s.

(c) *Extraction solution.*—Mix 300 mL methyl alcohol, 100 mL pyridine, 100 mL H_2O, and 10 mL CH_3COOH. (Proportionate amounts may be prepared.)

C. Preparation of Sample Solution

(Throughout all stages, protect solutions from undue exposure to light and keep at pH <7.0. Where directed to filter through paper, use paper known not to adsorb riboflavin [ash-free papers have been found satisfactory].)

Place measured amount of sample in suitable size flask and proceed by one of following methods:
(**a**) *For dry or semidry materials containing no appreciable amount of basic substances.*—Add volume $0.1N$ HCl equal in mL to ≥ 10 times dry weight sample in grams; resulting solution must contain ≤ 0.1 mg riboflavin/mL. If material is not readily soluble, comminute so that it may be evenly dispersed in liquid. Then agitate vigorously and wash down sides of flask with $0.1N$ HCl.

Heat mixture in autoclave 30 min at 121–123° and cool. If lumping occurs, agitate until particles are evenly dispersed. Adjust, with vigorous agitation, to pH 6.0–6.5 with NaOH solution; then immediately add dilute HCl until no further precipitation occurs (usually ca pH 4.5, isoelectric point of many proteins).

Dilute mixture to measured volume containing >0.1 μg riboflavin/mL and filter through paper. (In case of mixture difficult to filter, centrifuging and/or filtering through fritted glass, using suitable analytical filter-aid, may often be substituted for, or may precede, filtering through paper. Ash-free filter paper pulp and Celite Analytical Filter-Aid have been found satisfactory.) Take aliquot of clear filtrate and check for dissolved protein by adding dropwise, first dilute HCl, and if no precipitate forms, then, with vigorous agitation, NaOH solution, and proceed as follows:

(*1*) If no further precipitation occurs, add, with vigorous agitation, NaOH solution to pH 6.8, dilute solution to final measured volume containing ca 0.1 μg riboflavin/mL, and if cloudiness occurs, filter again.

(*2*) If further precipitation occurs, adjust solution again to point of maximum precipitation, dilute to measured volume containing >0.1 μg riboflavin/mL, and then filter. Take aliquot of clear filtrate and proceed as in (*1*).

If riboflavin content of sample is so low that these requirements cannot be met, concentrate clear filtrate obtained at ca pH 4.5 to suitable volume with heat under reduced pressure. Filter if necessary and proceed as in (*1*).

(**b**) *For dry or semidry materials containing appreciable amounts of basic substances.*—Adjust mixture to pH 5.0–6.0 with dilute HCl. Add amount of H_2O such that total volume liquid is equal in mL to ≥ 10 times dry weight sample in g. (Resulting solution must contain ≤ 0.1 mg riboflavin/mL.) Then add equivalent of 1.0 mL $10N$ HCl/100 mL liquid and proceed as in (**a**), beginning with second sentence.

(**c**) *For liquid materials.*—Adjust pH to 5.0–6.0 with dilute HCl or, with vigorous agitation, NaOH solution, and proceed as in (**b**), beginning with second sentence.

(**d**) *For concentrates, premixes, and multivitamin supplements.*—Place measured amount of sample in flask and add volume extraction solution equal in mL to ≥ 10 times dry weight sample in grams; resulting solution must contain ≤ 0.1 mg riboflavin/mL. If sample is not readily soluble, comminute so that it may be dispersed evenly in liquid. Then agitate vigorously and wash down sides of flask with extraction solution.

Reflux mixture 1 h and cool. If lumping occurs, agitate mixture until particles are dispersed evenly. Dilute mixture to measured volume with extraction solution and let any undissolved particles settle, or filter or centrifuge, if necessary. Take aliquot of clear solution and dilute with H_2O to measured volume containing ca 0.1 μg riboflavin/mL and filter if solution is not clear. Proceed with determination, **970.65E**.

D. Determination

To each of ≥ 4 tubes (or reaction vessels) add 10 mL sample solution. (If fluorometer is type that requires tubular cuvets, all reactions may be carried out in matched set of these cuvets.) To each of ≥ 2 tubes add 1 mL standard riboflavin working solution I, **B(a)**(*3*), and mix, and to each of ≥ 2 remaining tubes, add 1 mL H_2O and mix. To each tube add 1 mL CH_3COOH and mix; add, with mixing, 0.5 mL 4.0% $KMnO_4$ solution (volume may be increased for sample solutions that contain excess of oxidizable material, but ≤ 0.5 mL in excess of that required to complete oxidation of foreign material should be added). Let stand

443

2 min; then to each tube add, with mixing, 0.5 mL 3.0% H_2O_2 solution; permanganate color must be destroyed within 10 s. Shake vigorously until excess O is expelled. If gas bubbles remain on sides of tubes after foaming stops, remove by tipping tubes so that solution flows slowly from end to end.

In fluorometer, measure fluorescence (X) of sample solution containing 1 mL added standard riboflavin working solution I. Next, measure fluorescence (B) of sample solution containing 1 mL added H_2O. Add, with mixing, 20 mg *powdered $Na_2S_2O_4$* to ≥ 2 tubes, measure minimum fluorescence (C) within 5 s. Calculate on basis of aliquots taken as follows:

$$\text{mg Riboflavin/mL final sample solution} = [(B - C)/(X - B)] \times 0.10 \times 0.001$$

(Value of $(B - C)/(X - B)$ must be ≥ 0.66 and ≤ 1.5.)

Note: Quantity of $Na_2S_2O_4$ appreciably >20 mg may reduce foreign pigments and/or foreign fluorescing substances, thereby causing erroneous results.

E. Alternative Determination

(Applicable to high potency samples)

Add 10 mL sample solution to ≥ 2 cuvets. Add 10 mL working standard solution II, **B(a)**(*4*), to each of another set of ≥ 2 cuvets. Add 1 mL CH_3COOH to each tube and mix. Measure fluorescence of sample and standard solutions in fluorometer. Add, with mixing, 20 mg *powdered $Na_2S_2O_4$* to 1 tube each of standard and sample and measure minimum fluorescence within 5 s. Calculate on basis of aliquots taken as follows:

$$\text{mg Riboflavin/mL final sample solution} = [(I - Q)/(I' - Q')] \times (0.1 \times 0.001)$$

where I and I' = fluorescence intensities of sample and standard, respectively, and Q and Q' = fluorescences of sample and standard, respectively, after $Na_2S_2O_4$ addition.

References: JAOAC **23**, 346(1940); **24**, 413(1941); **25**, 459(1942); **26**, 81(1943); **27**, 540(1944); **30**, 392(1947); **31**, 701(1948); **32**, 108, 461(1949); **33**, 88, 632(1950); **37**, 770(1954); **43**, 42(1960); **53**, 542(1970). CAS-83-88-5 (riboflavin)

31.4   981.15—Riboflavin in Foods and Vitamin Preparations

Automated Method
First Action 1981
Final Action 1982
AACC-AOAC Method

[Applicable to products for which manual method, **970.65** (*see* 31.3), is applicable and which contain ≥ 0.1 µg/g.]

(*Caution: See Appendix* for safety notes on permanganates.)

A. Apparatus

(a) *Automatic analyzer.*—Technicon AutoAnalyzer II system with flow scheme as in Fig. **981.15** (Technicon Instruments Corp.), or equivalent. Prepare in accordance with manufacturer's directions.

(b) *Fluorometer.*—Technicon Fluoronephelometer with LY-013-B008-01-C flow cell or Aminco Fluoro-Colorimeter with J4-7413 flow cell and J4-7125 4 watt lamp.

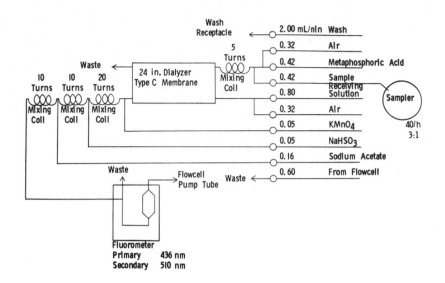

Figure 981.15.—Flow diagram for automated determination of riboflavin.

(c) *Filters.*—Primary: with band pass of 50% *T* at 430 nm (Technicon 518-7004); secondary: sharp cut 37% *T* at 513–527 nm and 80% *T* at 557 nm (Technicon 518-7032).

(d) *Glass electrode.*—Small diameter for adjusting pH in volumetric flask.

(e) *Filter medium.*—Glass fiber paper, Whatman GF/A, or equivalent, shown not to adsorb riboflavin.

B. Reagents

(a) *Wetting agent.*—30% aqueous Brij 35 solution (Atlas Chemical Industries, Wilmington, DE 19899).

(b) *Metaphosphoric acid solution.*—Dissolve 15 g HPO_3 in 1 L H_2O and adjust pH to 1.9 with NaOAc solution. Add 30 g NaCl and 1 mL wetting agent, and filter. Prepare fresh weekly.

(c) *Sodium acetate solution.*—1.25M. Dissolve 345 g $NaOAc \cdot 3H_2O$ in and dilute to 2 L with H_2O.

(d) *Metaphosphoric acid buffer.*—pH 4.3. Dissolve 15 g HPO_3 in 1 L H_2O and adjust to pH 4.3 with crystalline NaOAc. Prepare fresh daily.

(e) *Wash solution.*—Adjust pH of 2 L 0.1M HCl to 4.3 with 1.25M NaOAc (ca 240 mL). Add pH 4.3 HPO_3 buffer, (d), to make 4 L and add 4 mL wetting agent. Prepare fresh daily.

(f) *Dialysate receiving solution.*—Mix equal volumes wash solution and HPO_3 solution, (b).

(g) *Sodium acetate solution.*—0.4%. Dissolve 4.0 g $NaOAc \cdot 3H_2O$ and dilute to 1 L with H_2O.

(h) *Potassium permanganate solution.*—1%. Dissolve 2.0 g $KMnO_4$ in 200 mL H_2O by magnetic stirring 30 min, and filter through glass fiber GF/A filter. Store in dark bottle and prepare fresh weekly.

(i) *Sodium bisulfite solution.*—Dissolve 1.1 g $NaHSO_3$ in 50 mL pH 7 phosphate buffer (4.55 g KH_2PO_4 and 9.45 g Na_2HPO_4/L). In use, adjust $NaHSO_3$ solution concentration visually in continuous flow system so that there is ca 10% excess over that required to reduce $KMnO_4$. Avoid large excess of $NaHSO_3$. Once $NaHSO_3$ level is determined, it is not necessary to repeat adjustment unless pump tubes are changed.

(j) *Sodium hydrosulfite solution.*—Dissolve 2.0 g $Na_2S_2O_4$ in 100 mL 0.4% NaOAc solution. Keep solution in ice bath when in use (stable ca 2 h).

(**k**) *Riboflavin standard solutions.*—(*1*) *Stock solution.*—50 µg/mL. Dissolve 50.0 mg riboflavin (stored in dark in desiccator) in ca 800 mL 0.1M HCl (overnight magnetic stirring required) and dilute to 1 L with 0.1M HCl. Store under toluene in dark. Prepare fresh every 2 weeks. (*2*) *Intermediate solution.*—10 µg/mL. Dilute 40 mL stock solution to 200 mL with 0.1M HCl. (*3*) *Working solution.*—1 µg/mL. Dilute 10 mL intermediate solution to 100 mL with 0.1M HCl. Prepare solutions (*2*) and (*3*) fresh daily. Prepare standards to accompany sample solutions by pipetting 1, 3, 5, 10, and 15 mL working standard solution into 100 mL amber volumetric flasks and adding 49, 47, 45, 40, and 35 mL 0.1M HCl, respectively, to obtain concentrates of 0.01, 0.03, 0.05, 0.10, and 0.15 µg riboflavin/mL in determination. Autoclave and treat samples and standards alike.

C. Preparation of Sample

Grind representative portion to pass No. 40 sieve.

D. Determination

Transfer accurately weighed portion (1.5 g maximum) of ground sample containing ca 10 µg riboflavin to 100 mL amber volumetric flask, and add 50.0 mL 0.1M HCl, washing down sides of flask and dispersing sample. Cover flasks with foil and autoclave 30 min at 121°. Exhaust autoclave slowly to prevent bumping. Let cool to room temperature. (Solutions may be stored at this point.) For products which spatter during hydrolysis, use erlenmeyer and transfer to volumetric flask after autoclaving.

Add predetermined aliquot of 1.25M NaOAc with swirling. [Reproducible dispensing unit is convenient for this step. Adjust unit so that when aliquot of 1.25M NaOAc solution is added to 50.0 mL 0.1M HCl, pH is 4.3 ± 0.1 (ca 6.0 mL).] Add ca 35 mL pH 4.3 HPO_3 buffer. Check pH with meter and adjust any sample hydrolysate differing from standards by ≥0.1 pH unit. (If solution is also to be used for thiamin determination, add 5.0 mL Takadiastase solution (5% in pH 4.3 CH_3COOH) and incubate overnight at 37° before diluting to volume. Enzyme hydrolysis will not affect riboflavin determination, but enzyme solution must also be added to standards because enzyme contains small amount of riboflavin.) Dilute solutions to volume with pH 4.3 HPO_3 buffer solution, add drop of wetting agent, and filter through glass fiber paper.

Pump high standard solution (0.15 µg/mL) through system and set recorder pen at 100% with standard calibration adjustment on fluorometer. Aspirate and pump set of standards and sample filtrates through system. Use one 0.10 µg/mL standard with every series of 20 samples to correct for any drift. If sample is more concentrated than highest standard, dilute with wash solution to bring peak height into range of standards. After all samples have been run, replace NaOAc solution with $Na_2S_2O_4$. Let run to stable baseline, adjust to original baseline, and resample filtrates to obtain corresponding blanks.

Standards provide linear standard curve passing through origin. Subtract peak height of blank from peak height of sample and determine concentration, *C,* µg/mL, from standard curve.

$$\text{mg Riboflavin/100 g} = C \times 10/W$$

where *W* = g sample.

References: J. Agric. Food Chem. **23,** 815(1975). JAOAC **62,** 1041(1979).
CAS-83-88-5 (riboflavin)

31.5   985.31—Ribloflavin in Ready-to-Feed Milk-Based Infant Formula
Fluorometric Method
First Action 1985
Final Action 1988

See **970.65** (*see* 31.3).

Reference: JAOAC **68,** 514(1985).

Chapter 32
Sodium

32.1

985.35—Minerals in Ready-to-Feed
Milk-Based Infant Formula
Atomic Absorption Spectrophotometric Method
First Action 1985
Final Action 1988

See Chapter 12.14.

32.2

956.01—Potassium and/or Sodium in Plants
Flame Photometric Method
Final Action 1965

See Chapter 27.2.

32.3

953.01—Metals in Plants
General Recommendations
for Emission Spectrographic Methods
First Action 1988

See Chapter 12.5.

32.4

980.03—Metals in Plants
Direct Reading Spectrographic Method
Final Action 1988

See Chapter 12.3.

32.5   966.16—Sodium in Fruits and Fruit Products
Flame Spectrophotometric Method
First Action 1966
Final Action 1968

(*Caution: See Appendix* for safety notes on flame photometers.)

A. Reagents and Apparatus

(**a**) *Sodium standard solutions.*—Dry reagent grade NaCl at 100° overnight and dilute 2.5422 g to 1 L with H_2O. (Solution contains 1000 ppm Na.) Dilute 10 mL to 100 mL, and further dilute 1, 2, 4, 6, 8, and 10 mL diluted solution to 100 mL to make standard solutions containing, respectively, 1, 2, 4, 6, 8, and 10 ppm Na. Store in clean, dry poly(ethylene) bottles.

(**b**) *Flame spectrophotometer.*

B. Determination

Prepare sample solution as in **920.149**. Dilute, if necessary, to reduce Na concentration to range covered by flame photometer (preferably 4–10 ppm Na). Aspirate sample solution (diluted or undiluted) directly into flame.

    I. **920.149** (Preparation of Fruit Sample)

Transfer samples received in open packages (i.e., not sterile) without delay to glass-stoppered containers and keep in cool place. To avoid effects of fermentation, make prompt determinations of alcohol, total and volatile acids, solids, and sugars, particularly in case of fruit juices and fresh fruits. (Portions for determination of sucrose and reducing sugars may be weighed and kept several days without fermenting if the slight excess of neutral $Pb(OAc)_2$ solution required in determination is added. *Note:* $Pb(OAc)_2$ is toxic. Label samples to show its addition.) Prepare various products for analysis as follows:

(**a**) *Juices.*—Mix thoroughly by shaking to ensure uniform sample, and filter through absorbent cotton or rapid paper. Prepare fresh juices by pressing well pulped fruit and filtering. Express juice of citrus fruits by commercial device, and filter.

(**b**) *Jellies and sirups.*—Mix thoroughly to ensure uniform sample. Prepare solution by weighing 300 g thoroughly mixed sample into 2 L flask and dissolve in H_2O, heating on steam bath if necessary. Apply as little heat as possible to minimize inversion of sucrose. Cool, dilute to volume, mix thoroughly by shaking, and use aliquots for the various determinations. If insoluble material is present, mix thoroughly and filter first.

(**c**) *Fresh fruits, dried fruits, preserves, jams, and marmalades.*—Pulp by passing through food chopper, or by use of soil dispersion mixer, Hobart mixer, or other suitable mechanical mixing apparatus, or by grinding in large mortar, and mixing thoroughly, completing operation as quickly as possible to avoid loss of moisture. With dried fruits, pass sample through food chopper 3 times, mixing thoroughly after each grinding. Set burrs or blades of food chopper as close as possible without crushing seeds. Grind entire contents of No. 10 or smaller container. Mix contents of larger containers thoroughly by stirring and remove portion for grinding. With stone fruits, remove pits and determine their proportion in weighed sample.

Prepare solution by weighing into 1.5–2 L beaker 300 g fresh fruit, or equivalent of dried fruit, preserves, jams, and marmalades, well-pulped and mixed in blender or other suitable type of mechanical grinder; add ca 800 mL H_2O; and boil 1 h replacing at intervals H_2O lost by evaporation. Transfer to 2 L volumetric flask, cool, dilute to volume, and filter. With unsweetened fruit, ashing is facilitated by addition of sugar before boiling; therefore weigh 150 g fruit, add 150 g sugar and 800 mL H_2O, and proceed as above.

(d) *Canned fruits.—See* **968.30**. Carefully invert by hand all fruits having cups or cavities if they fall on sieve with cups or cavities up. Cups or cavities in soft products may be drained by tilting sieve, but no other handling of these products while draining is permissible. Examination of sirup in which fruits are preserved is often enough. Separate liquor by draining, **968.30B**, and treat as in (a).

II. **968.30** (Canned Vegetables, Drained Weight)

A. Sieves

See "Definition of Terms and Explanatory Notes" in *Official Methods of Analysis* (1990) 15th Ed. Use 8″ (20 cm) diameter for containers ≤3 lb (1.36 kg) or 12″ (30 cm) diameter for containers >3 lb.

B. Determination

Weigh full can, open, and pour entire contents on No. 8 sieve (use 7/16″ sieve for canned tomatoes). Without shifting product, incline sieve at ca 17–20 angle to facilitate drainage. Drain 2 min, directly weigh either drained solids or free liquid, and weigh dry empty can. From weights obtained, determine % liquid and % drained solid contents.

Determine $\%T$ for standards and plot curve of $\%T$ against ppm Na. Determine $\%T$ for sample and use standard curve to determine ppm Na in sample or follow instructions of manufacturer, making check determinations as necessary. If internal standard instrument is used, add appropriate amount of LiCl to both standard and sample solutions.

Report as mg Na_2O/100 g sample. Na × 1.3480 = Na_2O.

Reference: JAOAC **49,** 617(1966).
CAS-7440-23-5 (sodium)

32.6   990.23—Sodium and Potassium in Dried Milk
Flame Emission Spectrometric Method
First Action 1990
IDF-ISO-AOAC Method

See Chapter 27.8.

32.7   969.23—Sodium and Potassium in Seafood
Flame Photometric Method
First Action 1969
Final Action 1971

See Chapter 27.9.

32.8   976.25—Sodium in Foods for Special Dietary Use
Ion Selective Electrode Method
First Action 1976
Final Action 1977

(Applicable to foods containing ≤ 100 mg Na/100 g)

A. Apparatus

(**a**) *Electrode.*—Sodium combination ion selective electrode (Model 96-11, replacement Model 8611), Orion Research, Inc., or equivalent).

(**b**) *Graph paper.*—Gran's plot paper, 10% volume corrected (No. 90-00-90, Orion Research, Inc., or equivalent).

(**c**) *Magnetic stirrer.*—with 4 cm (1½ in.) Teflon-coated stirring bar. Use mat to insulate sample from motor heat.

(**d**) *pH meter.*—With expanded mV scale (Model 701/701A, (replacement Model SA 720), Orion Research, Inc., or equivalent).

B. Reagents

(**a**) *Buffer solution.*—pH 10.2. Total ionic strength adjustment buffer (TISAB), $0.5M$ triethanolamine. Dissolve 74.6 g triethanolamine in ca 900 mL H_2O, adjust pH to 10.2 with HCl, and dilute to 1 L with H_2O.

(**b**) *Sodium standard solutions.*—(*1*) *Stock solution.*—10 mg/mL. Accurately weigh 2.5421 g NaCl, previously dried overnight at 100°, into 100 mL volumetric flask. Dissolve and dilute to volume with H_2O, and mix. (*2*) *Working solutions.*— 0.1, 1.0, and 2.0 mg/mL. Pipet 1, 10, and 20 mL stock solution into separate 100 mL volumetric flasks, dilute each to volume with buffer solution, and mix.

C. Preparation of Sample

Blend entire contents of can, including H_2O. Weigh 10.0 g sample and dilute to 100 mL with buffer solution. Mix and transfer to 150 mL beaker.

D. Determination

(**a**) *For foods with 0–5 mg declared Na/100 g.*—Immerse electrode in sample beaker and stir magnetically 2–5 min to equilibrate. Record mV potential on expanded mV scale. From 10 mL buret, add five 1.0 mL portions 0.1 mg Na/mL working standard solution to beaker, stirring magnetically 30 s after each addition. Plot mV reading for 0, 1, 2, 3, 4, and 5 mL on graph paper, (**b**). Plot *E* directly for both blank and sample descending 5 mV for each major line crossing vertical axis. Plot most positive mV reading at top of vertical axis. Draw best straight line through points, extrapolate line to horizontal axis, and read mg Na in sample.

Perform blank determination on 100 mL buffer solution, adding five 1.0 mL portions 0.1 mg Na/mL working standard solution, as above. Plot mV readings on graph paper, omitting 0 mL reading, such that 5 mL reading falls near top of paper. Draw best straight line through points, extrapolate line to horizontal axis, and read mg Na in blank.

$$\text{mg Na/100 g food} = [(S - B) \times 100]/W$$

where S = mg Na in sample, B = mg Na in blank, and W = g sample.

(b) *For foods with 5–50 mg declared Na/100 g.*—Proceed as in (a), except use 1.0 mg Na/mL working standard solution.

(c) *For foods with 50–100 mg declared Na/100 g.*— Proceed as in (a), except use 2.0 mg Na/mL working standard solution.

Reference: JAOAC **59,** 1131(1976).
CAS-7440-23-5 (sodium)

32.9 984.27—Calcium, Copper, Iron, Magnesium, Manganese, Phosphorus, Potassium, Sodium, and Zinc in Infant Formula
Inductively Coupled Plasma Emission Spectroscopic Method
First Action 1984
Final Action 1986

See Chapter 12.13.

Chapter 33
Sugars (Mono & Di)

33.1

982.14—Glucose, Fructose, Sucrose, and Maltose in Presweetened Cereals
Liquid Chromatographic Method
First Action 1982
Final Action 1983

A. Apparatus

(a) *Chromatography equipment.*—See **980.13A(a)** through (d) (*see* 33.2), but change capacity factor in **980.13A(b)** to 1.5; include automatic injectors, 410 differential refractometer (Waters Associates, Inc., WISP 710B and R1 410, respectively, or equivalents) 100 × 4.6 (id) mm Spheri-5 amino cartridge (Brownlee Labs, or equivalent) and use specific injection volume in 10–50 μL range in **980.13A(c)**.

(b) *Filter cartridge.*—100 × 2 (id) mm (Waters Assoc., Inc.), or 15 × 3.2 (id) mm 7 μm amino guard cartridge (Brownlee Labs, or equivalent.).

(c) *Guard column packing.*—Optional. C_{18} Corasil, 100 × 2 (id) mm (Waters Associates, Inc.), or 15 × 3.2 (id) mm, 7 μm amino guard cartridge (Brownlee Labs, Inc.), or equivalent, as long as overall LC system meets column criteria of **980.13A(b)**.

B. Reagents

(a) *Sugar standard solution.*—Dry individual sugar standards (fructose, glucose, sucrose, and maltose; available from Sigma Chemical Co.) 12 h at 60° under vacuum. Dissolve in alcohol–H_2O (1 + 1) to obtain concentrations of 3 mg/mL each for fructose, glucose, and maltose and 15 mg/mL for sucrose. After LC injection, compare peak response of sample and standard, and adjust concentrations of standard solution proportionately to obtain standard response within 10% of sample responses.

(b) *Mobile phase.*—CH_3CN (LC grade) and H_2O (purified via Milli-Q System, or equivalent) (80 + 20). Filter through Whatman GF/F 0.7 μm glass fiber filter or through 0.45 μm Pall nylon 66 filter. Optionally, filter CH_3CN and H_2O separately through 0.45 μm PTFE and cellulose ester membranes, respectively. Degas in ultrasonic bath before use. Vary CH_3CN-H_2O ratio and flow rate if necessary to meet column criteria.

C. Preparation of Sample

(a) *Fat extraction.*—Weigh 2.00–10.00 g finely ground cereal into ≥100 mL centrifuge bottle. If sample does not warrant fat extraction, proceed to step (b). Add 50 mL petroleum ether and centrifuge ca 10 min at 2000 rpm. Aspirate and discard petroleum ether without siphoning off solid material. Repeat extraction. Evaporate residual petroleum ether with gentle stream of N and break up solid material with glass rod.

(b) *Sugar extraction.*—Add 100 mL alcohol–H_2O (1 + 1) and weigh. Place in 80–85° H_2O bath 25 min and stir occasionally. Cool to room temperature and add alcohol to original weight. Filter portion of extract through 0.45 μm nylon syringe filter (Nalge Co., 75 Panorama Creek Dr, PO Box 20365, Rochester, NY

14602-0365, or equivalent). If cloudy, centrifuge 10 min at ≥ 2000 rpm. If still cloudy, recentrifuge portion of extract 5 min at ≥ 3500 rpm and filter through 0.45 μm nylon syringe filter. If guard column is used, omit step (c) and save filtered extract for LC analysis.

(c) *Cleanup*.—Fill C_{18} Sep-Pak cartridge with mobile phase and force through filter, leaving liquid above packing. Repeat with sample extract twice, collecting eluate from second pass for LC analysis. Filter through 0.45 μm nylon syringe filter if necessary.

D. Determination

Inject sample solution (10–50 μL) into column with flow rate of mobile phase at 1.5–2.5 mL/min. Inject same volume of standard solution that will give peak response $\pm$ 10% of sample peak response. Two injections each of sample and standard solution are required for adequate precision.

Measure areas or peak heights of each sugar peak in sample and standard, but only measure peak height for components which are near detection limit and have adjacent interfering peak.

$$\% \text{ Component} = (R/R') \times (C'/W) \times V \times 100$$

where R and R' = area or peak height of sample sugar and standard sugar, respectively; V = mL alcohol–H_2O added to sample = 100; W = g sample; C' = concentration of sugar standard in g/mL.

Elimination of interfering peak from possible presence of NaCl.—(1) Prepare blank solution of ca 2 mg NaCl/mL in same injection solvent used for sugar standard solutions, and inject blank solution immediately after sugar standards and before samples. (2) If NaCl interferes with peaks of sugars being analyzed, wash column with solution of 0.1% TEPA (Cat. No. T5902, Eastman Kodak Co.) in CH_3CN–H_2O (80 + 20). Adjust pH of TEPA solution to ca 7 with CH_3COOH, and then wash column 2 h at 1.5 mL/min. Flush column with ca 100 mL mobile phase before continuing analyses. This remedy provides only temporary cure (10 injections). (3) Alternatively, add 2 drops of concentrated CH_3COOH/L of mobile phase to eliminate NaCl interference in elution of fructose or glucose. *Note:* This step, (3), should be used only as an alternative to and not in addition to step (2).

Reference: JAOAC **65**, 256(1982); **66**, 197(1983); **67**, 379(1984); **68**, 259(1985); **72**, 85(1989).
CAS-57-48-7 (fructose)
CAS-50-99-7 (glucose)
CAS-69-79-4 (maltose)
CAS-57-50-1 (sucrose)

33.2

980.13—Fructose, Glucose, Lactose, Maltose, and Sucrose in Milk Chocolate
Liquid Chromatographic Method
Final Action

(*Caution: See Appendix* for safety notes on acetonitrile.)

A. *Apparatus*

(a) *Liquid chromatograph.*—With Waters Associates, Inc. M6000A pump, R401 refractive index detector, or equivalent, and 10 mV recorder.

(b) *Column packing.*—Waters Associates, Inc. μ-Bondapak carbohydrate column, 300 $\times$ 4 (id) mm. Column must meet following criteria:

$$\text{Capacity factor for fructose} = K' = (t_R - t_0)/t_0 \geq 5$$

where t_R = retention time for fructose = time from injection to maximum peak height of fructose; t_0 = retention time for solvent = time from injection to maximum peak height of first baseline distortion or solvent peak.

Resolution factor (distance between 2 band centers divided by average band width) =

$$R_s = (t_2 - t_1)/0.5(t_{w1} + t_{w2})$$

where t_2 and t_1 = times from injection to maximum peak heights of second peak (glucose) and first peak (fructose), respectively; and t_{w1} and t_{w2} = baseline widths (in time units) of first and second peaks, respectively. For fructose:glucose ratios of 2.0–0.5, $R_s \geq 1.0$; for ratios ≥ 2, $R_s \geq 1.25$. Replace column when either or both criteria are not met.

(c) *Injection valve.*—Waters Associates, Inc. 7120 LC injector with 50 μL loop, or equivalent.

(d) *Ancillary equipment.*—Bransonic 12 ultrasonic bath (Branson Ultrasonics Corp., Eagle Rd, Danbury CT 06810-1961), or equivalent, to degas solvents; Corning PC 353 stirrer; and filtration apparatus for solvent purification.

B. *Reagents*

(a) *Sugar standard solution.*—10 μg/mL. Dry individual sugar standards (fructose, glucose, sucrose, lactose, and maltose; available from Sigma Chemical Co.) 12 h at 60° under vacuum. Dissolve in H_2O and serially dilute to concentration of 10 μg/mL. Prepare daily.

(b) *Mobile phase.*—CH_3CN (Mallinckrodt Nanograde, or equivalent) + H_2O (charcoal filtered) (80 + 20). Filter through Whatman GF/F 0.7 μm glass fiber filter, and degas in ultrasonic bath before use.

C. *Preparation of Sample*

Weigh 10.0 g finely divided milk chocolate into $\geq$ 100 mL centrifuge bottle and add 50 mL petroleum ether. Centrifuge ca 15 min at ca 1800 rpm. Decant and discard supernate. Repeat extraction.

Pulverize residue with glass rod, add 100 g H_2O, and weigh. Place in 85–90° H_2O bath 25 min. Cool to room temperature and add H_2O to original weight. Centrifuge 10 min at 2000 rpm, withdraw portion of clear supernate, and filter through 0.45 μm Swinney syringe filter.

D. Determination

Fill 50 μL injection loop with sample solution and inject into column with mobile solvent flowing at 1.5–2.0 mL/min. Calculate concentrations of each sugar by comparing peak heights or areas of each sugar peak from sample with corresponding height or area of standard. Use same method of measurement (area or height) throughout.

Reference: JAOAC **63**, 595(1980).
CAS-57-48-7 (fructose)
CAS-50-99-7 (glucose)
CAS-63-42-3 (lactose)
CAS-69-79-4 (maltose)
CAS-57-50-1 (sucrose)

33.3   984.17—Sugars in Licorice Extracts
Liquid Chromatographic Method
First Action 1984

(Applicable to paste or spray-dried products)

A. Principle

Sample is dissolved in H_2O, filtered, and subjected to column cleanup. Aliquot is injected into LC apparatus equipped with differential refractometer detector. Response is compared with that of standard solution.

B. Apparatus

(**a**) *Liquid chromatograph.*—Model M6000A solvent delivery system, Model U6K universal injector, Model R401 differential refractometer, and 30 cm × 4 mm μBondapak/carbohydrate column (Waters Associates, Inc.), or equivalent.

(**b**) *Computing integrator.*—Model 3390A (Hewlett Packard), or equivalent.

(**c**) *Guard column.*—Packed with 37–50 μm AX/Corasil (Waters Associates, Inc.), or equivalent.

(**d**) *Sample and solvent clarification kit.*—Aqueous and organic (Waters Associates, Inc.), or equivalent.

(**e**) *Cartridge.*—Sep-Pak™ C_{18} (Waters Associates, Inc.), or equivalent. Condition just before use by passing 10 mL mixture followed by 10 mL H_2O through cartridge.

C. Reagents

(**a**) *Mobile phase.*—Use LC grade reagents, CH_3CN–H_2O (83 + 17). Filter and degas mobile phase with solvent clarification kit. Flow rate 2.0 mL/min.

(**b**) *Sugar standard solution.*—2.5 mg/mL each fructose, glucose, sucrose, and maltose (Sigma Chemical Co.). Accurately weigh 250 mg each fructose, glucose, sucrose, and maltose into 100 mL volumetric flask and dilute to volume with H_2O, heating gently until dissolved. Using aqueous sample clarification kit, filter through 0.45 μm filter, followed by preconditioned C_{18} cartridge.

D. Sample Preparation

Accurately weigh 1.0 g licorice product into 250 mL erlenmeyer and add 100.0 ML H_2O. Place flask in 85–90° H_2O bath until sample dissolves, then cool to room temperature. Filter through 0.45 μm filter. Pass 5 mL sample through preconditioned C_{18} cartridge, and collect eluate. Sugars in sample should pass through C_{18} cartridge and any nonpolar components in sample will be retained.

E. Liquid Chromatography

Let LC column equilibrate 30 min at flow rate of 2.0 mL/min. Inject 10 μL mixed sugar standard solution. Approximate retention times are fructose, 6.6 min; glucose, 7.7 min; sucrose, 12.4 min; and maltose, 15.2 min (retention times vary from one column to another). Inject 60 μL sample solution. If samples are analyzed in series, re-inject standard solution at regular intervals.

Calculate concentration of each sugar by comparing either peak heights or peak areas of standard with corresponding peak heights or peak areas of sample. Calculate amount of each sugar by the following equation:

$$\% \text{ Sugar} = (C'/C) \times (Ar/Ar') \times (V'/V) \times 100$$

where C' and C = concentration of standard and sample in mg/mL; Ar' and Ar = average peak area of standard and sample, respectively (Ht'/Ht could be used for height instead of area); V' and V = μL injected of standard and sample, respectively.

Reference: JAOAC **67**, 764(1984).

33.4   977.20—Separation of Sugars in Honey
Liquid Chromatographic Method
Final Action

A. Apparatus

(a) *Chromatograph.*—Waters Associates Model ALC/GPC, or equivalent, with Model 6000A solvent delivery system and Model U6K injector.

(b) *Detector.*—Waters Associates R-401 refractive index detector, or equivalent.

(c) *Recorder.*—Varian Aerograph Model A-25 dual pen recorder, or equivalent.

(d) *Column.*—300 × 4 (id) mm μ-Bondapak/Carbohydrate (Waters Associates, No. 84038).

(e) *Sample clarification kit.*—Available in kit form from Waters Associates (No. 26865), or equivalent; 0.45 μm filters stable in organic solvents are suitable.

(f) *Syringes.*—10 μL No. 701-N point style No. 1, 2 × 0.020″ od, 25 gage needle (Hamilton Co.).

B. Reagents

(a) *Mobile phase.*—Nonspectro acetonitrile (Burdick & Jackson Laboratories, Inc.) diluted with H_2O (83 + 17). Degas mobile phase daily by magnetic stirring 15 min under vacuum.

(b) *Sugar standard solution.*—Place 3.804 g fructose (Mallinckrodt Chemical Works), 3.010 g glucose (Mallinckrodt Chemical Works), and 0.602 g sucrose into 100 mL volumetric flask, dissolve in 50 mL

H_2O, and add CH_3CN to volume. Composition of standard approximates 5 g honey dissolved in 50 mL aqueous CH_3CN (1 + 1).

C. Operating Conditions

Fructose, glucose, and sucrose are baseline separated and quantitated in 20 min under following conditions: flow rate, 1.0 mL/min (ca 500 psig; 3.45 MPa); temperature, ambient (ca 23°); detector (R-401), 8× (fructose and glucose) and 2× (sucrose); attenuation, 10 mV on recorder, detector set so that 380 μg fructose gives full-scale deflection of pen; and chart speed, 0.1″/min. Mono-, di-, and trisaccharides are eluted from column in order of MW.

D. Preparation of Sample

Weigh 5.000 g sample in small beaker and transfer to 50 mL volumetric flask with 25 mL H_2O. Immediately dilute to volume with CH_3CN and filter through 0.45 μm filter, using sample clarification kit.

E. Chromatography

Inject 10 μL standard solution into chromatograph. Establish retention times, measure peak heights, and check reproducibility. Repeat for sample solution. Calculate glucose, fructose, and sucrose from integrator values or from peak heights as follows:

$$\text{Weight \% sugar} = 100 \times (PH/PH') \times (Volume/volume') \times (W'/W)$$

where PH and PH' = peak heights (or integrator values) of sample and standard, respectively; V and V' = mL sample and standard (50 and 100) solutions, respectively; and W and W' = g sample (5.000) and standard, respectively.

References: JAOAC **60**, 838(1977); **62**, 515(1979).
CAS-57-48-7 (fructose)
CAS-50-99-7 (glucose)
CAS-57-50-1 (sucrose)

33.5   983.22—Saccharides (Minor) in Corn Sugar
Liquid Chromatographic Method
First Action 1983
Corn Industries Research Foundation-AOAC Method

A. Principle

Polysaccharides in high (98 + %) dextrose corn sugar are quantitated vs maltose standard and calculated as disaccharides (DP_2) and tri- and higher saccharides (DP_{3+}).

B. Determination

Proceed as in **979.23** (*see* 33.6), except use only Aminex Q15-S resin column (**979.23B[g]**), or equivalent, and use ca 3 g maltose·H_2O standard/25 mL instead of mixed sugar standard, **979.23C(e)**. Compute dry basis concentration of maltose by multiplying by 0.94. Determine response factor for maltose dry basis by injecting 10 μL standard solution and proceeding as in **979.23F**. Prepare sample as in **979.23G**. Complete determination as in **979.23H**, but inject 50 μL diluted sample.

C. Calculations

Results are computed automatically when using **979.23B(c)**. List DP_2 results and combine all tri- and higher saccharides and list sum as DP_{3+}. Subtract sum of DP_2 and DP_{3+} from 100 to obtain glucose (dextrose) (DP_1) value. Report results on ash-free, carbohydrate dry substance basis. In absence of computing integrator, list areas for DP_2 and sum for DP_{3+}, multiply each by maltose response factor and by 100 to obtain $\%DP_2$ and $\%DP_{3+}$. Subtract sum of $\%DP_2$ and $\%DP_{3+}$ from 100 to obtain $\%DP_1$.

Reference: JAOAC **65,** 1366(1982).

33.6   979.23—Saccharides (Minor) in Corn Sirup
Liquid Chromatagraphic Method
First Action 1979
Corn Industries Research Foundation-AOAC Method

A. Principle

Corn sirup solution is passed through cation exchange column. Sugars are separated by molecular exclusion and selective adsorption, and detected wih differential refractometer. Peaks are quantitated against appropriate standard with digital computing integrator. Psicose, fructose, dextrose, maltulose, other disaccharides (DP_2), DP_3, DP_4, etc. are determined in corn sirup with 50W-X4 resin. Alternative Q15-S column is suitable for determination of psicose, fructose, dextrose, total DP_2, DP_3, and DP_{4+}.

B. Apparatus

(**a**) *Liquid chromatograph.*—Waters Associates Model 201 equipped with Model 6000 pump and Model R-401 refractive index detector (Waters Associates, Inc.), or equivalent.

(**b**) *Recorder.*—Hewlett-Packard Model 7100B recorder with Model 17505A input module, or equivalent.

(**c**) *Digital integrator.*—Spectra-Physics Autolab System I Computing Integrator with calculation capability, used according to manufacturer's "Method 1" (Spectra-Physics, 3333 N First St, San Jose, CA 95134), or equivalent.

(**d**) *Circulating bath.*—45 $\pm$ 0.005°. Haake, Model FK (replacement Model D8L) (Haake Buchler Instruments, Inc., 244 Saddle River Rd, Saddle Brook, NJ 07662-6001), or equivalent.

(**e**) *Circulating bath.*—78 $\pm$ 0.05°. Haake Model FS, or equivalent. Dow Corning 200, 5cS viscosity silicone oil may be used as bath medium.

(**f**) *Syringe.*—100 μL Precision Sampling, Series B, Model 01-9264, PRESSURE-LOK (Precision Sampling Corp., 8275 West El Cajon, PO Box 15886, Baton Rouge, LA 70895), or equivalent.

(**g**) *LC column.*—610 × 7 (id) mm (24 × 3/8″[od]) stainless steel column packed with Aminex 50W-X4, 20–30 μm, Ca resin (or, alternatively, Aminex Q15-S, 19–25 μm, Ca resin), and fitted with Waters Associates Model 98764 column temperature control block and 3/8″, 10 μm frit, end fittings.

C. Reagents

(a) *Mobile phase.*—Degassed H_2O, filtered through 0.22 μm Millipore filter before use. Keep at ca 65° and stir slowly on hot plate-stirrer to remove dissolved gas.

(b) *Column packing.*—Aminex 50W-X4, 20-30 μm, or Q15-S, 19-25 μm, Ca form resin. Slurry required amount of Aminex 50W-X4, H form, or Q15-S, Na form cation exchange resin (Bio-Rad Laboratories) with H_2O, transfer to 350 mL medium porosity fritted glass funnel, and remove H_2O with vacuum. Wash each 10 g resin with 300 mL filtered (Whatman No. 4 paper, or equivalent) $0.3M$ $Ca(OAc)_2$ solution adjusted to pH 6.2 with CH_3COOH. Wash each 10 g resin with 200 mL H_2O. Remove H_2O from treated resin with vacuum and store in nonactinic bottle at room temperature.

(c) *Mixed ion exchange resin.*—Exhaust (2 L $1.5N$ NaOH) and regenerate (2 L $1.5N$ HCl) ca 600 mL bed volume Duolite C-3 (Diamond Shamrock Corp., PO Box 348, Painesville, OH 44077) cation resin. Repeat twice. Exhaust (2 L $1.5N$ HCl) and regenerate (once each with 2 L $1.5N$ NaOH, and 2 L $2N$ Na_2CO_3) ca 600 mL bed volume Duolite ES-561 weak base anion exchange resin. Repeat twice. Wash final regenerated resins with H_2O to pH ranges of 4-5 (C-3) and 6-7 (ES-461). Air dry resins, combine equal weights of each, and mix. Avoid strong base resins which may promote alkaline isomerization of sample.

(d) *Carbohydrate standards.*—Glucose (NIST); fructose (Pfanstiehl Laboratories, Inc., 1219 Glen Rock Ave., Waukegan, IL 60085); maltose·H_2O, Grade HHH (Hayashibara Co., Ltd, 2-3 Shimoishii, 1-CHOME, Okayama 700, Japan); maltotriose (United States Biochemical Corp., 21000 Miles Pkwy, Cleveland, OH 44128); acid converted 42 Dextrose Equivalent (DE) corn sirup (available from ADM Corn Sweeteners, PO Box 1470, Decatur, IL 62525, or CPC International, Inc., International Plaza, PO Box 8000, Englewood Cliffs, NJ 07632); psicose (Carb. Res. **16**, 383[1971]); maltulose (Cereal Science Today **17**, 180[1972]).

Estimate corn sirup composition by determining level of each saccharide shown for given DE in CRA, Inc. Critical Data Tables, pp. 8–13. Determine DE as in **923.09C** (*see* 33.14), and **941.14B**. Purity of given sugar may be determined by normalized LC analysis.

941.14 (Moisture in Corn Sirups and Sugars)

(Applicable to corn sirups and crude corn sugars)

A. Material and Apparatus

(a) *Diatomaceous earth.*—Filter-Cel, or equivalent. Preferably analytical grade. If commercial grade is used, wash with HCl, then with H_2O to remove acid, and dry in oven at ca 105°. (Material should give negative test for acid when moistened.)

(b) *Moisture dish.*—Al dish 25 mm high × 75 mm diameter, with cover.

(c) *Pestle.*—Flat-end glass stirring rod ca 60 mm long.

B. Determination

Place 10 g Filter-Cel in moisture dish containing pestle and dry to constant weight. Weigh ca 5 g corn sirup or sugar in nickel scoop, dilute with ca 5 mL H_2O, and add to Filter-Cel. Wash scoop with three 2 mL portions H_2O and add washings to Filter-Cel. Thoroughly incorporate solution with Filter-Cel by means of pestle, yielding *damp* workable mass. Dry to constant weight in vacuum oven at 100° for corn sirup or 70° for crude corn sugars.

Reference: Ind. Eng. Chem. Anal. Ed. **13**, 858(1941).

(e) *Mixed sugar standard.*—Prepare standard sugar solution to contain ca 3 g dry carbohydrate substance/25 mL. Make dry basis % of each standard sugar equivalent to level in typical sample of given type. Use 42

DE corn sirup to represent DP_{4+} fraction, adding dry weights of mono-, di-, and trisaccharide from 42 DE sirup to dry weights of pure glucose, maltose, and maltotriose used for standard preparation. Add appropriate dry weight of each standard sugar to tared 50 mL beaker. Record weight to fifth place. Add 20 mL H_2O, cover, and place on steam bath to dissolve. Transfer quantitatively to 25 mL volumetric flask, dilute to volume, and mix. Add several drops toluene as preservative. Store at room temperature. Avoid toluene layer when drawing up solution for standard injection. Compute dry basis concentration of each sugar:

% sugar, dry basis = weight sugar $\times$ 100/(weight glucose + a + b) + (weight fructose + c)
+ [(weight maltose $\times$ 0.94) + d + e] + [(weight maltotriose $\times$ 0.94) + f + g + h] + weight DP_{4+}

where maltose and maltotriose weights are multiplied by 0.94 to account for H_2O of hydration and trace impurities; a and b = weight glucose from 42 DE sirup and maltulose; c = weight fructose from maltulose; d and e = weights of DP_2 from 42 DE sirup and maltulose; and f, g, and h = DP_3 weights from 42 DE sirup, maltulose, and maltose.

D. Preparation of Column

Place empty column vertically, and attach 380 $\times$ 7.7 (id) mm (15 $\times$ ⅜" [od]) stainless steel precolumn, using ⅜" union. Attach end fitting to bottom of column and vacuum line to end fitting. Attach open-ended vessel (ca 500 mL) to precolumn with Tygon tubing and secure vessel in same plane as column. Slowly fill column, precolumn, and ca ⅓ of vessel with H_2O. Slurry ca 50 mL bed volume of resin and add to vessel, using vacuum. Bring column to 78°. Pull vacuum on column until resin level in vessel is constant. Discontinue vacuum, disconnect vessel from precolumn, and pump solvent through precolumn and column at 0.5 mL/min (0.7 mL/min for Q15-S resin) overnight. Disconnect end fitting from precolumn and precolumn from column. Fill end fitting with ca 5 mm resin and attach to column. Cap end with fittings when storing column.

E. Operating Conditions

Flow rate 0.4 mL/min (0.6 mL/min for Q15-S resin); column temperature 78°; detector temperature 45°; detector attenuation 8$\times$; detector output 10 mV; recorder attenuation 1$\times$; recorder range 10 mV; chart speed 2 in./h. Program integrator to obtain trapezoidal baseline correction for each peak and to prevent erroneous baseline at valley point between fused peaks or on plateau created by fused peak cluster.

F. Standardization

Inject 30 μL (ca 3.5 mg solids) of standard solution. Integrate standard sugar peaks in normalized mode. Sum DP_{4+} fractions obtained from normalized printout to obtain DP_{4+} normalized response. Divide known dry basis concentration by normalized response for each component to obtain ratios. Divide each component ratio by glucose ratio to obtain System I KF values (calibration factors). Program component KF values in System I, **979.23B(c)**, using Method 1 and glucose as reference ($KF_{glucose}$ = 1). Enter DP_3 KF at both DP_3 retention time and at time 100 s less than DP_3 time, to provide KF for panose, isomaltotriose, and linear DP_4 when 50W-X4 resin is used. List DP_{4+} KF as default KF for DP_{5+} calculation when 50W-X4 resin is used.

G. Preparation of Sample

Determine approximate dry substance as in **943.05C**. Dilute sample by weight to ca 12% dry substance with H_2O. Add ca 0.3 g mixed exchange resin to ca 6 g diluted sample and shake 10 min to remove possible interfering ionic material that elutes in DP_{4+} region.

943.05 (Dry Substance in Corn Sirups and Sugars)
C. Method II—By Refractometer
(Applicable only to liquid samples containing no undissolved solids)
Determine refractometer reading at 45°. Circulate H_2O through jackets of refractometer long enough to let temperature of prisms and of sample reach equilibrium, continuing circulation during observation, and taking care that temperature is held constant. From Tables **943.05B** and **C** obtain commercial Baumé corresponding to observed refractive index. From Table **943.05A** obtain corresponding dry substance.
References: Ind. Eng. Chem. Anal. Ed. **16,** 161(1944). J. Agric. Food Chem. **32,** 971(1984). JAOAC **68,** 259(1985).

Table 943.05A. Commercial Baumé Table for Dry Substance in Corn Syrup and High Fructose Corn Syrup (Commerical Baumé = Bé 140°F/60°C + 1° Bé)

	Dextrose Equiv. (top); Maltose, %DB (bottom)								Fructose, %DB		
	28	32	42	42	50	55	63	95	42	55	90
		15	13	33	50	18	30				
Commercial Baumé	Dry Substance,[a] %										
36	66.46	66.61	66.99	67.00	67.43	67.53	68.24	69.88	70.02	70.12	70.13
37	68.37	68.52	68.91	68.91	69.34	69.47	70.19	71.88	72.02	72.14	72.15
38	70.28	70.44	70.84	70.83	71.27	71.41	72.15	73.90	74.05	74.17	74.19
39	72.20	72.36	72.78	72.76	73.21	73.36	74.11	75.92	76.09	76.20	76.24
40	74.13	74.31	74.73	74.70	75.15	75.33	76.09	77.95		78.26	76.29
41	76.09	76.25	76.69	76.65	77.10	77.31	78.08	80.00		80.32	80.36
42	78.05	78.22	78.67	78.60	79.06	79.29	80.07	82.04			82.44
43	80.02	80.20	80.66	80.58	81.04	81.31	82.08				
44	82.01	82.18	82.65	82.56	83.03	83.32	84.09				

[a]Dry substances are left blank whenever the carbohydrate solutions are supersaturated with respect to dextrose and, therefore, do not exist as one (liquid) phase.

Table 943.05B.—Commercial Baumé Table of Refractive Index of Corn Syrups and High Fructose Corn Syrups at 45° (Commercial Baumé = Bé 140°F/60°C + 1° Bé)

Commercial Baumé	Dextrose Equiv. (top); Maltose, %DB (bottom)								Fructose, %DB		
	28	32	42	42	50	55	63	95	42	55	90
		15	13	33	50	18	30				
	Refractive Index[a] at 45°										
36	1.4588	1.4585	1.4579	1.4585	1.4583	1.4575	1.4579	1.4571	1.4566	1.4565	1.4561
37	1.4637	1.4633	1.4626	1.4632	1.4630	1.4622	1.4627	1.4618	1.4613	1.4613	1.4607
38	1.4686	1.4683	1.4675	1.4681	1.4678	1.4671	1.4675	1.4666	1.4661	1.4661	1.4654
39	1.4733	1.4732	1.4725	1.4730	1.4728	1.4720	1.4724	1.4715	1.4710	1.4709	1.4703
40	1.4784	1.4784	1.4775	1.4781	1.4778	1.4771	1.4775	1.4765		1.4758	1.4752
41	1.4837	1.4836	1.4827	1.4832	1.4829	1.4822	1.4826	1.4816		1.4810	1.4803
42	1.4890	1.4890	1.4880	1.4885	1.4881	1.4874	1.4878	1.4867			1.4854
43	1.4944	1.4945	1.4934	1.4939	1.4935	1.4928	1.4932				
44	1.5001	1.5001	1.4990	1.4994	1.4990	1.4983	1.4986				

[a]Refractive indices are left blank whenever the carbohydrate solutions are supersaturated with respect to dextrose and, therefore, do not exist as one (liquid) phase.

Table 943.05C. Refractive Index Table for Dry Substance in Corn Syrups and High Fructose Corn Syrups

Refractive Index at 45°	Dextrose Equiv. (top); Maltose, %DB (bottom)								Fructose, %DB		
	28	32	42	42	50	56	63	95	42	55	90
		15	13	33	50	18	30				
	Dry Substance,[a] %										
1.4550	64.93	65.18	65.83	65.60	66.09	66.50	66.99	68.95	69.30	69.42	69.68
1.4600	66.92	67.19	67.86	67.62	68.13	68.56	69.07	71.11	71.46	71.59	71.86
1.4650	68.93	69.16	69.86	69.62	70.14	70.59	71.42	73.23	73.60	73.72	74.00
1.4700	70.92	71.11	71.82	71.58	72.13	72.58	73.14	75.29	75.69	75.82	76.11
1.4750	72.83	73.02	73.76	73.52	74.07	74.55	75.12	77.34	77.76	77.89	78.20
1.4800	74.73	74.90	75.67	75.43	75.99	76.48	77.08	79.37		79.93	80.24
1.4850	76.58	76.76	77.56	77.31	77.88	78.40	79.01	81.37		81.94	82.27
1.4900	78.42	78.59	79.40	79.16	79.75	80.27	80.91				84.26
1.4950	80.22	80.39	81.22	80.96	81.69	82.12	82.78				

465

Table 943.05C. Refractive Index Table for Dry Substance in Corn Syrups and High Fructose Corn Syrups

	Dextrose Equiv. (top); Maltose, %DB (bottom)								Fructose, %DB		
	28	32	42	42	50	56	63	95	42	55	90
		15	13	33	50	18	30				
Refractive Index at 45°	Dry Substance,[a] %										
1.5000	82.00	82.16	83.02	82.78	83.40	83.95	84.63				
1.5050	83.76	83.90	84.79	84.56	85.19	85.75	86.45				

[a]Dry substances are left blank whenever the carbohydrate solutions are supersaturated with respect to dextrose and, therefore, do not exist as one (liquid) phase.

H. Determination

Rinse syringe with diluted sample 4 times before injection. Inject 30 μL diluted sample, **979.23G**. Best accuracy is obtained when dry substance solids injected for sample and standard are equivalent. Integrate eluted peaks, using System I and Method I. After injection, wash syringe 4 times with warm tap H_2O, allowing air bubbles to scrub syringe walls. Wash syringe twice with H_2O.

I. Calculations

Results are computed automatically when using **979.23B(c)**. List fructose, glucose, maltulose, and other DP_2 results. Combine maltotriose, panose-isomaltotriose, and linear DP_4 results, and list sum as DP_{3-4}. Sum remaining results and list as DP_{5+}. Report results on ash-free, carbohydrate dry substance basis. In absence of computing integrator, list areas for fructose (f), glucose (g), maltulose, other DP_2, sum of maltotriose, panose-isomaltotriose and linear DP_4, and sum of DP_{5+}, and compute result by equation:

$$\%\text{Component} = [(\text{Area component})(\text{KF component})] \times 100/\{[(\text{Area}_f)(\text{KF}_f)] + [(\text{Area}_g)(\text{KF}_g)]$$
$$+ \dots + [(\text{Area}_{5+})(\text{KF}_{5+})]\}$$

References: JAOAC **62,** 527(1979); **69,** 258(1986).
CAS-50-99-7 (dextrose)
CAS-57-48-7 (fructose)
CAS-50-99-7 (glucose)
CAS-17606-72-3 (maltulose)
CAS-23140-52-5 (psicose)

33.7   **971.18—Carbohydrates in Fruit Juices**
Gas Chromatographic Method
First Action 1971
Final Action 1980

A. Apparatus

Gas chromatograph.—Varian Model 1520 (replaced by Model 3720), with dual column and thermal detectors operated at 250° and 200 mA. GC conditions: 1.8 m × 6 mm (6′ × ¼″) stainless steel column packed with 3.8% SE-30 on 60–80 mesh silanized Diatoport S (replaced by Chromosorb W-HP, Analabs, Inc.), programmed at 4°/min from 190 to 275° (for sharper separation of sorbitol and glucose peaks, program at 2°/min until complete invert sugar pattern appears, and then at 4°/min); injector temperature 225°; He gas flow 40 mL/min; sample size and attenuation adjusted to give 50% full scale deflection for fructose peak.

B. Reagents

(*Note:* Tri-Sil reagent and pyridine may be harmful. *Caution:* Protect skin and eyes when using. Use effective fume removal device.)

(**a**) *Neutral lead acetate solution.*—Dissolve 8 g Pb(OAc)$_2$·3H$_2$O in H$_2$O and dilute to 100 mL with H$_2$O.

(**b**) *Tri-Sil reagent.*—Pyridine solution of trimethylchlorosilane (TMS) and hexamethyldisilazane (10 + 1 + 2) (available as Tri-Sil 48999, Pierce Chemical Co.). Use to prepare TMS derivatives.

C. Determination

Place 2.0 mL single-strength fruit juice in 15 mL capped centrifuge tube, add 0.5 mL Pb(OAc)$_2$ solution and 10 mL alcohol, mix, and centrifuge. Decant clear supernate into small porcelain dish. Wash residue once with 5 mL 80% alcohol, mix, centrifuge, and add clear supernate to porcelain dish. Evaporate to dryness on steam bath and keep on bath 15 min after apparent dryness. Extract sugars with five 2 mL portions hot pyridine, thoroughly mixing each portion with residue and heating on steam bath during mixing. Filter each hot extract through small glass wool plug into small flask. Cool combined extracts and transfer 0.5 mL to 5 mL vial with Teflon-lined cap. Add few pieces of Drierite to vial; then add 2.0 mL Tri-Sil reagent. Let stand 1 h at 37° and inject volume solution such that fructose peak is ca half scale. (Turbidity in final solution does not affect GC determination.) Compare curve with authentic sample prepared in same way. Order of appearance is fructose, α-glucose, sorbitol, β-glucose, and sucrose.

Reference: JAOAC **53**, 1193(1970).
CAS-57-48-7 (fructose)
CAS-50-99-7 (glucose)
CAS-50-70-4 (sorbitol)
CAS-57-50-1 (sucrose)

33.8   **973.28—Sorbitol in Food**
                                            Gas Chromatographic Method
                                            First Action 1973
                                            Final Action 1974

(Apple and apple by-products contain naturally occurring sorbitol.)
(*Caution: See Appendix* for safety notes on distillation, acetic anhydride, and methanol.)

A. Principle

Sorbitol is extracted with methyl alcohol, and acetate derivative is formed in presence of pyridine, extracted with $CHCl_3$, and determined by GC.

B. Apparatus

(a) *Soxhlet extractor.*—Medium size (Corning No. 3740, Kimble No. 24071, or equivalent), with 33 × 80 mm extraction thimble.

(b) *Gas chromatograph.*—Equipped with flame ionization detector, 1 mv strip chart recorder, and 1.8 m (6') × 4 mm id U-shaped glass column packed with 10% DC-200 on 100–120 mesh Gas-Chrom Q (Applied Science). Operating conditions: temperatures (°)—column 200 (or such that retention time of sorbitol acetate is 9–10 min), injector 230, detector 210; flow rates (mL/min)—N carrier gas 120, air 350–400, H optimal; sensitivity 0.4×10^{-9} amp for full scale deflection; or equivalent conditions so that acetate equivalent to 2.5 µg sorbitol will give ½ scale deflection.

C. Reagents

(a) *Diatomaceous earth.*—Celite 545, acid-washed.

(b) *Sorbitol.*—Reagent grade, or equivalent (Fisher Scientific Co. S-459).

D. Extraction

Place moist products in 60° forced-draft oven until dry (overnight drying is convenient). Chop dry sample in Hobart mixer. Weigh sample containing ca 400 mg sorbitol (usually ca 10 g), mix with 5 g Celite, and place in extraction thimble. Place piece of glass wool on top of sample. Add 125 mL anhydrous methyl alcohol to extraction flask, and extract 2 h at rapid boil. Quantitatively transfer methyl alcohol extract to 200 mL volumetric flask with methyl alcohol and dilute to volume with methyl alcohol.

E. Preparation of Standard Curve

Accurately weigh ca 20, 40, 60, and 80 mg sorbitol into separate 125 mL ⊺ 24/40 erlenmeyer. Add 3 mL pyridine and 10 mL Ac_2O. Fit flask with air condenser and reflux 1 h on steam bath. Add 60–80 mL H_2O, mix, and cool. Extract with four 20 mL and one 15 mL portion $CHCl_3$. Dilute to 100 mL with $CHCl_3$ in volumetric flask. Inject ca 5 µL into gas chromatograph.

Prepare standard curve by plotting response (sq mm/µL injected) against mg sorbitol initially weighed.

F. Determination

Pipet 25 mL methyl alcohol extract into 125 mL ⊺ 24/40 erlenmeyer. Evaporate extract to dryness on steam bath with current of air. Proceed as in **973.28E**, beginning "Add 3 mL pyridine ... ", dissolving

468

residue as completely as possible. Calculate % sorbitol as follows:

$$\% \text{ Sorbitol} = (\text{mg from standard curve} \times 0.8)/\text{g sample}$$

Reference: JAOAC **56,** 66(1973).
CAS-50-70-4 (sorbitol)

33.9 954.11—Separation of Sugars in Honey
Charcoal Column Chromatographic Method I
Final Action 1977

A. Principle

By adsorption of honey sample on charcoal column, followed by elution into monosaccharide, disaccharide, and higher sugar fractions, interference of disaccharides in glucose and fructose determinations is eliminated. Elution is by progressively higher alcohol concentrations, followed by determination of individual monosaccharides, sucrose, and reducing disaccharides collectively as maltose, and trisaccharides and higher sugars collectively after hydrolysis.

B. Preparation and Standardization of Adsorption Column

Column is 22 mm od × 370 mm long, with 1 L spherical section and ᵀ 35/20 spherical joint at top. Adsorbent is 1 + 1 mixture of Darco G-60 charcoal and rapid filter-aid (Celite 545 or Dicalite 4200). Insert glass wool plug, wet from below, and add enough dry adsorbent to dry tube (23–26 cm) to compress to 17 cm when vacuum is applied with *gentle* tapping of column. Remove excess charcoal from walls of tube, and add filter-aid layer at top with *gentle* packing (1–1.5 cm). Wash column with 500 mL H_2O and 250 mL 50% alcohol, and let stand overnight with 50% alcohol on it. Flow rate should be 5.5–8.0 mL/min with H_2O at 9 lb/sq in. (62 kPa) pressure. Slower flow rates delay analyses excessively.

Alcohol content of eluting solutions must be adjusted to retentive power of charcoal used. Wash column alcohol-free with 250 mL H_2O, quantitatively add 10 mL solution of 1.000 g anhydrous glucose to top, and draw it into column with suction (do not let dry). Add 300 mL H_2O to top, break suction, apply pressure (≤10 lb/sq in.; 69 kPa), and collect eluate in five 50 mL portions in tared beakers. Include 10 mL from sample introduction in first 50 mL fraction. Evaporate fractions on steam bath, dry in vacuum oven at 80–100°, and weigh.

Decant remaining H_2O from top of column, pass 50 mL 50% alcohol and then 250 mL H_2O through column, and repeat chromatography, using 1.000 g anhydrous glucose in 10 mL 1% alcohol, washing with 250 mL 1% alcohol as above. Select as *solvent 1* that which removes glucose in 150 mL. Repeat chromatography with 2% alcohol, if necessary.

Wash column with 250 mL H_2O and then 20 mL 5% alcohol. To top, add 10 mL 5% alcohol solution containing 100 mg maltose and 100 mg sucrose. Elute as above with 250 mL 5% alcohol, weighing evaporated 50 mL portions of filtrate. Repeat, if necessary, with 7, 8, and 9% alcohol to find *solvent 2* that will elute ≥98% disaccharides in 200 mL. *Solvent 1* previously selected must not elute disaccharides. Combinations found satisfactory with various charcoals are 1%, 7%, 2%, 8%; 2%, 9%. At conclusion, pass 100 mL 50% alcohol through column, and store under layer of this solvent.

C. Preparation of Fractions

Wash column with 250 mL H_2O and decant any supernate. Pass 20 mL *solvent 1* through column, and discard. Dissolve 1 g sample in 10 mL *solvent 1* in 50 mL beaker. Transfer sample (using long-stem funnel) onto column, and force into column. Use 15 mL *solvent 1* to rinse beaker and funnel, and add to column. Collect all eluate, beginning with sample introduction, in 250 mL volumetric flask. Add 250 mL *solvent 1*, and collect exactly 250 mL total (fraction *1*, monosaccharides). Decant excess solvent from top, add 265–270 mL *solvent 2*, and collect 250 mL in volumetric flask (fraction *2*, disaccharides). Decant excess, add 110 mL 50% alcohol (*solvent 3*), and collect 100 mL in volumetric flask (fraction *3*, higher sugars). Mix each fraction thoroughly. Column may be stored indefinitely, outlet closed, under 50% alcohol. Discard after 8 uses.

Fructose

D. Reagents

Use reagents in **959.11A** (*see* 33.29) and following:

(**a**) *Iodine solution.*—0.05*N*. Dissolve 13.5 g pure I in solution of 24 g KI in 200 mL H_2O, and dilute to 2 L. Do not standardize.

(**b**) *Sodium sulfite solution.*—1%. Dissolve 1 g Na_2SO_3 in 100 mL H_2O. Make fresh daily.

(**c**) *Brom cresol green solution.*—Dissolve 150 mg brom cresol green in 100 mL H_2O.

E. Determination

Pipet 20 mL fraction *1* into 200 mL volumetric flask. Add 40 mL 0.05*N* I solution by pipet; then with vigorous mixing, add 25 mL 0.1*N* NaOH over 30 s period, and immediately place flask in 18 $\pm$ 0.1° H_2O bath. Exactly 10 min after alkali addition, add 5 mL 1*N* H_2SO_4 and remove from bath. Exactly neutralize I with Na_2SO_3 solution, using 2 drops starch solution, **959.11A(d)**, near end point. Back-titrate with dilute I if necessary. Add 5 drops brom cresol green and exactly neutralize solution with 1*N* NaOH; then make just acid to indicator. Dilute to volume and determine reducing value of 5 mL aliquots by Shaffer-Somogyi method, **959.11B** (*see* 33.29).

Make duplicate blanks and determinations. Deduct titration from that of blank and calculate fructose:

% Fructose = 500[(titer $\times$ 0.1150) + 0.0915] $\times$ 100/mg sample

Fructose correction for glucose determination = f.c. = [(titer $\times$ 0.1150) + 0.0915] $\times$ 40. Bracketed quantity is mg fructose in 5 mL aliquot, valid between 0.5 and 1.75 mg fructose.

Glucose

F. Reagent

Sodium thiosulfate solution.—0.05*N*. Prepare from standardized stock 0.1000*N* solution, **942.27**.

942.27 (Standard Solutions of Sodium Thiosulfate)

A. Preparation of Standard Solution

Dissolve ca 25 g $Na_2S_2O_3 \cdot 5H_2O$ in 1 L H_2O. Boil gently 5 min and transfer while hot to storage bottle previously cleaned with hot chromic acid cleaning solution and rinsed with warm boiled H_2O. (Temper bottle, if not heat-resistant, before adding hot solution.) Store solution in dark, cool place; do not return unused portions to stock bottle. If solutions less concentrated than 0.1*N* are desired, prepare by dilution with boiled H_2O. (More dilute solutions are less stable and should be prepared just before use.)

B. Standardization

Accurately weigh 0.20–0.23 g $K_2Cr_2O_7$ (NIST SRM 136 dried 2 h at 100°) and place in glass-stoppered I flask (or glass-stoppered flask). Dissolve in 80 mL Cl-free H_2O containing 2 g KI. Add, with swirling, 20 mL ca $1N$ HCl and immediately place in dark 10 min. Titrate with $Na_2S_2O_3$ solution, **942.27A**, adding starch solution after most of I has been consumed.

$$\text{Normality} = \text{g } K_2Cr_2O_7 \times 1000/\text{mL } Na_2S_2O_3 \times 49.032$$

Refs.: JAOAC **25**, 659(1942); **27**, 557(1944); **28**, 594(1945); **38**, 382(1955); **47**, 43, 46(1964); **48**, 103(1965).

G. Determination

Pipet 20 mL fraction *1* into duplicate 250 mL erlenmeyers. Evaporate to dryness on steam bath in air current. Add 20 mL H_2O, pipet in 20 mL $0.05N$ I, and slowly add 25 mL $0.1N$ NaOH, as in fructose determination. Immediately place in $18 \pm 0.1°$ H_2O bath. Exactly 10 min after alkali addition, add 5 mL $2N$ H_2SO_4, remove from bath, and titrate with $0.05N$ $Na_2S_2O_3$, using starch solution, **959.11A(d)**.

Make duplicate blanks, using H_2O, subtract titration value from that of blank, and calculate glucose:

$$\% \text{ Glucose} = 56.275[\text{titer} - (0.01215 \times \text{f.c.})] \times 100/\text{mg sample}$$

where f.c. = fructose correction from fructose determination. Equation is valid over range 10–15 mg glucose in 20 mL. In presence of glucose, 1 mg fructose requires 0.01215 mL $0.05N$ $Na_2S_2O_3$, in range 15–60 mg fructose.

Reducing Disaccharides as Maltose

H. Determination

Pipet 5 mL aliquots of fraction *2* into 25 × 200 mm test tubes, and determine reducing value as in **959.11B**, except boil tubes 30 min. Value for 15 min H_2O blank may be used here. Calculate % reducing disaccharides as maltose:

$$\% \text{ ''Maltose''} = 50[(\text{titer} \times 0.2264) + 0.075] \times 100/\text{mg sample}$$

Maltose correction for sucrose determination = m.c. = maltose titer × 0.92. Bracketed quantity is mg maltose in 5 mL aliquot, valid between 0.15 and 3.80 mg maltose. Reducing value of maltose at 15 min is 92% of final value.

Sucrose

I. Determination

Pipet 25 mL fraction *2* into 50 mL volumetric flask. Add 5 mL $6N$ HCl and 5 mL H_2O. Mix, let stand 17 min in 60° H_2O bath, cool, and neutralize to brom cresol green with $5N$ NaOH (103 g/500 mL). (Polyethylene squeeze bottle is excellent for holding and delivering alkali.) Adjust to acid color of indicator, using $2N$ H_2SO_4 to correct over-run. Dilute to volume and determine reducing value of 5 mL aliquots by Shaffer-Somogyi determination, **959.11B**. Subtract titration from blank, and calculate sucrose by reference to curve constructed from following table:

Sucrose in 5 mL Aliquot Oxidized, mg	0.005N Na$_2$S$_2$O$_3$ Required, mL
0.255	1.75
0.502	3.95
1.004	8.72
1.260	11.28

From curve obtain S_1 = sucrose equivalent to maltose correction, **954.11H**, and S_2 = sucrose equivalent of sucrose titer.

$$\% \text{ Sucrose} = 50(2S_2 - S_1) \times 100/\text{mg sample}$$

Higher Sugars or "Dextrin"

J. Determination

Pipet 25 mL aliquots of fraction 3 into 50 mL volumetric flasks. Add 5 mL 6N HCl and 5 mL H$_2$O, and heat 45 min in boiling H$_2$O bath. Cool, neutralize as for sucrose, dilute to volume, and determine reducing value by Shaffer-Somogyi determination, **959.11B**. Subtract titration value from blank and obtain glucose equivalent from curve constructed from following table:

Glucose, mg	Titer, mL
0.05	0.20
0.10	0.60
0.25	1.85
0.50	4.00
1.00	8.50
2.00	7.60

$$\% \text{ Higher sugars} = 40(\text{glucose equivalent}) \times 100/\text{mg sample}$$

Notes: For most accurate work, Shaffer-Somogyi values must check within 0.04 mL. Calibration of all operations, including column, using known synthetic mixtures of glucose, fructose, sucrose, maltose, and raffinose (corrected for moisture) is recommended for critical work. Sugar:mL Na$_2$S$_2$O$_3$ relations [(titer × 0.1150) + 0.0915] in equation for % fructose, and [(titer × 0.2264) + 0.075] in equation for % maltose, are obtained by analyzing known mixtures of glucose and fructose for fructose, and known amounts of maltose, respectively, by method.

Efficiency of column separation may be checked by paper chromatography of fractions *1, 2,* and *3* as in **959.12C**.

References: JAOAC **37**, 466(1954); **39**, 1016(1956); **42**, 341(1959); **43**, 774(1960).
CAS-9004-53-9 (dextrin)
CAS-57-48-7 (fructose)
CAS-50-99-7 (glucose)
CAS-69-79-4 (maltose)
CAS-57-50-1 (sucrose)

33.10   **979.21—Separation of Sugars in Honey**
Charcoal Column Chromatographic Method II
Final Action

A. Principle

For use when sucrose is sugar of primary interest. Sugars are separated by charcoal column, **954.11B** and **C**, (*see* 33.9). Glucose is determined in disaccharide fraction *2* by glucose oxidase before and after invertase hydrolysis and calculated to sucrose. Other sugars are determined by weighing residues of separated fractions.

B. Reagents

(**a**) *Column.*—Prepare as in **954.11B**. Alternatively, use slurry preparation: Place glass wool plug at bottom of column and add ca 1 cm dry filter aid (Dicalite 4200, or equivalent). Wet filter aid layer from below. With outlet open, add slurry of 20 g adsorbent mixture in 200 mL H_2O from top. Let drain 5 min and apply 27.6 kPa (4 psi) pressure until surface is stabilized. Then apply 69 kPa (10 psi) pressure, release, and remove excess adsorbent beyond 17 cm depth by suction from above. Add ca 1 cm filter aid. Wash column as in **954.11B**.

(**b**) *Acetate buffer solution.*—0.1M, pH 4.5. Add 5.72 mL CH_3COOH to 500 mL H_2O, adjust to pH 4.5 with 1M NaOH, and dilute to 1 L.

(**c**) *Tris buffer solution.*—pH 7.6. To 48.44 g tris(hydroxymethyl)aminomethane (available as Trizma base, No. T 1503, Sigma Chemical Co.) in 500 mL H_2O, add 384 mL 0.8M HCl, adjust to pH 7.6 if necessary, and dilute to 1 L.

(**d**) *Glucose oxidase-peroxidase reagent (GOP).*—Dissolve 120 mg glucose oxidase (Type II: purified, 15,000–20,000 units/g; Sigma Chemical Co. G 6125, or equivalent) and 32 mg peroxidase (Type I: from horseradish, salt-free powder; Sigma Chemical Co. P 8125, or equivalent) in 400 mL tris buffer, (**c**). Add solution of 270 mg *o*-tolidine·2HCl (available from Fisher Scientific Co. as Fisher certified T-320) in 520 mL H_2O. Refrigerate in brown bottle. Filter before use, if necessary. Stable ≥6 weeks.

(**e**) *Invertase reagent.*—Dissolve 12.5 mg invertase (Grade VI, from baker's yeast, essentially melibiase-free, activity ca 200 units/mg; Sigma Chemical Co. I 5875, or equivalent) in 50 mL pH 4.5 acetate buffer solution, (**b**).

(**f**) *Glucose standard solution.*—0.1 mg/mL. Dissolve 25.0 mg glucose (SRM 41, NIST) in 25 mL H_2O in 250 mL volumetric flask. Boil 2 min and dilute to volume or dilute to volume and hold final solution 2 h before use.

C. Preparation of Fractions

Proceed as in **954.11C**.

D. Determination of Sugars

(**a**) *Glucose.*—Dilute 5.00 mL fraction *1* to 100 mL and pipet 2 mL portions into each of two 18 × 150 mm test tubes. Place tube with 2 mL H_2O in rack, follow with 1 tube containing 2 mL standard glucose solution (100 μg/mL), the 2 sample tubes, then 1 standard. Repeat sequence if additional determinations are to be made. At intervals appropriate to measuring technique to be used (i.e., 30 or 60 s with flow-through cells; longer as needed for manual cells), add 5.00 mL glucose oxidase reagent at room temperature to each tube, beginning with H_2O tube, which will be reagent blank. After 60 min from addition of reagent, add 0.15 mL 4N HCl to first tube and mix thoroughly with vortex mixer.

Continue same timing with other solutions. Zero instrument with blank tube and determine A at 530 nm of each successive tube 1 min after addition of acid. Average A for each pair of sample tubes and calculate glucose concentration, using average A' of standards before and after corresponding sample tubes.

$$\mu g \text{ Glucose in tube} = (A/A') \times \mu g \text{ glucose in standard tube}$$

$$\% \text{ Glucose in honey} = \mu g \text{ glucose in tube} \times 2.5/\text{mg sample}$$

where factor 2.5 = 20 (dilution factor) × 250 (volume fraction)/(1000 μg/mg) × 2 (volume in tube).
(b) *Sucrose.*—Pipet 2 mL fraction *2* into each of four 18 × 150 mm test tubes. Prepare 2 series, one control, other inverted. For each series, arrange in rack tube with 2 mL H_2O, 2 sample tubes, tube with 2 mL glucose standard, 2 sample tubes, etc., finishing with 2 mL glucose standard. To all tubes in control series add 0.50 mL H_2O; to all tubes in inverted series add 0.50 mL invertase reagent (or 0.50 mL pH 4.5 acetate buffer may be added to standard tubes). Hold all tubes 30 min at room temperature. Continue as in (**a**), beginning "At intervals appropriate . . .", beginning with inverted series followed by control series.

$$\mu g \text{ Glucose} = (\mu g \text{ glucose in standard tube}) \times (A/A')$$

$$\% \text{ Sucrose in honey} = 0.02375 \, (\mu g \text{ glucose in inverted tube} - \mu g \text{ glucose in control tube})/\text{g sample}$$

where 0.02375 = μg glucose × 1.9 × 10^{-6} × (1/2) × 250 × 100; μg glucose × 1.9 = μg sucrose; 10^{-6} = μg/g; 1/2 = 2 mL analyzed; 250 = mL dilution of sample; 100 = to convert to %.

E. Distribution of Sugars

Filter fractions if filter aid is visible. Evaporate to dryness, on steam bath with current of air or N, 50.0 mL fraction *1*, 100 mL fraction *2*, and entire fraction *3*, finally transfering each fraction to separately weighed 50 mL beakers. Dry to constant weight in vacuum oven at ≤95°.

$$\% \text{ Monosaccharides} = \text{g fraction } 1 \times 500/\text{g sample}$$

$$\% \text{ Disaccharides} = \text{g fraction } 2 \times 250/\text{g sample}$$

$$\% \text{ Higher sugars} = \text{g fraction } 3 \times 100/\text{g sample}$$

References: JAOAC **62**, 515(1979); **62**, 966(1979); **63**, 269(1980).
CAS-50-99-7 (glucose)
CAS-57-50-1 (sucrose)

33.11   969.39—Glucose in Corn Sirups and Sugars
Glucose Oxidase Method
First Action 1969
Final Action 1970

A. Principle

Glucose is enzymatically oxidized with glucose oxidase to form H_2O_2, which reacts with a dye in presence of peroxidase to give stable colored product proportional to glucose concentration.

B. Reagents

(a) *Glucose test solution.*—Consists of (1) *Glucose oxidase.*—1000 glucose oxidase units/mL; purified (Miles Laboratories, Inc., or equivalent). (2) *Horseradish peroxidase.*—Available from Worthington Biochemical Co., Halls Mill Rd, Freehold, NJ 07728. (3) *Chromogen.*—o-Dianisidine·2HCl. (4) *Acetate buffer solution.*—pH 5.5, 0.1M. Dissolve 13.608 g NaOAc·3H₂O and dilute to 1 L with H_2O. Add 2.7 mL CH₃COOH and adjust pH with NaOAc or CH₃COOH, if necessary.

Dissolve 40 mg chromogen, 40 mg horseradish peroxidase, and 0.4 mL glucose oxidase in 0.1M acetate buffer and dilute to 100 mL with buffer solution.

(b) *Glucose standard solution.*—1 mg/mL. Dissolve 1.000 g NIST D-glucose, SRM 917 (previously dried 4 h at 70° under vacuum) in H_2O and dilute to 1 L in volumetric flask. Mix and let stand 2 h to permit mutarotation to occur. Prepare fresh on day of use.

C. Apparatus

(a) *Spectrophotometer.*—Suitable for measuring A at 540 nm, with matching 1 cm cells.
(b) *Water bath.*—Capable of maintaining temperature at $30 \pm 1°$.

D. Preparation of Standard Curve

Pipet 1, 2, 3, and 4 mL aliquots standard glucose solution into separate 50 mL volumetric flasks and dilute to volume with H_2O. Mix and pipet 2 mL of each diluted standard into 18 × 150 mm test tubes (0.04, 0.08, 0.12, 0.16 mg glucose). Use 2 mL H_2O as blank. Place all tubes in 30° H_2O bath 5 min. At 0 time, start reaction by adding 1.0 mL glucose test solution to first tube. Allow 30–60 s interval between enzyme addition to each subsequent tube. Mix tubes and let react exactly 30 min at 30°. Immediately stop reaction (30–60 s intervals) by pipetting 10 mL H_2SO_4 (1 + 3) into each tube. Mix, cool to room temperature, and measure A against reagent blank at 540 nm, using 1 cm cells. Plot A at 540 nm against mg glucose on linear coordinate paper.

E. Determination

Weigh 1–5 g sirup sample to nearest 0.1 mg, using weighing bottle to prevent moisture loss during weighing. Dilute successively with H_2O to concentration of 2.5–7.5 mg glucose/100 mL. Pipet 2 mL diluted sample into 18 × 150 mm test tube. Proceed as in **969.39D**, beginning ''Place all tubes in 30° H_2O bath 5 min.'' Determine mg glucose from standard curve and calculate % glucose in sample.

For results on dry substance basis, determine sample dry substance as in **943.05**.

Reference: JAOAC **52**, 556(1969).
CAS-50-99-7 (glucose)

33.12

984.15—Lactose in Milk
Enzymatic Method
First Action 1984
Final Action 1985

A. Principle

Lactose is hydrolyzed to glucose and β-galactose in presence of β-galactosidase and H_2O. β-Galactose is then oxidized by NAD to galactonic acid in presence of β-galactose dehydrogenase; amount of NADH formed, stoichiometric with lactose content, is measured by A at 340 nm.

B. Apparatus

(a) *Spectrophotometer.*—Any spectrophotometer with slit width ≤ 10 nm.

(b) *Cuvets.*—Glass or disposable plastic cuvets (1 cm light path).

(c) *Pipets.*—Capillary pipets for transfer of volumes < 1 mL. Use transfer or measuring pipets for transfer of volumes > 1 mL.

(d) *Stirrer.*—Plastic or glass rod, 1 mm diameter.

C. Reagents

(a) *Carrez I solution.*—3.60 g $K_4[Fe(CN)_6] \cdot 3H_2O$/100 mL H_2O.

(b) *Carrez II solution.*—7.20 g $ZnSO_4 \cdot 7H_2O$/100 mL H_2O.

(c) *Assay reagents.*—Kits are available from Boehringer-Mannheim, Diagnostics Div., 9115 Hague Rd, PO Box 50100, Indianapolis, IN 46250-0100. (*1*) *Solution 1.*—610 mg lyophilisate consisting of citrate buffer (pH 6.6), NAD (35 mg), $MgSO_4$, and stabilizers. Dissolve lyophilisate in 7.0 mL redistilled H_2O (Reagent Grade I quality) before use. (*2*) *Solution 2.*—About 1.7 mL enzyme suspension of β-galactosidase (ca 100 U). (*3*) *Solution 3.*—34 mL solution consisting of potassium diphosphate buffer (0.51 mol/L, pH 8.6) and stabilizers. (*4*) *Solution 4.*—About 1.7 enzyme suspension of galactose dehydrogenase (ca 35 U).

D. Determination

(a) *Sample preparation.*—Accurately weigh ca 2 g milk into 100 mL volumetric flask, add ca 60 mL redistilled H_2O, and mix. Add 5 mL Carrez I solution and mix. Add 5 mL Carrez II solution and mix. Add 10 mL 0.1M NaOH solution and mix vigorously. Dilute to volume with redistilled H_2O, mix, and filter through paper. Use clear filtrate for assay. This procedure breaks emulsions, absorbs some colors, and precipitates proteins.

(b) *Assay.*—Label one cuvet "blank" and one cuvet "sample." Pipet 0.20 mL solution 1 into each cuvet. Pipet 0.05 mL solution 2 into each cuvet. Pipet 0.10 mL sample solution (filtrate) into sample cuvet. Mix both cuvets with stirrer, and hold 10 min at 20–25°. Pipet 1.00 mL solution 3 into each cuvet. Pipet 2.00 mL redistilled H_2O into blank cuvet and 1.90 mL redistilled H_2O into sample cuvet. Mix and hold ca 2 min at 20–25°. Determine A (A_1) of each solution at 340 nm. Add 0.05 mL solution 4 to each cuvet. Mix and hold at 20–25° until reaction has stopped (ca 10–15 min). Determine A (A_2) of both solutions. If reaction has not stopped after 15 min, continue to read at 2 min intervals until A remains constant 2 min.

Convert A readings to anhydrous lactose, C, by the following equation:

$$C(\text{g/L sample solution}) = (V \times MW \times \Delta A)/(\epsilon \times d \times v \times 1000)$$

where V = final volume (mL); v = sample volume (mL); MW = molecular weight of anhydrous lactose (342.3); d = light path (cm); ϵ = absorption coefficient of NADH at 340 nm = 6.3 (1 $\times$ mmol^{-1} $\times$

cm^{-1}); $\Delta A = (A_{S2} - A_{S1}) - (A_{B2} - A_{B1})$, i.e., absorption differences for blank and samples. Thus, for anhydrous lactose, equation becomes:

$$C(g/L) = (3.30 \times 342.3)/(6.3 \times 1 \times 0.1 \times 1000) = 1.793 \times \Delta A$$

Since sample was diluted before analysis, multiply result by dilution factor, F. In general case, 2 g to 100 mL, F = 50.

Reference: JAOAC **67,** 637(1984).

33.13   906.03—Invert Sugar in Sugars and Sirups
Munson-Walker General Method
Final Action
Surplus 1989

See Official Methods of Analysis (1984) 14th Ed., **31.037–31.044.**

33.14   923.09—Invert Sugar in Sugars and Sirups
Lane-Eynon General Volumetric Method
Final Action

A. Reagents

Soxhlet modification of Fehling solution.—Prepare by mixing equal volumes of (**a**) and (**b**) immediately before use.

(**a**) *Copper sulfate solution.*—Dissolve 34.639 g $CuSO_4 \cdot 5H_2O$ in H_2O, dilute to 500 mL, and filter through glass wool or paper. Determine Cu content of solution [preferably by electrolysis, **929.09F** (*see* 33.15)], and adjust so that it contains 440.9 mg Cu/25 mL.

(**b**) *Alkaline tartrate solution.*—Dissolve 173 g KNa tartrate·4H$_2$O (Rochelle salt) and 50 g NaOH in H_2O, dilute to 500 mL, let stand 2 days, and filter through prepared asbestos, **906.03A** (*see* 33.13).

(**c**) *Invert sugar standard solution.*—1%. To solution of 9.5 g pure sucrose, add 5 mL HCl and dilute with H_2O to ca 100 mL. Store several days at room temperature (ca 7 days at 12–15° or 3 days at 20–25°); then dilute to 1 L. (Acidified 1% invert sugar solution is stable for several months.) Neutralize aliquot with ca 1N NaOH and dilute to desired concentration immediately before use.

B. Standardization

Accurately pipet 10 or 25 mL mixed Soxhlet reagent, or 5 or 12.5 mL each of Soxhlet solutions **923.09A(a)** and (**b**), into 300–400 mL erlenmeyer. (Amount of Cu taken differs slightly between 2 methods of pipetting, and method used must be consistent in standardization and determination.) Prepare standard solution of pure sugar of such concentration that >15 mL and <50 mL is required to reduce all the Cu. Dispense from buret with offset tip to keep tube out of steam. To determine mg sugar required to completely reduce Cu at different concentrates, consult **930.44** and **930.45.** Add sugar solution within

0.5–1.0 mL of total required, heat cold mixture to bp on wire gauze over burner, and maintain moderate boiling 2 min (coarse grains of C or other suitable inert material may be used to prevent bumping). Without removing flame add 1 mL *0.2% aqueous methylene blue solution* (or 3–4 drops 1% solution) and complete titration within total boiling time of ca 3 min by small additions (2–3 drops) of sugar solution to decoloration of indicator. (Maintain continuous evolution of steam to prevent reoxidation of Cu or indicator.) After complete reduction of Cu, methylene blue is reduced to colorless compound and solution resumes orange Cu_2O color which it had before addition of indicator.

Multiply titer by mg/mL standard solution to obtain total sugar required to reduce the Cu. Compare with tabulated value in **930.44** or **930.45** to determine correction, if any, to be applied to table. Small deviations from tabulated values may arise from variations in technique or composition of reagents. If only approximate results (within 1%) are required, standardization may be omitted, provided specifications of analysis are rigidly observed.

C. Determination

(**a**) *Incremental method.*—If approximate concentration of sugar in sample is unknown, proceed by incremental method of titration. To 10 or 25 mL mixed Soxhlet solution, add 15 mL sugar solution and heat to bp over wire gauze. Boil ca 15 s and rapidly add further amounts of sugar solution until only faintest perceptible blue remains. Then, add 1 mL 0.2% aqueous methylene blue solution (or 3–4 drops 1% solution) and complete titration by adding sugar solution dropwise. (Error resulting from this titration will generally be ≤1%.)

(**b**) *Standard method.*—For higher precision repeat titration, adding almost entire sugar solution required to reduce all Cu and proceed as in **923.09B**. From **930.44** or **930.45** find total reducing sugar corresponding to titer and apply correction previously determined. Calculate as follows: total reducing sugar required × 100/titer = mg sugar in 100 mL.

930.44.—Total reducing sugar required for complete reduction of 10 ml Soxhlet solution to be used in conjunction with Lane-Eynon general volumetric method

Titer	Invert Sugar, No Sucrose	g Sucrose/100 mL Invert Sugar				Glu-cose	Fruc-tose	Maltose		Lactose	
		1	5	10	25			Anhyd.	$C_{12}H_{22}O_{11}$ ·H_2O	Anhyd.	$C_{12}H_{22}O_{11}$ ·H_2O
						Required for Reduction of 10 ml Soxhlet Soln					
15	50.5	49.9	47.6	46.1	43.4	49.1	52.2	77.2	81.3	64.9	68.3
16	.6	50.0	.6	.1	.4	.2	.3	.1	.2	.8	.2
17	.7	.1	.6	.1	.4	.3	.3	.0	.1	.8	.2
18	.8	.1	.6	.1	.3	.3	.4	.0	.0	.7	.1
19	.8	.2	.6	.1	.3	.4	.5	76.9	80.9	.7	.1
20	.9	.2	.6	.1	.2	.5	.5	.8	.8	.6	.0
21	51.0	.2	.6	.1	.2	.5	.6	.7	.7	.6	.0
22	.0	.3	.6	.1	.1	.6	.7	.6	.6	.6	.0

930.44.—Total reducing sugar required for complete reduction of 10 ml Soxhlet solution to be used in conjunction with Lane-Eynon general volumetric method

Titer	Invert Sugar, No Sucrose	g Sucrose/100 mL Invert Sugar				Glu-cose	Fruc-tose	Maltose		Lactose	
		1	5	10	25			Anhyd.	$C_{12}H_{22}O_{11}$ ·H_2O	Anhyd.	$C_{12}H_{22}O_{11}$ ·H_2O
						Required for Reduction of 10 ml Soxhlet Soln					
23	.1	.3	.6	.1	.0	.7	.7	.5	.5	.5	67.9
24	.2	.3	.6	.1	.9	.8	.8	.4	.4	.5	.9
25	.2	.4	.5	.0	.8	.8	.8	.4	.4	.5	.9
26	.3	.4	.6	.0	.8	.9	.9	.3	.3	.5	.9
27	.4	.4	.6	.0	.7	.9	.9	.2	.2	.4	.8
28	.4	.5	47.7	.0	.7	50.0	53.0	.1	.1	.4	.8
29	.5	.5	.7	.0	.6	.0	.1	.0	.0	.4	.8
30	.5	.5	.7	.0	.5	.1	.2	.0	.0	.4	.8
31	.6	.6	.7	45.9	.5	.2	.2	75.9	79.9	.4	.8
32	.6	.6	.7	.9	.4	.2	.3	.9	.9	.4	.8
33	.7	.6	.7	.9	.3	.3	.3	.8	.8	.4	.8
34	.7	.6	.7	.8	.2	.3	.4	.8	.8	.4	.9
35	.8	.7	.7	.8	.2	.4	.4	.7	.7	.5	.9
36	.8	.7	.7	.8	.1	.4	.5	.6	.6	.5	.9
37	.9	.7	.7	.7	.0	.5	.5	.6	.6	.5	.9
38	.9	.7	.7	.7	.0	.5	.6	.5	.5	.5	.9
39	52.0	.8	.7	.7	41.9	.6	.6	.5	.5	.5	.9
40	.0	.8	.7	.6	.8	.6	.6	.4	.4	.5	.9
41	.1	.8	.7	.6	.8	.7	.7	.4	.4	.6	68.0
42	.1	.8	.7	.6	.7	.7	.7	.3	.3	.6	.0
43	.2	.8	.7	.5	.6	.8	.8	.3	.3	.6	.0
44	.2	.9	.7	.5	.5	.8	.8	.2	.2	.6	.0
45	.3	.9	.7	.4	.4	.9	.9	.2	.2	.7	.1
46	.3	.9	.7	.4	.4	.9	.9	.1	.1	.7	.1
47	.4	.9	.7	.3	.3	51.0	.9	.1	.1	.8	.2
48	.4	.9	.7	.3	.2	.0	54.0	.1	.1	.8	.2

930.44.—Total reducing sugar required for complete reduction of 10 ml Soxhlet solution to be used in conjunction with Lane-Eynon general volumetric method

Titer	Invert Sugar, No Sucrose	g Sucrose/100 mL Invert Sugar				Glu-cose	Fruc-tose	Maltose		Lactose	
		1	5	10	25			Anhyd.	$C_{12}H_{22}O_{11}$ ·H_2O	Anhyd.	$C_{12}H_{22}O_{11}$ ·H_2O
					Required for Reduction of 10 ml Soxhlet Soln						
49	.5	.0	.7	.2	.1	.0	.0	.0	.0	.8	.2
50	.5	.0	.7	.2	.0	.1	.0	.0	.0	.9	.3

930.45.—Total reducing sugar required for complete reduction of 25 ml Soxhlet solution to be used in conjunction with Lane-Eynon general volumetric method

Titer	Invert Sugar, No Sucrose	1 g Sucrose/100 mL Invert Sugar	Glucose	Fructose	Maltose		Lactose	
					Anhyd	$C_{12}H_{22}O_{11}$· H_2O	Anhyd	$C_{12}H_{22}O_{11}$· H_2O
				Required for Reduction of 25 mL Soxhlet Soln				
15	123.6	122.6	120.2	127.4	197.8	208.2	163.9	172.5
16	.6	.7	.2	.4	.4	207.8	.5	.1
17	.6	.7	.2	.5	.0	.4	.1	171.7
18	.7	.7	.2	.5	196.7	.1	162.8	.4
19	.7	.8	.3	.6	.5	206.8	.5	.1
20	.8	.8	.3	.6	.2	.5	.3	170.9
21	.8	.8	.3	.7	195.8	.1	.0	.6
22	.9	.9	.4	.7	.5	205.8	161.8	.4
23	.9	.9	.4	.8	.1	.4	.6	.2
24	124.0	.9	.5	.8	194.8	.1	.5	.0
25	.0	123.0	.5	.9	.5	204.8	.4	169.9
26	.1	.0	.6	.9	.2	.4	.2	.7
27	.1	.0	.6	128.0	193.9	.1	.0	.5
28	.2	.1	.7	.0	.6	203.8	160.8	.3
29	.2	.1	.7	.1	.3	.5	.7	.2
30	.3	.1	.8	.1	.0	.2	.6	.0
31	.3	.2	.8	.1	192.8	202.9	.5	168.9

930.45.—Total reducing sugar required for complete reduction of 25 ml Soxhlet solution to be used in conjunction with Lane-Eynon general volumetric method

Titer	Invert Sugar, No Sucrose	1 g Sucrose/100 mL Invert Sugar	Glucose	Fructose	Maltose		Lactose	
					Anhyd	$C_{12}H_{22}O_{11} \cdot H_2O$	Anhyd	$C_{12}H_{22}O_{11} \cdot H_2O$
32	.4	.2	.8	.2	.5	.6	.4	.8
33	.4	.2	.9	.2	.2	.3	.2	.6
34	.5	.3	.9	.3	191.9	.0	.1	.5
35	.5	.3	121.0	.3	.7	201.8	.0	.4
36	.6	.3	.0	.4	.4	.5	159.8	.2
37	.6	.4	.1	.4	.2	.2	.7	.1
38	.7	.4	.2	.5	.0	.0	.6	.0
39	.7	.4	.2	.5	190.8	200.8	.5	167.9
40	.8	.4	.2	.6	.5	.5	.4	.8
41	.8	.5	.3	.6	.3	.3	.3	.7
42	.9	.5	.4	.6	.1	.1	.2	.6
43	.9	.5	.4	.7	189.8	199.8	.2	.6
44	125.0	.6	.5	.7	.6	.6	.1	.5
45	.0	.6	.5	.8	.4	.4	.0	.4
46	.1	.6	.6	.8	.2	.2	.0	.4
47	.1	.7	.6	.9	.0	.0	158.9	.3
48	.2	.7	.7	.9	188.9	198.9	.8	.2
49	.2	.7	.7	129.0	.8	.7	.8	.2
50	.3	.8	.8	.0	.7	.6	.7	.1

References: J. Soc. Chem. Ind. **42,** 32T(1923). JAOAC **9**, 35(1926); **12,** 38(1929).
CAS-8013-17-0 (invert sugar)

33.15   929.09—Invert Sugar in Sugars and Sirups
Determination of Reduced Copper
Final Action
Surplus 1989

See Official Methods of Analysis (1984) 14th Ed., **31.039–31.044**.

33.16   945.59—Invert Sugar in Sugars and Sirups
Ofner Volumetric Method
Final Action
Surplus 1970

(For materials containing small amounts of invert sugar in presence of sucrose)

See Official Methods of Analysis (1984) 14th Ed., **29.046–29.047**.

33.17   945.60—Invert Sugar in Sugars and Sirups
Meissl-Hiller Gravimetric Method
Final Action
Surplus 1970

(For materials containing $>1.5\%$ invert sugar and $<98.5\%$ sucrose)

See Official Methods of Analysis (1965) 10th Ed., **29.048**.

33.18   950.56—Invert Sugar in Sugars and Sirups
Quisumbing-Thomas Method
First Action
Surplus 1970

See Official Methods of Analysis (1970) 11th Ed, **31.048–31.049**.

33.19 **955.36—Invert Sugar in Sugars and Sirups**
Berlin Institute Method
First Action

(Applicable to dark-colored solutions without defecation)

A. Reagent

Müller's solution.—Dissolve 35 g $CuSO_4 \cdot 5H_2O$ in 400 mL boiling H_2O. Separately dissolve 173 g KNa tartrate·$4H_2O$ (Rochelle salt) and 68 g Na_2CO_3 in 500 mL boiling H_2O. Cool, mix the 2 solutions, and dilute to 1 L. Shake with small amount of C and filter. If precipitate forms on storage, refilter.

B. Determination

Select amount of sample (10 g or less) containing ≤30 mg invert sugar. Pipet 10 mL Müller's solution and 100 mL sugar solution into 300 mL flask and cover. Mix thoroughly and heat exactly 10 min in H_2O bath boiling so vigorously that immersion of flask does not interrupt boiling. Place flask so that H_2O level is ≥2 cm above surface of liquid in flask. After heating period, cool flask rapidly without agitation. Add 5 mL $5N$ CH_3COOH to cooled solution, mix, and immediately add excess $0.0333N$ I solution (20–40 mL) from buret. After all Cu_2O precipitate dissolves, titrate excess I with $0.0333N$ $Na_2S_2O_3$.

Apply following corrections to mL I solution consumed: (1) mL I required in blank with H_2O instead of sugar solution; (2) mL I required by sugar solution in determination conducted without heating; (3) 2.0 mL I for reducing action of 10 g sucrose or proportionate correction for smaller amount of sucrose. After these corrections 1 mL $0.0333N$ I = 1 mg invert sugar.

Reference: JAOAC **38,** 594(1955).
CAS-8013-17-0 (invert sugar)

33.20 **970.58—Invert Sugar in Molasses**
Final Action

A. Preparation of Sample Solution

Proceed as in **968.28C** (*see* 33.64). Then, pipet 100 mL filtrate into 200 mL volumetric flask, dilute to volume with H_2O, and mix well.

B. Titration of Sample

Proceed as in **968.28F–G**, except use aliquot of prepared sample solution without inversion as indicated in Table **970.58**.

Table 970.58.—Aliquots for Cane Sirups and Molasses (Without Inversion)

mL H$_2$O	mL Aliquot	g Sample in Aliquot	Total Sugar as Invert, %	
			Max.	Min.
40	10	0.16	61.00	40.00
35	15	0.24	40.00	30.00
30	20	0.32	30.00	24.00
25	25	0.40	24.00	20.00
20	30	0.48	20.00	15.00
10	40	0.64	15.00	12.00
—	50	0.80	12.00	8.00

33.21   931.07—Glucose and Sucrose in Eggs
Sugar Inversion Method
Final Action

A. Preparation of Solution

(a) *Liquid eggs.*—Accurately weigh, by difference, ca 25 g well-mixed sample, **925.29(a)** or **(b)**, into 250 mL volumetric flask containing 1 g CaCO$_3$ and 50 mL 5% NaCl solution. Add 130 mL alcohol with continuous mixing. Let stand few minutes for gas bubbles to rise to surface, cool to room temperature, dilute to volume with H$_2$O, mix, and filter (18.5 cm folded paper). Transfer 150 mL filtrate to 250 mL beaker and evaporate to 20–30 mL to remove alcohol. Cool, and wash with H$_2$O into 100 mL volumetric flask, holding volume to 80–90 mL. Add dry powdered *phosphotungstic acid* in small amounts in slight excess to precipitate any protein, mix, let stand few minutes for gas bubbles to rise to surface, dilute to volume with H$_2$O, mix, and filter. To filtrate add, in very small portions, enough dry powdered KCl to precipitate any excess phosphotungstic acid, filter if necessary, and test filtrate for complete precipitaten.

To correct for error due to volume occupied by precipitate in samples containing added sucrose, repeat determination, weighing same amount of sample into 500 mL volumetric flask containing 1 g CaCO$_3$ and 100 mL 5% NaCl solution. Add 260 mL alcohol with continuous mixing. Let stand few minutes for gas bubbles to rise to surface, cool to room temperature, dilute to volume with H$_2$O, mix, and filter through 18.5 cm folded paper. Transfer 300 mL filtrate to 400 mL beaker, evaporate to 20–30 mL, and proceed as above. To obtain amount of sucrose, subtract % sucrose obtained in 250 mL dilution determination from twice the % obtained in 500 mL dilution determination.

(b) *Dried eggs.*—From well-mixed sample, **925.29(c)**, transfer 2.5 g whites or 10 g yolks or whole eggs to 250 mL volumetric flask containing 1 g CaCO$_3$ and 50 mL 5% NaCl solution, and let stand 1 h mixing every 5 min. Add 130 mL alcohol with continuous mixing, and proceed as in (a), beginning with third sentence.

925.29 (Sampling of Eggs, Collection and Preparation of Sample)

No simple rules can be made for collection of sample representative of average of any particular lot of egg material, as conditions may differ widely. Experienced judgment must be used in each instance. For large lots, preferably draw several samples for separate analyses rather than attempt to get one composite representative sample. Sampling for microbiological examination, if required, should be performed first; *see* **939.14A–B** (*Official Methods of Analysis* [1990] 15th Ed.).

(a) *Liquid eggs.*—Obtain representative container or containers. Mix contents of container thoroughly and draw ca 300 g. (Long-handle dipper or ladle serves well.) Keep sample in hermetically sealed jar in freezer or with solid CO_2. Report odor and appearance.

(b) *Frozen eggs.*—Obtain representative container or containers. Examine contents as to odor and appearance. (Condition of contents can be determined best by drilling to center of container with auger and noting odor as auger is withdrawn. If impossible to secure individual containers, samples may consist of composite of borings from contents of each container.) Take borings diagonally across can from ≥ 3 widely separated parts, starting 2–5 cm in from edge and extending to opposite side as near to bottom as possible. Pack shavings tightly into sample jar and fill it completely to prevent partial dehydration of sample. Seal jar tightly and store in freezer or with solid CO_2. Before analyzing, warm sample in bath held at $<50°$, and mix well.

(c) *Dried eggs.*—Obtain representative container or containers. For small packages, take entire parcel or parcels for sample. For boxes and barrels, remove top layer to depth of ca 15 cm (6″) with scoop or other convenient instrument. Draw small amounts of sample totaling 300–500 g from accessible parts of container and place in hermetically sealed jar. Report odor and appearance. Prepare sample for analysis by mixing 3 times through domestic flour sifter to thoroughly break up lumps. (Grind flake albumen samples to pass entirely through No. 60 sieve. Mix well.) Keep in hermetically sealed jar in cool place.

References: JAOAC **8**, 599(1925); **53**, 439(1970); **58**, 314(1975).

B. Determination

(a) *Reducing sugars direct.*—Transfer 25 mL prepared filtrate to 400 mL beaker, and proceed as in **906.03B** (*see* 33.13). Report as % glucose.

(b) *Reducing sugars invert.*—Transfer 50 mL prepared filtrate to 100 mL volumetric flask, and invert sucrose as in **925.48(b)** or (c) (*see* 33.72). Neutralize with NaOH solution, cool to room temperature, and dilute to volume with H_2O. Transfer ≤ 50 mL to 400 mL beaker, and proceed as in **906.03B**. Deduct % invert sugar obtained before inversion from that obtained after inversion, multiply difference by 0.95, and report as % sucrose.

References: JAOAC **14**, 397(1931); **16**, 305(1933); **22**, 302(1939).
CAS-50-99-7 (glucose)
CAS-57-50-1 (sucrose)

33.22　　　　　**936.06—Glucose in Cacao Products**
Sichert-Bleyer Method
First Action

A. Reagents

(a) *Ferric ammonium sulfate solution.*—Dissolve 120 g $Fe_2(SO_4)_3 \cdot (NH_4)_2SO_4 \cdot 24H_2O$ and 100 mL H_2SO_4 in H_2O and dilute to 1 L.

(b) *Potassium permanganate solution.*—0.1N. Prep as in **940.35**.

> **940.35** (Standard Solution of Potassium Permanganate)
>
> *A. Preparation of Standard Solution*
>
> Dissolve slightly more than desired equivalent weight (3.2 g for 0.1N) of $KMnO_4$ in 1 L H_2O. Boil solution 1 hr. Protect from dust and let stand overnight. Thoroughly clean 15 cm glass funnel, perforated porcelain plate from Caldwell crucible, and glass-stoppered bottle (preferably of brown glass) with warm chromic acid cleaning solution. Digest asbestos for use in gooches on steam bath 1 hr with ca 0.1N $KMnO_4$ that has been acidified with few drops H_2SO_4 (1 + 3). Let settle, decant, and replace with H_2O. To prepare glass funnel, place porcelain plate in apex, make pad of asbestos ca 3 mm thick on plate, and wash acid-free. (Pad should not be too tightly packed and only moderate suction should be applied.) Insert stem of funnel into neck of bottle and filter $KMnO_4$ solution directly into bottle without aid of suction.
>
> *B. Standardization*
>
> For 0.1N solution, transfer 0.3 g dried (1 hr at 105°) Na oxalate (NIST SRM 40) to 600 mL beaker. Add 250 mL H_2SO_4 (5 + 95), previously boiled 10–15 min and then cooled to 27 ± 3°.
>
> Stir until $Na_2C_2O_4$ dissolves. Add 39–40 mL $KMnO_4$ solution at rate of 25–35 mL/min, stirring slowly. Let stand until pink disappears (ca 45 sec). If pink persists because $KMnO_4$ solution is too concentrated, discard and begin again, adding few mL less of $KMnO_4$ solution. Heat to 55–60°, and complete titration by adding $KMnO_4$ solution until faint pink persists 30 sec. Add last 0.5–1 mL dropwise, letting each drop decolorize before adding next.
>
> Determine excess of $KMnO_4$ solution required to turn solution pink by matching with color obtained by adding $KMnO_4$ solution to same volume of boiled and cooled dilute H_2SO_4 at 55–60°. This correction is usually 0.03–0.05 mL. From net volume $KMnO_4$, calculate normality:
>
> Normality = g $Na_2C_2O_4$ × 1000/mL $KMnO_4$ × 66.999
>
> Refs.: JAOAC **23**, 543(1940); **31**, 568(1948). J. Research NBS **15**, 493(1935), Research Paper No. 843.

B. Standardization

To obtain factor for 0.1N $KMnO_4$ make analysis as in **936.06C** on 10 mL solution containing 50 mg pure glucose. From Table **936.06**, titer of 15.38 mL corresponds to 50 mg glucose; 15.38 divided by titer obtained gives correction factor for $KMnO_4$ solution. Multiply all titers by this factor before referring to Table **936.06**. Redetermine factor each day analyses are made.

Table 936.06.—Sichert-Bleyer Table for Determination of Glucose[a]

Titer, *mL* 0.1*N* Permanganate	Glucose, mg									
	0	0.1	0.2	0.3	0.4	0.5	0.6	0.7	0.8	0.9
10	26.5	26.8	27.1	27.4	27.8	28.1	28.4	28.7	29.0	29.3
11	29.7	30.0	30.4	30.7	31.1	31.5	31.8	32.2	32.6	32.9
12	33.3	33.7	34.1	34.5	34.9	35.4	35.8	36.2	36.6	37.0
13	37.4	37.9	38.4	38.8	39.3	39.8	40.3	40.7	41.2	41.7
14	42.2	42.7	43.2	43.8	44.3	44.9	45.4	46.0	46.5	47.0
15	47.6	48.2	48.8	49.4	50.1	50.7	51.3	51.9	52.5	53.2
16	53.8	54.5	55.2	55.9	56.6	57.3	58.0	58.7	59.4	60.2
17	60.9	61.7	62.5	63.3	64.1	64.9	65.7	66.5	67.4	68.2
18	69.0	69.9	70.9	71.9	72.8	73.8	74.8	75.7	76.7	77.6
19	78.6	79.6	80.7	81.7	82.7	83.7	84.8	85.8	86.8	87.8
20	88.9	90.0	91.2	92.3	93.5	94.7	96.0	97.2	98.5	99.7

[a] Table may be interpolated for each 0.01 mL, but should not be extrapolated.

C. Determination

Proceed as in **938.02C** (*see* 33.24), through ''. . . immerse in briskly boiling H_2O bath exactly 20 min.'' Filter Cu_2O precipitate through gooch prepared as in **906.03A**, and wash flask and crucible 3 times with hot H_2O. (It is not necessary to remove all precipitate from flask.)

Transfer asbestos mat and crucible to 150 mL beaker marked at 60 mL. Wash flask with exactly 20 mL $FeNH_4(SO_4)_2$ solution in 3 portions and transfer quantitatively to beaker containing crucible. (All precipitate must be dissolved.) Finally wash flask and crucible with hot H_2O and remove crucible. Add hot H_2O to 60 mL mark. Heat to bp on hot plate, let stand 3 min, and titrate with 0.1*N* $KMnO_4$. Addition of 1 mL H_3PO_4 toward end of titration facilitates reading of end point. Pink-gray end point persists ca 20 s. Multiply titer by factor and obtain mg glucose from Table **936.06**.

References: Z. Anal. Chem. **107**, 328(1936). Z. Spiritusind. **56**, 64(1933).
CAS-50-99-7 (glucose)

33.23   938.18—Glucose in Cacao Products
Zerban-Sattler Method
First Action

A. Reagents

    (a) *Soxhlet modification of Fehling copper solution.*—See **923.09A(a)** (*see* 33.14).

    (b) *Sodium acetate solution.*—Dissolve 500 g NaOAc.3H$_2$O in ca 800 mL hot H$_2$O, cool, and dilute to 1 L.

    (c) *Potassium iodide-iodate solution.*—Dissolve 5.4 g KIO$_3$ and 60 g KI in H$_2$O, add 0.25 g NaOH dissolved in little H$_2$O, and dilute to 1 L.

    (d) *Sulfuric acid.*—Approximately 2N. Dilute 57 mL H$_2$SO$_4$ to 1 L.

    (e) *Saturated potassium oxalate solution.*—Dissolve 165 g K$_2$C$_2$O$_4$.H$_2$O in 500 mL hot H$_2$O, and cool.

    (f) *Sodium thiosulfate standard solution.*—0.1N Use standard solution, **942.27** (*see* 33.9), 1 mL 0.1N Na$_2$S$_2$O$_3$ = 6.354 mg Cu.

    (g) *Sugar solution.*—Dissolve amount of sample containing ca 10 g solids in H$_2$O and dilute to 1 L.

B. Determination

Transfer 10 mL Soxhlet solution, 20 mL NaOAc solution, 10 mL sugar solution, and 10 mL H$_2$O to 250 mL erlenmeyer. Mix, close flask with rubber stopper provided with Bunsen valve, and immerse in briskly boiling H$_2$O bath exactly 20 min. Immerse in cold running H$_2$O, venting valve to prevent boiling caused by vacuum. Cool, add 25 mL KI-KIO$_3$ solution by pipet, and mix by gentle shaking. Rapidly add 40 mL 2N H$_2$SO$_4$ from graduate; then, add 20 mL K$_2$C$_2$O$_4$ solution from graduate. Shake until precipitate completely dissolves, and titrate excess I with 0.1N Na$_2$S$_2$O$_3$.

    Determine blank, substituting H$_2$O for sugar solution. Difference between titer of blank and that of sample is direct measure of Cu$_2$O precipitated. From Table **938.18** obtain glucose equivalent corresponding to titer of 0.1N Na$_2$S$_2$O$_3$.

    Correction for reducing effect of maltose.—If maltose is present, correct observed titer of 0.1N Na$_2$S$_2$O$_3$ for reducing effect of maltose by subtracting correction obtained from Table **938.18** by interpolation.

Table 938.18.—Zerban-Sattler Table for Determination of Glucose with Copper Acetate Reagent[a]

	Glucose, mg										Maltose Corrections (Subtracted from Observed Titer) Maltose Present, mg		
Titer	0.0	0.1	0.2	0.3	0.4	0.5	0.6	0.7	0.8	0.9	200	100	50
10	25.7	26.0	26.3	26.6	26.9	27.2	27.5	27.8	28.1	28.4	2.5	1.4	0.6
11	28.7	29.0	29.3	29.6	29.9	30.3	30.6	30.9	31.2	31.5	2.3	1.2	0.4
12	31.8	32.2	32.5	32.9	33.2	33.6	34.0	34.3	34.7	35.9	2.2	1.1	0.4
13	35.4	35.8	36.1	36.5	36.8	37.2	37.6	37.9	38.3	38.6	2.0	1.0	0.3

Table 938.18.—Zerban-Sattler Table for Determination of Glucose with Copper Acetate Reagent[a]

| Titer | Glucose, mg | | | | | | | | | | Maltose Corrections (Subtracted from Observed Titer) | | |
| | | | | | | | | | | | Maltose Present, mg | | |
	0.0	0.1	0.2	0.3	0.4	0.5	0.6	0.7	0.8	0.9	200	100	50
14	39.0	39.4	39.9	40.3	40.7	41.2	41.6	42.0	42.4	42.9	1.9	1.0	0.3
15	43.3	43.8	44.2	44.7	45.1	45.6	46.1	46.5	47.0	47.4	1.8	1.0	0.3
16	47.9	48.4	49.0	49.5	50.1	50.6	51.1	51.7	52.2	52.8	1.7	1.0	0.3
17	53.3	53.9	54.5	55.2	55.8	56.4	57.0	57.6	58.3	58.9	1.6	0.9	0.3
18	59.5	60.2	60.9	61.6	62.3	63.1	63.8	64.5	65.2	65.9	1.4	0.8	0.3
19	66.6	67.4	68.2	69.0	69.8	70.6	71.4	72.2	73.0	73.8	1.2	0.7	0.3
20	74.6	75.6	76.5	77.5	78.4	79.4	80.3	81.3	82.2	83.2	1.0	0.6	0.2
21	84.4	85.2	86.3	87.4	88.5	89.6	90.6	91.7	92.8	93.9	0.6	0.4	0.2
22	95.0										0.4	0.3	0.1

[a] Table may be interpolated for each 0.01 mL, but should not be extrapolated.

References: Ind. Eng. Chem. Anal. Ed. **10**, 669(1938). Z. Spiritusind. **56**, 64(1933).
CAS-50-99-7 (glucose)

33.24   938.02—Glucose in Cacao Products

First Action

Prepare clarified and deleaded sample solution as in **920.82**, except use only 10 g. Proceed as in **938.18B** or **936.06C**.

I. **920.82** (Sucrose in Cacao Products)

Transfer 26 g prepared sample, **970.20**, to 250 mL centrifuge bottle, add ca 100 mL petroleum ether, shake 5 min, and centrifuge. Decant clear solvent carefully and repeat extraction with petroleum ether. Place bottle containing defatted residue in warm place until petroleum ether is expelled. Add 100 mL H_2O and shake until most of chocolate is detached from sides and bottom of bottle. Loosen stopper and carefully immerse bottle 15 min in H_2O bath kept at 85–90°, shaking occasionally to remove all chocolate from sides of bottle. Remove from bath, cool, and add *basic Pb(OAc)₂ solution* (specific gravity 1.25) to complete precipitation (5 mL is usually enough). Add H_2O to make total of 110 mL added liquid. Mix thoroughly, centrifuge, and decant supernate through small filter. Precipitate excess Pb with powdered dry $K_2C_2O_4$ and filter. Dilute

10 or 20 mL filtrate with equal volume H_2O, mix, and polarize in 200 mm tube at 20°. Obtain invert reading as in **925.48(b)** (*see* 33.72). Multiply both readings by 2 to obtain direct and invert polarizations *"P"* and *"I."* From data obtained, calculate % sucrose (*S*) from following formulas:

$$S = \frac{(P - I)(110 + X)}{143 - t/2}$$

where

$$X = \frac{0.2244(P - 21d)}{1 - 0.00204(P - 21d)}$$

where

$$d = \frac{P - I}{143.0 - t/2}$$

References: JAOAC **16,** 564(1933); **17,** 377(1934).
CAS-57-50-1 (sucrose)

II. **970.20** (Cacao Products, Preparation of Sample)
(**a**) *Powdered products.*—Mix thoroughly and preserve in tightly stoppered bottles.
(**b**) *Chocolate products.*—(*1*) Chill ca 200 g sweet or bitter chocolate until hard, and grate or shave to fine granular condition. Mix thoroughly and preserve in tightly stoppered bottle in cool place. Alternatively—
(*2*) Melt ca 200 g bitter, sweet, or milk chocolate by placing in suitable container and partly immersing container in bath at ca 50°. Stir frequently until sample melts and reaches temperature of 45–50°. Remove from bath, stir thoroughly, and while still liquid, remove portion for analysis, using glass or metal tube, 4–10 mm diameter, provided with close-fitting plunger to expel sample from tube, or disposable plastic syringe.
Reference: JAOAC **53,** 388(1970).

References: Ind. Eng. Chem. Anal. Ed. **10,** 669(1938). JAOAC **28,** 531(1945).

33.25   925.37—Glucose (Commercial) in Fruits and Fruit Products
Procedure

See **930.37B** (*see* 33.81).

33.26   933.02—Glucose in Plants
Micro Method
Final Action

See **959.11B** (*see* 33.29).

33.27   935.62—Glucose in Sugars and Sirups
Chemical Methods
Final Action

A. *Lane-Eynon General Volumetric Method*

Proceed as in **923.09C** (*see* 33.24), referring titer to **930.44** or **930.45** (*see* 33.14).

B. *Munson-Walker General Method*

Proceed as in **906.03B** (*see* 33.13), and obtain weight glucose from **940.39** (*Official Methods of Analysis* [1990] 15th Ed., pp 1286–1294).

C. *Folin and Wu Micro Method*

See **31.054–31.055**, *Official Methods of Analysis* (1975) 12th Ed.

33.28   945.67—Glucose in Corn Sirups and Sugars
Steinhoff Methods
First Action
Surplus 1974

A. *Zerban-Sattler Modification*

See **31.206–31.207**, *Official Methods of Analysis* (1975) 12th Ed.

B. *Sichert-Bleyer Modification*

See **31.208–31.209**, *Official Methods of Analysis* (1975) 12th Ed.

33.29   959.11—Glucose in Sugars and Sirups
Shaffer-Somogyi Micro Method
First Action 1959
Final Action 1960

A. Reagents

(a) *Shaffer-Somogyi carbonate 50 reagent, 5 g KI.*—Dissolve 25 g each of anhydrous Na_2CO_3 and KNa tartrate·$4H_2O$ (Rochelle salt) in ca 500 mL H_2O in 2 L beaker. Add through funnel with tip under surface, with stirring, 75 mL of solution of 100 g $CuSO_4$·$5H_2O$/L. Add 20 g $NaHCO_3$, dissolve, and add 5 g KI. Transfer solution to 1 L volumetric flask, add 250 mL $0.100N$ KIO_3 (3.567 g dissolved and diluted to 1 L), dilute to volume, and filter through fritted glass. Age overnight before use.

(b) *Iodide-oxalate solution.*—Dissolve 2.5 g KI and 2.5 g $K_2C_2O_4$ in H_2O and dilute to 100 mL. Prepare fresh weekly.

(c) *Thiosulfate standard solution.*—$0.005N$. Prepare daily from standardized stock $0.1N$ solution, **942.27** (*see* 33.9).

(d) *Starch indicator.*—Rub 2.5 g soluble starch and ca 10 mg HgI_2 in little H_2O. Dissolve in ca 500 mL boiling H_2O.

B. Determination

Pipet 5 mL solution containing 0.5–2.5 mg glucose into 25 × 200 mm test tube. Add 5 mL reagent, (**a**), and mix well by swirling. Prepare blank, using 5 mL H_2O and 5 mL reagent. Place tubes, capped with bulb or funnel, in boiling H_2O bath 15 min. Carefully remove tubes without agitation to running H_2O cooling bath 4 min. Remove caps and add down side of each tube 2 mL KI-$K_2C_2O_4$ solution and then 3 mL $2N$ H_2SO_4 (56 mL/L). (Do not agitate solutions while alkaline.) Mix thoroughly to ensure that all Cu_2O is dissolved, and let stand in cold H_2O bath 5 min, mixing twice during that time. Titrate with $0.005N$ $Na_2S_2O_3$, using starch indicator, (**d**). Subtract titration of test solution from that of blank and determine amount glucose in 5 mL solution from Table **959.11**.

Table **959.11.**—Shaffer-Somogyi Dextrose-Thiosulfate Equivalents

	mg glucose = (0.1099) (mL 0.005 N $Na_2S_2O_3$) + 0.048									
	Tenths mL $0.005N$ thiosulfate									
	0	0.1	0.2	0.3	0.4	0.5	0.6	0.7	0.8	0.9
mL 0.005 N $Na_2S_2O_3$	mg Dextrose in 5 mL of solution									
3	0.378	0.389	0.400	0.411	0.422	0.432	0.444	0.455	0.466	0.477
4	0.488	0.499	0.510	0.521	0.532	0.543	0.554	0.565	0.576	0.587
5	0.598	0.608	0.619	0.630	0.641	0.652	0.663	0.674	0.685	0.696
6	0.707	0.718	0.729	0.740	0.751	0.762	0.773	0.784	0.795	0.806
7	0.817	0.828	0.839	0.850	0.861	0.872	0.883	0.894	0.905	0.916

Table **959.11**.—Shaffer-Somogyi Dextrose-Thiosulfate Equivalents

	mg glucose = (0.1099) (mL 0.005 N Na$_2$S$_2$O$_3$) + 0.048									
	Tenths mL 0.005N thiosulfate									
	0	0.1	0.2	0.3	0.4	0.5	0.6	0.7	0.8	0.9
mL 0.005 N Na$_2$S$_2$O$_3$	mg Dextrose in 5 mL of solution									
8	0.927	0.938	0.949	0.960	0.971	0.982	0.993	1.004	1.015	1.026
9	1.037	1.048	1.059	1.070	1.081	1.092	1.103	1.114	1.125	1.136
10	1.147	1.158	1.169	1.180	1.191	1.202	1.213	1.224	1.235	1.246
11	1.257	1.268	1.279	1.290	1.301	1.312	1.323	1.334	1.345	1.356
12	1.367	1.378	1.389	1.400	1.411	1.422	1.433	1.444	1.455	1.466
13	1.477	1.488	1.499	1.510	1.521	1.532	1.543	1.554	1.565	1.576
14	1.587	1.598	1.609	1.620	1.631	1.642	1.653	1.664	1.675	1.686
15	1.697	1.707	1.718	1.729	1.740	1.751	1.762	1.773	1.784	1.795
16	1.806	1.817	1.828	1.839	1.850	1.861	1.872	1.883	1.894	1.905
17	1.916	1.927	1.938	1.949	1.960	1.971	1.982	1.993	2.004	2.015
18	2.026	2.037	2.048	2.059	2.070	2.081	2.092	2.103	2.114	2.125
19	2.136	2.147	2.158	2.169	2.180	2.191	2.202	2.213	2.224	2.235
20	2.246	2.257	2.268	2.279	2.290	2.301	2.312	2.323	2.334	2.345
21	2.356	2.367	2.378	2.389	2.400	2.411	2.422	2.433	2.444	2.455
22	2.466	2.477	2.488	2.499	2.510	2.521	2.532	2.543	2.554	2.565

J. Biol. Chem. **100**, 695(1933); **160**, 61(1945); JADAC **42**, 341(1959); **43**, 645(1960).

Make control determinations with known amounts of glucose and apply corrections for any deviations from tabulated equivalents.

CAS-50-99-7 (glucose)

33.30   **935.63—Fructose in Sugars and Sirups**
Chemical Methods
Final Action

A. Lane-Eynon General Volumetric Method
Proceed as in **923.09C** (*see* 33.14) referring titer to **930.44** or **930.45** (*see* 33.14).

B. Munson-Walker General Method

Proceed as in **906.03B** (*see* 33.13) and **929.09F** (*see* 33.15), and obtain weight fructose equivalent to weight Cu from **940.39** [*Official Methods of Analysis* (1990) 15th Ed., pp 1286–1294].

33.31   932.15—Fructose in Sugars and Sirups
Jackson-Mathews
Modification of Nyns Selective Method
Final Action

A. Reagent

Ost solution.—Dissolve 250 g anhydrous K_2CO_3 in ca 700 mL hot H_2O, add 100 g pulverized $KHCO_3$, and agitate mixture until completely dissolved. Cool, and add, with very vigorous agitation, solution of 25.3 g $CuSO_4 \cdot 5H_2O$ in 100–150 mL H_2O. Dilute to 1 L and filter.

B. Determination

Transfer 50 mL Ost solution to 125 mL erlenmeyer and pipet in volume sample solution containing ≤92 mg fructose or its equivalent of fructose-glucose mixture (glucose has ca ½ reducing power of fructose). Add H_2O to 70 mL. Immerse in H_2O bath regulated at 55°, preferably within 0.1°. Digest exactly 75 min, swirling at 10 or 15 min intervals.

Filter precipitated Cu_2O on closely packed asbestos-mat gooch, and wash flask and precipitate thoroughly without attempting to transfer precipitate quantitatively. Determine Cu by one of methods described in **929.09** (*see* 33.15). As it is usually difficult to transfer Cu precipitate quantitatively from erlenmeyer, select method of Cu analysis in which total Cu is dissolved in HNO_3 and determined by electrolysis or $Na_2S_2O_3$ titration, or in $Fe_2(SO_4)_3$ solution followed by $KMnO_4$ titration as in **929.09E**.

See Table **932.15** for fructose equivalent. If sample contained glucose in addition to fructose, analytical result is not true but "apparent" fructose, as glucose has appreciable reducing action under conditions of analysis. To determine correction for glucose, analyze sample also for total reducing sugars and compute true glucose and fructose by series of approximations. Calculate % reducing sugars in original sample and similarly % "apparent" fructose. Difference between these 2 percentages is "apparent" glucose. Divide apparent glucose by factor 12.4 and deduct result from apparent fructose to obtain new approximation to true fructose. Deduct new fructose % from total reducing sugar % to obtain more nearly correct value for true glucose and again divide by 12.4. Deduct quotient from original value of "apparent" fructose and continue approximation in same manner until % fructose remains essentially unaltered by 2 successive approximations.

Table 932.15.—Copper-Fructose Equivalents According to Jackson and Mathews Modification of Nyns Selective Method for Fructose; Values Expressed in mg

(Linear interpolation yields accurate results)			
Cu	Fructose	Cu	Fructose
5	2.5	130	39.3
10	4.5	140	42.0
15	6.2	150	44.7
20	7.9	160	47.4
25	9.5	170	50.0
30	11.0	180	52.6
35	12.5	190	55.2
40	13.9	200	57.9
45	15.4	210	60.6
50	16.8	220	63.4
55	18.3	230	66.4
60	19.7	240	69.4
65	21.2	250	72.5
70	22.5	260	75.7
80	25.4	270	79.0
90	28.1	280	82.4
100	30.9	290	85.9
110	33.7	300	89.5
120	36.5	310	93.2

If original sample contained sucrose, determine by means of Clerget method, **925.48**. Correct Cu for reducing action of sucrose before referring to table. One, 2, 3, 4, and 5 g sucrose under conditions of analysis precipitate 3.3, 5.7, 7.4, 8.5, and 9.0 mg Cu, respectively.

Reference: JAOAC **15,** 79, 198(1932).
CAS-57-48-7 (fructose)

33.32   33.32   960.06—Fructose in Plants
Somogyi Micro or Munson-Walker Method
First Action 1960
Final Action 1961

A. Reagents

(a) *Glucose oxidase preparation.*—Add slowly, stirring constantly, 100 mL H_2O to 5 g glucose oxidase preparation (''DeeO L-750'' code 4633000, Miles Laboratories, Inc., 1127 Myrtle St, Elkhart, IN 46514). Stir ca 1 min and centrifuge or filter to obtain clear solution. Add ca 1 mL $CHCl_3$ and refrigerate. Solution is stable ≥ 1 month.

(b) *McIlvaine's citrate-phosphate buffer.*—Dissolve 214.902 g $Na_2HPO_4 \cdot 12H_2O$ and 42.020 g citric acid in H_2O and dilute to 1 L.

B. Determination

To suitable aliquot add 1/4 its volume of buffer to give pH ca 5.8. Add 30% as much glucose oxidase preparation as estimated glucose content (for 500 mg glucose add 150 mg glucose oxidase, *i.e.,* 3 mL solution), and few drops 30% H_2O_2 (omit if Somogyi method is to be used in determination). Let stand overnight at room temperature.

Determine fructose by Somogyi micro method, **959.11B** (*see* 33.29), or by MunsonWalker method, **906.03** (*see* 33.13), using Table **960.06**. Check equivalents in range of interest, using pure fructose as standard, and correct as necessary.

Table 960.06.—Abbreviated Munson and Walker Table for Calculating Fructose (From *Official and Tentative Methods of Analysis*, AOAC, 5th Ed., 1940)

Cuprous Oxide, mg	Fructose, mg	Cuprous Oxide, mg	Fructose, mg
10	4.5	300	148.6
50	23.5	350	174.9
100	47.7	400	201.8
150	72.2	450	229.2
200	97.2	490	253.9
250	122.7	--	--

References: JAOAC **41**, 307, 681(1958); **42,** 650(1959); **43,** 512(1960); **44,** 267(1961).

33.33   **950.57—Arabinose, Galactose, and Xylose
and Other Sugars in Sugars and Sirups**
First Action

Proceed as in **959.11B** (*see* 33.29), using appropriate heating time and equation for calculation from Table **950.57**. Make control determinations with known amounts of sugar and apply corrections for any deviations from equations.

Table 950.57.—Shaffer-Somogyi Sugar-Thiosulfate Equivalents (y = mg sugar in 5 mL; x = mL 0.005 N $Na_2S_2O_3$)

Sugar	Heating Time, min	Equation
L-Arabinose	30	$y = 0.1234x + 0.060$
Fructose	15	$y = 0.1113x + 0.079$
D-Galactose	30	$y = 0.1332x + 0.033$
Glucose	15	$y = 0.1099x + 0.048$
Lactose	35	$y = 0.2031x + 0.030$
Maltose	30	$y = 0.2199x + 0.072$
D-Mannose	35	$y = 0.1148x + 0.084$
D-Ribose	25	$y = 0.1381x + 0.098$
L-Sorbose	15	$y = 0.1244x + 0.116$
D-Xylose	30	$y + 0.1103x + 0.044$

CAS-147-81-9 (arabinose)
CAS-59-23-4 (galactose)
CAS-58-86-6 (xylose)

33.34   **920.139—Sucrose in Lemon, Orange, and Lime Extracts**
Final Action

Neutralize normal weight of sample, evaporate to dryness, wash several times with ether, dissolve in H_2O, and proceed as in **925.47B** (*see* 33.70), **925.48** (*see* 33.72), or **930.36** (*see* 33.41).

33.35   902.02—Sucrose in Vanilla Extract
Final Action

See **925.47B** (*see* 33.70), **925.48** (*see* 33.72), or **930.36** (*see* 33.41).

Reference: J. Am. Chem. Soc. **24,** 1133(1902).

33.36   920.184—Sucrose in Honey
Final Action

Proceed as in **930.36** (*see* 33.41). To determine reducing sugars after inversion, invert 50 mL solution, **920.182(a)**, as in **925.47B(b)** or **(c)** (*see* 33.70), or **925.48(b)** or **(c)** (*see* 33.72), dilute 10 mL this solution with small amount of H$_2$O, neutralize with Na$_2$CO$_3$, and dilute to 250 mL with H$_2$O. Use 50 mL of this solution, making determination as in **920.183(a)** (*see* 33.52).

    920.182 (Polarization [Direct] of Honey)
        (a) *Immediate direct polarization.*—Transfer 26 g honey to 100 mL volumetric flask with H$_2$O, add 5 mL alumina cream, **925.46B(b)** (*see* 33.71), dilute to volume with H$_2$O at 20°, filter, and polarize immediately in 200 mm tube.

33.37   920.189—Sucrose in Maple Products
Final Action

A. Polarimetric Methods
    Proceed as in **925.47B** (*see* 33.70), or **925.48** (*see* 33.72), or calculate from results of **920.188A** and **920.188B(a)**, using appropriate formula from **925.47B** or **925.48**.

        920.188 (Polarization of Maple Products)
            A. Direct Polarization
            See **925.47B(a)**.
            B. Invert Polarization
            (a) *At 20°.*—Proceed as in **925.47B(b)** or **(c)** or **925.48(b)** or **(c)**.

B. By Reducing Sugars Before and After Inversion
    See **930.36** (*see* 33.41).

33.38   925.35—Sucrose in Fruits and Fruit Products
Final Action

A. By Polarization

Determine by polarizing before and after inversion. *See* **925.47B** (*see* 33.70), **925.48** (*see* 33.72), or **896.02** (*see* 33.62).

B. By Reducing Sugars Before and After Inversion

Transfer sample representing (if possible) ca 2.5 g total sugars to 200 mL volumetric flask; dilute to ca 100 mL and add excess of saturated neutral $Pb(OAc)_2$ solution, **925.46B(d)** (ca 2 mL is usually enough). Mix, dilute to volume, and filter, discarding first few milliliters filtrate. Add dry K or Na oxalate to precipitate excess Pb used in clarification, mix, and filter, discarding first few milliliters filtrate. Take 25 mL filtrate or aliquot containing (if possible) 50–200 mg reducing sugars and proceed as in **906.03** (*see* 33.13).

For inversion at room temperature transfer 50 mL aliquot clarified and deleaded solution to 100 mL volumetric flask, add 10 mL HCl (1 + 1), and let stand at room temperature ($\geq 20°$) 24 h; exactly neutralize with concentrated NaOH solution, using phenolphthalein, and dilute to 100 mL. Take aliquot and determine total sugars as invert as in **906.03**. Calculate sucrose as in **930.36** (*see* 33.41).

33.39   925.44—Sucrose in Food Dressings
Final Action

Subtract percent invert sugar obtained before inversion, **925.42** (*see* 33.56), from that obtained after inversion, **925.43** (*see* 33.57), and multiply difference by 0.95.

33.40   930.07—Sucrose in Plants
Inversion Methods
Final Action

A. Hydrochloric Acid Inversion

Using aliquot of cleared solution, **931.02B** (*see* 33.59), proceed as in **925.05**.

925.05 (Sucrose in Animal Feed)

Place 10 g sample in 250 mL volumetric flask. If material is acid, neutralize by adding 1–3 g $CaCO_3$. Add 125 mL 50% alcohol by volume, mix thoroughly, and boil on steam bath or by partially immersing flask in H_2O bath 1 h at 83–87°, using small funnel in neck of flask to condense vapor. Cool and let mixture stand several h, preferably overnight. Dilute to volume with neutral 95% alcohol, mix thoroughly, let settle or centrifuge 15 min at 1500 rpm, and decant closely. Pipet 200 mL supernate into beaker and evaporate on steam bath to 20–30 mL. Do not evaporate to dryness. Little alcohol in residue does no harm.

Transfer to 100 mL volumetric flask and rinse beaker thoroughly with H_2O, adding rinsings to flask. Add enough *saturated neutral $Pb(CH_3COO)_2$ solution* (ca 2 mL) to produce flocculent precipitate, shake thoroughly, and let stand 15 min. Dilute to volume with H_2O, mix thoroughly, and filter through dry paper. Add enough anhydrous Na_2CO_3 or potassium oxalate to filtrate to precipitate all Pb, again filter through dry paper, and test filtrate with little anhydrous Na_2CO_3 or potassium oxalate to make sure that all Pb has been removed.

Place 50 mL prepared solution in 100 mL volumetric flask, add piece of litmus paper, neutralize with HCl, add 5 mL HCl, and let inversion proceed at room temperature as in **925.48(c)** (*see* 33.72). When inversion is complete, transfer solution to beaker, neutralize with Na_2CO_3, return solution to 100 mL flask, dilute to volume with H_2O, filter if necessary, and determine reducing sugars in 50 mL solution (representing 2 g sample) as in **906.03B** (*see* 33.13). Calculate results as invert sugar.

% Sucrose = [% total sugar after inversion
− % reducing sugars before inversion
(both calculated as invert sugar)] × 0.95

Because insoluble material of grain or cattle food occupies some space in flask as originally made up, correct by multiplying all results by factor 0.97, as results of large number of determinations on various materials show average volume of 10 g material to be 7.5 mL.

References: USDA Bur. Chem. Circ. **71**. JAOAC **41**, 276(1958); **42**, 39(1959).
CAS-57-50-1 (sucrose)

B. Invertase Inversion

(**a**) *For plants giving hydrolysis end point within 2 hours.*—Pipet aliquot of cleared solution, **931.02B**, into 400 mL Pyrex beaker and make slightly acid to methyl red with CH_3COOH. Add 3 drops 1% solution of *Wallerstein invertase scales*. Let mixture stand at room temperature 2 h. Add reagents as in **923.09B** (*see* 33.14), and determine reducing power. Calculate results as invert sugar. Deduct reducing power of original solution, also expressed as invert sugar, and multiply difference by 0.95.

(**b**) *For plants giving slower hydrolysis end point.*—Place aliquot of solution, **931.02B**, in small volumetric flask. Make slightly acid to methyl red with CH_3COOH. Add 3 drops 1% solution of *Wallerstein invertase scales* and few drops toluene. Stopper flask and let stand overnight or longer at room temperature. Dilute to volume with H_2O and use aliquot for reducing power as above.

CAS-57-50-1 (sucrose)

33.41   930.36—Sucrose in Sugars and Sirups
From Reducing Sugars Before and After Inversion
Final Action

Determine reducing sugars as in **906.03B** (*see* 33.13) [clarification having been effected with neutral $Pb(OAc)_2$ as in **925.46(d)** (*see* 33.71)] and calculate to invert sugar from **940.39** (*Official Methods of Analysis* [1990] 15th Ed.). Invert solution as in **925.47B(b)** or **(c)** (*see* 33.70), or **925.48(b)** or **(c)** (*see* 33.72); exactly neutralize acid; and again determine reducing sugars, but calculate them to invert sugar from table, **940.39**, using invert sugar alone column. Deduct % invert sugar obtained before inversion from that obtained after inversion and multiply difference by 0.95 to obtain % sucrose. Dilute solutions in both determinations so that ≤230 mg invert sugar is present in amount taken for reduction. It is important that all Pb be removed from solution with anhydrous powdered K oxalate before reduction.

33.42   950.51—Sucrose in Nuts and Nut Products
Final Action

See **22.049**, *Official Methods of Analysis* (1965) 10th Ed.

33.43   927.07—Lactose in Meat
Benedict Solution Method
First Action

A. Reagents

    (a) *Acclimated yeast suspension (for use in presence or absence of maltose).*—Macerate 2 cakes (0.6 oz [17 g] each) bakers yeast and wash with 3 ca 50 mL portions H_2O, centrifuging between washings. Prepare medium containing 1.0 g anhydrous $MgSO_4$, 2.0 g NH_4Cl, 1.0 g anhydrous K_2HPO_4, 0.5 g KCl, 0.02 g $FeSO_4 \cdot 7H_2O$, 0.7 g peptone, and 20.0 g technical maltose. Dissolve each ingredient in small amount H_2O and add, in order given, to flask containing ca 500 mL H_2O. Dilute to 1 L. Warm, filter, bring filtrate to rolling boil, and let cool to room temperature. Add washed yeast to 1 L medium and incubate ca 24 h at 30°, stirring frequently first few hours. Separate yeast by decanting and centrifuging, wash twice with H_2O, add to 1 L fresh medium, and incubate additional 24 h with agitation first few hours. Separate yeast from medium, wash thoroughly ≥4 times with H_2O, dilute to 100 mL, and refrigerate. Yeast remains active 2–3 weeks. (Yeast may remain active longer if frozen.)

    (b) *Washed yeast suspension (for use in absence of maltose).*—Mix 2 cakes bakers yeast to smooth suspension with ca 150 mL H_2O. Centrifuge 5 min and discard aqueous layer. Repeat mixing with H_2O and centrifuging 4 more times, or until supernate after centrifuging is practically clear. Again suspend yeast in H_2O and dilute with H_2O to 100 mL. Store in refrigerator at ca 4° and shake well before using. Discard after 2 weeks.

(c) *Benedict solution.*—Dissolve 16 g $CuSO_4 \cdot 5H_2O$ in 125–150 mL H_2O. Dissolve 150 g Na citrate·$2H_2O$, 130 g anhydrous Na_2CO_3, and 10 g $NaHCO_3$ in ca 650 mL hot H_2O. Combine the 2 solutions, cool, dilute to 1 L, and filter.

(d) *Lactose standard solution.*—1.5 mg anhydrous lactose/mL. Dissolve 1.5789 g lactose·H_2O in H_2O and dilute to 1 L.

(e) *Iodine standard solution.*—Mix 5.08 g I with 10.2 g KI, dissolve in small volume of H_2O, filter, and dilute to 1 L.

(f) *Sodium thiosulfate standard solution.*—Dissolve 9.92 g $Na_2S_2O_3 \cdot 5H_2O$ in H_2O and dilute to 1 L.

(g) *Dilute acetic acid.*—Dilute 240 mL CH_3COOH to 1 L with H_2O.

(h) *Dilute phosphoric acid.*—Dilute 240 mL H_3PO_4 to 1 L with H_2O.

(i) *Citric acid-phosphate buffer.*—pH 4.8. Mix solutions in proportions of 10.14 mL 0.1M citric acid (19.21 g/L) and 9.86 mL 0.2M Na_2HPO_4 (28.4 g anhydrous/L), and adjust to pH 4.8, using pH meter. Store in refrigerator and discard if solution becomes turbid.

(j) *Starch solution.*—Rub 2.5 g soluble starch and ca 10 mg HgI_2 in little H_2O. Dissolve in ca 500 mL boiling H_2O.

B. Determination (in Presence of Maltose)

Place 10 g sample in 100 mL volumetric sugar flask, add small volume of H_2O, and break up sample by agitation. Add ca 50 mL H_2O and warm on steam bath ca 30 min. Cool to room temperature, add 2 mL HCl, and dilute to volume, using bottom of fat layer as meniscus. Add 5.0 mL *20% phosphotungstic acid solution*, mix well, let stand few minutes, and filter through moist paper. Pipet 40 mL filtrate into 50 mL volumetric flask and neutralize just to acid side of chlorophenol red or other indicator which shows change at ca pH 4.8. Add 5 mL pH 4.8 buffer solution, dilute to volume, and mix.

Transfer ca 40 mL of this solution to centrifuge tube to which 5 mL yeast suspension, (a), has been added and from which H_2O has been separated. Mix yeast and sample well and incubate 3 h at 30°, stirring frequently. Centrifuge and determine reducing sugars:

Pipet 10 mL clear solution into 300 mL erlenmeyer, add 20 mL Benedict solution, (c), bring to bp in 3–5 min, and boil slowly exactly 3 min. Remove from heat, cool, and add 100 mL H_2O and 10 mL dilute CH_3COOH, (g), slowly while swirling. Add ca 30% excess standard I, (e) (15 mL for ca 1.5% lactose), and agitate to dissolve Cu_2O. Let flask stand ≥ 5 min, add 20 mL dilute H_3PO_4, (h), and titrate excess I with standard $Na_2S_2O_3$ solution, (f), using starch indicator.

Determine lactose:I ratio by using 10 mL standard lactose solution and carrying through determination as above, beginning " ... add 20 mL Benedict solution, ... " Determine I:$Na_2S_2O_3$ ratio by using 10 mL H_2O and carrying through determination as above, beginning " ... add 20 mL Benedict solution, ... "

% Lactose = 100 KV/W, where K = g lactose/mL I solution, V = volume I solution consumed, and W = g sample in aliquot, considering volume original sample solution as 100 mL rather than 105 mL, to correct for volume occupied by meat.

C. Determination (in Absence of Maltose)

Prepare solution as in **927.07B**, first paragraph. Place 5 mL washed yeast suspension, (a) or (b), in lipless centrifuge tube, centrifuge, and drain and discard supernate. Add 40 mL prepared solution to yeast residue in centrifuge tube, stopper, and shake vigorously to dislodge and suspend yeast. Let stand with occasional shaking 1 h. Centrifuge and determine lactose in clear solution as in **927.07B**, third paragraph.

References: J. Biol. Chem. **75**, 33(1927); **79**, 649(1928). J. Dairy Res. **7**, 41(1936). Conn. Agric. Exp. Stn. Bull. **401**, 869(1937); **415**, 695(1938); **426**, 14(1939). JAOAC **23**, 811(1940); **40**, 770(1957); **41**, 293(1958). CAS-63-42-3 (lactose)

33.44 930.32—Lactose in Process Cheese
Final Action

Prepare suspension as in **928.05C** through addition of $Na_2C_2O_4$ solution. Shake vigorously 1 min; add 25 g powdered Na_2SO_4 and shake 2 min; add 10 mL H_2SO_4 (1 + 1) and shake; then add 25 mL *20% phosphotungstic acid solution* and shake vigorously. Transfer contents of bottle to 500 mL volumetric flask, cool at once to 20°, and dilute to volume with H_2O. Mix thoroughly, let stand 10 min, and filter through dry folded paper. Transfer 150 mL filtrate to each of two 250 mL volumetric flasks, add 10% NaOH solution to one flask until mixture is alkaline to litmus, and then add 5 g solid KCl and mix thoroughly. Cool to 20° and dilute to volume with H_2O. Mix well, let stand 10 min, and filter through dry folded paper.

    I. **928.05** (Tartaric Acid in Cheese, Quantitative Method)

        B. Reagents

        (**a**) *Potassium chloride wash solution.*—Dissolve 15 g KCl in 100 mL H_2O and add 20 mL alcohol.

        (**b**) *Tartaric acid solution.*—Dissolve 1.5 g pure tartaric acid in previously boiled and cooled H_2O and dilute to 100 mL at 20°. Titrate with $0.1N$ NaOH to determine weight tartaric acid in 10 mL solution.

        (**c**) *Hydrochloric acid solution.*—2%. Dilute 47 mL HCl to 1 L with H_2O.

        C. Determination

        Weigh 25 g prepared sample, **955.30**, into 500 mL wide-mouth bottle and add, 25 mL at time, 100 mL H_2O at 50–60°, shaking vigorously after each addition. Continue shaking until cheese is thoroughly broken up. Add 25 mL *2% $Na_2C_2O_4$ solution* and shake vigorously 1 min. Add 100 mL 2% HCl, 25 mL at time, shaking vigorously after each addition. Add 50 g powdered KCl and shake 5 min. To avoid churning, keep mixture warm (ca 50°) during shaking. Transfer mixture with aid of H_2O, to 300 mL volumetric flask, cool to 20°, and dilute to volume with H_2O. Mix thoroughly; let stand 10 min, with occasional shaking, and filter through dry folded paper, discarding first few milliliters filtrate. Disregard any opalescence and transfer 200 mL filtrate to 250 mL volumetric flask. Neutralize with $1N$ NaOH, using phenolphthalein and add 5.2 mL in excess. Dilute to volume with H_2O, mix thoroughly, let stand few minutes, and filter through dry folded paper, discarding first few mL filtrate.

        To 100 mL filtrate in 250 mL beaker add, with constant stirring, 10 mL of the tartaric acid solution, 2 mL CH_3COOH, and 23 mL alcohol. Cool in ice bath, stir vigorously until cream of tartar begins to crystallize, and let stand in refrigerator overnight. Prepare Caldwell crucible with pad of asbestos ca 10 mm thick. (*Caution: See Appendix* for safety notes on asbestos.) Decant most of liquid through this filter, wash precipitate into crucible with KCl wash solution, and wash beaker and precipitate 3 times, using total of 20–30 mL wash solution. Place asbestos and precipitate in beaker in which precipitation was made and wash crucible with ca 50 mL hot H_2O. Heat solution to bp and titrate while hot with $0.1N$ NaOH, using phenolphthalein. Calculate % tartaric acid in cheese by formula:

$$X = 14.26[0.015(B + 1.5) - C]$$

where C = g tartaric acid in 10 mL of the tartaric acid reagent; and B = mL $0.1N$ NaOH required for titration. In factor 14.26, concentration caused by insoluble solids of cheese of average composition is taken into consideration.

Reference: JAOAC **11**, 287(1928).

CAS-526-83-0 (tartaric acid)

II. 955.30 (Cheese, Preparation of Samples)

Cut wedge sample into strips and pass 3 times through food chopper. Grind plugs in food chopper (preferable method), or cut or shred very finely and mix thoroughly.

With creamed cottage and similar cheeses, place 300–600 g sample at $<15°$ in 1 L (1 qt) cup of high-speed blender and blend for minimum time (2–5 min) required to obtain homogeneous mixture. Final temperature should be $≤25°$. This may require stopping blender frequently after channeling and spooning cheese back into blades until blending action starts. (Use of variable transformer in line to permit slow speed at first minimizes channeling when speed is increased later.)

Determine lactose in 50 mL aliquot as in **906.03B** (*see* 33.13). Treat the 150 mL in second flask as in **925.48(c)** (*see* 33.72), using 10 mL HCl, etc. Add 10% NaOH solution until alkaline to litmus, and add 5 g solid KCl. Mix thoroughly, cool to 20°, and dilute to volume with H_2O. Let stand 10 min. Filter if necessary through dry paper. Determine lactose in 50 mL aliquot as before. Agreement between amounts of Cu_2O reduced before and after inversion establishes absence of sucrose.

Since insoluble material of cheese and phosphotungstic acid precipitate occupy some space in flask as originally prepared, it is necessary to correct for this volume. From average composition of cheese, volume of precipitate was calculated to be 14 mL. To obtain true amount lactose present, multiply all results by factor 0.97.

References: JAOAC **13**, 243(1930); **16**, 484(1933).

CAS-63-42-3 (lactose)

33.45   933.04—Lactose in Milk Chocolate
Final Action

(In absence of other reducing sugars)

Determine reducing sugars before inversion as in **906.03B** (*see* 33.13), in aliquot (usually 20 mL) of the Pb-free filtrate obtained in **920.82** (*see* 33.24). Determine reduced Cu as Cu_2O by volumetric thiosulfate method, **929.09C** (*see* 33.15). Correct for Cu_2O due to sucrose as follows: Obtain approximate % lactose, using data obtained in **920.82**, as follows: Approximate lactose = $[P(1.1 + X/100) - S]/0.79$

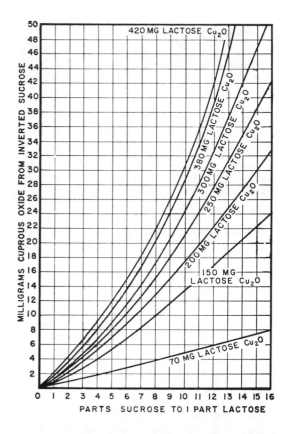

Figure 933.04. Graph used in correcting cuprous oxide for effect of sucrose.

From calculated polarimetric sucrose/lactose ratio and total Cu_2O obtained as above, determine amount of Cu_2O to be subtracted from total Cu_2O found, using graph, Fig. **933.04**. Convert corrected Cu_2O to g lactose (L), using table, **940.39** (*Official Methods of Analysis* [1990] 15th Ed.). Then obtain % lactose from following relationship:

$$\% \text{ lactose} = L(110 + X)/0.26C$$

where X = value obtained in polarimetric sucrose determination and C = volume solution (mL) used in above lactose determination.

References: JAOAC **16**, 564(1933); **17**, 377(1934). CAS-63-42-3 (lactose)

33.46   **935.65—Lactose in Sugars and Sirups**
Chemical Methods
Final Action

A. Lane-Eynon General Volumetric Method
    Proceed as in **923.09C** (*see* 33.14), referring titer to **930.44** (*see* 33.14), or **930.45** (*see* 33.14).

B. Munson-Walker General Method
    Proceed as in **906.03B** (*see* 33.13), and **929.09A** (*see* 33.15), and obtain weight lactose equivalent to weight of Cu_2O from **940.39** (*Official Methods of Analysis* [1990] 15th Ed.).

33.47   945.48K—Evaporated Milk (Unsweetened)
Final Action

B. Preparation of Sample—Procedure
IDF-ISO-AOAC Method

(a) Temper unopened can in H_2O bath at ca 60°. Remove and vigorously shake can every 15 min. After 2 h remove can and let cool to room temperature. Remove entire lid and thoroughly mix by stirring contents in can with spoon or spatula. (If fat separates, sample is not properly prepared.)

(b) Dilute 40 g prepared mixture (a) with 60 g H_2O and mix thoroughly.

References: JAOAC **28,** 207(1945); **52,** 239(1969).

K. Lactose

Proceed as in **896.01B** (*see* 33.67), or **930.28** (*see* 33.84), using diluted sample, **945.48B(b)**, and correct result for dilution.

33.48   952.05—Lactose in Bread
Titrimetric Method
First Action

A. Apparatus

(a) *Rack.*—Metal rack so constructed as to prevent agitation of tubes while in boiling H_2O bath.

(b) *Titration stirrer.*—For stirring solution during titration; rod made from glass tubing, sealed and flared at lower end to form button-like foot, is convenient. Make side arm consisting of several layers adhesive tape attached near enough to top of tube to prevent breaking bottom of titration tube.

B. Reagents

(a) *Yeast suspension.*—Wash 25 g fresh commercial bakers yeast with five 100 mL portions H_2O or until last washings are clear. Centrifuge and decant after each wash. Suspend in 100 mL H_2O and store 24 h at 0–4° before use. Discard after 1 week.

(b) *Yeast nutrient solution.*—Dissolve 1.7 g Bacto peptone (Difco Laboratories), 0.50 g K_2HPO_4, and 0.33 g $MgSO_4 \cdot 7H_2O$ in H_2O, and dilute to 100 mL with H_2O.

(c) *Protein precipitant.*—Dissolve 50 g Na tungstate and 6 g Na_2HPO_4 in 200 mL H_2O. Slowly add 220 mL 2N HCl, mix, and dilute to 500 mL with H_2O.

(d) *Somogyi reagent.*—Dissolve 12 g Rochelle salt, 20 g Na_2CO_3, and 25 g $NaHCO_3$ in ca 500 mL H_2O and pour into solution, with stirring, 6.5 g $CuSO_4 \cdot 5H_2O$ dissolved in ca 100 mL H_2O; add solution of 10 g KI, 0.80 g KIO_3, and 18 g $K_2C_2O_4 \cdot H_2O$, and dilute to 1 L. (Only KIO_3 need be weighed accurately.) Let stand few days; then filter off any small amount of precipitate.

(e) *Sodium thiosulfate solution.*—0.005N. Prepare daily by diluting 0.1N solution, **942.27** (*see* 33.9).

C. Determination

Weigh 10 g air-dried bread, add 5 g Filter-Cel, and mix well. Transfer mixture to extraction thimble (ca 30 × 77 mm), cover with cotton pad, place in Soxhlet extractor, add 150 mL alcohol-H_2O mixture (126 mL alcohol + 61 mL H_2O), and extract overnight on hot plate set at medium heat. Transfer extract to 250 mL beaker (previously marked at 40 mL), evaporate on steam bath with aid of weak air current to ca 40 mL, and transfer to 100 mL volumetric flask, rinsing well. Cool, dilute to volume, and mix well. Pipet 10 mL aliquot into 50 mL erlenmeyer; add 6 mL yeast suspension and 5 mL yeast nutrient solution. Prepare blank test, using 10 mL H_2O in place of sample extract. Stopper flask with 1-hole rubber stopper fitted with piece of 6 mm (not smaller) glass tubing ca 10 cm long. Shake at moderate rate 2.5 h in constant temperature H_2O bath at 30°.

Transfer to 50 mL centrifuge tube and centrifuge ca 10 min at ca 1000 rpm. Decant supernate into 50 mL volumetric flask. Rinse erlenmeyer with 10 mL H_2O, decanting onto residue in centrifuge tube. Mix residue and H_2O with glass rod. Centrifuge and combine washing with previous supernate in 50 mL volumetric flask. Repeat washing, using 10 mL H_2O. Add, with shaking, 2.5 mL protein precipitant. Dilute to volume, mix well, and filter, discarding first few mL filtrate. (This is convenient stopping point; stopper flask for continuation next day.)

Pipet 5.0 mL clear filtrate into Pyrex test tube (22 × 175 mm) and neutralize to phenol red end point with 0.5N NaOH. Add 5.0 mL Somogyi reagent, mix by rotary motion, and add 2 drops benzene. Cap tube with glass bulb and place in metal rack. Immerse rack containing tubes in vigorously boiling H_2O bath exactly 15 min. Cool, avoiding agitation, to ca 35° in H_2O bath. Add 2.5 mL 2N H_2SO_4, shake with rotary motion, let stand 1–2 min, and titrate excess I with 0.005N $Na_2S_2O_3$, adding 6 drops 1% starch indicator near end of titration. (Titrations should be finished in 30 min.) From difference between titration value of blank (H_2O, yeast suspension, and yeast nutrient) and that of sample, determine weight lactose present from standard curve. This value in mg lactose represents amount in 100 mg air-dry bread or % lactose.

Prepare standard curve, using 0–4.5 mg pure *lactose hydrate* (0, 0.2, 0.5, 1.0, 2.0, 3.0, 4.0, and 4.5 mg from portions of solution containing 1.0 mg/mL) in enough H_2O to make 5 mL. Add 5.0 mL Somogyi reagent, mix by rotary motion, and add 2 drops benzene. Proceed as above from ''Cap tube … '' Plot difference between titration value for 0 mg lactose and that for each lactose solution against corresponding lactose concentration in milligrams.

Reference: JAOAC **35**, 56, 697(1952).
CAS-63-42-3 (lactose)

33.49   935.64—Maltose in Sugars and Sirups
Chemical Methods
Final Action

A. Lane-Eynon General Volumetric Method
Proceed as in **923.09C** (*see* 33.14), referring titer to **930.44** (*see* 33.14), or **930.45** (*see* 33.14).

B. Munson-Walker General Method
Proceed as in **906.03B** (*see* 33.13), and **929.09A** (*see* 33.15), and obtain weight maltose equivalent to weight Cu_2O from **940.39** (*Official Methods of Analysis* [1990] 15th Ed.).

33.50   906.01—Sugars (Reducing) in Plants
Munson-Walker General Method
Final Action

See **906.03** (*see* 33.13).

33.51   920.190—Sugars (Reducing) in Maple Products as Invert Sugar
Final Action

(**a**) *Before inversion.*—Proceed as in **923.09C** (*see* 33.14), or **906.03B** (*see* 33.13), using aliquot of solution used for direct polarization, **920.188A** (*see* 33.37). If solution is clarified, only neutral Pb(OAc)$_2$ solution may be used, and excess of Pb must be removed with dry Na oxalate.

(**b**) *After inversion.*—Proceed as in **923.09C** or **906.03B**, using aliquot of solution used for invert polarization, **920.188B(a)**. If solution is clarified, only neutral Pb(OAc)$_2$ solution may be used, and excess of Pb must be removed with dry Na oxalate.

33.52   920.183—Sugars (Reducing) in Honey
Final Action

(**a**) *Munson-Walker method.*—Dilute 10 mL solution, **920.182(a)** (*see* 33.36), to 250 mL and determine reducing sugars in 25 mL of this solution by **906.03B** (*see* 33.13). Calculate result to % invert sugar.

(**b**) *Lane-Eynon method.*—Dilute 10 mL solution, **920.182(a)**, to 500 mL and determine reducing sugars by constant volume method:

Standardize Fehling solutions, **923.09A** (*see* 33.14), so that 5.00 mL solution (**a**) and 5 mL solution (**b**) will react completely with 50 mg invert sugar standard solution, **923.09A(c)**, added as 25 mL of dilution to 2 g/L.

Pipet 5 mL of each Fehling solution into 250 mL erlenmeyer. Add 7 mL H$_2$O, few boiling chips, and 15 mL diluted honey solution from buret with offset tip. Heat to bp over wire gauze, and maintain moderate boil 2 min. Add 1 mL 0.2% methylene blue solution, or 3–4 drops 1% solution, while still boiling and complete titration within total boiling time of 3 min by repeated small additions of diluted honey solution until indicator is decolorized. (Observe color of supernate.) Note volume honey solution used (x mL).

Repeat titration, using 5 mL of each Fehling solution, $(25 - x)$ mL H$_2$O, and all but 1.5 mL diluted honey solution (from buret) determined in preliminary titration. Add honey solution to end point within 3 min and note volume diluted honey solution used (y mL). Duplicate titrations should agree within 0.1 mL.

$$\% \text{ Invert sugar} = 25000/(\text{g honey sample} \times y)$$

References: JAOAC **53**, 390(1970); **70**, 392(1987).
CAS-8013-17-0 (invert sugar)

33.53   **921.03—Sugars (Reducing) in Plants**
Quisumbing-Thomas Method
Final Action
Surplus 1970

See **31.048–31.049**, *Official Methods of Analysis* (1970) 11th Ed.

33.54   **925.15—Sugars in Roasted Coffee**
Final Action

Weigh 10 g prepared sample, **920.91**, into 250 mL volumetric flask, add 1 g powdered NH_4NaHPO_4, and proceed as in **925.05** (*see* 33.40), paragraph 1 and 2, beginning with addition of 50% alcohol, and **906.03B** (*see* 33.13). Determine Cu in Cu_2O precipitate either volumetrically, **929.09C** (*see* 33.15), or electrolytically, **929.09F**.

920.91 (Roasted Coffee, Preparation of Sample)
Grind sample to pass No. 30 sieve and store in tightly stoppered bottle.

Reference: JAOAC **3**, 498(1920).

33.55   **925.36—Sugars (Reducing) in Fruits and Fruit Products**
Inversion Method
Final Action

Proceed as in **925.35B** (*see* 33.38), paragraph 1. Express results as invert sugar.

33.56   **925.42—Sugars (Reducing) Before Inversion in Food Dressings**
Final Action

Weigh 20 g sample into wide-mouth 4 oz (120 mL) bottle and extract oil by adding ca 80 mL petroleum ether, shaking, and centrifuging. Draw off as much as possible of petroleum ether solution (conveniently done by using suction and short-stem pipet), and repeat treatment with petroleum ether until all oil is removed (indicated by absence of color in solvent; usually 4 extractions are required). Reserve ether solution for identification of oil. Remove petroleum ether from residue with air current and transfer residue with H_2O to 100 mL volumetric flask. Add 5–10 mL *fresh solution of HPO_3* (remove any white coating on HPO_3 by rinsing with H_2O, dissolve 5 g transparent lumps or sticks in cold H_2O, and dilute to 100 mL), mix thoroughly, dilute to volume, and filter. Transfer 80 mL filtrate, or as large aliquot as possible, to 100 mL volumetric flask; neutralize with NaOH solution

509

(1 + 1), using phenolphthalein; cool, dilute to volume, and determine reducing sugars on aliquot as in **906.03B** (*see* 33.13). Calculate to invert sugar.

With dressings, particularly those containing starch, that cannot be clarified by above method, remove oil as in **905.02**, using 1 mL NH_4OH and 5 mL alcohol/g sample; transfer residue to 250 mL volumetric flask with 50% alcohol, and proceed as in **925.05** (*see* 33.40), and **906.03B**.

I. 905.02 (Fat in Milk, Roese-Gottlieb Method)

(Details of this method comply with method which has been agreed upon by International Dairy Federation, International Organization for Standardization, and AOAC for publication by each organization and which is published as international standard in *FAO/WHO Code of Principles Concerning Milk and Milk Products and Associated Standards.*)

(*Caution: See Appendix* for safety notes on distillation, flammable solvents, diethyl ether, and petroleum ether.)

Prepare as in **925.21** and weigh, to nearest mg, ca 10 g sample into fat-extraction flask or tube. Add 1.25 mL NH_4OH (2 mL if sample is sour) and mix thoroughly. Add 10 mL alcohol and mix well. Add 25 mL ether (all ether must be peroxide-free), stopper with cork or stopper (synthetic rubber) unaffected by usual fat solvents, and shake very vigorously 1 min. Cool, if necessary; add 25 mL petroleum ether (boiling range 30–60°) and repeat vigorous shaking. Centrifuge flask at ca 600 rpm or let it stand until upper liquid is practically clear. Decant ether solution into suitable flask or metal dish. Wash lip and stopper of extraction flask or tube with mixture of equal parts of the 2 ethers and add washings to weighing flask or dish. Repeat extraction of liquid remaining in flask or tube twice, using 15 mL of each solvent each time and adding H_2O if necessary, but omitting rinsing with mixed solvents after final extraction. (Third extraction is not necessary with skim milk.)

Evaporate solvents completely on steam bath at temperature that does not cause spattering or bumping (boiling chips may be added). Dry fat to constant weight in oven at $102 \pm 2°$ or vacuum oven at 70–75° under pressure <50 mm Hg (6.7 kPa). Weigh cooled flask or dish, without wiping immediately before weighing. Remove fat completely from container with 15–25 mL warm petroleum ether, dry, and weigh as before. Loss in weight = weight fat. Correct weight fat by blank determination on reagents used. If blank is >0.5 mg, purify or replace reagents. Difference between duplicate determinations obtained simultaneously by same analyst should be ≤0.03 g fat/100 g product.

References: Z. Nahr. Genussm. **9**, 531(1905). JAOAC **34**, 237(1951); **52**, 235(1969).

II. 925.21 (Preparation of Milk Sample, Procedure)

Bring sample to ca 20°, mix until homogeneous by pouring into clean receptacle and back repeatedly, and promptly weigh or measure test portion. If lumps of cream do not disperse, warm sample in H_2O bath to ca 38° and keep mixing until homogeneous, using policeman, if necessary, to reincorporate any cream adhering to container or stopper. Where practical and fat remains dispersed, cool warmed samples to ca 20° before transferring test portion.

When Babcock method, **989.04C** (*see* Chapter 18.12), is used, adjust both fresh and composite samples to ca 38°, mix until homogeneous as above, and immediately pipet portions into test bottles.

33.57 **925.43—Sugars (Reducing) After Inversion in Food Dressings**
Final Action

Invert aliquot of solution, **925.42** (*see* 33.56), as in **925.48(b)** or (**c**) (*see* 33.72), nearly neutralize with NaOH solution (1 + 1), and determine reducing sugars in inverted solution as in **906.03B**. Calculate to invert sugar from **940.39**, *Official Methods of Analysis* (1990) 15th Ed.

33.58 **925.52—Sugars in Canned Vegetables**
Final Action

A. Reducing Sugars Before Inversion

Weigh 20 g sample into 200 mL volumetric flask, dilute with ca 100 mL H_2O, clarify with slight excess of neutral $Pb(OAc)_2$ solution, **925.46B(d)** (*see* 33.71), dilute to volume, and filter. Remove excess Pb with anhydrous Na_2SO_4 or with dry Na or K oxalate. Filter, and determine reducing sugars as in **906.03B** (*see* 33.13). Express result as % invert sugar.

B. Reducing Sugars After Inversion

Transfer 50 mL filtrate, **925.52A**, to 100 mL volumetric flask, add 5 mL HCl, and let stand overnight, as in **925.48(c)** (*see* 33.72). Nearly neutralize with NaOH solution, cool, dilute to volume, and determine reducing sugars in aliquot as in **906.03B**. Express result as % invert sugar.

C. Sucrose

See **930.36** (*see* 33.41).

33.59 **931.02—Sugars in Plants**
Preparation of Sample
Final Action

A. Preparation of Solution

(**a**) *General method.*—Prepare fresh sample as in **922.02(b)**. Pour alcohol solution through filter paper or extraction thimble, catching filtrate in volumetric flask. Transfer insoluble material to beaker, cover with 80% alcohol, warm on steam bath 1 h, let cool, and again pour alcohol solution through same filter. If second filtrate is highly colored, repeat extraction. Transfer residue to filter, let drain, and dry. Grind residue so that all particles will pass through 1 mm sieve, transfer to extraction thimble, and extract 12 h in Soxhlet apparatus with 80% alcohol. Dry residue and save for starch determination. Combine alcohol filtrates and dilute to volume at definite temperature with 80% alcohol.

922.02(b) (Plants, Preparation of Sample)

(**b**) *For carbohydrates.*—Thoroughly remove all foreign matter and rapidly grind or chop material into fine pieces. Add weighed sample to hot redistilled alcohol to which enough precipitated $CaCO_3$ has been added to neutralize acidity, using enough alcohol so that final concentration, allowing for H_2O content of sample, is ca 80%. Heat nearly to bp on steam or H_2O bath 30 min, stirring frequently. (Samples may be stored until needed for analysis.)

References: Botan. Gaz. **73**, 44(1922). Proc. Am. Soc. Hort. Sci. 1927, p. 191. JAOAC **13**, 224(1930); **16**, 71(1933); **19**, 70(1936).

For dried materials, grind samples finely, and mix well. Weigh sample into beaker, and continue as above, beginning '' ... cover with 80% alcohol, ... ''

(**b**) *Applicable when starch is not to be determined.*—Prepare fresh sample as in **922.02(b)**, but boil on steam bath 1 h. Decant solution into volumetric flask, comminute solids in high-speed blender with 80% alcohol. Boil blended material on steam bath 0.5 h, cool, transfer to volumetric flask, dilute to mark with 80% alcohol at room temperature, filter, and take aliquot for analysis.

Grind dry material to pass No. 20 sieve or finer, transfer weighed sample to volumetric flask, and add 80% alcohol and enough $CaCO_3$ to neutralize any acidity. Boil 1 h on steam bath, cool, adjust volume at room temperature with 80% alcohol, filter, and take aliquot for analysis.

B. Clarification with Lead (1)

Place aliquot alcohol extract in beaker on steam bath and evaporate off alcohol. Avoid evaporation to dryness by adding H_2O if necessary. When odor of alcohol disappears, add ca 100 mL H_2O and heat to 80° to soften gummy precipitates and break up insoluble masses. Cool to room temperature and proceed as in (**a**) or (**b**):

(**a**) Transfer solution to volumetric flask, rinse beaker thoroughly with H_2O, and add rinsings to flask. Add enough *saturated neutral $Pb(CH_3COO)_2$ solution* to produce flocculent precipitate, shake thoroughly, and let stand 15 min. Test supernate with few drops of the $Pb(CH_3COO)_2$ solution. If more precipitate forms, shake and let stand again; if no further precipitate forms, dilute to volume with H_2O, mix thoroughly, and filter through dry paper. Add enough solid sodium oxalate to filtrate to precipitate all the Pb, and refilter through dry paper. Test filtrate for presence of Pb with little solid sodium oxalate.

(**b**) Add twice minimum amount of saturated neutral $Pb(CH_3COO)_2$ solution required to cause complete precipitation, as found by testing portion of supernate with few drops dilute sodium oxalate solution. Let mixture stand only few minutes; then filter into beaker containing estimated excess of sodium oxalate crystals. Let Pb precipitate drain on filter and wash with cold H_2O until filtrate no longer gives precipitate in oxalate solution. Assure excess of oxalate by testing with 1 drop $Pb(CH_3COO)_2$. Filter and wash precipitated lead oxalate, catching filtrate and washings in volumetric flask. Dilute to volume with H_2O and mix.

C. Clarification with Ion-Exchange Resins (2)

Place aliquot alcohol extract, **931.02A**, in beaker and heat on steam bath to evaporate alcohol. Avoid evaporation to dryness by adding H_2O. When odor of alcohol disappears, add ca 15–25 mL H_2O and heat to 80° to soften gummy precipitates and break up insoluble masses. Cool to room temperature. Prepare thin mat of Celite on filter paper in buchner or on fritted glass filter and wash until H_2O comes through clear. Filter sample through Celite mat, wash mat with H_2O, dilute filtrate and washings to appropriate volume in volumetric flask, and mix well.

Place 50.0 mL aliquot in 250 mL Erlenmeyer; add 2 g *Amberlite IR-120(H)* analytical grade cation (replaced by REXYN 101[H] resin, Fisher Scientific Co.) and 3 g *Duolite A-4(OH)* anion ion exchange resins. Let stand 2 h with occasional swirling. Take 5 mL aliquot deionized solution and determine reducing sugars as glucose as in **959.11B** (*see* 33.29).

References: (1) JAOAC **14,** 73, 225(1931); **15,** 71(1932). (2) JAOAC **36,** 402(1953).

33.60 935.39—Baked Products
Final Action

(Other than bread; not containing fruit)

G. Sugars—Final Action 1976
See **975.14** (*see* 33.65).

33.61 945.29—Sugars (Total Reducing) in Brewing Sugars and Sirups
Final Action

A. Munson-Walker General Method

Transfer 50 mL "10% solution," **945.22A(a)**, to 250 mL volumetric flask. Clarify, if necessary, with alumina cream or neutral Pb(OAc)$_2$ solution only (never basic Pb[OAc]$_2$), and dilute to volume at 20° with H$_2$O. Mix thoroughly and either centrifuge or filter until clear. If Pb(OAc)$_2$ solution was used for clarification, remove excess Pb with dry Na$_2$C$_2$O$_4$. Filter, and determine reducing sugars on 10 mL aliquot as in **906.03B** (*see* 33.13); **929.09A** (*see* 33.15); **935.62B** (*see* 33.27); or **935.64B** (*see* 33.49). Calculate results in terms of invert sugar for invert sirups and sugars; glucose for corn sugars and sirups; and maltose for malt sirups. If character of sample is in doubt, express reducing sugars as glucose.

$$\% \text{ Reducing sugar, as-is} = 25M/W$$

where *M* is mg sugar from appropriate column of **940.39**, *Official Methods of Analysis* (1990) 15th Ed., and *W* is g sample used to prepare "10% solution."

945.22 (Extract of Brewing Sugars and Sirups)
A. Extract
(a) *Preparation of "10% solution."*—Accurately weigh ca 50 g well mixed representative sample, dissolve in warm H$_2$O, transfer quantitatively to 500 mL volumetric flask, and dilute to volume at 20°. Mix thoroughly.

B. Lane-Eynon General Volumetric Method

Dilute 50 mL solution, clarified as in **945.29A**, to 100 mL and proceed as in **923.09, 935.62,** or **935.64,** referring titer to **930.44** (*see* 33.14), or **930.45** (*see* 33.14). Calculate results as in **945.29A.**

C. Glucose

To 5 mL aliquot of solution prepared as in **945.29A**, add 15 mL H_2O and proceed as in **938.02C** (*see* 33.24), or **936.06C** (*see* 33.22).

Reference: ASBC: Adjunct Materials; Sugars and Syrups 14.
CAS-50-99-7 (glucose)

33.62   945.66—Total Reducing Sugars
First Action

(**a**) *Lane-Eynon General Volumetric Method.*—See **923.09** (*see* 33.14). Use glucose as standard.
(**b**) *Munson-Walker General Method.*—See **906.03B** (*see* 33.13). Prepare dilution containing ca 1% reducing sugar.

33.63   950.50—Sugars (Reducing) in Nuts and Nut Products
Munson-Walker Method
Final Action

Prepare sample as in 1st and 2nd paragraphs of **22.049**, *Official Methods of Analysis* (1965) 10th Ed. Proceed as in **906.03B** (*see* 33.13), using 25 mL aliquot (representing 2 g sample). Express results as glucose or invert sugar.

References: JAOAC **33,** 753(1950); **34,** 357(1951).

33.64   968.28—Total Sugars in Molasses as Invert Sugar
Lane-Eynon Constant Volume Volumetric Method
First Action 1968
Final Action 1969

A. Apparatus

(**a**) *Electric heater.*—With white top and continuous temperature control over range 110–600°; attaining maximum temperature within 5 min.
(**b**) *Buret.*—50 mL, graduated in 0.1 mL, with stopcock or pinchcock and offset delivery tube.

B. Reagents

(**a**) *Soxhlet modification of Fehling solution.*—Prepare as in **923.09A(a)** and (**b**) (*see* 33.14).
(**b**) *Invert sugar standard solutions.*—(*1*) *Stock solution.*—10 mg/mL. Prepare as in **923.09A(c)**, using 5 mL HCl (specific gravity 1.18 at 20/4°) and letting stand 3 days at room temperature (20–25°). (*2*)

Working solution.—5 mg/mL. Pipet 100 mL stock solution into 200 mL volumetric flask, add few drops phenolphthalein, and neutralize with 20% NaOH. Dilute to volume and mix well. Prepare fresh daily.

C. Preparation of Sample Solution

(**a**) *Dried products containing not less than 30% total sugars.*—Weigh 8.00 g sample and transfer with 250 mL H_2O, preheated to 60 ± 5°, into 500 mL volumetric flask. Mechanically shake flask 30 min. Let stand additional 30 min and cool to 20°. Dilute to volume with H_2O. Mix well and filter, using filter aid (Hyflo Super-Cel, or equivalent) and loose texture paper (Whatman No. 1, or equivalent). Discard first 25 mL filtrate. Cover funnel during filtration with watch glass to prevent evaporation.

(**b**) *Liquids.*—Weigh 8.00 g sample and transfer with H_2O to 500 mL volumetric flask. Dissolve, and dilute to volume with H_2O. Proceed as in (**a**), beginning "Mix well ... "

D. Standardization of Soxhlet Reagent

Fill 50 mL buret with working standard solution containing 5 mg invert sugar/mL.

Accurately pipet 10 mL each Soxhlet solution, (**a**) and (**b**), into 300 mL erlenmeyer, mix, and add 30 mL H_2O. Add from buret almost all standard working solution (ca 19 mL) necessary to reduce the Cu. Add few boiling chips. Place cold mixture on heater, regulate heat so that boiling will begin in ca 3 min, and maintain at moderate boil exactly 2 min, reducing heat, if necessary, to prevent bumping. Without removing flask from heater, add ca 4 drops *1% aqueous methylene blue solution* and complete titration within total boiling time of ca 3 min by dropwise addition of working standard solution at intervals of ca 10 s until boiling mixture resumes bright orange appearance which it had before indicator was added. Maintain continuous evolution of steam to prevent reoxidation by air. Repeat standardization several times. Factor *F* is average number milliliters standard sugar solution required to completely reduce 20 mL Soxhlet solution. Use average of ≥3 titrations.

E. Inversion with Acid at Room Temperature

Pipet 100 mL filtrate, **968.28C**, into 200 mL volumetric flask, and add 5 mL HCl (specific gravity 1.18 at 20/4°). Let stand 24 h at 20–25° or 10 h at >25°. Add few drops phenolphthalein and neutralize with 20% NaOH solution. Add few drops 0.5*N* HCl until red disappears. Dilute to volume with H_2O and mix well.

F. Approximate Titration of Sample

Determine approximate sugar content of sample as follows: Accurately pipet 10 mL each Soxhlet solution, (**a**) and (**b**), into 300 mL erlenmeyer, mix, and add 10 mL aliquot inverted sample solution. Add 40 mL H_2O so that volume H_2O plus volume sample solution is 50 mL, as in **968.28D**. Mix without heating by swirling. Add few boiling chips. Place flask on heater, regulating heat so that boiling begins in ca 3 min. After liquid boils 10–15 s, observe change in color of solution. If blue color persists, add working standard sugar solution 0.5–1.0 mL at time, with few s actual boiling after each addition until unsafe to add more without risk of passing end point. Add 3–4 drops methylene blue solution and continue adding sugar solution, ca 1 mL at time, at intervals of ca 10 s, until indicator is completely decolorized. Calculate approximate % invert sugar in sample.

G. Titration of Sample

Pipet 10 mL each of Soxhlet solution, (**a**) and (**b**), into 300 mL erlenmeyer, mix, and add aliquot inverted sample solution as indicated in Table **968.28**. Add mL H_2O specified in table so that volume H_2O plus volume sample solution is 50 mL, as in **968.28D**, and mix without heating by swirling. Add few boiling chips. Place flask on heater, regulate heat so that boiling begins in ca 3 min, and during boiling, rapidly add working standard invert sugar solution from buret, so that 0.5–1.0 mL is required to complete titration. Continue as in **968.28D**, beginning ''Without removing flask ... '' Maintain moderate boiling.

$$\% \text{ Sugar as invert} = (F - M) \times I \times 100/W$$

where F is Cu factor (mL standard sugar solution required to reduce 20 mL mixed Soxhlet reagent); M is mL standard sugar solution used in back-titration of sample; I is g invert sugar in 1 mL working standard sugar solution; and W is g sample in aliquot used. Report total sugars, expressed as invert.

Table 968.28.—Aliquots for Cane Sirups and Molasses

| mL H$_2$O | mL Aliquot | g Sample in Aliquot | Total Sugar as Invert, % | |
			Max.	Min.
40	10	0.08		73.00
35	15	0.12	82.00	58.00
30	20	0.16	61.00	41.00
25	25	0.20	49.00	35.00
20	30	0.24	41.00	29.00

References: JAOAC **51**, 755(1968); **52**, 564(1969); **53**, 347(1970).
CAS-8013-17-0 (invert sugar)
CAS-57-50-1 (sucrose)

33.65   975.14—Sugars in Bread
Final Action

(a) *Reducing sugars.*—Prepare sample as in **925.05** (*see* 33.40), paragraphs 1 and 2. Proceed as in **906.03B** (*see* 33.13), using 25 mL aliquot (representing 2 g sample). Express results as glucose or invert sugar.
(b) *Sucrose.*—Proceed as in **925.05**.

33.66   939.03—Sugars (Reducing and Nonreducing) in Flour
Titrimetric Method
Final Action

A. Reagents

(a) *Acetate buffer solution.*—Dilute 3 mL CH$_3$COOH, 4.1 g anhydrous NaOAc, and 4.5 mL H$_2$SO$_4$ to 1 L with H$_2$O.

(**b**) *Sodium tungstate solution.*—12%. Dilute 12.0 g $Na_2WO_4 \cdot 2H_2O$ to 100 mL with H_2O.

(**c**) *Alkaline ferricyanide solution.*—0.1N. 33.0 g pure dry $K_3Fe(CN)_6$ and 44.0 g Na_2CO_3/L.

(**d**) *Acetic acid-salts solution.*—Dilute 200 mL CH_3COOH, 70 g KCl, and 40 g $ZnSO_4 \cdot 7H_2O$ to 1 L with H_2O.

(**e**) *Soluble starch-potassium iodide solution.*—Add 2 g soluble starch to small amount cold H_2O and pour slowly into boiling H_2O with constant stirring. Cool thoroughly (or resulting mixture will be dark colored), add 50 g KI, and dilute to 100 mL with H_2O. Add 1 drop NaOH solution (1 + 1). Use 1 mL.

(**f**) *Thiosulfate standard solution.*—0.1N. 24.82 g $Na_2S_2O_3 \cdot 5H_2O$ and 3.8 g $Na_2B_4O_7 \cdot 10H_2O$/L. Make blank determination with each day's series of sugar determinations to guard against changes in the $K_3Fe(CN)_6$ solution and correct for any reducing impurities in reagents as follows:

Combine 5 mL alcohol, 50.0 mL acetate buffer solution, and 2 mL Na tungstate solution. To 5 mL of this mixture (used in place of 5 mL flour extract) add 10.0 mL $K_3Fe(CN)_6$ solution and proceed as in **939.03C(a)**. (10.0 mL $Na_2S_2O_3$ solution should discharge the blue starch-I color.) If titration falls within 10 ± 0.05 mL do not discard reagents but correct in subsequent sugar calculations by using $Na_2S_2O_3$ equivalent of 10 mL $K_3Fe(CN)_6$ solution (*i.e.*, mL $Na_2S_2O_3$ solution required in above titration) instead of 10.0 as basis for subtraction.

B. Preparation of Extract

Place 5.675 g flour in 100 or 125 mL erlenmeyer. Tip flask so that all flour is at one side; then wet flour with 5 mL alcohol. Tip flask so that wet flour is at upper side and add 50.0 mL acetate buffer solution, keeping solution from coming in contact with flour until all is added to flask. Then shake flask to bring flour into suspension. Immediately add 2 mL Na tungstate solution and again mix thoroughly. Filter at once (Whatman No. 4, or equivalent), discarding first 8–10 drops filtrate.

C. Determination

(**a**) *Reducing sugars.*—Pipet 5 mL flour extract into ca 75 mL test tube (Pyrex 25 × 200 mm). Add exactly 10 mL $K_3Fe(CN)_6$ solution to test tube, mix, and immerse in vigorously boiling H_2O bath so that liquid in tube is 3–4 cm below surface of boiling H_2O.

After exactly 20 min in boiling H_2O bath, cool tube under running H_2O, and pour at once into 100 or 125 mL erlenmeyer. Rinse test tube with 25 mL CH_3COOH-salts solution, (**d**), add to erlenmeyer, and mix thoroughly. Then add 1 mL starch-KI solution. Titrate with 0.1N $Na_2S_2O_3$ solution until blue completely disappears (10 mL micro buret recommended). Subtract mL 0.1N $Na_2S_2O_3$ used in titration from 10.00. In case of slight blank in $K_3Fe(CN)_6$-$Na_2S_2O_3$ titration, correct by subtracting from $Na_2S_2O_3$ equivalent of $K_3Fe(CN)_6$ solution. This difference represents definite amount of reducing sugar/10 g flour, calculated as maltose from Table **939.03**.

Table 939.03. 0.1N Ferricyanide Maltose-Sucrose Conversion Table[a]

0.1N Ferricyanide Reduced, mL	Maltose/10 g Flour, mg	Sucrose/10 g Flour, mg	0.1N Ferricyanide Reduced, mL	Maltose/10 g Flour, mg	Sucrose/10 g Flour, mg
0.10	5	5	4.50	237	214
0.20	10	10	4.60	244	218
0.30	15	15	4.70	251	223
0.40	20	19	4.80	257	228
0.50	25	24	4.90	264	233

Table 939.03.—0.1N Ferricyanide Maltose-Sucrose Conversion Table[a]

0.1N Ferricyanide Reduced, mL	Maltose/10 g Flour, mg	Sucrose/10 g Flour, mg	0.1N Ferricyanide Reduced, mL	Maltose/10 g Flour, mg	Sucrose/10 g Flour, mg
0.60	31	29	5.00	270	238
0.70	36	34	5.10	276	242
0.80	41	38	5.20	282	247
0.90	46	43	5.30	288	251
1.00	51	48	5.40	295	256
1.10	56	52	5.50	302	261
1.20	60	57	5.60	308	266
1.30	65	62	5.70	315	270
1.40	71	67	5.80	322	275
1.50	76	71	5.90	328	280
1.60	80	76	6.00	334	285
1.70	85	81	6.10	341	290
1.80	90	86	6.20	347	294
1.90	96	91	6.30	353	299
2.00	101	95	6.40	360	304
2.10	106	100	6.50	367	309
2.20	111	104	6.60	373	313
2.30	116	109	6.70	379	318
2.40	121	114	6.80	385	323
2.50	126	119	6.90	392	328
2.60	130	123	7.00	398	333
2.70	135	128	7.10	406	337
2.80	140	133	7.20	412	342
2.90	145	138	7.30	418	347
3.00	151	143	7.40	425	352
3.10	156	148	7.50	431	357
3.20	161	152	7.60	438	362
3.30	166	157	7.70	445	367
3.40	171	161	7.80	451	372
3.50	176	166	7.90	458	377
3.60	182	171	8.00	465	382
3.70	188	176	8.10	472	387
3.80	195	181	8.20	478	392
3.90	201	186	8.30	485	397
4.00	207	190	8.40	492	402
4.10	213	195	8.50	499	407
4.20	218	200	8.60	505	-
4.30	225	204	8.70	512	-
4.40	231	209	8.80	519	-

[a]These values are arbitrarily given for 10 g flour altho detn is made on only 0.5 g flour.

(b) *Nonreducing sugars.*—Pipet 5 mL flour extract into 20 cm test tube and immerse in vigorously boiling H_2O bath. After boiling 15 min, cool under running H_2O and add exactly 10 mL $K_3Fe(CN)_6$ solution.

Proceed as in (**a**). $K_3Fe(CN)_6$ reduced after hydrolysis $-$ $K_3Fe(CN)_6$ reduced by maltose in flour = nonreducing sugars calculated as sucrose and determined from Table **939.03**.

References: JAOAC **22**, 535(1939). Cereal Chem. **14**, 603(1937).
CAS-69-79-4 (maltose)
CAS-57-50-1 (sucrose)

33.67
896.01—Lactose in Milk
Polarimetric Method
Final Action

A. Reagents

(**a**) *Acid-mercuric nitrate solution.*—Dissolve Hg in twice its weight HNO_3 and dilute with 5 volumes H_2O.
Or—
(**b**) *Mercuric iodide solution.*—Dissolve 33.2 g KI and 13.5 g $HgCl_2$ in 200 mL CH_3COOH and 640 mL H_2O.

B. Determination

Weigh 65.8 g (2 normal wt) milk into each of 2 volumetric flasks, 100 and 200 mL, respectively. To each flask add 20 mL acid-$Hg(NO_3)_2$ solution or 30 mL HgI_2 solution. To 100 mL flask add *5% phosphotungstic acid solution* to mark, and to the 200 mL flask add 15 mL 5% phosphotungstic acid solution and dilute to mark with H_2O. Shake both flasks frequently during 15 min, filter through dry filter, and polarize. (It is preferable to read solution from 200 mL flask in 400 mm tube to reduce error of reading; solution from 100 mL flask may be read in 200 mm tube.) Calculate % lactose in sample as follows: (1) Subtract reading of solution from 200 mL flask (using 400 mm tube) from reading of solution from 100 mL flask (using 200 mm tube); (2) multiply difference by 2; (3) subtract result from reading of solution from 100 mL flask; (4) divide result by 2.

References: Analyst **21**, 182(1896). JAOAC **25**, 603(1942); **27**, 232(1944).
CAS-63-42-3 (lactose)

33.68   896.02—Sucrose in Sugars and Sirups
Double Dilution Method
Final Action 1970

(Applicable to substances in which volume of combined insoluble matter and precipitate from clarifying agents is >1 mL from 26 g)

Weigh 13 g sample and dilute to 100 mL, using appropriate clarifier (basic Pb(OAc)$_2$ for dark-colored confectionery or molasses, and alumina cream for light-colored confectionery). Also weigh 26 g sample and dilute this second solution with clarifier to 100 mL. Filter both solutions, and obtain direct polariscopic readings. Invert each solution as in **925.47B(b)** or (**c**) or **925.48(b)** or (**c**) and obtain respectively invert readings.

    True direct polarization of sample = 4 times direct polarization of diluted solution minus direct polarization of undiluted solution. True invert polarization = 4 times invert polarization of diluted solution minus invert polarization of undiluted solution. Calculate sucrose from true polarizations thus obtained, using formula in **925.47B(b)** (*see* 33.70), or **925.48(b)** or (**c**) (*see* 33.72), corresponding to method of inversion used.

Reference: Analyst **21**, 182(1896).

33.69   920.115—Sweetened Condensed Milk
Final Action

A. Sampling—Final Action 1974
    See **968.12** (*see* Chapter 18.17), and **970.27** (*see* Chapter 18.17).

B. Preparation of Sample—Procedure
    (**a**) Temper unopened can in H$_2$O bath at 30–35° until warm. Open, scrape out all milk adhering to interior of can, transfer to dish large enough to permit stirring thoroughly, and mix until whole mass is homogeneous.

    (**b**) Weigh 100 g thoroughly mixed sample into 500 mL volumetric flask, dilute to volume with H$_2$O, and mix thoroughly. If sample will not emulsify uniformly, weigh out separate portion of (**a**) for each determination.

C. Lactic Acid
    See **937.05** [*see Official Methods of Analysis* (1990) 15th Ed.].

D. Total Solids
    Transfer 10 mL prepared solution, **920.115B(b)**, to weighed flat-bottom dish, ≥5 cm diameter, containing 15–20 g previously dried sand or asbestos fiber. Heat on steam bath 30 min and then in vacuum oven at 100° to constant weight. Cool in desiccator and weigh quickly to avoid absorption of H$_2$O. Correct result for dilution.

E. Ash

Evaporate 10 mL prepared solution, **920.115B(b)**, to dryness on H_2O bath and ignite residue as in **900.02A** or **B** (*see* Chapter 10.1). Correct result for dilution.

IDF-ISO-AOAC Method

F. Fat—Roese-Gottlieb Method

Accurately weigh 2–2.5 g prepared sample, **920.115B(a)**, into fat-extraction flask or tube; dilute with H_2O to ca 10.5 mL, and proceed as in **945.48G** (*see* Chapter 18.14).

References: JAOAC **28,** 207(1945); **52,** 239(1969).

G. Protein

Determine N as in **920.105** (*see* Chapter 28.18), using 10 mL prepared solution, **920.115B(b)**, and correct result for dilution.

$$\% \text{ N} \times 6.38 = \% \text{ total "protein."}$$

H. Lactose

Dilute 100 mL prepared solution, **920.115B(b)**, in 250 mL volumetric flask to ca 200 mL; add 6 mL $CuSO_4$ solution, **923.09A(a)** (*see* 33.14), and alkali solution of concentration and in proportion as in **930.28** (*see* 33.84). Dilute to volume and mix thoroughly. Filter through dry filter and determine lactose as in **906.03B** (*see* 33.13). Correct result for dilution.

Sucrose
IDF-ISO-AOAC Method

I. Reagent

(*Caution*: *See Appendix* for safety notes on mercury salts and toxic dusts.)
Mercuric nitrate solution.—To 220 g yellow HgO, add 300–400 mL H_2O and enough (but with minimum excess) HNO_3 to form clear solution (ca 140 mL), being careful to use least possible excess of acid. Dilute to 800–900 mL and slowly add 10% NaOH solution with constant shaking until slight permanent precipitate forms. Dilute to 1 L and filter. As solution tends to become acid with age owing to deposition of basic Hg salts, add dilute alkali occasionally until slight permanent precipitate forms, and refilter.

J. Determination

Place 50 mL prepared solution, **920.115B(b)**, in 100 mL volumetric flask; add 25 mL H_2O, mix, add 5 mL $Hg(NO_3)_2$ solution, and shake thoroughly. Without delay and with constant shaking, neutralize to litmus paper with $0.5N$ NaOH, but avoid alkaline reaction (12–13 mL). Dilute to 100 mL with H_2O, mix thoroughly, and filter through dry paper. Polarize filtrate in 200 mm tube; then invert at room temperature as in **925.48(c)** (*see* 33.72), and polarize inverted solution. Correct both readings for volume occupied by protein, **920.115G**, and fat, **920.115F**; 1 g protein occupies 0.8 mL and 1 g fat, 1.075 mL. Calculate % sucrose by following formula, using corrected direct and invert readings obtained above:

$$S = [100(a - b)/(142.35 - (t/2))] \times (26/W)$$

where S = % sucrose in sample; a = corrected direct polarization; b = corrected invert polarization; t = temperature of solution polarized; and W = weight sample taken (10 g).

CAS-57-50-1 (sucrose)

33.70   925.47—Sucrose in Sugars and Sirups
Polarimetric Method
Before and After Inversion with Invertase
Final Action 1970

(In the absence of raffinose)

A. Reagent

Invertase solution.—Commercial invertase preparations are available (without melibiase) (Wallerstein Co.). If desired to prepare solution in laboratory, see **31.024** (*Official Methods of Analysis* [1980] 13th Ed.).

B. Determination

(**a**) *Direct reading.*—Dissolve double normal weight of sample (52 g), or fraction thereof, in H_2O in 200 mL volumetric flask; add necessary clarifying agent, **925.46B(a)**, (**b**), or (**d**) (*see* 33.71), avoiding excess; shake, dilute to volume with H_2O, mix well, and filter, keeping funnel covered with watch glass. Reject first 25 mL filtrate.

If Pb clarifying agent was used, remove excess Pb from solution when enough filtrate collects by adding anhydrous Na_2CO_3, little at time, avoiding excess; mix well and refilter, rejecting first 25 mL filtrate. (Instead of weighing 52 g into 200 mL flask, two 26 g portions may be diluted to 100 mL each, and treated exactly as described. Depending on color of product, multiples or fractions of normal weight may be used, and results calculated to basis of 26 g/100 mL.)

Pipet one 50 mL portion Pb-free filtrate into 100 mL volumetric flask, dilute to volume with H_2O, mix well, and polarize in 200 mm tube. Result, multiplied by 2, is direct reading (*P* of formula given below) or polarization before inversion. (If 400 mm tube is used, reading equals *P*.) If there is possibility of mutarotation, proceed as in **925.46D**.

(**b**) *Invert reading.*—First determine volume of CH_3COOH necessary to make 50 mL of the Pb-free filtrate distinctly acid to methyl red; then to another 50 mL Pb-free solution in 100 mL volumetric flask add requisite volume of acid and 5 mL invertase solution, fill flask with H_2O nearly to 100 mL, and let stand overnight (preferably at $\geq 20°$).

Cool, and dilute to 100 mL at 20°. Mix well and polarize at 20° in 200 mm tube. If in doubt as to completion of hydrolysis, let portion of solution remain several h and again polarize. If there is no change from previous reading, inversion is complete. Carefully note reading and temperature of solution. If it is necessary to work at temperature other than 20°, which is permissible within narrow limits, complete volumes and make both direct and invert readings at same temperature. Correct polarization for optical activity of invertase solution and multiply by 2. Calculate % sucrose, *S*, by following formula:

$$ S = \frac{100\ (P - I)}{132.1 - 0.0833(13 - m) - 0.53(t - 20)} $$

where *P* = direct reading, normal solution; *I* = invert reading, normal solution; *t* = temperature at which readings are made; and *m* = g total solids from original sample in 100 mL inverted solution. To obtain *m* for liquids, determine total solids in original sample as % by weight, as in **932.14C** [*see Official Methods of Analysis* (1990) 15th Ed.], and multiply this figure by weight original sample in 100 mL invert solution.

(c) *For rapid inversion at 55–60°.*—If more rapid inversion is desired, proceed as follows: Prepare sample as in (a) and to 50 mL Pb-free filtrate in 100 mL volumetric flask add enough CH_3COOH to render solution distinctly acid to methyl red, **925.47A** (*see* 33.70). Determine volume of CH_3COOH required before pipetting 50 mL portion as in (b). Add 10 mL invertase solution, mix thoroughly, place flask in H_2O bath at 55–60°, and let stand at that temperature 15 min, shaking occasionally.

Cool, add Na_2CO_3 until distinctly alkaline to litmus paper, dilute to 100 mL at 20°, mix well, and determine polarization at 20° in 200 mm tube. Let solution remain in tube 10 min and again determine polarization. If there is no change from previous reading, mutarotation is complete. Carefully note reading and temperature of solution. Correct polarization for optical activity of invertase solution and multiply by 2. Calculate % sucrose by formula given in (b).

If solution has been made so alkaline as to cause destruction of sugar, polarization, if negative, will in general decrease, since decomposition of fructose ordinarily is more rapid than that of other sugars present. If solution has not been made alkaline enough to complete mutarotation quickly, polarization, if negative, will in general increase. As analyst gains experience he may omit polarization after 10 min if he has satisfied himself that he is adding enough Na_2CO_3 to complete mutarotation at once without causing any destruction of sugar during period intervening before polarization.

Reference: JAOAC **8**, 256, 258(1925).
CAS-57-50-1 (sucrose)

33.71   925.46—Sucrose in Sugars and Sirups
Polarimetric Methods

A. General Procedure—Final Action 1970

(Rules of International Commission for Uniform Methods of Sugar Analysis [ICUMSA])

(a) *Standardization of saccharimeter scale.*—Saccharimeter scale must be graduated in conformity with International Sugar Scale adopted by ICUMSA. Rotations on this scale are designated as degrees sugar (°S).

Basis of calibration of 100° point on International Sugar Scale is polarization of normal solution of pure sucrose (26.000 g/100 mL) at 20° in 200 mm tube, using white light and dichromate filter defined by Commission, (b). This solution, polarized at 20°, must give saccharimeter reading of exactly 100°S. Temperature of sugar solution during polarization must be kept constant at 20°.

Following rotations hold for normal quartz plate of International Sugar Scale: Normal Quartz Plate = 100°S = 40.690° ± 0.002° (λ = 5461 Å) at 20°
$$1° (\lambda = 5461 A) = 2.4576°S$$
Normal Quartz Plate = 100°S = 34.620° ± 0.002° (λ = 5892.5 Å) at 20°
$$1° (\lambda = 5892.5 Å) = 2.8885°S$$

For existing saccharimeters graduated on Herzfeld-Schönrock scale, either change saccharimeter scale or use weight w of 26.026 g in 100 mL.

(b) *Directions for raw sugars.*—In general, make all polarizations at 20°. For countries where mean temperature is >20°, saccharimeters may be adjusted at 30° or any other suitable temperature, under conditions specified above, provided sugar solution is diluted to final volume and polarized at this same temperature.

In determining polarization of substances containing sugar, use only half-shade instruments, either single- or double-wedge, and either 200 or 400 mm instruments. During observation, keep apparatus in fixed position and so far removed from source of light that polarizing nicol is not warmed. As sources of light, use lamps that give strong white illumination or Na lamp. Whenever there is any irregularity in source of light, place thin ground-glass plate between source of light and polariscope so as to render illumination uniform.

Before and after each set of observations, determine correct adjustment of saccharimeter, using standardized quartz plates; use calibrated weights, polarization flasks, and observation tubes and cover glasses. (Scratched or stained cover glasses must not be used.) Make several readings and take mean thereof but do not reject any reading.

Quartz plates are standardized to second decimal place. Instrument and plate must be at same temperature (preferably 20°). Different points of scale, preferably 20°, 50°, 80°, and 100°S, should be tested against the plates.

In determining polarization, use whole normal weight (26 ± 0.002 g) for 100 mL or multiple for any corresponding volume. Bring solution exactly to mark at proper temperature and after wiping out neck of flask with filter paper, add minimum amount of *dry basic Pb(OAc)$_2$*, **925.46B(c)**, shake to dissolve, and pour all clarified sugar solution on rapid, air-dry filter. Cover funnel at start of filtration. Reject first 25 mL filtrate and use remainder (must be perfectly clear) for polarization. In no case return whole solution or any part to filter. If filtrate is cloudy after 25 mL has been rejected, begin new determination. Polarize in 200 mm tube. If, after all means have been used to effect proper decolorization, solution is too dark to read, use 100 mm tube and multiply reading by 2.

Other permissible clarifying and decolorizing agents are alumina cream, **925.46B(b)**, or concentrated alum solution. Do not use boneblack or decolorizing powders.

Whenever white light is used, it must be filtered through solution of $K_2Cr_2O_7$ of such concentration that % $K_2Cr_2O_7$ × length of column of solution in cm = 9. Double this concentration in polarizing carbohydrate materials of high rotation dispersion, such as commercial glucose, etc.

(c) *Normal weights and conversion factors of different saccharimeter scales.—(1) Herzfeld-Schönrock scale.*—Normal weight = 26.026 g/100 mL solution. 1° = 0.34657° Angular Rotation D.*

(2) *International sugar scale.*—Normal weight = 26.000 g/100 mL solution. 1° = 0.34620° Angular Rotation D.*

(3) *French sugar scale.*—Normal weight = 16.269 g/100 mL solution. 1° = 0.21667° Angular Rotation D.*

*D = Na light of 589.2 nm

References: Z. Ver. Deut. Zucker-Ind. **50,** (N.F. 37), 357(1900); **63,** (N.F. 50), 25(1913). J. Ind. Eng. Chem. **5,** 167(1913). JAOAC **18,** 162(1935). NIST Circular C **440,** 1942, pp. 768, 774. Int. Sugar J. **35,** 19(1933); **39,** 32S(1937).

CAS-57-50-1 (sucrose)

B. Preparation and Use of Clarifying Reagents

—Final Action 1970

(*Caution: See Appendix* for safety notes on toxic dusts.)

(a) *Basic lead acetate solution.*—Activate litharge by heating 2.5–3 h at 650–670° in furnace (cooled product should be lemon color). Boil 430 g neutral Pb(OAc)$_2$·3H$_2$O, 130 g freshly activated litharge, and 1 L H$_2$O 30 min. Let mixture cool and settle; then dilute supernate to specific gravity of 1.25 with recently boiled H$_2$O. (Solid basic Pb(OAc)$_2$ may be substituted for the normal salt and litharge in preparation of solution. Because of error caused by volume of precipitate, this reagent is not recommended for clarifying products of low purity.)

(**b**) *Alumina cream.*—Prepare cold saturated solution of alum in H_2O. Add NH_4OH with constant stirring until solution is alkaline to litmus, let precipitate settle, and wash by decantation with H_2O until wash H_2O gives only slight test for sulfates with $BaCl_2$ solution. Pour off excess H_2O and store residual cream in glass-stoppered bottle. (Alumina cream is suitable for clarifying light-colored sugar products or as adjunct to other agents when sugars are determined by polariscopic or reducing sugar methods.)

(**c**) *Dry basic lead acetate ACS.*—$3Pb(OAc)_2 \cdot 2PbO$. Of this salt, ca 0.3 g = 1 mL basic $Pb(OAc)_2$ solution, (**a**). In making clarification, add small amount of dry salt to sugar solution after diluting to volume, and shake; then add more salt and shake again, repeating addition until precipitation is complete, but avoiding any excess. When molasses or any other substance producing heavy precipitate is being clarified, add some dry, coarse sand to break up pellets of basic $Pb(OAc)_2$ and precipitate. (Unless in excess, dry basic $Pb(OAc)_2$ does not cause volume error.)

(**d**) *Neutral lead acetate solution.*—Prepare saturated solution of neutral $Pb(OAc)_2$ and add to sugar solution before diluting to volume. (This reagent may be used for clarifying light-colored sugar products when sugars are determined by polariscopic methods, and its use is imperative when reducing sugars are determined in solution used for polarization.)

To remove excess Pb used in clarification, add anhydrous K or Na oxalate to clarified filtrate in small amounts until test for Pb in filtrate is negative; then refilter.

References: JAOAC **16**, 78(1933); **17**, 74(1934).

C. Temperature Corrections for Polarization of Sugars
.—First Action 1970

(**a**) *Refined sugars.*—Polarizations of sugars testing ≥ 99, when made at temperature other than 20°, may be calculated to polarizations at 20° by following formula:

$$P_{20} = p_t[1 + 0.0003 (t - 20)]$$

where p_t = polarization at temperature read, t. (May be applied to beet sugar and raw cane sugars polarizing $\geq 96°S$ without appreciable error.)

(**b**) *Raw sugars.*—Polarization of raw cane sugars $<96°S$ when made at temperatures other than 20°, may be calculated to polarizations at 20° by following formula:

$$P_{20} = p_t + 0.0015 (p_t - 80) (t - 20)$$

where p_t and t are same as in (**a**).

When % fructose in the sugar is known (in case of honeys and sugar cane products = ca 1/2 reducing sugars), use following formula:

$$P_{20} = p_t + 0.0003S (t - 20) - 0.00812F (t - 20)$$

where p_t *and* t are same as in (**a**); S = % sucrose; and F = % fructose.

These formulas give results agreeing closely with polarizations obtained at 20° if sugar is of average normal composition.

Reference: Browne and Zerban, "Sugar Analysis," 1941, p. 395.

D. Mutarotation—Procedure

Products, such as honey and commercial glucose, that contain glucose or other reducing sugars in crystalline form or in solution at high density may show mutarotation under conditions prevailing during analysis. Only constant rotation should be used in polarimetric methods. To obtain this, let solution prepared for polarization stand overnight before making reading. If it is desired to make reading immediately, heat neutral solution (pH ca 7.0) to bp or add few drops NH_4OH, before diluting to volume;

or, if solution has been made to volume, add dry Na_2CO_3 until just distinctly alkaline to litmus paper. (Do not let slightly alkaline solutions stand at such high temperatures or for such lengths of time as to cause destruction of fructose.) Determine completion of mutarotation by making readings at 15–30 min intervals until constant.

33.72   925.48—Sucrose in Sugars and Sirups
Polarimetric Method Before and After Inversion with Hydrochloric Acid
Final Action 1970

(a) *Direct reading.*—Prepare solution as in **925.47B(a)** (*see* 33.70). Pipet 50 mL Pb-free filtrate into 100 mL volumetric flask; add 2.315 g NaCl and 25 mL H_2O. Dilute to volume with H_2O at 20° and polarize in 200 mm tube at 20°. Multiply reading by 2 to obtain direct reading.

(b) *Invert reading.*—Pipet 50 mL portion Pb-free filtrate into 100 mL volumetric flask and add 20 mL H_2O. Add, little by little, while rotating flask, 10 mL HCl (specific gravity 1.1029 at 20/4° or 24.85° Brix at 20°). Heat H_2O bath and adjust heater to keep bath at 60°. Place flask in H_2O bath, agitate continuously ca 3 min, and leave flask in bath exactly 7 min longer. Place flask at once in H_2O at 20°.

When contents cool to ca 35°, dilute almost to mark. Leave flask in bath at 20° at least 30 min longer and finally dilute to mark. Mix well and polarize solution in 200 mm tube provided with lateral branch and H_2O jacket, keeping temperature at 20°. This reading must be multiplied by 2 to obtain invert reading. If it is necessary to work at temperature other than 20°, which is permissible within narrow limits, volumes must be completed and both direct and invert polarizations must be made at exactly same temperature.

Calculate % sucrose, S, by following formula:

$$S = \frac{100\,(P - I)}{132.56 - 0.0794(13 - m) - 0.53(t - 20)}$$

where P = direct reading, normal solution; I = invert reading, normal solution; t = temperature at which readings are made; and m = g total solids from original sample in 100 mL inverted solution. To obtain m for liquids, determine total solids in original sample as % by weight as in **932.14C** [*see Official Methods of Analysis* (1990) 15th Ed.], and multiply this figure by weight original sample in 100 mL invert solution.

(c) *Inversion at room temperature.*—Inversion may also be accomplished as follows: (*1*) Pipet 50 mL Pb-free filtrate into 100 mL volumetric flask, add 20 mL H_2O and 10 mL HCl (specific gravity 1.1029 at 20/4° or 24.85° Brix at 20°), and set aside 24 h at ≥22°; or (*2*) set aside 10 h if >28°. Dilute to 100 mL at 20° and polarize as in (b). Under these conditions formula must be changed to following:

$$S = \frac{100\,(P - I)}{132.66 - 0.0794(13 - m) - 0.53(t - 20)}$$

Reference: JAOAC **8,** 400(1925).
CAS-57-50-1 (sucrose)

33.73 926.13—Sucrose and Raffinose in Sugars and Sirups
Polarimetric Method Before and After Treatment with Two Enzyme Preparations
Final Action 1970

A. Reagents

(**a**) *Invertase solution (top yeast extract).*—Commercially available. This solution should be free from enzyme melibiase. Its invertase activity should be at least as great as that used for determination of sucrose in absence of raffinose, **31.024(4)**★, 13th ed.

(**b**) *Invertase-melibiase solution (bottom yeast extract).*—Prepare as in **925.47A**, using bottom fermenting brewers yeast instead of bakers yeast. Invertase activity should be at least as great as in (**a**). Obtainable only from brewers as a liquid. Compress by filtering on buchner.

Test melibiase activity of solution as follows: Add 2 mL solution to be tested to 20 mL weakly acid melibiose solution polarizing $+20.0°S$ and let stand 30 min at ca 20°. Add enough Na_2CO_3 to make solution slightly alkaline to litmus paper. Preparation suitable for overnight hydrolysis of solutions containing ≤ 0.2 g raffinose in 100 mL should have hydrolyzed 35% of melibiose present under conditions mentioned; preparation suitable for overnight hydrolysis of solutions containing ≤ 0.65 g raffinose in 100 mL should have produced 50% hydrolysis of melibiose; and preparation suitable for overnight hydrolysis of solutions containing 0.65–1.3 g raffinose in 100 mL should have hydrolyzed at least 70% of melibiose present under above conditions. Preparations of melibiose solution that polarize $+20°S$ before hydrolysis will polarize $+16.4°$, $+14.9°$, and $+12.9°S$ after 35, 50, and 70% hydrolysis, respectively.

B. Determination

With sugar beet products, weigh material specified in Table **926.13**, transfer to 300 mL volumetric flask, add volume basic $Pb(OAc)_2$ solution, **925.46B(a)** (*see* 33.71), indicated in table, and dilute to volume at 20°. Mix thoroughly and filter through fluted paper in closely covered funnel, rejecting first 25 mL filtrate. When enough filtrate collects, remove Pb from solution by adding $NH_4H_2PO_4$ in as small excess as possible, Table **926.13**. This condition is readily determined after little practice by appearance of $Pb_3(PO_4)_2$ precipitate, which usually flocculates and settles rapidly in presence of slight excess of the salt. Mix well and filter, again rejecting at least first 25 mL filtrate.

Table 926.13.—Amounts of Sample and Reagents Required for Clarification and Deleading of Beet Sugar-House Products

Material	Amount per 100 mL, g	Basic Lead Acetate (55° Brix), mL	Ammonium Dihydrogen Phosphate, g
Cossettes[a]	13	3	0.2
Pulp	100 mL[b]	2-4	0.2
Lime cake or sewer[c]	26.5	1.5	....[d]
Thin juice	52	2	0.2-0.3
Thick juice	26	4	0.3-0.4
White massecuite	13 or 26	3 or 6	0.3-0.7
High wash sirup	13 or 26	3 or 6	0.3-0.7

Table 926.13.—Amounts of Sample and Reagents Required for Clarification and Deleading of Beet Sugar-House Products

Material	Amount per 100 mL, g	Basic Lead Acetate (55° Brix), mL	Ammonium Dihydrogen Phosphate, g
High green sirup	13 or 26	5 or 10	0.3-0.7
Raw or remelt massecuite	13	6	0.3-0.4
Raw or remelt sugar	26	3-4	0.3-0.4
Sugar melter	26	2-3	0.3-0.4
Low wash sirup	13	8-10	0.4-0.5
Low green sirup or molasses	13	10	0.4-0.5
Saccharate cakes and milk (carbonated)	26	4-6	0.3-0.4
Steffen waste and wash watersR	78 or 50 mL	2-3	0.2

[a] Usual method of extn, 26 g in 201.2 mL.
[b] Dil. to 110 mL.
[c] Neutralize with HAOc before adding basic $Pb(OAc)_2$.
[d] As Ca in soln will be partly pptd by the phosphate, it is necessary to add enough phosphate to complete pptn of both Pb and Ca salts, and no definite quantity can be specified.

Make direct polarization in 200 mm tube at 20° unless solution contains appreciable amount of invert sugar, in which case pipet 50 mL portion Pb-free filtrate into 100 mL flask, dilute with H_2O to volume, mix well, and polarize at 20°, preferably in 400 mm tube. This reading, calculated to normal weight of 26 g in 100 mL and 200 mm tube length, is direct reading (P) of formula given below for polarization before inversion.

Transfer two 50 mL portions of the Pb-free filtrate to 100 mL volumetric flasks. To one add 5 mL invertase solution (top yeast extract) and to other 5 mL invertase-melibiase solution (bottom yeast extract); let stand overnight at room temperature (preferably ≥20°), dilute to volume, mix well, and polarize at 20°, preferably in 400 mm jacketed tube.

If rapid hydrolysis is desired, add 10 mL of each of the enzyme solutions to 50 mL portions Pb-free filtrate in 100 mL volumetric flasks and place in H_2O bath 40 min at 50–55°. Then add Na_2CO_3 until solution is slightly alkaline to litmus paper, dilute to volume at 20°, mix well, and polarize at 20°, preferably in 400 mm tube. Correct invert readings for optical activity of enzyme solution and calculate polarization to that of normal weight solution of 26 g/100 mL; also calculate reading to 200 mm tube length, if necessary.

Calculate % of anhydrous raffinose, R, and sucrose, S, from following formulas:

$$R = 1.354(X - Y)$$

$$S = \frac{(P - 2.202X + 1.202Y)100}{132.12 - 0.00718[132.12 - (P - 2.202X + 1.202Y)]}$$

where P = direct polarization, normal solution; X = corrected polarization after top yeast hydrolysis, normal solution; and Y = corrected polarization after bottom yeast hydrolysis, normal solution. Quantities X and Y are treated algebraically.

Reference: JAOAC **9**, 33(1926).

33.74   926.14—Sucrose and Raffinose in Sugars and Sirups
Polarimetric Method Before and After Inversion with Hydrochloric Acid
Final Action 1970
Surplus 1989

(Of value chiefly in analysis of beet products)

See **31.029**, *Official Methods of Analysis* (1984) 14th Ed.

33.75   970.57—Sucrose in Molasses
Polarimetric Methods
Final Action

Polarimetric methods (when required by law). *See* **925.46** (*see* 33.71), **925.47** (*see* 33.70), **926.13** (*see* 33.73), **926.14** (*see* 33.74), **896.02** (*see* 33.68).

33.76   942.20—Sucrose in Sugar Beets
First Action

A. Hot Water Digestion Method I
(*Caution: See Appendix* for safety notes on vacuum.)
Pass sample (usually in form of cossettes) through meat grinder fitted with plate having 6 mm (¼″) perforations and mix thoroughly. Weigh 26 g prepared sample and rinse into 201.0 mL Kohlrausch flask, using ca 100 mL H_2O. Place flask under good vacuum 5–10 min to remove air, carefully avoiding mechanical loss when vacuum is first applied. Add H_2O to ca 175 mL, and digest in H_2O bath at 80°, supporting flask so that body is entirely immersed but is not in contact with heating element. Remove flask 2 or 3 times during digestion, swirl contents, and after each agitation wash down pulp adhering to walls of flask with little H_2O at 80°.

    After exactly 30 min digestion, fill flask to within 2–5 mL of mark with H_2O at 80° and continue digestion exactly 10 min longer. Cool to room temperature in H_2O bath. Add 6 mL basic $Pb(OAc)_2$

solution, **925.46B(a)** (*see* 33.71), and H_2O to fill to mark. (Previous additions of H_2O and reagents should be so adjusted that ≤ 4 mL H_2O is required to dilute to volume.) Mix well by shaking, let stand 5 min, shake again, and filter. Let stand near saccharimeter at least 5 min, and polarize in 400 mm glass tube. If volume adjustment and polariscopic observation are made at 20°, reading gives % sucrose directly; if at other temperatures, apply formula in **925.46C(a)**.

Notes: The 1 mL >200 mL volume is the determined volume of marc for beets grown in Colorado and neighboring states. It should be determined for other localities. Beets of abnormally low purity may require 8–10 mL basic $Pb(OAc)_2$ solution for clarification. If foaming causes trouble, flask may be put under vacuum second time after cooling, or few drops ether or 1 drop *amyl alcohol* may be added before solution is diluted to volume.

Reference: JAOAC **25,** 98(1942).

CAS-57-50-1 (sucrose)

B. Hot Water Digestion Method II

Use Ni-plated sheet Fe vessels, 11 cm high, 6 cm body diameter, and 4 cm mouth diameter; use stoppers covered with Sn foil to fit.

Weigh 26 g prepared beet pulp, **942.20A**, on watch glass (small enough to go into neck of beaker) and transfer to metal beaker; add 177 mL dilute basic $Pb(OAc)_2$ solution (5 parts basic $Pb(OAc)_2$ solution, **925.46B(a)**, to 100 parts H_2O); shake, and stopper lightly. Submerge beaker in H_2O bath 30 min at 75–80°, shaking intermittently. When all air is expelled (generally after 5 min), tighten stopper. After 30 min, shake, cool to standard temperature, filter, add drop CH_3COOH to filtrate, and polarize in 400 mm tube. Reading is % sugar in beet pulp.

Reference: USDA Bur. Chem. Bull. **146,** p. 19.

33.77   945.55—Sucrose in Gelatin
Final Action 1969

A. Reagents

(a) *Tannin solution.*—Dissolve 5 g tannin in 100 mL cold H_2O.

(b) *Lead acetate solution.*—Dissolve 100 g $Pb(OAc)_2 \cdot 3H_2O$ in 200 mL H_2O. (This makes 30° Bé. solution.)

B. Determination

Place 13 g sample in 300 or 400 mL beaker, add 2 g $CaCO_3$ and 2 g Filter-Cel, and mix well with glass rod. Add 175 mL boiling H_2O, creaming mixture with little of the H_2O at first. Stir thoroughly and let stand few min to ensure solution. Cool under cold H_2O to 30°, slowly add 25 mL tannin solution with stirring, and let stand 5 min. (This volume tannin solution is enough for most powders; if 30 mL is required, use 170 mL H_2O instead of 175 mL.) Slowly add 10 mL $Pb(OAc)_2$ solution with stirring, and filter on 18.5 cm Whatman No. 2 paper. (Total volume liquid used in each case is 210 mL, which yields 200 mL after evaporation and concentration. If precipitation has been conducted properly, solution will filter readily and filtrate will be clear.) Read optical rotation of this solution in 200 mm tube at 20°.

If sample contains reducing sugar, delead with $K_2C_2O_4$, add Filter-Cel, and filter. Invert by placing 50 mL filtrate in 100 mL volumetric flask with 5 mL HCl and letting stand overnight. After inversion, neutralize with concentrated NaOH solution, using phenolphthalein. Discharge color of indicator with $0.1N$

HCl. Cool to 20°, dilute to volume, and read optical rotation in 200 mm tube. Use following Clerget formula modified for % sucrose in gelatin dessert powders:

$$S = \frac{100 \ (4P - 8I)}{142.66 + 0.0676(m - 13) - t/2}$$

where S = % sucrose; P = direct reading; I = invert reading; t = temperature at which readings are made (20°); and m = g total solids from original sample/100 mL invert solution (3.25 g). Simplified:
$$S = 100(4P - 8I)/132$$
Reference: Annual Report Dept. Farms and Markets, New York, 1926, Legislative Document No. 15, p. 78 (1927).
CAS-50-99-7 (glucose)
CAS-57-50-1 (sucrose)

C. Glucose

Determine polarization due to glucose (D) by subtracting % sucrose (S) as found in **945.55B** from direct reading of polariscope in circular degrees (P) multiplied by 4: $D = 4P - S$.
$$\% \ \text{Glucose} = D \times 66.5/52.5 = 1.267D$$
where D = polarization due to glucose; 66.5 = specific rotation of sucrose; and 52.5 = specific rotation of glucose.

33.78   950.29—Sucrose in Nonalcoholic Beverages
Final Action

A. By Polarization

Determine by polarizing before and after inversion as in **925.47** (*see* 33.70), or **925.48** (*see* 33.72).

B. By Reducing Sugars Before and After Inversion

See **930.36** (*see* 33.41).

33.79   950.30—Sugars (Reducing) in Nonalcoholic Beverages
Final Action

Use value obtained for reducing sugars before inversion, **950.29B** (*see* 33.78).

33.80   950.31—Glucose (Commercial) in Nonalcoholic Beverages
Procedure

See **930.37B** (*see* 33.81).

33.81   930.37—Glucose (Commercial) in Sugars and Sirups
Polarimetric Methods
Procedure (Approximate)

A. Substances Containing Little or No Invert Sugar

Commercial glucose cannot be determined accurately, since amounts of dextrin, maltose, and dextrose present vary. However, in sirups in which amount of invert sugar is too small to appreciably affect result, commercial glucose may be estimated approximately by following formula:

$$G = (a - S)100/211$$

where G = % commercial glucose solids; a = direct polarization, normal solution; and S = % cane sugar.

Express results in terms of commercial glucose solids polarizing + 211°S. (Result may be recalculated in terms of commercial glucose of any polarization desired.)

B. Substances Containing Invert Sugar

Prepare inverted half-normal solution of substance as in **925.48(b)** (*see* 33.72), except cool solution after inversion, make neutral to phenolphthalein with NaOH solution, slightly acidify with HCl (1 + 5), and treat with 5–10 mL alumina cream, **925.46B(b)** (*see* 33.71), before diluting to volume. Filter, and polarize at 87° in 200 mm jacketed metal tube. Multiply reading by 200 and divide by factor 196 to obtain amount of commercial glucose solids polarizing + 211°S. (Result may be recalculated in terms of commercial glucose of any polarization desired.)

33.82   972.16—Fat, Lactose, Protein, and Solids in Milk
Mid-Infrared Spectroscopic Method
First Action 1972

See Chapter 28.23.

33.83   **975.19—Lactose in Milk**
                                        Infrared Method
                                        First Action

See **972.16H** and **I**, Chapter 28.23.

33.84   **930.28—Lactose in Milk**
                                        Gravimetric Method
                                        Final Action

Dilute 25 g sample with 400 mL H_2O in 500 mL volumetric flask. Add 10 mL $CuSO_4$ solution, **923.09A(a)**, and ca 7.5 mL KOH solution of such concentration that 1 volume is just enough to completely precipitate the Cu as hydroxide from 1 volume of the $CuSO_4$ solution. (Instead, 8.8 mL 0.5N NaOH may be used. After addition of alkali solution, mixture must still be acid and contain Cu in solution.) Dilute to volume, mix, filter through dry filter, and determine lactose in aliquot of filtrate as in **906.03B** (*see* 33.13). From **940.39** [*see Official Methods of Analysis* (1990) 15th Ed., PP. 1286–1294] , obtain weight lactose equivalent to weight Cu_2O.

33.85   **920.110—Lactose in Cream**
                                        Gravimetric Method
                                        Final Action

See **930.28** (*see* 33.84).

Chapter 34
Thiamine

34.1   **942.23—Thiamine (Vitamin B₁) in Foods**
Fluorometric Method
Final Action

(Methods not applicable in presence of materials that adsorb thiamine or which contain extraneous materials which affect thiochrome fluorescence)

A. Reagents and Apparatus

(a) *Double-normal sodium acetate.*—Dissolve 272 g NaOAc·3H₂O in enough H₂O to make 1 L.

(b) *Bromocresol green pH indicator.*—Dissolve 0.1 g indicator by triturating in agate mortar with 2.8 mL 0.05N NaOH, and dilute to 200 mL with H₂O. Transition range: 4.0 (green)–5.8 (blue).

(c) *Bromophenol blue indicator.*—Dissolve 0.1 g indicator by triturating in agate mortar with 3.0 mL 0.05N NaOH, and dilute to 250 mL with H₂O. Transition range: 3.0 (yellow)–4.6 (blue).

(d) *Enzyme solution.*—Prepare, on day on which it is to be used, 10% aqueous solution of enzyme preparation potent in diastatic and phosphorolytic activity. (Among enzymes available for this purpose are Mylase 100 [U.S. Biochemical Corp.], Takadiastase [Pfalz and Bauer 375 Fairfield Ave, Stamford CT 06902], and α-amylase [Miles Laboratories, Inc., 1127 Myrtle St, PO Box 70, Elkhart, IN 46514].) Check each batch for performance against thiamine mono-, di-, and triphosphate. Evaluate % recovery compared with USP Reference Standard Thiamine. If recovery is >85%, enzyme preparation is suitable.

(e) *Bio-Rex 70 (hydrogen form).*—50–100 mesh. Add 300 mL 2N HCl to 50 g Bio-Rex 70 (Bio-Rad Laboratories), stir 15 min, decant, and repeat. Add 300 mL H₂O, stir 1 min, decant, and repeat until pH of H₂O is 4.5–7.0. H₂O should be free of suspended resin when allowed to settle 15 s. If not, repeat H₂O washing until clear.

(f) *Chromatographic columns.*—Use glass chromatographic tubes (ca 275 mm overall length, with reservoir capacity ca 60 mL) consisting of 3 parts fused together with following approximate dimensions (od × length, mm): (*1*) reservoir at top, 35 × 95, (*2*) adsorption tube in middle, 8 × 145, drawn into (*3*) capillary at bottom 35 mm long and of such diameter that when tube is filled, rate of flow will be ≤1 mL/min. Prepare tubes for use as follows: Over upper end of capillary, with aid of glass rod, place pledget of fine glass wool. To adsorption tube, add H₂O suspension resin to height of approximately 100 mm, taking care to wash down all silicate from walls of reservoir. To keep air out of adsorption column, keep layer of liquid above surface of silicate during adsorption process. (Prevent tube from draining by placing rubber cap, filled with H₂O to avoid inclusion of air, over lower end of capillary.)

(g) *Neutral potassium chloride solution.*—Dissolve 250 g KCl in H₂O to make 1 L.

(h) *Acid potassium chloride solution.*—Add 8.5 mL HCl to 1 L of the neutral KCl solution.

(i) *Sodium hydroxide solution.*—15%. Dissolve 15 g NaOH in H₂O to make 100 mL.

(**j**) *Potassium ferricyanide solution.*—1%. Dissolve 1 g $K_3Fe(CN)_6$ in H_2O to make 100 mL. Prepare solution on day it is used.

(**k**) *Oxidizing reagent.*—Mix 4.0 mL of the 1% $K_3Fe(CN)_6$ solution with the 15% NaOH solution to make 100 mL. Use solution within 4 h.

(**l**) *Isobutyl alcohol.*—Redistilled in all-glass apparatus. Use redistilled product as anhydrous or H_2O-saturated.

(**m**) *Quinine sulfate stock solution.*—Use quinine sulfate solution to govern reproducibility of fluorometer. Prepare stock solution by dissolving 10 mg quinine sulfate in $0.1N$ H_2SO_4 to make 1 L. Store in light-resistant containers.

(**n**) *Quinine sulfate standard solution.*—Dilute 1 volume quinine sulfate stock solution with 39 volumes $0.1N$ H_2SO_4. (Solution fluoresces to ca same degree as does isobutanol extract of thiochrome obtained from 1 µg thiamine·HCl.) Store solution in light-resistant containers.

(**o**) *Thiamine hydrochloride standard solutions.*—(*1*) *Stock solution.*—100 µg/mL. Accurately weigh 50–60 mg USP Thiamine Hydrochloride Reference Standard that has been dried to constant weight over P_2O_5 in desiccator. (Reference standard is hygroscopic; avoid absorption of moisture.) Dissolve in 20% alcohol adjusted to pH 3.5–4.3 with HCl, and dilute to 500 mL with the acidified alcohol. Add enough additional acidified alcohol to make concentration exactly 100 µg thiamine·HCl/mL. Store at ca 10° in glass-stoppered, light-resistant bottle. (*2*) *Intermediate solution.*—10 µg/mL. Dilute 100 mL stock solution to 1 L with 20% alcohol adjusted to pH 3.5–4.3 with HCl. Store at ca 10° in glass-stoppered, light-resistant bottle. (*3*) *Working solution.*—1 µg/mL. To 10 mL intermediate solution, add ca 50 mL ca $0.1N$ HCl, digest or autoclave as in **942.23B(a)(*1*)**, cool, and dilute to 100 mL with the $0.1N$ HCl. Prepare fresh solution for each assay.

For materials containing free thiamine, dilute 20 mL working solution to 100 mL with $0.1N$ HCl. Designate as assay standard solution and proceed directly to oxidation, **942.23E**.

For materials containing thiamine pyrophosphate, take 20 mL working solution and proceed as in **942.23C**, beginning ". . . dilute to ca 65 mL . . . ." Designate final 25 mL eluate (equivalent to 5 µg USP Thiamine·HCl Reference Standard) from **942.23D** as assay standard solution and proceed as in **942.23E**.

B. Extraction

(**a**) *For materials containing free thiamine (not applicable in presence of thiamine pyrophosphate).*—Place measured amount of sample in flask of suitable size, prepare sample by (*1*), (*2*), or (*3*), and proceed directly to oxidation, **942.23E**.

(*1*) *For dry or semidry materials containing no appreciable quantity of basic substances.*—Add volume $0.1N$ HCl equal in mL to ≥10 times dry weight sample in grams. Comminute and evenly disperse material in liquid if it is not readily soluble. If lumping occurs, agitate vigorously so that all particles come in contact with liquid; then wash down sides of flask with $0.1N$ HCl. Digest 30 min at 95–100° in steam bath, or in boiling H_2O, with frequent mixing; or autoclave mixture 30 min at 121–123°. Cool, and if lumping occurs, agitate mixture until particles are evenly dispersed. Dilute with $0.1N$ HCl to measured volume containing ca 0.2 µg thiamine/mL. Designate as Assay Sample Solution.

(*2*) *For dry or semidry materials containing appreciable amounts of basic substances.*—Add dilute HCl to adjust mixture to ca pH 4.0. Add amount of H_2O such that total volume liquid is equal in mL to ≥10 times dry weight sample in grams. Add equivalent of 1 mL $10N$ HCl/100 mL liquid and proceed as in (*1*), beginning with second sentence.

(*3*) *For liquid materials.*—Adjust material to ca pH 4.0 with dilute HCl, or, with vigorous agitation, NaOH solution, and proceed as in (*2*), beginning with second sentence.

(b) *For materials containing thiamine pyrophosphate.*—Proceed as in (**a**)(*1*), but dilute with 0.1*N* HCl to measured volume containing 0.2–5.0 μg thiamine/mL, followed by enzyme hydrolysis and purification, **942.23C–D**.

C. Enzyme Hydrolysis

Take aliquot containing ca 10–25 μg thiamine, dilute to ca 65 mL with 0.1*N* HCl, and adjust pH to 4.0–4.5 with ca 5 mL 2*N* NaOAc, using pH meter or bromocresol green indicator and spot plate. End point should be definitely on blue side of color change. Add 5 mL enzyme solution, mix, and incubate 3 h at 45–50°. Cool, adjust to ca pH 3.5, using bromophenol blue indicator or pH meter, dilute to 100 mL with H_2O, and filter through paper known not to adsorb thiamine (ash-free papers have been found satisfactory).

D. Purification

Pass aliquot of filtered solution containing ca 5 μg thiamine through prepared chromatographic column, and wash column with three 5 mL portions of almost boiling H_2O. Do not permit surface of liquid to fall below surface of resin.

Elute thiamine from resin by passing five 4.0–4.5 mL portions almost boiling (>60°) acid-KCl solution through column. Do not permit surface of liquid to fall below surface of resin until final portion of acid-KCl solution has been added. Collect eluate in 25 mL volumetric flask, cool, and dilute to volume with acid-KCl solution. Designate this as Assay Sample Solution.

E. Oxidation of Thiamine to Thiochrome

To each of ≥4 ca 40 mL tubes (or reaction vessels) add ca 1.5 g NaCl or KCl and 5 mL assay standard solution. (*Precision and accuracy of results depend upon uniform technique in conducting following oxidation.* Protect solution from light, which destroys thiochrome. Use pipet that delivers 3 mL in 1–2 s for addition of oxidizing reagent.) Place tip of pipet containing oxidizing reagent in neck of tube and hold it so that stream of solution does not hit side of tube. Gently swirl tube to produce rotary motion in liquid and immediately add 3 mL oxidizing reagent. Remove pipet and swirl tube again to ensure adequate mixing. *Immediately* add 13 mL isobutanol, stopper, and shake tube vigorously ≥15 s. Similarly treat ≥1 tube and treat each of ≥2 remaining tubes (standard blanks) similarly except replace oxidizing reagent with 15% NaOH solution.

To each of ≥4 similar tubes add 5 mL Assay Sample Solution. Treat these tubes in same manner as directed for tubes containing working standard solution.

After isobutanol has been added to all tubes, shake again ca 2 min. (Tubes may be placed in shaker box for this additional shaking.) Centrifuge tubes at low speed until clear supernate can be obtained from each. Pipet or decant ca 10 mL isobutanol extract (upper layer) from each tube into cell for thiochrome fluorescence measurement.

F. Thiochrome Fluorescence Measurement

(Thiamine content of oxidized Assay Solution is determined by comparing intensity of fluorescence of extract of this solution with that from oxidized standard solution. Intensity of fluorescence is proportional to amount of thiamine present and may be measured with suitable fluorometer. Input filter of narrow *T* range with maximum ca 365 nm and output filter of narrow *T* range with maximum ca 435 nm have been found satisfactory. Use quinine sulfate standard solution to govern reproducibility of fluorometer.)
(*Caution: See Appendix* for safety notes on photofluorometers.)

Measure fluorescence (*I*) of isobutanol extract from oxidized Assay Sample Solution. Next measure fluorescence (*b*) of extract from Assay Sample Solution, which has been treated with 3 mL 15% NaOH solution. Then measure fluorescence (S) of extract from oxidized assay standard solution. Finally, measure fluorescence (d) of extract from assay standard solution, which has been treated with 3 mL 15% NaOH solution (standard blank).

G. Calculation

Calculate as follows:

$$\mu g \text{ Thiamine·HCl in 5 mL Assay Solution} = (I - b)/(S - d)$$

References: JAOAC **25**, 456(1942); **27**, 534(1944); **28**, 554(1945); **31**, 455(1948); **43**, 45, 55(1960); **64**, 1336(1981).

CAS-67-03-8 (thiamine hydrochloride)

34.2   957.17—Thiamine (Vitamin B$_1$) in Bread
Fluorometric Method
Final Action 1960

A. Reagents and Apparatus

Use reagents and apparatus as in **942.23A** (*see* 34.1), and the following:

(a) *Thiamine hydrochloride working solution.*—1 μg/mL. Pipet 20 mL thiamine·HCl intermediate solution, **942.23A(o)(2)**, into 200 mL volumetric flask and dilute to volume with ca 0.1N HCl. Prepare fresh daily.

(b) *Procedural standard solution.*—Pipet 40 mL working solution, (a), into one of the acid digestion containers, dilute to ca 150 mL with ca 0.1N HCl, and continue as under sample treatment (1 mL = 0.2 μg thiamine·HCl in final volume). (To be used for recovery experiments to test efficiency of method.)

(c) *Direct standard solution.*—0.2 μg/mL. Pipet 40 mL working solution, (a), into 200 mL volumetric flask, add ca 16 mL H$_2$O, and dilute to volume with eluting acid KCl solution, **942.23A(h)**.

B. Acid and Enzyme Digestions

Weigh ($\pm$ 0.05 g) amount of air-dried bread, **960.24**, containing ca 40 μg thiamine and transfer to 250 mL digestion flask or centrifuge bottle. Add 150 mL ca 0.1N HCl, stirring with glass rod to provide homogeneous mixture with ca 1/2 of acid and using remainder to wash down side of container. Digest 30 min in boiling H$_2$O bath. Stir enough to prevent lumping or clotting, especially during first 5–10 min. Cool to room temperature and adjust pH to 4.5 by adding 2N NaOAc, **942.23A(a)**, using pH meter or bromocresol green indicator, **942.23A(b)**, and spot plate; end point should be definitely on blue side of green-blue change. Alternatively, use constant amount of hydrolyzing acid and previously determined amount of NaOAc solution required to adjust to pH 4.5.

Add 5 mL enzyme solution, **942.23A(d)**, mix, warm to 45°, and digest in H$_2$O bath 1 h at 45–50°. Stir at 10–15 min intervals. Cool, transfer to 200 mL volumetric flask, and dilute to volume with 0.1N HCl. Mix, and filter through paper known not to adsorb thiamine. (Paper can be tested by comparing filtered and nonfiltered procedural standard solution, **957.17A(b)**. Ash-free papers have been found satisfactory.) Check pH of filtrate, using bromophenol blue indicator, **942.23A(c)**, and spot plate, or pH meter (should be ca 3.5 for subsequent base-exchange separation), and purify as in **942.23D**.

960.24 (Vitamins in Enriched Bread, Preparation of Sample)

Determine fresh weight of entire sample taken for drying, usually 6 loaves of 1 lb size or alternate slices from 6 loaves of 1.5 lb size. Slice unsliced bread into slices ca 1 oz each. Spread slices on coarse screens, elevated to provide good air circulation, and let air dry until crisp enough for efficient grinding. (If riboflavin is also to be determined, drying should be done in absence of light.) Weigh air-dried bread and grind entire amount to pass No. 20 sieve. Mix well, and store in air-tight glass jars at ca 10°. Determine air-dry weight:fresh weight ratio for subsequent use in calculation of results to fresh basis.

Proceed as in chapter on vitamins.

C. Oxidation of Thiamine to Thiochrome

Pipet duplicate 5 mL aliquots of direct standard solution, **957.17A(c)**, and duplicate 5 mL aliquots of Assay Sample Solution into ca 40 mL tubes or reaction vessels, and proceed as in **942.23E**.

D. Thiochrome Fluorescence Measurement

Thiamine content of oxidized Assay Solution is determined by comparing intensity of fluorescence of extract of this solution with that from oxidized direct standard solution, **957.17A(c)**, correcting for blank fluorescence of each of these solutions. Intensity of fluorescence is linear in range 0–2 μg thiamine and may be measured with fluorometer as in **942.23F**.

Correct for blank of Assay Solutions giving extremely high blank fluorescence readings with 15% NaOH solution by alternative technique, **953.17D**.

$$\text{mg Thiamine·HCl/lb (fresh basis)} = (I/B) \times (40 \times 454 \times F/W \times 1000)$$

if specified aliquots have been used, where I = corrected reading of assay solution; B = corrected reading of standard solution; W = grams air-dried bread sample; and F = air-dry weight:fresh weight ratio.

References: JAOAC **40,** 843(1957); **41,** 603(1958); **43,** 47(1960).
CAS-67-03-8 (thiamine hydrochloride)

34.3   953.17—Thiamine (Vitamin B₁) in Grain Products
Fluorometric (Rapid) Method
Final Action

(Applicable to determination of thiamine in enriched flour, farina, corn meal, macaroni, and noodle products, or where bound thiamine or thiamine pyrophosphate is not significant)

A. Reagents

See **942.23A(c), (i), (j), (k), (l), (m), (n),** and **(o)** (*see* 34.1).

B. Preparation of Standard Solution

Dilute 5 mL thiamine·HCl intermediate solution, **942.23A(o)(2)**, to 250 mL with ca 0.1N HCl (1 mL = 0.2 μg thiamine·HCl). Designate this as working standard solution. If NaCl is to be added to sample for extraction, add NaCl to working standard solution, before final dilution, to give final concentration of ca 5% (weight/volume). Proceed as in **953.17D**.

C. Extraction

Weigh enough sample to give final Assay Solution with thiamine concentration of ca 0.2 μg/mL (e.g., 4.54 g enriched flour for 100 mL or 9.07 g for 200 mL final volume) and proceed by one of following methods: (**a**) *95–100° Digestion*.—Place measured amount of sample in bottle or flask of suitable size. (Addition of NaCl to give final concentration of ca 5% (weight/volume) aids in subsequent separation of sample solution. Thoroughly mix flour and salt with stirring rod before adding 0.1N HCl.) Add in 2 portions, with vigorous stirring, volume ca 0.1N HCl in proportion ca 15 mL acid to 1 g sample, using part of acid to wash down sides of vessel. Place vessel in H$_2$O bath previously heated to 95–100°. Stir at frequent intervals to keep solids in suspension during thickening stage (5–8 min) and occasionally during balance of total heating time of 30 min.

After hydrolysis has proceeded ca 10 min, place drop of solution on spot plate and test with thymol blue. Solution should be distinctly red (pH 1.0–1.2). If not enough (indicating presence of basic substances in sample), add ca 1N HCl in 1.0 mL portions until desired acidity is reached. Note volume of 1N acid required to supplement the 0.1N acid and *repeat digestion* with new sample weight and necessary mixture of 1N and 0.1N acids. Cool, and dilute with 0.1N HCl to measured volume containing ca 0.2 μg thiamine/mL.

Centrifuge mixture until supernate is clear or practically so and/or filter through paper known not to adsorb thiamine (ash-free papers have been found satisfactory), or filter through fritted glass funnel, using suitable analytical filter-aid (ash-free filter pulp and Celite Analytical Filter-Aid have been found satisfactory). Discard first 1/10 part of filtrate. Designate remainder of filtrate as Assay Sample Solution. (**b**) *Autoclaved digestion*.—Proceed as in (**a**) without addition of NaCl, except to autoclave 20 min at 5 lb (34.5 kPa) pressure (108–109°) with total heating time ≤35 min including 5–10 min to attain desired pressure and ca 5 min to reduce pressure. (It may be necessary to preheat autoclave to ca 100° before inserting samples.)

D. Oxidation

Proceed as in **942.23E**, except add ca 2.5 g NaCl or KCl to each tube (or reaction vessel) before addition of 5 mL working standard solution, **953.17B**, or 5 mL Assay Sample Solution, **953.17C**. After addition of working standard solution or Assay Sample Solution, gently swirl each tube until most of salt is dissolved. Measure fluorescence of isobutanol extracts as in **942.23F**, and calculate thiamine·HCl content as in **942.23G**.

Alternative blank reading.—Use following technique on samples giving extremely high blank readings with 15% NaOH solution: After reading fluorescence of all tubes, add 1 drop (0.05 mL) HCl (1 + 1) to each tube of isobutanol extract from oxidized Assay and Standard Solutions, swirl, and take additional reading. This quenches thiochrome fluorescence and provides blank reading for each tube. Use average values obtained for Standard and Assay Solutions in place of *b* and *d* in **942.23G**.

References: JAOAC **36**, 837(1953); **37**, 122, 757(1954); **38**, 722(1955).
CAS-67-03-8 (thiamine hydrochloride)

34.4   986.27—Thiamine (Vitamin B₁) in Milk-Based Infant Formula

Fluorometric Method
First Action 1986
Final Action 1988

A. Principle

Thiamine content of extract is estimated by oxidizing thiamine to thiochrome and measuring fluorescence. Intensity of fluorescence is proportional to thiamine concentration.

B. Apparatus

(**a**) *Photofluorometer.*—Equipped with narrow transmittance range filters with input filter maximum at ca 365 nm and output filter maximum at ca 435 nm.

(**b**) *Chromatographic tubes.*—Glass chromatographic tubes (ca 275 mm overall length with reservoir capacity ca 60 mL) consisting of 3 parts described below fused together and having approximate measurements listed (inside diameter): Top: reservoir 95 mm long and 30 mm diameter, converging into middle part. Middle part: adsorption tube 145 mm long and 6 mm diameter, converging into lower part. Lower part: tube drawn into capillary 35 mm long and of such diameter that, when tube is charged, rate of flow will not be >1 mL/min.

C. Reagents

(**a**) *Chromatographic resin.*—Add 300 mL 2N HCl to 50 g Bio-Rex 70 (H form) (Bio-Rad Laboratories), stir 15 min, decant, and repeat. Add 300 mL H_2O, stir 1 min, decant, and repeat until pH of H_2O is 4.5–7.0. H_2O should be free of suspended resin when allowed to settle 15 s. If not, repeat H_2O washing until clear.

(**b**) *Sodium acetate, 2N.*—Dissolve 272 g NaOAc·3H₂O in enough H_2O to make 1 L.

(**c**) *Bromcresol green indicator.*—Dissolve 0.1 g indicator by triturating in agate mortar with 2.8 mL 0.05N NaOH, and dilute to 200 mL with H_2O.

(**d**) *Enzyme solution, 10% weight/volume.*—Dissolve 10 g Takadiastase (Pfaltz and Bauer, 375 Fairfield Ave, Stamford, CT 06902) in H_2O and dilute to 100 mL. Prepare fresh daily.

(**e**) *Potassium chloride solution, 25% weight/volume.*—Dissolve 250 g KCl in sufficient H_2O to make 1 L.

(**f**) *Acid potassium chloride solution.*—Add 8.5 mL HCl to 1 L neutral KCl solution.

(**g**) *Potassium ferricyanide solution, 1%.*—Dissolve 1 g $K_3Fe(CN)_6$ in sufficient H_2O and dilute to 100 mL. Prepare fresh daily.

(**h**) *Oxidizing reagent.*—Mix 4.0 mL 1% $K_3Fe(CN)_6$ solution with sufficient 15% NaOH solution to make 100 mL. Use this reagent within 4 h after preparation.

(**i**) *Isobutly alcohol.*—Redistilled in all-glass apparatus.

(**j**) *Quinine sulfate stock solution.* Use quinine sulfate solution to monitor reproducibility of fluorometer. Prepare stock solution by dissolving 10 mg quinine sulfate in 0.1N H_2SO_4 sufficient to make 1 L. Store stock solution in red or amber container.

(**k**) *Quinine sulfate standard solution.*—Dilute 5.0 mL quinine sulfate stock solution with sufficient 0.1N H_2SO_4 to make 200 mL. This solution fluoresces to about same degree as does isobutyl alcohol extract of thiochrome obtained from 1 μg thiamine·HCl. Store this solution in red or amber container.

(**l**) *Acidified alcohol, 20% weight/volume.*—Dilute 250 mL alcohol with H_2O to make 1 L. Add HCl dropwise to adjust to pH 3.5–4.3.

(**m**) *Acetic acid, 3%.*—Dilute 30 mL glacial acetic acid with H_2O to 1 L.

D. Tube Preparation

Prepare chromatographic tubes for use as follows: With aid of glass rod, place pledget of fine glass wool over upper end of capillary. Taking care to wash down all resin from walls of reservoir, add H_2O suspension of 1.0–2.0 g resin to adsorption tube. To keep air out of adsorption tube, keep layer of liquid above surface of resin during adsorption process. Place rubber cap, filled with H_2O to avoid inclusion of air, over lower end of capillary to prevent tube from draining.

E. Preparation of Thiamine·HCl Standard Solutions

(a) *Stock standard solution, 100 μg/mL.*—Accurately weigh 50.0 mg USP Thiamine·HCl Reference Standard previously dried by storing over P_2O_5 in desiccator. Since reference standard is hygroscopic, take precautions to avoid moisture absorption during weighing. Transfer 50.0 mg standard to 500 mL volumetric flask. Dissolve in acidified 20% alcohol, and dilute to 500.0 mL with additional acidified alcohol. Store in red or amber glass-stoppered bottle in refrigerator. Solution is stable several months.

(b) *Working standard solution, 3 μg/mL.*—Dilute 3.0 mL stock standard solution with 0.1N HCl to make 100 mL. Prepare fresh daily.

F. Preparation of Sample

(a) Pipet into 100 mL centrifuge tube (or 125 mL erlenmeyer) amount of sample estimated to contain ca 15 μg thiamine·HCl. Add 65 mL 0.1N HCl. Continue as in (c) below.

(b) Pipet 5 mL working standard solution (3 μg/mL) into 100 mL centrifuge tube (or 125 mL erlenmeyer). Add 65 mL 0.1N HCl. Continue as in (c) below.

(c) Evenly disperse any solid material in liquid. If lumping occurs, agitate vigorously so that all particles come in contact with liquid. Digest 30 min at 95–100° in steam bath or in boiling H_2O bath with frequent mixing, or autoclave mixture at 121° for 30 min.

Cool, and, if lumping occurs, agitate mixture until particles are evenly dispersed.

G. Enzyme Hydrolysis

Quantitatively transfer cooled sample and standard extracts to respective 100 mL volumetric flasks. Adjust pH of each solution to 4.0–4.5 with ca 5 mL 2N NaOAc solution using bromcresol green indicator on spot plate. Add 5 mL enzyme solution, mix, and incubate 3 h at 45–50°. Cool, dilute to 100 mL with 0.1N HCl, and filter through paper known not to absorb thiamine. (Ash-free paper has been found satisfactory.)

H. Purification

Pass 10 mL aliquot of filtered standard and sample solutions (containing ca 1.5 μg thiamine·HCl) through respective prepared chromatographic tubes. Then wash each tube with three 5 mL portions of almost-boiling H_2O, taking care to prevent surface of liquid from falling below surface of resin.

Elute thiamine from resin by passing five 4.0–4.5 mL portions of almost-boiling acid KCl solution through each tube. Take care to prevent surface of liquid from falling below surface of resin until final portion of acid KCl solution has been added. Collect eluate thus obtained from hydrolysis and purification of standard in 25 mL volumetric flask. Cool and dilute to volume with acid KCl solution. Designate this as *standard solution*. Collect eluate thus obtained from hydrolysis and purification of aliquot of sample in 25 mL volumetric flask. Cool and dilute to volume with acid KCl solution. Designate this as *assay solution*.

I. Oxidation of Thiamine to Thiochrome

Precision and accuracy of results depend on uniform technique in conducting following oxidation procedure:

To each of 4 or more 40 mL tubes or reaction vessels, add ca 1.5 g NaCl or KCl and 5 mL standard solution. (Protect these solutions from light; thiochrome is light-sensitive.)

Use pipet that delivers 3 mL in 1–2 s for addition of oxidizing reagent. Place tip of pipet, containing oxidizing reagent, in neck of tube and hold it so that stream of oxidizing reagent does not hit side of tube. Swirl tube gently to produce rotary motion in liquid and immediately add 3 mL oxidizing reagent. Remove pipet and swirl tube again to ensure adequate mixing. Let stand 9.0 min. *Immediately* add 13 mL redistilled isobutyl alcohol, stopper tube, and shake vigorously 15 s. Treat one or more additional tubes similarly. Treat each of 2 or more of remaining tubes (standard blanks) in same manner except replace oxidizing reagent with 3 mL 15% NaOH solution.

To each of 4 or more similar tubes, add 5 mL assay solution. Treat these tubes in same manner as directed for tubes containing standard solution (including addition of 1.5 g NaCl or KCl).

After isobutyl alcohol has been added to all tubes shake again ca 2 min. Centrifuge tubes at low speed until clear supernate can be obtained from each. Pipet or decant ca 10 mL isobutyl alcohol extract (upper layer) from each tube into cell for measurement of thiochrome fluorescence.

J. Thiochrome Fluorescence Measurement

Measure fluorescence of isobutyl alcohol extract from oxidized assay solution and call this reading "U". Measure fluorescence of extract from assay solution which has been treated with 3 mL 15% NaOH solution (assay blank) and call this reading "b". Measure fluorescence of extract from standard solution, which has been treated with 3 mL 15% NaOH solution (standard blank) and call this reading "d".

Thiamine·HCl, mg/L "as fed" formula = $[(U - b)/(S - d)] \times [15/(A \times 1000)] \times R$

where U = reading of assay sample; b = reading of assay sample blank; S = reading of standard sample; d = reading of standard sample blank; R = reconstitution value expressed as weight or volume of sample required to make 1 L "as fed" formula; A = amount of sample, in grams or mL.

K. Notes and Precautions

Thiochrome is stable in isobutyl alcohol but it is desirable to make readings promptly. Ordinarily, delays up to 20 min will not alter results, providing solutions are not exposed to bright daylight.

Duplicate samples simultaneously carried through assay procedure should give values agreeing $\pm 2.5\%$ of mean. Assays of homogenous material made on different days should agree $\pm 5\%$ of mean.

Between readings of thiochrome samples, check photofluorometer with working quinine solution.

Reference: JAOAC **69,** 777(1986).
CAS-67-03-8 (thiamine·HCl)
CAS-59-43-8 (thiamine)

Chapter 35
Tryptophan

35.1

960.46—Vitamin Assays
Microbiological Methods
Final Action

See Chapter 15.1.

35.2

988.15—Tryptophan in Foods and Food and Feed Ingredients
Ion Exchange Chromatographic Method
First Action 1988

A. *Principle*

Protein is hydrolyzed under vacuum with 4.2N NaOH. After pH adjustment and clarification, tryptophan is separated by ion exchange chromatography with measurement of ninhydrin chromophore or by reverse phase liquid chromatography with UV detection.

B. *Apparatus*

(a) *Amino acid analyzer.*—Dionex D-500, or equivalent, operated in accordance with manufacturer's instructions. Column, 50 cm × 1.75 mm id stainless steel, packed with DC5A cation exchange resin (Dionex Corp., 1228 Titan Way, Sunnyvale, CA 94088). Operating conditions: flow rate 8 mL/h. Column temperature: hold at 59° for 0 to 50:00 min, then increase to 65° for 50:00 to 90:00 min. Pump regenerant 0.2N NaOH for 0 to 5:35 min. Elution buffers: Na citrate elution buffer 1, pH 4.25, 0.2N, 5:35 to 50:00 min; then Na citrate elution buffer 2, pH 5.3, 0.14N with 4% 2-Propanol, 50:00 to 90:00 min.

(b) *Modified micro-Kjeldahl flasks.*—25 mL micro-Kjeldahl flasks fitted with 12 mm id × 15 cm long neck. Constrict neck to ca 6 mm id 5 cm above bulb of flask (available as special order from Ace Glass, Inc.). These modifications can be made easily by experienced glass blower.

(c) *LC system.*—Waters 6000 instrument, or equivalent, operated according to manufacturer's instructions. Column: 25 cm × 4.6 mm id stainless steel μBondapak C_{18} (Waters Chromatography Div., Millipore Corp.). Operating conditions: flow rate 1.5 mL/min; mobile phase 0.0085M NaOAc (adjusted to pH 4.0 with CH_3COOH)-methyl alcohol (95 + 5); UV at 280 nm, 0.01 AUFS.

(d) *Vacuum pump.*—Capable of 10 μm (Sargent-Welch DuoSeal Model No. 1400 equipped with diffusion pump head, or equivalent).

(e) *Membrane filter.*—0.45 μm.

C. Reagents

(a) *Water.*—Purified by Milli-Q system (Millipore Corp.), or equivalent. Use throughout method.

(b) *Tryptophan standard solution.*—*(1) Stock solution:* 1 mg/mL. Dissolve 250 mg L-tryptophan (Calbiochem, 10933 N. Torrey Pines Rd, LaJolla, CA 92037) in 100 mL H_2O with 6 drops HCl. Add 3 drops "pHix" buffer preservative (Pierce Chemical Co.), and dilute to 250 mL with H_2O. *(2) Working solution I:* 0.1 mg/ mL. Dilute 10 mL stock solution to 100 mL with H_2O. *(3) Working solution II:* 0.04 mg/mL. Dilute 4 mL stock solution to 100 mL with H_2O. Refrigerate standard solutions when not in use. Prepare solutions fresh monthly.

(c) *Na citrate loading buffer.*—pH 4.25, 0.2N (Pierce Chemical Co.). Filter twice through 0.45 μm filter.

(d) *Na citrate eluting buffer.*—pH 5.3, 0.14N, 4% 2-propanol. Dilute 262 mL pH 4.95 buffer and 40 mL 2-propanol to 1 L with H_2O. Filter twice through 0.45 μm filter.

(e) *Regenerant solution.*—0.2N NaOH with EDTA. Dissolve 32 g NaOH and 3 g Na_2EDTA in H_2O and dilute to 4 L with H_2O. Filter twice through 0.45 μm filter.

D. Preparation of Samples

Grind test sample in centrifugal mill fitted with 1 mm screen, and mix thoroughly. Weigh test portion containing 100 mg protein ($\leq$300 mg) into modified micro-Kjeldahl flask.

(a) *Test samples with >5% lipids.*—Add 10 mL petroleum ether to weighed sample in flask. Swirl gently to mix and sonicate 20 min. Let settle. Centrifuge if necessary. Siphon off as much petroleum ether as possible, taking care not to remove any solids. Evaporate remaining petroleum ether under gentle stream of N. Continue as under *Preparation of Hydrolysates.*

(b) *Test samples with <5% lipids.*—Continue as under *Preparation of Hydrolysates.*

E. Preparation of Hydrolysates

Deaerate 4.2N NaOH by bubbling with N for 10 min. Add 10 mL deaerated 4.2N NaOH to each flask. Add 3 drops 1-octanol. Immediately freeze treated solution in dry ice-ethyl alcohol bath. Then remove flask from bath and evacuate to 10 μm. Turn off vacuum and seal neck of flask at constriction with dual head O/natural gas flame. Place sealed flask in beaker containing H_2O at room temperature until sample solution is melted. Place flask in 110° oven for 20 h.

Let flasks cool to room temperature. Etch neck of each flask with glass knife and break seal by touching white-hot glass rod to etch mark. Tap neck of flask to break off tip into clean 50 mL beaker. Rinse neck of flask with 1 mL pH 4.25 Na citrate buffer solution, collecting rinse in beaker. Quantitatively transfer hydrolysate to same 50 mL beaker, rinsing flask with two 2 mL portions of pH 4.25 Na citrate buffer solution. Neutralize solution with 3.5 mL HCl, and stir vigorously. Adjust pH to 4.25 $\pm$ 0.05.

Quantitatively transfer solution to 25 mL volumetric flask, and dilute to volume with H_2O. Pour into 40 mL centrifuge tube and centrifuge 20 min at 1150 × *g*. Filter supernate through glass fiber paper (Whatman GF/A). Transfer filtrate to centrifuge tube and centrifuge 10 min at 23 000 × *g*.

F. Determination

Load 40 μL test or standard solution into amino acid analyzer. Operate system according to manufacturer's instructions. Inject standards at beginning and end of run and after every 5 or 6 test solutions.

For LC separation, inject 15 μL test or standard solution. Measure *A* at 280 nm.

G. Calculations

Measure peak areas for tryptophan in test samples and standards. Calculate % tryptophan as follows:

$$\text{Tryptophan, g/100 g} = [(PA/PA') \times C \times (V/W)] \times 100$$

where PA and PA' = peak areas of sample and standard, respectively; C = g standard/mL; V = volume of final dilution, mL; W = weight sample, g.

Reference: JAOAC **71,** 603(1988).
CAS-73-22-3 (L-tryptophan)

Chapter 36
Vitamin A

36.1   **974.29—Vitamin A in Mixed Feeds, Premixes, and Foods**
Colorimetric Method
First Action 1974

(Not applicable to products containing provitamin A [carotene] as predominant source of vitamin A activity nor to high potency vitamin A concentrates used for feed, premix, and food manufacture.)

A. Apparatus

(**a**) *Photoelectric colorimeter.*—Evelyn or similar low-light transmitting colorimeter or spectrophotometer with direct-reading deflecting-type galvanometer and optical mechanism or filter for 620 nm wavelength (vitamin A) and 440 nm (carotene). Use matched absorption tubes. Instrument providing linearity between *A* and concentration is preferable.

(**b**) *Carr-Price reagent dispenser.*—9 or 10 mL all-glass apparatus with 3–4 mm diameter opening for rapid reagent delivery. Hypodermic syringe, pipet, automatic pipet, or glass cylinder may be used. Keep apparatus clean and moisture-free.

(**c**) *Chromatographic tubes.*—(*1*) *For margarine and butter.*—Join 9 × 100–120 mm glass tube to 20 × 40–50 mm reservoir at 1 end and 5 × 60 mm tube, fitted into stopper, at other end. (*2*) *For other products.*—18 (ca 12 mm id) × 200 mm glass tube sealed to 5 × 100 mm tube.

(**d**) *Eluate receiver.*—Fraction collector, or 100 mL lipless graduate fitted with 2-hole stopper, with stem of chromatographic tube inserted through one hole and bent glass tube connected to vacuum source through other. Use H_2O aspirator for vacuum.

(**e**) *Alkaline digestion (hydrolysis) apparatus.*—H_2O-cooled refluxing apparatus connected to *long-neck* Ts boiling flask, 250 or 500 mL. Calibrate at convenient volume in neck (e.g., 250 mL flask at 260 mL). Heat on boiling H_2O or steam bath, or hot plate with magnetic stirrer. For margarine and butter use 125 mL long-neck boiling flask calibrated at convenient volume in neck (e.g., 135 or 140 mL).

(**f**) *Extraction apparatus.*—50–60 mL heavy duty centrifuge tube, glass-stoppered or screw-cap *with Teflon liner* (check for leakage). For extracting larger volume needed for low potency samples, use 125 or 250 mL separator (no rubber stoppers). For margarine and butter, use special 65 mL centrifuge tube available from Kontes Glass Co. as Cat. No. K411050-9018, special no caps, with Teflon-lined caps Cat. No. K410120-1024, or from Lab Glass, Inc., 1172 N West Blvd, Vineland, NJ 08360, Cat. No. 45212-type tube, special order, length 165 mm.

(**g**) *Ultraviolet light.*—Longwave, 360 nm. Use *only* low-intensity lamp.

(**h**) *Evaporation assemblies.*—Modify 2 arms of Y-tube to U-shape, and attach stoppers wrapped with tinfoil or Teflon ribbon (pipe seal). Connect top arm to H_2O aspirator. Use back-flow safety bottle, and manometer or gage for measuring vacuum, and 2-way stopcock in system to open and close vacuum. Heat colorimeter tubes containing ≤10 mL vitamin A solution, attached 2 at a time to apparatus, in H_2O

bath at 60–65°, shaking gently to prevent bumping and speed evaporation. Optionally use partial vacuum and N. To concentrate larger volume extract, use simple 50–200 mL vacuum apparatus consisting of 3-way stopcock, single arm to flask, second to vacuum through trap, and third sealed to small vertical reservoir made from test tube for adding solvent when vacuum is broken, or use rotary evaporation apparatus.

B. Reagents

(*Caution: See Appendix* for safety notes on distillation, toxic solvents, flammable solvents, chloroform, and hexane.)

(**a**) *Adsorbent.*—Alumina, neutral, activity grade 1 (No. A-950, Fisher Scientific). Place 5 g H_2O in small glass-stoppered bottle, add 95 g alumina, and mix by shaking until no lumps are observed. Let stand and cool ≥2 h before use. Adjust activity if necessary as in **974.29C**. Store in small, well filled, tightly closed bottles. Moisture content must be controlled; do not expose original or prepared alumina to air.

(**b**) *Chloroform.*—Reagent grade. If not clear, purify by distillation, discarding first and last 10%. Discard distilled $CHCl_3$ after 1 week.

(**c**) *Hexane.*—Reagent, or high quality, commercial grade, redistilled from all-glass apparatus, saving 64–68° fraction. Must be free of alcohols, esters, and ketones.

(**d**) *Alcohol.*—95%. SDA No. 3-A, or No. 30; aldehyde-free by Schiff's test.

(**e**) *Acetone in hexane solution.*—4 and 15%. Dilute reagent grade acetone with hexane, (**c**).

(**f**) *Solution for removing antimony trichloride from colorimeter tubes.*—Wash tubes with HCl, or soak in 10% Rochelle salt solution to which small amount detergent is added. Wash thoroughly in hot detergent solution.

(**g**) *Potassium hydroxide solution.*—Dissolve 70 g reagent grade KOH in 70 mL H_2O, mix, and cool. Prepare fresh each time.

(**h**) *Color reagents.*—(*1*) *Antimony trichloride (Carr-Price reagent).*—20%. (*Caution:* $SbCl_3$ is toxic and corrosive; avoid contact.) Use reagent grade $SbCl_3$ crystals from unopened, tightly sealed bottle. Do not use if bottle contains fluids or colored products, or if crystals are moist and sticky. Add 100 g $SbCl_3$ crystals to $CHCl_3$ and dilute to 500 mL. Warm and shake to dissolve. Cool, and add 15 mL Ac_2O. If solution is not clear, filter, centrifuge, or let settle and decant. Work rapidly with minimum exposure of crystals or prepared reagent to atmosphere. Reagent is stable ≥2 months when stored in tight glass-stoppered brown bottle. (*2*) *Trifluoroacetic acid (TFA) solution.*—Prepare 1 + 2 (volume/volume) solution of CF_3COOH (Eastman Kodak Co.) in $CHCl_3$, CH_2Cl_2, or $C_2H_2Cl_2$. Prepare calibration curve as in **974.29F(d)**, with specific combination used for samples. Discard after 1 week.

(**i**) *Vitamin A reference solution.*—Use USP Reference Standard Solution which contains crystalline all-*trans* retinyl acetate in cottonseed oil, equivalent to 30 mg retinol (vitamin A alcohol)/g oil (or as stated when purchased).

(**j**) *Carotene reference crystals.*—Pure α- and β-carotene are available from Sigma Chemical Co. Crystals should dissolve in hexane without residue and have characteristic spectrophotometeric curve. Determine concentration as in **941.15D**, using spectrophotometer.

941.15D (Carotenes in Fresh Plant Materials and Silages, Spectrophotometric Method)
D. Determination
Determine *A* of solution as soon as possible with spectrophotometer at 436 nm or with instrument having suitable filter system, such as Klett photo-meter with No. 44 filter, or Evelyn photoelectric colorimeter with 440 nm filter. Calibrate these instruments first with solutions of high purity β-carotene as shown by characteristic absorption curve (J. Biol.

Chem. **144,** 21(1942)). Prepare calibration chart and convert *A* of solution to be determined to carotene concentration from chart.

When determinations are made with properly calibrated spectrophotometer at 436 nm,

$$C = (A \times 454)/(196 \times L \times W)$$

where *C* = concentration carotene (mg/lb) in original sample, *L* = cell length in cm, and *W* = g sample/mL final dilution. Report results as mg *β*-carotene/lb. Multiply by 2.2 to give ppm or by 1667 to give International Units/lb.

References: Ind. Eng. Chem. Anal. Ed. **13,** 600(1941); **15,** 18(1943); **16,** 513(1944); **19,** 170(1947). J. Biol. Chem. **164,** 2(1946). JAOAC **25,** 573, 886(1942); **26,** 77(1943); **27,** 542(1944); **28,** 563(1945); **29,** 18(1946); **30,** 412(1947); **31,** 459, 621, 623, 633, 776(1948); **32,** 480, 766, 775, 804(1949); **33,** 647(1950); **34,** 387, 460(1951); **35,** 736, 826(1952); **36,** 857(1953); **37,** 753, 756, 880, 887, 894(1954); **38,** 694(1955); **39,** 139(1956); **40,** 865(1957); **41,** 600(1958); **42,** 528(1959); **45,** 219(1962); **48,** 168(1965); **53,** 181, 186(1970).
CAS-36-88-4 (carotene)

C. Adsorption Column

Place *small* glass wool or cotton plug at bottom of chromatographic tube. Pack with adsorbent added in small portions, tamping lightly, to height 5–6 cm. (Vacuum helps in packing.) Top with 0.5 cm powdered, anhydrous Na_2SO_4, level, and pack lightly. Use immediately; do not expose to air flow.

Test column for recovery of vitamin A as follows: Hydrolyze and extract 100–200 mg USP Vitamin A Reference Standard as in **974.29F(a)(2)** and **(b)**. Prepare solution to contain 30–40 *μ*g extracted vitamin A and 50–100 *μ*g carotene, diluted to 15 mL with hexane. Wash prepared column with 20 mL hexane and adjust vacuum (only slight vacuum required) for elution rate of ca 2 drops/s. Add vitamin A-carotene mixture before top of column runs dry. Elute carotene with 4% acetone in hexane (20–30 mL normally required). Locate vitamin A band by brief inspection with UV light. Band should be ≤2 cm below top of alumina. (*Caution:* Avoid looking at radiations. Use only low-intensity UV lamp.)

Elute vitamin A with 15% acetone in hexane (30–35 mL normally required). Inspect last few mL eluate for vitamin A fluorescence. If necessary, elute with more solvent until fluorescence no longer is observed in eluate. If vitamin A elutes too slowly, prepare adsorbent using 1–2% more H_2O, **974.29B(a)**, and test again; if vitamin A elutes too rapidly, use less H_2O. Evaporate suitable aliquot of eluate to dryness under vacuum or N, add 1 mL $CHCl_3$ to dissolve residue, and determine vitamin A as in **974.29F(d)**. Compare result with that for hydrolyzed vitamin A not chromatographed. Recovery should be ≥90%.

D. Standardization

Determine blank on all reagents, including cottonseed oil. *A* of blank should be almost 0.

(**a**) *Preparation of standard vitamin A curve.*—Cut tip from capsule containing USP Reference Standard Solution of vitamin A and express oil into small tared beaker or watch glass. Weigh accurately. Transfer oil to volumetric flask and dilute to volume with $CHCl_3$. Use solution as soon as possible; discard after 8 h. Work in subdued light or use low-actinic glassware. Make ≥5 dilutions of vitamin A solution with $CHCl_3$ so that 1 mL aliquots treated as in **974.29F(d)** give *T* in 20–85% range (*A*, 0.7–0.07) at 620 nm. Plot *T* or *A* against *μ*g vitamin A. If plot of *A* is straight line, factor may be calculated for determining vitamin A in samples.

(**b**) *Preparation of standard carotene curve.*—Prepare series of dilutions of carotene in hexane. Plot A at 440 nm against μg carotene. Use curve or factor to determine carotene concentration of samples.
(**c**) *Determination of correction factor for yellow pigment in vitamin A eluate.*—Monohydroxy carotenoids (e.g., cryptoxanthol) elute with hydrolyzed vitamin A (vitamin A alcohol). Correct for pigment when present in more than traces, as follows: Hydrolyze 30–40 g ground yellow corn as in **974.29F(a)(***1***)**. Extract 50 mL solution with two 50 mL portions hexane in separator. Wash extract with H_2O, dry with anhydrous Na_2SO_4, and concentrate to 15–20 mL. Chromatograph as in **974.29F(c)**, and save fraction eluting with 15% acetone in hexane. Make $\geq$5 dilutions so that A values at 440 nm are in 0.1–0.6 range (concentrate solution if necessary). Evaporate 10 mL of each solution in colorimeter tubes as in **974.29A(h)**, dissolve residue in 1 mL $CHCl_3$, and develop and read blue color at 620 nm as in **974.29F(d)**. Plot A at 440 nm against A at 620 nm. Use this curve to calculate A of carotenoid pigment-$SbCl_3$ (or TFA reagent) product in vitamin A determination at 620 nm, based on A of carotenoid at 440 nm. If plot is linear, calculate factor to correct for vitamin A equivalent to pigment in vitamin A determination.

E. Storage and Preparation of Sample

(**a**) *Dry mixed feed and premixes.*—Collect 600–800 g bulk sample. Refrigerate in dark in tightly closed glass or plastic containers. Immediately before analysis, warm to room temperature, grind entire sample so that $\geq$95% passes No. 20 sieve, mix by rolling on paper, or by equivalent method, regrind, and remix. (Grinding helps fracture and disperse high-potency beadlet-type vitamin A products in sample.) Sample, avoiding loss of fine particles. Some high-potency products (e.g., $\geq$30 μg vitamin A/g) containing stabilized vitamin A are sampled better if diluted with freshly ground cereal grain before initial grinding and sampling. Do not store ground sample >1 week.
(**b**) *Foods.*—Proceed as in (**a**), except bulk sample of 400 g is enough for products not containing stabilized vitamin A. Sticky pastries, prepared drink mixes, canned pet foods, etc., may require special sampling, e.g., use of sections of crushed pastry, individual pack of food, or as directed for official tests.
(**c**) *Liquid feed supplements and premixes.*—Store in cool place, but at $\geq$8°, in tightly closed glass or plastic containers. Warm to 35–40° immediately before analysis. Mix thoroughly by repeated pouring or stirring before sampling.
(**d**) *Margarine and butter.*—Store in refrigerator. Do not expose to light or heat. Just before analysis, soften 2 or more 0.25 lb (100 g) sticks, or equivalent, to be able to cut lengthwise. Remove sample from each piece by cutting small sections at random locations, or by pushing plastic syringe, with end cut off and beveled, into cut sticks at random locations. Prepare tub margarine by making 2 or 3 horizontal cuts and sampling resulting slabs. Do not mix butter or margarine before sampling. Mixing causes H_2O to separate from some samples which cannot be worked back in. To retain sample, wrap without mixing and refrigerate.

F. Determination

(Work in subdued light; avoid high laboratory temperature. Complete all steps of method as rapidly as consistent with careful following of directions. Use explosion-proof centrifuge when centrifuging solvent containing ether or hexane.)
(*1*) *For products containing less than 5000 USP units vitamin A/lb* (ca 1500 μg/lb or 3000 μg/kg), weigh $\geq$40 g sample prepared as in **974.29E**, into 500 mL long-neck boiling flask. (*2*) *For products containing 5000–20,000 unit/lb,* use 20–40 g sample and 250–500 mL flask. (*3*) *For products containing 20,000–80,000 unit/lb,* use 10–20 g sample and 250 mL flask. (*4*) *For margarine and butter,* weigh 10.0 g sample into 125 mL boiling flask.

To low-fat products, add 1 g *fresh* cottonseed or peanut oil to boiling flask before alkaline digestion. Proceed as in (**a**)(*1*) or (*2*).

(**a**) *Alkaline digestion (hydrolysis).*—(*1*) *Mixed dry samples, premixes, and semimoist foods.*—Add volume (mL) alcohol equal to 4 times weight (g) sample, but ≥ 40 mL. Mix thoroughly. Slowly add, with mixing, volume KOH solution equal to g sample, but ≥ 10 mL. Place stirring bar in flask. Reflux 30 min at ca 2 drops/s. Agitate flasks ≥ 3 times during refluxing to disperse any aggregates formed, or use hot plate with magnetic stirring. (Hand agitation with stirring bar gives better dispersion on some samples than does magnetic stirring.) Cool rapidly to room temperature. Add alcohol-H_2O solution (3 + 1) up to 20–30 mL below calibration mark. Shake to mix thoroughly. Add alcohol-H_2O solution to calibration mark, and mix again. (Use size flask to have vitamin A concentration convenient for further steps of method; do not over-dilute.) Let suspended matter settle. After standing, if solution in flask is single, homogeneous phase, proceed to (**b**); if not, *see* (**b**)(*2*). (Sticky film on walls of flask when sample has high sugar content apparently causes no difficulty if contents are well mixed.)

(*2*) *Liquid samples (supplements containing molasses, liquid breakfast drinks, etc.).*—If sample is viscous, mix thoroughly with equal volume warm H_2O. Add slowly, with mixing, volume (mL) KOH solution equal to weight (g) sample. Add slowly, with mixing, volume (mL) alcohol equal to 4 times weight (g) sample. Digest sample as in (*1*), beginning with "Place stirring bar in flask."

(*3*) *For margarine and butter.*—Add volume alcohol and KOH solution, reflux, cool, and dilute as in (**a**)(*1*). Diluted hydrolyzed sample should be homogeneous and clear, with little if any material separating on standing.

(**b**) *Extraction.*—(*1*) *For products containing more than 1500 μg vitamin A/lb.*—Transfer 5.0–15.0 mL solution, depending on vitamin A concentration, free of suspended matter, to the 50–60 mL centrifuge tube. Add 2 mL H_2O for each 5 mL solution, and add 20.0 mL hexane. Extract vitamin A by shaking vigorously ≥ 1 min. Let phases separate and centrifuge briefly. If amount of vitamin A in extract is < 1 mg and if hexane layer is clear, with only traces of yellow color, draw lower layer from bottom of centrifuge tube with pipet and filler bulb, and discard; if hexane layer is yellow, proceed to (**c**). Wash extract in tube once with 20 mL H_2O, let layers separate, and centrifuge briefly. Transfer 1.0–10.0 mL hexane extract, as required for satisfactory color development, to colorimeter tube and proceed to vitamin A determination, (**d**). Avoid loss of hexane by evaporation. If vitamin A recovery is low, again extract solution containing vitamin A, and combine extracts before washing.

(*2*) *For solutions of (a)(1) separating into two liquid phases.*—Shake vigorously and remove portion for extraction before separation occurs, and proceed as in (*1*), or transfer total contents, without dilution with alcohol-H_2O, to separator. Add volume (mL) H_2O equal to 2 times weight (g) sample; extract once with volume (mL) hexane equal to 3 times weight (g) sample and again with 2 volumes hexane. Combine extracts and wash with two 100 mL portions H_2O, or until free of alkali. Dilute to smallest suitable volume. Centrifuge portion, or dry with anhydrous Na_2SO_4 and dilute to previous volume. Proceed to (**c**) or transfer 1.0–10.0 mL to colorimeter tube and proceed to (**d**) if no pigments are present.

(*3*) *For products containing less than 1500 μg vitamin A/lb that require extraction of more than 15 mL hydrolyzed solution, or those with measurable carotenoid pigments.*—Use separator, increasing H_2O and hexane volumes proportionally. Extract twice, combine extracts, dilute to volume, wash, and centrifuge or dry as in (*2*). Proceed to (**c**), or transfer 1.0–10.0 mL to colorimeter tube and proceed to (**d**) if no pigments are present.

(*4*) *For margarine and butter.*—Transfer 10.0 mL solution to 65 mL special centrifuge tube, add 10.0 mL H_2O, and mix. Add 30 mL ether-hexane (2 + 1). Extract by shaking vigorously ≥ 1 min. Centrifuge briefly to hasten separation. Draw lower layer from bottom of centrifuge tube with pipet and filler bulb and transfer to another centrifuge tube. Add 15 mL ether-hexane (2 + 1) and shake ≥1 min. Centrifuge briefly. Draw off upper layer completely and combine with solution in first centrifuge tube.

Wash combined extracts with 15 mL cool ether-saturated H_2O. Centrifuge briefly, draw off and discard lower wash solution. Repeat washing and centrifuging. Mark on centrifuge tube position of upper and lower menisci of ether-hexane layer, for volume correction due to loss of solvent.

If yellow pigments are not present, remove 10.0 mL upper layer containing vitamin A and proceed as in **974.29F(d)**, beginning "Evaporate solution as in **974.29A(h)** . . ." If yellow pigments are present, remove 30.0 mL upper layer containing vitamin A and carotene and proceed as in **974.29F(c)**. Correct results for volume changes due to loss of solvent during extraction.

(c) *Chromatography.*—If yellow pigments are present, chromatograph sample. If possible, use aliquot containing 25–60 μg vitamin A in 10–15 mL hexane extract. Concentrate portion hexane extract under vacuum, **974.29A(h)**, if necessary to obtain suitable vitamin A concentration. Wash packed column with 20 mL hexane, and add extract containing vitamin A just before top of column runs dry. Elute at ca 2 drops/s. Elute carotene with 4% acetone in hexane, and vitamin A with 15% acetone in hexane as in **974.29C**. Cryptoxanthin and related pigments elute with vitamin A.

(d) *Colorimetry.*—If carotene was separated during chromatography, determine concentration as in **941.15D**.

If vitamin A eluate in 15% acetone-hexane solution contains yellow pigment, read T (or A) as carotene with 440 nm filter. Calculate correction, **974.29D(c)**, to apply to A of blue-color reaction with vitamin A, using necessary dilution factor if 1:10 volume at 620 and 440 nm was not used.

Evaporate solution as in **974.29A(h)** under vacuum in H_2O bath at 60–65°. Dissolve residue in 1 mL $CHCl_3$. Adjust colorimeter to 100% T (or 0% A) at 620 nm, using 1 mL $CHCl_3$ and measured volume (9 or 10 mL) $SbCl_3$ (or TFA) reagent. (This point must remain constant for series of determinations; readjust as required.) Place tube containing 1 mL $CHCl_3$ solution of vitamin A in instrument. Add measured volume $SbCl_3$ (or TFA) reagent in 1–2 s. Read T (or A) as first transitory pause point (T should be in 20–85% range). Read quickly; color begins to fade and T increases slowly after 3–5 s. Instrument *cannot* be adjusted to make reading after $SbCl_3$ (or TFA) reagent is added. Examine tube contents within short time; solution should be blue, without turbidity, and blue should fade.

Determine recovery factor, R, for vitamin A determination by adding known amount vitamin A to samples (or blank feeds or foods when available) of general types analyzed, carrying analysis through entire method.

(e) *Calculation of vitamin A content.*—

$$\mu g \text{ Vitamin A/g} = (C_u - C_c) \times [V/(W \times R)]$$

or

$$\mu g \text{ Vitamin A/lb} = (C_u - C_c) \times V \times [454/(W \times R)]$$

where C_u = uncorrected concentration vitamin A from curve or factor; C_c = correction for yellow pigment in vitamin A eluate; V = final volume sample extract; W = g sample; and R = recovery factor for vitamin A.

(*Note*: If solids are present in flask after hydrolysis, results may be increased slightly. Ignore volume of solids unless sample is large and volume solution in flask is relatively small, in which case difference could be ≤5%. Correction for volume of solids is difficult because some samples leave considerable unhydrolyzed residue and others, none. Maximum correction is based on 10 g feed reducing volume in hydrolysis flask by 3 mL. Apply estimated correction, if necessary.)

(f) *To convert vitamin A and carotene contents in margarine and butter to vitamin A units and retinol equivalents.*—

$$\text{Vitamin A activity in units} = (\mu\text{g vitamin A} \times 3.33)$$
$$+ (\mu\text{g carotene} \times 1.67)$$

$$\text{Vitamin A activity in retinol equivalents}$$
$$= (\mu\text{g vitamin A}) + (\mu\text{g carotene/6})$$

References: JAOAC **33**, 615(1950); **34**, 370(1951); **35**, 706(1952); **36**, 812(1953); **37**, 742(1954); **38**, 692, 695(1955); **39**, 126(1956); **40**, 865(1957); **41**, 593(1958); **42**, 422, 520(1959); **43**, 30(1960); **49**, 250(1966); **57**, 897, 903(1974); **63**, 468(1980). Analyst **89**, 7(1964).
CAS-68-26-8 (vitamin A)

36.2 992.04—Vitamin A (Retinol Isomers) in Milk and Milk-Based Infant Formula
Liquid Chromatographic Method
First Action 1992

(Applicable to determination of all-*trans*-retinol and 13-*cis*-retinol in milk and milk-based infant formula.)
(Work in subdued artificial light)
(*Caution: See Appendix* for precautions on "Distillation, Extraction, and Evaporations," "Sodium and Potassium Hydroxides," "Safe Handling of Organic Solvents," "Diethyl Ether," and "Peroxides.")

Method Performance
    Mean recovery = 2730.3 IU vitamin A/L infant formula
    s_r = 98.8; s_R = 265.4; RSD$_r$ = 3.62%; RSD$_R$ = 9.72%

A. Principle

Sample is digested with ethanolic potassium hydroxide (KOH), and vitamin A is extracted into diethyl ether—hexane. Hexadecane is added to prevent destruction of the vitamin after evaporation. Residue is dissolved in heptane, and vitamin A isomers, all-*trans*-retinol and 13-*cis*-retinol, are determined by liquid chromatography on silica column.

B. Apparatus

(a) *Alkaline digestion apparatus.*—100 mL volumetric flask with Ts stopper (select flask with graduation mark low in neck), magnetic stirrer, and 25 mm × 8 mm (volume less than 1.5 mL) stirring bar.
(b) *Extraction apparatus.*—15 mL stoppered centrifuge tubes, Pasteur pipets with rubber bulbs, and water bath with clamps for evaporation of solvents under nitrogen.
(c) *Liquid chromatographic system (LC).*—Injector capable of 100 µL injections, pump capable of 3000 psi, 15 cm × 4.5 mm column packed with 3 µm silica (Apex 3 micron silica, Jones Chromatography, Columbus, OH is suitable), detector capable of measuring absorbance at 340 nm, and data recording system (chart recorder or integrator).
(d) *Spectrophotometer.*—Capable of measuring absorbance at 324.5 nm.

C. Reagents

(a) *Ethanolic pyrogallol solution.*—2% pyrogallol (1,3,5-trihydroxybenzene, 98%, Aldrich is suitable source) in 95% ethanol or SDA 3—A.

(b) *Ethanolic KOH solution.*—10% (w/v) KOH in 90% ethanol (prepared from absolute ethanol or SDA 3—A).

(c) *Extraction solution.*—Hexane–diethyl ether (85 + 15), HPLC grade hexane. Prepare fresh daily. Store ether in metal container under nitrogen.

(d) *Hexadecane solution.*—1 mL hexadecane in 100 mL hexane.

(e) *Mobile phase solution.*—Heptane–isopropanol, HPLC grade reagents, proportions are adjusted to obtain retention times specified in **D**, System Suitability Test.

(f) *Standard oil solution.*—*(1)* All-*trans*-retinol.—Dissolve 100 mg crystalline all-*trans*-retinol in 50 g cottonseed oil, stirring under nitrogen with magnetic stirrer. Store all-*trans*-retinol oil solution under nitrogen in low-actinic airtight container at 4°. Weigh ($\pm$ 0.1 mg) 3 drops of oil solution (ca 50 mg) into each of three 50 mL volumetric flasks; dissolve and dilute to volume with isopropanol. Read solution absorbance at least monthly at 324.5 nm, using 0.1% solution of cottonsed oil in isopropanol in reference cell. Calculate concentration of all-*trans*-retinol (ng/mL) in solutions by multiplying absorbance by 5460. Calculate mean content of oil (C_t) in ng/mg from weight of oil used.

(2) 13-cis-Retinol.—Prepare as in *(1)*, reading absorbance at 326 nm, and calculating concentration of 13-*cis*-retinol in solution by multiplying absorbance by 5930.

(g) *Standard working solutions.*—*(1)* All-*trans*-retinol.—Weigh ($\pm$ 0.1 mg) 3 drops of all-*trans*-retinol oil solution into each of three 50 mL volumetric flasks. Dissolve and dilute to volume with heptane containing 0.5% isopropanol. Prepare daily. Calculate concentration of all-*trans*-retinol (1–2 μg/mL) in standard working solution from weight of oil solution. Inject all-*trans*-retinol standard working solution to calibrate LC. Prepare standard solutions containing 50, 500, and 1000 ng/mL all-*trans*-retinol to verify linearity of standard curve by making appropriate dilutions of standard working solution in heptane containing 0.5% isopropanol. Verify by LC that ratio of all-*trans*-retinol to 13-*cis*-retinol in these solutions is >30.

(2) 13-cis-Retinol.—Prepare as *(1)*.

D. System Suitability Test

Inject 100 μL standard working solutions into LC. Adjust amount of isopropanol (1–5%) in LC solution, **C(e)**, and flow rate (1–2 mL/min) until 13-*cis*-retinol and all-*trans*-retinol elute ca 4.5 and 5.5 min, respectively. LC measurements should be <2% relative standard deviation when 100 ng/mL all-*trans*-retinol standard working solution is injected.

E. Digestion and Extraction of Sample

(a) *Powdered infant formula, powdered milk.*—Weigh 140 g powder into 1 L volumetric flask, add H_2O (boiled and cooled) almost to mark, flush with nitrogen, stopper flask, and mix. When foam collapses, dilute to volume with H_2O and mix.

(b) *Liquid infant formula, milk.*—Pipet 20 mL concentrated formula plus 20 mL H_2O, or 40 mL ready-to-use formula, or 40 mL preparation obtained in **(a)**, or 40 mL milk, into 100 mL digestion flask. Add 10 mL ethanolic pyrogallol solution, **C(a)**, and 40 mL ethanolic KOH solution, **C(b)**. Add ethanolic pyrogallol solution until liquid is ca 1 cm below graduation mark, stopper, shield contents from light by covering flask with Al foil, and stir 18 h. Dilute to volume with ethanolic pyrogallol solution, stopper, and stir to mix. Pipet 3 mL of digestate, using pipet filler safety bulb, into 15 mL centrifuge tube. Add 2 mL H_2O and 7 mL extraction solution, **C(c)**, and vortex 30 s, using gloves and safety glasses. Centrifuge 5 min at 2000 rpm. Transfer hexane (upper) layer, using Pasteur pipet with rubber bulb, to 25 mL volumetric flask. Transfer as much of hexane layer as possible with no more than trace of aqueous digest. Repeat extraction step 2× with 7 mL portions of extraction solvent, and pool hexane extracts in the 25 mL volumetric flask. Add 1 mL hexadecane solution, **C(d)**, and dilute to volume with hexane. Invert flask to mix, and then let stand ≥5 min to allow any aqueous digest to settle.

Pipet 15 mL of clear solvent from center of flask, avoiding contaminating aqueous digest, into 15 mL centrifuge tube, and evaporate under nitrogen. Dissolve residue immediately in 0.5 mL heptane, and transfer to sealable vials for LC determination.

F. Determination

Inject 100 μL standard working solutions into LC. Inject 100 μL sample extract, **E**. Measure peak areas for 13-*cis*- and all-*trans*-retinol.

G. Calculation

Calculate all-*trans*-retinol concentration, V_t, (ng/mL milk or diluted formula) as follows:

$$V_t = A_t/A_{st} \times W_t \times C_t \times 1/50 \times 25/15 \times 100/3 \times 1/2 \times 1/40$$
$$V_t = A_t/A_{st} \times W_t \times C_t \times 5/360$$

where A_t = peak area, all-*trans*-retinol in sample; A_{st} = peak area, all-*trans*-retinol in standard; W_t = weight, mg, oil solution used to prepare working standard solution; and C_t = concentration, ng/mg, all-*trans*-retinol in oil solution.

Calculate 13-*cis*-retinol concentration, V_c, (ng/mL milk or diluted formula) as follows:

$$V_c = A_c/A_{sc} \times W_c \times C_c \times 5/360$$

where A_c = peak area, 13-*cis*-retinol in sample; A_{sc} = peak area, 13-*cis*-retinol in standard; W_c = weight, mg, oil solution used to prepare working standard solution; and C_c = concentration, ng/mg, 13-*cis*-retinol in oil solution.

Ref.: J. AOAC Int.
CAS-68-26-8 (vitamin A)

36.3   992.06—Vitamin A (Retinol) in Milk-Based Infant Formula
Liquid Chromatographic Method
First Action 1992

(Applicable milk-based infant formulas containing >500 IU vitamin A per reconstituted quart.)

Method Performance (milk-based liquid, ready-to-feed, 3 manufacturers)
Mean recovery = 2658 IU vitamin A/L infant formula
s_r = 129.6; s_R = 279.0; RSD_r = 4.9%; RSD_R = 10.5%

A. Principle

Vitamin A in samples of infant formula is saponified, partitioned with organic solvent, separated from sample matrix, and quantified by liquid chromatography.

B. Apparatus

(a) *Liquid chromatograph (LC).*—Capable of pressures up to 3000 psi, with injector capable of 100 μL injections. Operating conditions: eluent flow rate 1.5 ± 0.2 mL/min; temperature ambient.

(b) *Detector.*—Capable of measuring absorbance at 336 nm, with sensitivity 0.1 AUFS.

(c) *Column.*—4.6 mm id × 15 cm stainless steel, packed with 5 μm silica-based cyano group stationary phase (Sepralyte CN, Analytichem International, Harbor City, CA is suitable).

(d) *Spectrophotometer.*—Capable of measuring absorbance at 325 nm.

(e) *Shaking water bath.*—Capable of maintaining 70 ± 2°, variable speed capable of 60 oscillations/min, with sample area ca 11 × 14" (Precision Scientific Model 25 is suitable).

(f) *Glassware.*—*(1)* 125 mL separatory funnels. *(2)* 5 mL volumetric flasks. *(3)* 100 mL low-actinic volumetric flasks.

C. Reagents

(a) *Mobile phase solution.*—Hexane–isopropyl alcohol (100 + 0.25, v/v), HPLC grade solvents. Degas 2–5 min under vacuum.

(b) *Wash solution.*—H_2O–absolute ethanol (3 + 2, v/v).

(c) *Extraction solution.*—Hexane–methylene chloride (3 + 1, v/v), HPLC grade solvents.

(d) *Saponification solution.*—10.5N potassium hydroxide (KOH). Dissolve 673 g KOH in 1 L H_2O.

(e) *Antioxidant solution.*—1% pyrogallol. Dissolve 5.0 g pyrogallol (1,3,5-trihydroxybenzene, 98%, Aldrich is suitable source) in 500 mL absolute ethanol.

(f) *Standard solutions.*—*(1) Stock standard solution.*—10 mg/mL retinyl palmitate in hexane. Quantitatively transfer contents of 1.0 g ampoule of retinyl palmitate (USP Reference Standard) with hexane (HPLC grade) into 100 mL low-actinic volumetric flask, dilute to volume with hexane, and shake well to dissolve. Make fresh every 2 weeks. Store at –20° in explosion-proof freezer when not in use.

(2) Intermediate standard solution.—Pipet 2 mL of stock standard solution, *(1)*, into 250 mL volumetric flask and dilute to volume with hexane.

(3) Working standard solution.—Approx. 1.6 μg/mL retinyl palmitate. Pipet 2 mL intermediate standard solution, *(2)*, into 100 mL low-actinic volumetric flask. Evaporate to dryness under nitrogen. Dissolve residue in antioxidant solution, **C(e)**, and dilute to volume. Prepare fresh daily.

D. Extraction of Standards and Samples

Pipet 10.0 mL working standard solution, **C(f)***(3)*, or sample volume containing ca 20 IU vitamin A activity (10 mL for ready-to-feed formulas) into 150 mL centrifuge tube. Bring sample volume to 10 mL with H_2O, if necessary. To standard tubes, add 10 mL H_2O, 20 mL antioxidant solution, **C(e)**, and 5 mL saponification solution, **C(d)**. To sample tubes, add 30 mL antioxidant solution and 5 mL saponification solution. Cap tubes and swirl briefly to mix. Place tubes in 70° shaking H_2O bath (ca 60 oscillations/min) for 25 min. Remove tubes and place in ice 5 min, or until contents cool to room temperature.

Quantitatively transfer contents to separate 125 mL separatory funnels. Wash remaining sample or standard from tube into funnel with 30 mL H_2O. Pipet 30.0 mL extraction solvent, **C(c)**, into funnel and shake ca 2 min. When layers separate, discard aqueous (lower) layer. Add 30 mL wash solution, **C(b)**, to funnel and shake very gently 30 s, venting frequently. Let phases separate and discard aqueous layer. Repeat wash step 3×. Pipet 20.0 mL portion from funnel to 50 mL tube and evaporate to dryness under nitrogen. Transfer residues quantitatively to separate 5 mL volumetric flasks and dilute to volume with mobile phase solution, **C(a)**.

E. Determination of Standard Concentration

Pipet 2 mL of intermediate standard solution, **C(f)**(2), into 50 mL volumetric flask and dilute to volume with hexane. Transfer portion of this solution into 1 cm cell path length cuvet and measure absorbance at 325 nm. Calculate concentration of working standard solution, C_{std}, as follows:

$$C_{std} = [A_{325}/(2 \times \Sigma \times b)] \times 10^4$$

where A_{325} = absorbance of working standard solution at 325 nm; Σ = 996, extinction coefficient of retinyl palmitate in hexane at 325 nm; and b = 1 cm, cell path length.

F. System Suitability Test

Inject 100 μL of saponified working standard solution into LC. Typical retention times for 13-*cis*-retinol and *trans*-retinol are 7.5 and 9.0 min, respectively. Calculate R factor between 13-*cis*-retinol and *trans*-retinol as follows:

$$R = 2(t_2 - t_1)/(W_1 + W_2)$$

where t_1 and t_2 = retention time measured from injection time to elution time of peak maximum of 13-*cis*-retinol and *trans*-retinol, respectively, and W_1 and W_2 = width of peak measured by extrapolating relatively straight sides to baseline of 13-*cis*-retinol and *trans*-retinol, respectively.

If R factor is <1.3, increase amount of isopropyl alcohol added per liter [mobile phase solution, **C(a)**] by ca 0.05%. Inject saponified working standard solution 5×. Calculate reproducibility of replicate injections in terms of standard deviations (per USP), which should be ≤2%. Typical relative standard deviation values for peak height are ± 1.3%.

G. Liquid Chromatography

Inject 100 μL standard or sample into LC.

H. Calculations

Since 13-*cis* vitamin A palmitate is not readily available, standard curve for all-*trans* vitamin A palmitate is used to determine biological potencies for both, correcting for 13-*cis* vitamin A palmitate, at 0.75 potency relative to all-*trans* vitamin A palmitate. This is based on assumption that relative molar absorptivities of both isomers are virtually equal at 336 nm.

Measure peak areas of *cis*- and *trans*-isomers of retinol in both sample and standard chromatograms. Multiply peak area under 13-*cis* vitamin A palmitate curve by 0.75. Sum the 2 areas to represent total peak area. Calculate IU per reconstituted quart of vitamin A activity (V) as follows:

$$V = (A_{sam}/A_{std}) \times C_{std} \times (1/0.55) \times 946.33$$

where A_{sam} = total peak area of sample; A_{std} = total peak area of standard; C_{std} = concentration of working standard solution, μg/mL; 1/0.55 = IU/μg retinyl palmitate; and 946.33 = mL/quart.

Ref.: J.AOAC Int.
CAS-68-26-8 (vitamin A)

Chapter 37
Vitamin C

37.1   **984.26—Vitamin C (Total) in Food**
Semiautomated Fluorometric Method
First Action 1984
Final Action 1985

A. Apparatus

(**a**) *Automatic analyzer.*—AutoAnalyzer II system equipped with flow scheme shown in Fig. **984.26** (Technicon Corp.).

(**b**) *Fluorometer.*—Aminco fluorocolorimeter equipped with flow cell and 4 watt lamp (SLM Instrument Inc., 810 W. Anthony Dr. Urbana, IL 61801), or equivalent.

(**c**) *Fluorometer filter.*—Primary 7-60, band pass 70% T at 356 nm; secondary Technicon No. 126-0077-01, band pass 40% T at 440 nm, or equivalent.

(**d**) *Rainin pipet.*—Model P-5000 (Rainin Instrument Co., Inc.), or equivalent.

(**e**) *Collection funnels.*—DisPo No. F-7501 (Scientific Products, Inc.), or equivalent.

(**f**) *Plastic cups.*—Falcon No. 4020 (Becton, Dickinson and Co., Oxnard, CA 93030), or equivalent.

(**g**) *Osterizer blender.*—Pulsematic 16 (Scientific Products, Inc.), or equivalent.

(**h**) *Magnetic stirrer.*—Thermolyne (Scientific Products, Inc.), or equivalent.

(**i**) *Mechanical shaker.*—Wrist-action shaker (Burrell Corp.), or equivalent.

(**j**) *Dispensing pipet.*—Kimax No. 37075-F (Ace Glass Co., Inc.), or equivalent.

B. Reagents

(**a**) *Brij solution.*—35% Brij in H_2O (Atlas Chemical, Wilmington, DE 19899).

(**b**) *Extraction solvent.*—4.0% metaphosphoric acid-methyl alcohol (3 + 1, pH 2.1). Prepare fresh weekly.

(**c**) *Wash solution.*—Add 1.5 mL Brij solution to 1 L extraction solvent, and filter.

(**d**) *Dialysate receiving solution.*—1.5 mL Brij solution/L H_2O.

(**e**) *Sodium acetate solutions.*—(*1*) Dissolve 302 g anhydrous sodium acetate in H_2O; dilute to 1 L with H_2O. Add 1.5 mL Brij solution, and filter. (*2*) Prepare solution as in (*1*); adjust pH to that of boric acid solution below (ca 6.9) with HCl.

(**f**) *Boric acid.*—Dissolve 5 g boric acid in 100 mL sodium acetate solution (*1*). Prepare fresh daily.

(**g**) *o-Phenylenediamine hydrochloride.*—0.5 mg/mL. Dissolve 50 mg *o*-phenylenediamine HCl (Eastman Kodak Co., No. 678) and dilute to 100 mL with H_2O. Prepare fresh daily.

(**h**) *Acid-washed Norit.*—Add 1 L 10% HCl (1 + 9) to 200 g Norit Neutral (Fisher Scientific Co., carbon, decolorizing, C-170), heat to bp, and filter with vacuum. Remove cake to large beaker. Add 1 L H_2O, stir, and filter. Repeat washing with H_2O and filtering. Dry overnight at 110–120°.

(**i**) *Norit slurry.*—Add 20 g acid-washed Norit to extraction solvent and dilute to 100 mL. Transfer slurry to 125 mL erlenmeyer equipped with magnetic stirrer apparatus. Mix slurry at rate to maintain homogeneity.

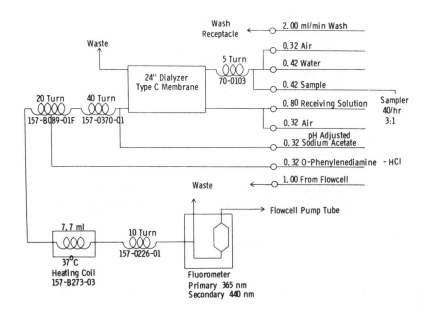

Figure 984.26.—Flow scheme for semiautomated method of analysis for total vitamin C.

(**j**) *Ascorbic acid standards.*—(*1*) *1.0 mg/mL.*—Accurately weigh 100 mg ascorbic acid (Mallinckrodt; stored in desiccator) into 100 mL volumetric flask, dissolve, and dilute to volume with extraction solvent. (*2*) *100 μg/mL.*—Pipet 10 mL of above solution into 100 mL volumetric flask and dilute to volume with extraction solvent. (*3*) *2, 10, 25 μg/mL.*—Pipet 2, 10, and 25 mL 100 μg/mL solution into separate 100 mL volumetric flasks, dilute to volume with extraction solvent.

C. Standard Curve

Add 1 mL (Rainin pipet) Norit slurry (0.2 g Norit) to each working standard solution (2, 10, 25 μg/mL). Shake and transfer contents of each volumetric flask to plastic cups and mechanically shake 10 min. Filter mixture (Whatman 2V), immediately transfer filtrate from DisPo funnels to AutoAnalyzer sampler, and pump through instrument. Adjust recorder so 25 μg/mL standard gives full scale peak. Pump other standard solutions through instrument.

D. Preparation of Sample

(**a**) *Low moisture samples.*—Grind to pass 40 mesh sieve. Accurately weigh portion of sample (maximum weight 5 g) containing ca 1.5 mg ascorbic acid into plastic cup and dispense 100 mL extraction solvent. Add 1 mL Norit slurry, cap, and shake 10 min. Filter and pump filtrate through AutoAnalyzer. Negligible error is introduced by moisture in sample.

(**b**) *High moisture samples (fruits and vegetables).*—Grind sample in blender. Weigh portion of slurry (maximum weight 5 g) containing ca 1.5 mg ascorbic acid into 100 mL volumetric flask and dilute to volume with extraction solvent. Add 1 mL Norit slurry, cap, shake, and transfer contents to cup. Continue as in (**a**), beginning ". . . cap, and shake 10 min."

(**c**) *Dehydroascorbic acid.*—Treat sample as in (**a**) except replace 1 mL Norit slurry with 1 mL extraction solvent.

(**d**) *Blank determination.*—Replace pH-adjusted sodium acetate line with boric acid solution. Pump standards and samples through flow scheme to obtain blank values.

E. Calculation

Plot peak height of standard minus blank vs. concentration. Obtain sample concentration in μg/mL by comparing blank-corrected peak heights for each sample with standard curve. No error is introduced by omitting 1 mL dilution from Norit slurry if it is omitted in both sample and standard calculations. Calculate total vitamin C or dehydroascorbic acid level in original sample as follows:

$$\text{Vitamin C, mg/100 g} = (C/W) \times 10$$

where C = concentration, μg/mL, of ascorbic or dehydroascorbic acid from calibration curve; W = sample weight, g; and 10 is a combined factor taking into account 100 mL extract, level reported per 100 g, and conversion of μg to mg.

Reference: JAOAC **66**, 1371(1983).

37.2   967.21—Vitamin C (Ascorbic Acid) in Vitamin Preparations and Juices
2,6-Dichloroindophenol Titrimetric Method
First Action 1967
Final Action 1968

(Applicable to determination of reduced ascorbic acid. Not applicable in presence of ferrous Fe, stannous Sn, cuprous Cu, SO_2, sulfite, or thiosulfate. *See Note.*)

A. Principle

Ascorbic acid reduces oxidation-reduction indicator dye, 2,6-dichloroindophenol, to colorless solution. At end point, excess unreduced dye is rose pink in acid solution. Vitamin is extracted and titration performed in presence of HPO_3-CH_3COOH or HPO_3-CH_3COOH-H_2SO_4 solution to maintain proper acidity for reaction and to avoid autoxidation of ascorbic acid at high pH.

B. Reagents

(**a**) *Extracting solutions.*—(*1*) *Metaphosphoric acid-acetic acid solution.*—Dissolve, with shaking, 15 g HPO_3 pellets or freshly pulverized stick HPO_3 in 40 mL CH_3COOH and 200 mL H_2O; dilute to ca 500 mL, and filter rapidly through fluted paper into glass-stoppered bottle. (HPO_3 slowly changes to H_3PO_4, but if stored in refrigerator, solution remains satisfactory 7–10 days.) (*2*) *Metaphosphoric acid-acetic acid sulfuric acid solution.*—Proceed as in (*1*), except use 0.3N H_2SO_4 in place of H_2O.

(**b**) *Ascorbic acid standard solution.*—1 mg/mL. Accurately weigh 50 mg USP Ascorbic Acid Reference Standard that has been stored in desiccator away from direct sunlight. Transfer to 50 mL volumetric flask. Dilute to volume *immediately before use* with HPO_3-CH_3COOH solution, (**a**)(*1*).

(**c**) *Indophenol standard solution.*—Dissolve 50 mg 2,6-dichloroindophenol Na salt (Eastman Kodak Co. No. 3463), that has been stored in desiccator over soda lime, in 50 mL H_2O to which has been added 42 mg $NaHCO_3$; shake vigorously, and when dye dissolves, dilute to 200 mL with H_2O. Filter through fluted paper into amber glass-stoppered bottle. Keep stoppered, out of direct sunlight, and store in refrigerator. (Decomposition products that make end point indistinct occur in some batches of dry indophenol and also develop with time in stock solution. Add 5.0 mL extracting solution containing excess ascorbic acid to 15 mL dye reagent. If reduced solution is not practically colorless, discard, and prepare new stock solution. If dry dye is at fault, obtain new supply.)

Transfer three 2.0 mL aliquots ascorbic acid standard solution to each of three 50 mL erlenmeyers containing 5.0 mL HPO_3-CH_3COOH solution, (a)(1). Titrate rapidly with indophenol solution from 50 mL buret until light but distinct rose pink persists ≥5 s. (Each titration should require ca 15 mL indophenol solution, and titrations should check within 0.1 mL.) Similarly titrate 3 blanks composed of 7.0 mL HPO_3-CH_3COOH solution, (a)(1), plus volume H_2O ca equal to volume indophenol solution used in direct titrations. After subtracting average blanks (usually ca 0.1 mL) from standardization titrations, calculate and express concentration of indophenol solution as mg ascorbic acid equivalent to 1.0 mL reagent. Standardize indophenol solution daily with freshly prepared ascorbic acid standard solution.

(d) *Thymol blue pH indicator.*—0.04%. Dissolve 0.1 g indicator by triturating in agate mortar with 10.75 mL 0.02N NaOH and dilute to 250 mL with H_2O. Transition range: 1.2 (red)–2.8 (yellow).

C. Preliminary Test for Appreciable Amount of Basic Substances

Grind representative sample or express contents from capsule and add ca 25 mL HPO_3-CH_3COOH solution, (a)(1). Test pH by placing drop thymol blue pH indicator on pestle or by using spot plate. (pH >1.2 indicates appreciable amounts of basic substances.) For liquid preparations, dilute representative sample ca two-fold with HPO_3-CH_3COOH solution, (a)(1), before testing with indicator.

D. Preparation of Sample Assay Solution

(a) *For dry materials containing no appreciable amount of basic substances.*—Pulverize sample by gentle grinding, add HPO_3-CH_3COOH solution, (a)(1), and triturate until sample is in suspension. Dilute with HPO_3-CH_3COOH solution, (a)(1), to measured volume. Designate this volume as V mL.

(Use ca 10 mL extracting solution/g dry sample. Final solution should contain 10–100 mg ascorbic acid/100 mL.)

(b) *For dry materials containing appreciable amounts of basic substances.*—Pulverize sample by gentle grinding, add HPO_3-CH_3COOH-H_2SO_4 solution, (a)(2), to adjust pH to ca 1.2, and triturate until sample is in suspension. Dilute with HPO_3-CH_3COOH solution, (a)(1), to measured volume. Designate this volume as V mL.

(Use ca 10 mL extracting solution/g dry sample. Final solution should contain 10–100 mg ascorbic acid/100 mL.)

(c) *For liquid materials.*—Take amount of sample containing ca 100 mg ascorbic acid. If appreciable amounts of basic substances are present, adjust pH to ca 1.2 with HPO_3-CH_3COOH-H_2SO_4 solution, (a)(2). Dilute with HPO_3-CH_3COOH solution, (a)(1), to measured volume containing 10–100 mg ascorbic acid/100 mL. Designate this volume as V mL.

(d) *For fruit and vegetable juices.*-Mix thoroughly by shaking to ensure uniform sample, and filter through absorbent cotton or rapid paper. Prepare fresh juices by pressing well pulped fruit and filtering. Express juice of citrus fruits by commercial device and filter. Add aliquots of ≥100 mL prepared juice to equal volumes of HPO_3-CH_3COOH solution, (a)(1). Designate total volume as V mL. Mix, and filter through rapid folded paper (Eaton-Dikeman No. 195, 18.5 cm, or equivalent).

E. Determination

Titrate 3 sample aliquots each containing ca 2 mg ascorbic acid and make blank determinations for correction of titrations as in **967.21B(c)**, using proper volumes of HPO_3-CH_3COOH solution, (a)(1), and

H_2O. If ca 2 mg ascorbic acid is contained in sample aliquot <7 mL, add HPO_3-CH_3COOH solution to give 7 mL for titration.

$$\text{mg Ascorbic acid/g, tablet, mL, etc.} = (X - B) \times (F/E) \times (V/Y)$$

where X = average mL for sample titration, B = average mL for sample blank titration, F = mg ascorbic acid equivalent to 1.0 mL indophenol standard solution, E = number of g, tablets, mL, etc. assayed, V = volume initial assay solution, and Y = volume sample aliquot titrated.

Note: Products containing ferrous Fe, stannous Sn, and cuprous Cu give values in excess of their actual ascorbic acid content by this method. Following are simple tests to determine whether these reducing ions are present in such amounts as to invalidate test: Add 2 drops *0.05% aqueous solution of methylene blue* to 10 mL freshly prepared mixture (1 + 1) of sample solution and HPO_3-CH_3COOH reagent and mix. Disappearance of methylene blue color in 5–10 s indicates presence of interfering substances. Stannous Sn does not give this test and may be tested for as follows: To another 10 mL sample solution to which 10 mL HCl (1 + 3) has been added, add 5 drops *0.05% aqueous solution of indigo carmine* and mix. Disappearance of color in 5–10 s indicates presence of stannous Sn or other interfering substance.

References: J. Biol. Chem. **103**, 687(1933); **112**, 625(1936); **116**, 409, 563(1936); **126**, 771(1938). Biochem. J. **27**, 580(1933); **30**, 2273(1936); **36**, 115(1942). Physiol. Rev. **16**, 238(1936). J. Am. Med. Assoc. **111**, 1290(1938). Biochemical Z. **301**, 229(1939). JAOAC 27, 537(1944); **28**, 559(1945); **29**, 69(1946); **30**, 673(1947); **32**, 479(1949); **34**, 380(1951); **36**, 1127(1953); **38**, 514(1955); **50**, 798(1967). CAS-50-81-7 (ascorbic acid)

37.3   967.22—Vitamin C (Ascorbic Acid) in Vitamin Preparations
Microfluorometric Method
First Action 1967
Final Action 1968

A. Principle

Ascorbic acid is oxidized to dehydroascorbic acid in presence of Norit. Oxidized form is reacted with *o*-phenylenediamine to produce fluorophor having activation maximum at ca 350 nm and fluorescence maximum at ca 430 nm. Fluorescence intensity is proportional to concentration.

Development of fluorescent derivative of vitamin is prevented by forming H_3BO_3-dehydroascorbic acid complex prior to addition of diamine solution. Any remaining fluorescence is due to extraneous materials. This serves as "blank."

Ascorbic plus dehydroascorbic acid is calculated by comparing corrected fluorescence reading for sample with that of standard similarly oxidized and treated.

B. Reagents

(a) *Extracting solutions.*—Prepare: (*1*) HPO_3-CH_3COOH and (*2*) HPO_3-CH_3COOH-H_2SO_4 solutions as in **967.21B(a)** (*see* 37.2).

(b) *Ascorbic acid standard solution.*—100 μg/mL. Dilute 10 mL ascorbic acid standard solution, **967.21B(b)**, to 100 mL with HPO_3-CH_3COOH solution, (a)(*1*).

(c) *o-Phenylenediamine solution.*—For each 100 mL solution required, weigh 20 mg *o*-phenylenediamine·2HCl (Eastman Kodak Co. No. 678). Dilute to volume with H_2O immediately before use.

(d) *Thymol blue pH indicator.*—Prepare as in **967.21B(d)**.

(e) *Sodium acetate solution.*—Dissolve 500 g NaOAc·$3H_2O$ in H_2O and dilute to 1 L.

(f) *Boric acid-sodium acetate solution.*—Dissolve 3 g H_3BO_3 in 100 mL NaOAc solution. Prepare fresh for each assay.

(g) *Acid-washed Norit.*—Add 1 L HCl (1 + 9) to 200 g Norit Neutral (Fisher Scientific Co., Carbon, decolorizing, C-170), heat to bp, and filter with vacuum. Remove cake to large beaker. Add 1 L H_2O, stir, and filter. Repeat washing with H_2O and filtering. Dry overnight at 110–120°.

C. Apparatus

(a) *Automatic pipetting machine.*—Brewer, Scientific Equipment Products (SEPCO), or equivalent. Calibrate to deliver 5 mL aliquots.

(b) *Vortex mixer.*—Scientific Industries, Inc., 70 Orville Dr, Bohemia, NY 11716, or equivalent.

(c) *Fluorometer.*—Aminco Fluoro-Microphotometer (SLM Instruments Inc., 810 W. Anthony Dr, Urbana, IL 61801) with lamp F4T4/BL and cuvet adapter B12-63019 to accept 18 × 150 mm test tubes, or equivalent. Use as primary filter Kopp Glass Co. Nos. C7380 and C5860 and as secondary filter Kopp Nos. C5113 and C3389. (C.S. No. 3-73). (*Caution: See Appendix* for safety notes on photofluorometers.)

(d) *Fluorescence reading tubes.*—Standardized 18 × 150 mm test tubes.

D. Preliminary Test for Appreciable Amount of Basic Substances

Proceed as in **967.21C**.

E. Preparation of Sample Assay Solution

(a) *For dry materials containing no appreciable amount of basic substances.*—Proceed as in **967.21D(a)**. Dilute with HPO_3-CH_3COOH solution, **967.21B(a)(*1*)**, to ca 100 μg ascorbic acid/mL. Designate this volume as *V* mL. Filter solutions containing large amounts of suspended solids through Whatman No. 12 paper, or equivalent. Designate as sample assay solution.

(b) *For dry materials containing appreciable amounts of basic substances.*—Proceed as in **967.21D(b)**. Then proceed as in (a), beginning "Dilute with . . . ."

(c) *For liquid materials.*—Proceed as in **967.21D(c)**. Then proceed as in (a), beginning "Dilute with . . . ."

(d) *For gelatin-encapsulated pharmaceutical products.*—Place sample in small beaker and heat gently with enough proper extracting solution, **967.21B(a)(*1*)** or (*2*), to cover. If capsules do not disintegrate readily, crush with glass rod. Cool rapidly to room temperature. If appreciable amounts of basic substances are present, adjust pH to ca 1.2 with HPO_3-CH_3COOH-H_2SO_4 solution, **967.21B(a)(*2*)**. Proceed as in (a), beginning "Dilute with . . . ."

Note: For samples difficult to filter, proceed as in applicable section, (a), (b), (c), or (d), except dilute sample assay solution with HPO_3-CH_3COOH solution to ca 50 μg ascorbic acid/mL. Compare with standard solution prepared by diluting 5 mL ascorbic acid standard solution, **967.21B(b)**, to 100 mL with HPO_3-CH_3COOH solution. (1 mL = 50 μg ascorbic acid.)

F. Determination

Following steps must be performed consecutively without delay.

Transfer 100 mL standard and sample assay solutions to 300 mL erlenmeyers. Add 2 g acid-washed Norit, shake vigorously, and filter through Whatman No. 12 paper, or equivalent, discarding first few mL. Transfer 5 mL each filtrate to separate 100 mL volumetric flasks, containing 5 mL H_3BO_3-NaOAc solution. Let stand 15 min, swirling occasionally. Designate as standard or sample blank solutions, respectively.

During 15 min period, transfer 5 mL of each filtrate to separate 100 mL volumetric flasks containing 5 mL NaOAc solution and ca 75 mL H_2O. Dilute to volume with H_2O. Transfer 2 mL of each solution to each of 3 fluorescence reading tubes. Designate as standard or sample tubes, respectively.

At appropriate time, dilute blank solutions to volume with H_2O. Transfer 2 mL of these solutions to each of 3 fluorescence reading tubes. Designate as standard or sample blank tubes, respectively.

Using automatic pipetting machine, add 5 mL o-phenylenediamine solution to all tubes. Use Vortex mixer to swirl tubes. Protect from light and let stand 35 min at room temperature.

G. Fluorometry

Measure fluorescence of standard tube (C), standard blank tube (B), sample tube (X), and sample blank tube (D).

$$\text{mg Ascorbic acid/g, tablet, mL, etc.} = [(\text{average } X - \text{average } D)/(\text{average } C - \text{average } B)] \times (20 \times S \times V/E)$$

where V = initial assay solution volume, E = number of g, tablets, mL, etc., and S = concentration of standard in mg/mL added to reading tube.

References: JAOAC **48,** 1248(1965); **50,** 798(1967).
CAS-50-81-7 (ascorbic acid)

37.4   985.33—Vitamin C (Reduced Ascorbic Acid) in Ready-to-Feed Milk-Based Infant Formula

2,6-Dichloroindophenol Titrimetric Method
First Action 1985
Final Action 1988

A. Principle

Ascorbic acid is estimated by titration with colored oxidation-reduction indicator, 2,6,dichloroindophenol. EDTA is added as chelating agent to remove Fe and Cu interferences.

B. Reagents

(a) *Precipitant solution.*—Dissolve with shaking 15 g glacial HPO_3 pellets in 40 mL glacial CH_3COOH and 150 mL H_2O. Dilute to 250 mL with H_2O and filter rapidly through folded qualitative paper (rapid, 18.5 cm, Whatman No. 541 or equivalent) into 500 mL beaker.

Dissolve with shaking 0.9 g EDTA in 200 mL H_2O and dilute to 250 mL. Mix equal volumes of HPO_3 and EDTA solutions immediately before use.

(**b**) *Ascorbic acid standard solution.*—1 mg/mL. Accurately weigh 50 mg USP Ascorbic Acid Reference Standard (stored in desiccator away from sunlight). Transfer to 50 mL volumetric flask. Dilute to volume with precipitant solution, (**a**). Prepare *immediately* before use in standardization of indophenol standard solution.

(**c**) *Indophenol standard solution.*—Dissolve 0.0625 g 2,6-dichloroindophenol Na salt (stored in desiccator over soda lime) in 50 mL H_2O in 250 mL volumetric flask to which has been added 0.0525 g reagent grade $NaHCO_3$. Shake vigorously; when dye dissolves, dilute to 250 mL with H_2O. Filter through rapid-flow folded paper into amber glass bottle. Store in refrigerator.

Transfer three 2.0 mL aliquots of ascorbic acid solution, (**b**), into each of three 50 mL erlenmeyers containing 5 mL precipitant solution, (**a**). Using 25 mL buret calibrated in 0.05 mL and with glass or Teflon stopcock, titrate rapidly with indophenol standard solution until light but distinct rose-pink persists for 5 s. (Each titration should require ca 15 mL and titrations should check ± 0.1 mL.) Titrate 3 blanks composed of 7 mL precipitant solution plus 15 mL H_2O. Average blank is 0.1 mL. Calculate dye equivalents: ascorbic acid equivalent to 1 mL indophenol standard solution = mg ascorbic acid/(mL dye − blank titration) = 2 mg/(mL dye − blank titration).

C. Preparation of Sample Assay Solution

Pipet 25–30 mL composite and equal volume of precipitant solution, (**a**), into 125 mL beaker. Designate total volume as V mL and volume of composite aliquoted as E mL. Filter through folded rapid qualitative paper, 18.5 cm (Whatman No. 541, or equivalent). Designate filtrate as assay solution.

D. Determination

Pipet three 10 mL aliquots of assay solution each into separate 50 mL erlenmeyers and titrate with indophenol standard solution. Similarly titrate 2 blanks composed of mL precipitant solution and H_2O equivalent to their respective volumes in assay solution aliquot titrated. Add volume of H_2O equivalent to mL indophenol standard solution used in titration of assay solution. Titrate with indophenol standard solution to same color end point observed in titration of standard aliquot.

$$\text{mg ascorbic acid/L ready-to-feed formula} = (X - B) \times (F/E) \times (V/Y) \times 1000$$

where X = average mL for assay solution titration; B = average mL for assay solution blank titration; F = mg ascorbic acid equivalent to 1.0 mL indophenol standard solution; E = volume composite aliquot; V = assay solution volume; Y = volume assay solution titrated = 10 mL; 1000 = conversion of mL to L.

Reference: JAOAC **68,** 514(1985).
CAS-50-81-7 (ascorbic acid)

Chapter 38
Vitamin D

38.1   982.29—Vitamin D in Mixed Feeds, Premixes, and Petroleum Foods
Liquid Chromatographic Method
First Action 1982
Final Action 1983

(Applicable to products containing <200 IU and >2 IU vitamin D/g. For products containing ≥200 IU vitamin D/g, use **980.26** [*Official Methods of Analysis* (1990) 15th Ed.].)

A. Principle

Samples are saponified and extracted, and unsaponifiable material is chromatographed successively on alumina to remove tocopherols and carotenes, if present, and on LC cleanup column to separate from interfering substances. Second LC column packed with silica separates vitamin D from impurities. Vitamin D is corrected for amount previtamin D formed during saponification. Vitamin D is sum of vitamin D and previtamin D.

B. Reagents

(a) *Solvents.*—methyl alcohol, alcohol, CH_3CN, toluene, peroxide- and acid-free ether, *n*-hexane (spectroquality). Dry *n*-hexane by passing through column 60 × 8 cm diameter containing 500 g 50–250 μm silica dried 4 h at 150°.

(b) *Sodium ascorbate solution.*—Dissolve 3.5 g ascorbic acid in 20 mL 1N NaOH. Prepare fresh daily.

(c) *Antioxidant solution.*—1 mg butylated hydroxytoluene (BHT)/mL hexane.

(d) *Petroleum ether.*—Reflux over KOH pellets and collect fraction distilling between 40° and 60°.

(e) *Ether–petroleum ether eluants.*—8 + 92 and 40 + 60.

(f) *Alumina.*—Neutral, type 1097 (E. Merck).

(g) *Mobile phase (for cleanup column).*—CH_3CN–methyl alcohol–H_2O (50 + 50 + 5).

(h) *Mobile phase (for analytical column).*—*n*-Hexane containing 0.35% (volume/volume) *n*-amyl alcohol.

(i) *Vitamin D standard solutions.*—USP Reference Standard Ergocalciferol (if sample labeled as containing vitamin D_2) or Cholecalciferol (if labeled as containing vitamin D or D_3). Accurately weigh ca 12.5 mg vitamin D standard (W'') in 100 mL amber volumetric flask. Dissolve without heat in toluene and dilute to volume with toluene (125 μg/mL, solution A). Dilute 10 mL solution A to 100 mL with mobile phase (h). Dilute 10 mL of this solution to 100 mL with toluene-mobile phase (h) (5 + 95) for vitamin D standard (solution B) (1.25 μg/mL; 50 IU/mL). Also dilute 10 mL solution A to 100 mL with mobile phase (g); dilute 20 mL of this solution to 100 mL with mobile phase (g) (2.5 μg/mL, solution C). Prepare fresh daily.

(j) *System suitability standard solution.*—Use USP Vitamin D Assay System Suitability Reference Standard, or prepare solution containing 2 mg vitamin D_3 and 0.2 mg trans-vitamin D_3/g in vegetable oil. Peaks of trans-vitamin D_3 and previtamin D_3 must have ca same peak heights. If necessary, increase previtamin D_3 content by warming oil solution ca 45 min at 90°. Store solution at 5°.

C. Alumina Column

Seal coarse fritted glass disk in lower end of 150 × 20 mm id tube and 250 mL bulb at upper end. Fit constricted portion at lower end with Teflon stopcock.

Heat 250 g alumina overnight at 750°. Cool and store in vacuum desiccator. Weigh 30 g dried alumina into 100 mL erlenmeyer. Pipet 2.7 mL H_2O into flask, and stopper. Heat 5 min on steam bath. Vigorously shake warm flask until powder is free-flowing. Cool and let stand 30 min.

Add 40 mL petroleum ether to deactivated alumina, swirl, and transfer to tube, using petroleum ether. Let packing settle. Maintain head of >0.5 cm liquid on column throughout assay (alumina column can be used for only 1 assay).

D. Liquid Chromatography

(a) *Liquid chromatograph.*—Hewlett-Packard 1010A, or equivalent, with 254 nm UV detector with 2 columns: cleanup and analytical.

(b) *Cleanup column.*—Stainless steel, 250 × 4.6 mm id, packed with 10 μm particle size Li-Chrosorb RP-18. Typical operating conditions: chart speed, 1 cm/min; eluant flow rate, 1.4 mL/min; detector sensitivity, 0.08 AUFS; temperature, ambient; valve injection volume, 500 μL; solvent system, CH_3CN-methyl alcohol-H_2O (50 + 50 + 5).

(c) *Analytical column.*—Stainless steel, 250 × 4.6 mm id, packed with 5 μm particle size Partisil-5, passing system suitability test. Typical operating conditions: chart speed, 1 cm/min; eluant flow rate, 2.6 mL/min (ca 1500 psi); detector sensitivity, 0.008 AUFS; temperature, ambient; valve injection volume, 200 μL; solvent system, n-hexane containing 0.35% (volume/volume) n-amyl alcohol.

E. System Suitability Test for Analytical Column

Dissolve 0.1 g system suitability standard solution in 100 mL toluene-mobile phase (5 + 95) and inject 200 μL. Determine peak resolution between previtamin D_3 and trans-vitamin D_3 as: $R = 2D/(B + C)$, where D = distance between peak maximum of previtamin D_3 and trans-vitamin D_3, B = peak width of previtamin D_3, and C = peak width of trans-vitamin D_3. Performance is satisfactory if R is ≥1.0.

F. Calibration

Inject 500 μL vitamin D standard solution (solution C) onto cleanup column through sampling valve and 200 μL solution B onto analytical column, and adjust operating conditions of detector to give largest possible on-scale peaks of vitamin D. Determine retention time of vitamin D on cleanup and analytical columns and peak height of vitamin D on analytical column. Retention time of vitamin D on clean-up column should be between 15 and 25 min; adjust H_2O content of mobile phase, if necessary, to achieve this situation. Retention time of vitamin D on analytical column should be between 15 and 20 min; adjust amyl alcohol content in mobile phase, if necessary, to achieve this situation.

G. Preparation of Sample

Isolation of unsaponifiable matter from powder.—Accurately weigh ca 25 g powdered sample (preferably particle size <1 mm) into saponification flask. Add 80 mL alcohol, 2 mL Na ascorbate solution, a pinch of Na_2EDTA, and 10 mL 50% aqueous KOH solution. Reflux 30 min on steam bath under N with magnetic stirring. Cool and extract with five 60 mL portions of ether in saponification flask; decant each time and transfer ether layer to 1 L separator containing 100 mL H_2O. Shake ether layer in separator (A), let separate, and transfer aqueous phase to 500 mL separator (B). Extract aqueous phase with 60 mL ether and transfer ether layer to separator (A). Wash combined ether extracts with 100 mL 0.5N KOH solution and then 100 mL portions of H_2O until last washing is neutral to phenolphthalein. Add 150 mL petroleum ether, wait 1/2 h, separate from last drops of H_2O, and add 2 sheets of 9 cm filter paper in strips to separator. Shake, add 1 mg BHT, and transfer to round-bottom flask, rinsing separator and paper with petroleum ether.

Evaporate solution by swirling (Rotavapor) under N stream in 40° H_2O bath. Dissolve residue immediately in 5 mL hexane.

H. Alumina Column Chromatography

Transfer sample solution to column with aid of three 10 mL portions of hexane. Discard eluate (contains carotenoids). Elute column with seven 10 mL portions of ether-hexane (8 + 92) and discard eluate (contains tocopherols and ethoxyquin).

Elute column with seven 10 mL portions of ether-hexane (40 + 60), discard first 20–25 mL, collecting rest of eluate in round-bottom flask (contains vitamins A and D) when front of fluorescent vitamin A band is located 3 cm from bottom of column. Examine column <1 s under UV light (360 nm) with portable UV lamp to verify elution of vitamin A. Evaporate solution by swirling (Rotavapor) under N stream in 40° H_2O bath. Transfer to centrifuge tube, rinsing flask with 2–3 mL ether, evaporate ether, and dissolve in 1.0 mL methyl alcohol with warming. Add 1.0 mL CH_3CN and cool. Centrifuge and use clear supernate for injection onto cleanup column.

I. Determination

(a) *Cleanup.*—Inject 500 μL sample solution onto cleanup column through sampling valve and adjust operating conditions of detector to give largest possible on-scale peaks for vitamin D. Collect fraction between 3 min before and 3 min after vitamin D peak in 10 mL volumetric flask. Add 1 mL antioxidant solution and evaporate to dryness under N stream. Dissolve residue immediately in 2.0 mL toluene-mobile phase (5 + 95). Use this solution for injection onto analytical column.

(b) *Assay.*—Inject 200 μL solution (a) onto analytical column through sampling valve, and adjust operating conditions of detector to give largest possible on-scale peaks of vitamin D. Measure peak height of vitamin D. Use same operating conditions and inject standard solution B. Measure peak height of vitamin D.

(c) *Calculation.*—

Vitamin D potency in IU/g sample = $(1.25 \times P \times W' \times V \times 40\,000)/(P' \times W \times V')$

where P = peak height of vitamin D in sample solution, 1.25 = correction factor for previtamin D formed during refluxing for saponification, P' = peak height of vitamin D in reference solution, W = grams sample weighed, W' = mg reference standard, V = total mL sample solution, V' = total mL reference standard solution, and 40 000 = IU vitamin D/mg USP Reference Standard.

Reference. JAOAC **66**, 751(1983).
CAS-67-97-0 (cholecalciferol; vitamin D_3)
CAS-50-14-6 (ergocalciferol; vitamin D_2)

38.2   936.14—Vitamin D in Milk, Vitamin Preparations, and Feed Concentrates
Rat Bioassay
Final Action

(Not applicable to products offered for poultry feeding)

A. Definitions

Assay group means group of rats to which assay sample (vitamin D sample) is administered during assay period. *Assay sample* means sample under examination for vitamin D potency. *Assay solution* means solution of sample in oil prepared for feeding after saponification. *Assay period* means interval in life of rat between last day of depletion period and eighth or eleventh day thereafter. *Assemble* means procedure by which rats are selected and assigned to groups for purposes of feeding, care, and observation. *Daily* means each of first 6 or 8 days of assay period. *Depletion period* means interval in life of rat between last day of preliminary period and first day of assay period. *Dose* means amount of reference oil or of assay milk or other supplement to be fed daily to rat during assay period. *Feed* means make readily available to rat or administer to rat by mouth. *Group* means 7 or more rats maintained on same required dietary regime during assay period. *Preliminary period* means interval in life of rat between seventh day after birth and first day of depletion period.

B. Reagents

(a) *Ground gluten.*—Clean, sound product made from wheat flour by almost complete removal of starch, containing ≤10% H_2O and, calculated on H_2O-free basis, ≥14.2% N, ≤15% N-free extract (using protein factor 5.7), and ≤5.5% starch (determined by diastase method, **974.06D**).

> I. **974.06** (Sugars [Total] in Animal Feed, Modified Fehling Solution Method)
>
> *D. Standardization*
>
> Fill 50 mL buret, with offset tip, with standard sugar solution (invert sugar for use with **974.06E(a)** and lactose with **974.06E(b)**). Proceed as in **968.28D**, paragraph 2, except use same type flask as used in **974.06E**, do not add H_2O, and start stirring after addition of indicator.
>
> *E. Determination*
>
> (a) *Difference method.*—Add reagents and stirring bar to 250 mL extraction flask (Corning Glass Works No. 5160, or equivalent) or to Erlenmeyer, as in **974.06D**. Transfer aliquot inverted solution, (a), to flask so that >1 but <5 mL standard solution will be required to reach end point, place on preheated mantle or hot plate, heat to bp, boil 2 min, add ca 1 mL indicator, and begin stirring. Complete determination by titrating with standard sugar solution to same end point used in standardization. Color change is not so sharp as in standardization, but under suitable light it is definite, discernible, and repeatable.
>
> (b) *Alternative method.*—Fill buret with sample solution, (b), or inverted sample solution, (a). As in **974.06D**, place reagents in flask, place on heater, add sample solution to within 2 mL of final titration (determined by trial), bring to bp, boil 2 min, and complete titration as in (a).

II. **968.28** (Total Sugars in Molasses as Invert Sugar, Lane-Eynon Constant Volume Volumetric Method)

B. Reagents

(a) *Soxhlet modification of Fehling solution.*—Prepare as in **923.09A(a)** and **(b)**.

(b) *Invert sugar standard solutions.*—*(1) Stock solution.*—10 mg/mL. Prepare as in **923.09A(c)**, using 5 mL HCl (specific gravity 1.18 at 20/4°) and letting stand 3 days at room temperature (20–25°). *(2) Working solution.*—5 mg/mL. Pipet 100 mL stock solution into 200 mL volumetric flask, add few drops phenolphthalein, and neutralize with 20% NaOH. Dilute to volume and mix well. Prepare fresh daily.

D. Standardization of Soxhlet Reagent

Fill 50 mL buret with working standard solution containing 5 mg invert sugar/mL.

Accurately pipet 10 mL each Soxhlet solution, **(a)** and **(b)**, into 300 mL erlenmeyer, mix, and add 30 mL H$_2$O. Add from buret almost all standard working solution (ca 19 mL) necessary to reduce the Cu. Add few boiling chips. Place cold mixture on heater, regulate heat so that boiling will begin in ca 3 min, and maintain at moderate boil exactly 2 min, reducing heat, if necessary, to prevent bumping. Without removing flask from heater, add ca 4 drops *1% aqueous methylene blue solution* and complete titration within total boiling time of ca 3 min by dropwise addition of working standard solution at intervals of ca 10 s until boiling mixture resumes bright orange appearance which it had before indicator was added. Maintain continuous evolution of steam to prevent reoxidation by air. Repeat standardization several times. Factor *F* is average number mL standard sugar solution required to completely reduce 20 mL Soxhlet solution. Use average of ≥3 titrations.

III. **923.09** (Invert Sugar in Sugars and Sirups, Lane-Eynon General Volumetric Method)

A. Reagents

Soxhlet modification of Fehling solution.—Prepare by mixing equal volumes of **(a)** and **(b)** immediately before use.

(a) *Copper sulfate solution.*—Dissolve 34.639 g CuSO$_4$·5H$_2$O in H$_2$O, dilute to 500 mL, and filter through glass wool or paper. Determine Cu content of solution (preferably by electrolysis, **929.09F**, *Official Methods of Analysis* [1984] 14th Ed., sec. **31.044**) and so adjust that it contains 440.9 mg Cu/25 mL.

(b) *Alkaline tartrate solution.*—Dissolve 173 g KNa tartrate·4H$_2$O (Rochelle salt) and 50 g NaOH in H$_2$O, dilute to 500 mL, let stand 2 days, and filter through prepared asbestos, **906.03A** (*see* Chapter 33.13).

(c) *Invert sugar standard solution.*—1%. To solution of 9.5 g pure sucrose, add 5 mL HCl and dilute with H$_2$O to ca 100 mL. Store several days at room temperature (ca 7 days at 12–15° or 3 days at 20–25°); then dilute to 1 L. (Acidified 1% invert sugar solution is stable for several months.) Neutralize aliquot with ca 1N NaOH and dilute to desired concentration immediately before use.

(b) *Reference oil.*—USP Ergocalciferol or Cholecalciferol Reference Standard.

(c) *Cottonseed oil.*—USP grade meeting following additional requirements: Saponify 10 g oil as in **936.14F**, and dissolve unsaponifiable residue in 10 mL petroleum ether. In separate container place 0.4 mL FeCl$_3$ solution (1 + 1000) and 12 mL solution of α,α-dipyridyl in absolute alcohol (1 + 6000), mix, and 5 min later read A in 1.0 cm cell at 520 nm, using suitable spectrophotometer, against absolute alcohol. Then add 0.2 mL solution of unsaponifiable residue in petroleum ether to entire colored solution, and after 5 min read A. Difference between first and second A values is ≥ 0.125.

(**d**) *Rachitogenic diet.*—Mix 76% whole yellow corn, ground to pass No. 30 sieve; 20% gluten, ground to pass No. 30 sieve; 3% $CaCO_3$; and 1% NaCl.

C. Preservation of Sample

Store samples so as to minimize exposure to heat, light, and air. Deliver milk samples in original container immediately after collection or store under refrigeration in iced container until delivered. After delivery to assayer, preserve in homogeneous state by refrigeration at $\leq 10°$ for ≤ 10 days, or for ≤ 30 days by addition of 2 drops 10% HCHO solution to 1 qt milk in addition to refrigeration at $\leq 10°$. Preserve evaporated and reconstituted milk in same manner as fluid milk. Soured or curdled sample is unsuitable for assay. Preserve sample of dried milk, after being opened by assayer, by refrigeration at $\leq 10°$.

D. Sample

Sample shall consist of ≥ 10 g food, 10 capsules or tablets, or sufficient volume of liquids to satisfy needs of entire assay.

If amount of vitamin D in sample is such that aliquot to be fed contains < 5 mg P, sample may be fed directly. If aliquot contains > 5 mg P, sample must be saponified.

All manipulations and dilutions of vitamin sample must be made with materials known to be free of vitamin D.

E. Preparation of Sample for Direct Feeding

(**a**) *Feed concentrates and tablets.*—Thoroughly grind weighed sample. Promptly weigh aliquot of ground powder and grind it again with equal weight of edible vegetable oil. To this add amount of powdered sucrose such that assay dose will be contained in 1–2 g. Mix thoroughly by grinding again and proceed as in assay period, **936.14K**.

(**b**) *Capsules.*—Open weighed capsules and transfer contents as completely as possible into container. Thoroughly mix combined contents and promptly weigh aliquot. Proceed as in (**a**). Obtain sample weight by subtracting weight empty ether-washed capsules from total weight capsules.

(**c**) *Oils.*—Add amount of edible vegetable oil that will produce dilution containing assay dose in volume equal to volume reference dilution.

(**d**) *Water-miscible liquids.*—Dilute as for oils, using H_2O, glycerol, or propylene glycol to facilitate feeding.

F. Preparation of Sample by Saponification

(*Caution: See Appendix* for safety notes on distillation, flammable solvents, and diethyl ether.)

Weigh sample and transfer to saponification flask. (For milk, *see* **936.14G**.)

In case of capsules or tablets, place ≥ 10 in small reflux flask, add 10 mL H_2O, and heat on steam bath ca 10 min. Crush each capsule or tablet with blunt glass rod and warm 5 min more. Add 2 mL cottonseed oil and volume of KOH (50% weight/volume) solution representing 2.5 mL for each gram total weight of sample plus cottonseed oil, but ≥ 15 mL. Add 50 mL alcohol and reflux vigorously 30 min in 100° bath. Cool solution and transfer to Squibb-type separator, using 50 mL H_2O. Extract with four 30 mL portions peroxide-free ether (USP anesthesia ether is suitable), using more H_2O or small portions alcohol to break any emulsions that may form. Wash combined ether extracts 4 times with H_2O as follows: (*1*) 100 mL with very gentle swirling; (*2*) 100 mL with gentle swirling; (*3*) 50 mL with gentle shaking;

(4) 50 mL with vigorous shaking. Dry ether extract with two 75 mL portions saturated NaCl solution, shaking vigorously both times. Transfer ether extract to beaker and evaporate on steam bath to convenient volume. If H_2O is present, dry with 3–5 g anhydrous Na_2SO_4. Decant into weighed container, rinse beaker and Na_2SO_4 with 3–5 additional portions ether, and combine all washings in weighed container. Evaporate ether on steam bath until no ether odor is detectable, and weigh fat. Multiply by 1.10 to determine volume, and add amount of edible vegetable oil that will produce convenient final dilution for feeding. Mix thoroughly (magnetic stirrer is desirable).

G. Preparation of Milk Samples

Proceed as in **936.14F** with following modifications: Use 50–100 mL alcohol and 10 g KOH pellets per 100 mL sample. Swirl until all KOH dissolves. Reflux 40–60 min. (To minimize bumping and scorching of sample, place several short pieces of glass stirring rod in saponification flask and use oil or H_2O bath at 100°.) Use 50–100 mL ether for first extraction. Only small part of butterfat is saponified, but fat may be fed without affecting results. Where unusually large amount (>0.5 g) of fat would have to be fed in every dose, extract from which ether has been evaporated may be resaponified as in **936.14F**.

H. Preliminary Period

Throughout preliminary period each rat must be raised under immediate supervision of, or according to directions specified by, assayer. Throughout preliminary period, keep rats on dietary regimen that provides for normal development in all respects, except to limit supply of vitamin D to such degree that rats weighing 40–60 g at age of 21–30 days and subsisting 18–25 days on suitable rachitogenic diet show evidence of severe rickets.

I. Depletion Period

Rat is suitable for depletion period when its age is ≤30 days, and its body weight is >44 g but ≤60 g, provided it shows no evidence of injury, disease, or anatomical abnormality that might hinder growth and development. Throughout depletion period provide each rat with rachitogenic diet and H_2O or USP H_2O *ad libitum,* and permit no other dietary supplement to be available.

J. Assembling Rats into Groups for Assay Period

Assemble rats that are suitable for assay period into groups. For each sample provide ≥1 assay group. In assay of one sample at least one reference group must be provided, but this reference group may be used for concurrent assay of ≥1 assay sample. (Where 2 reference groups are desired, dose levels must be selected so that ratio of higher to lower dose is not <1.5 or >2.5. Dosage levels for samples based upon single assumed potency for each sample may be equivalent to reference levels or at midlevel equal to square root of product of the 2 dosage levels of the reference). On any one day during interval of assembling rats into groups, total number of rats assigned to make up any one group must not exceed by >2 the number of rats that have been assigned to make up any other group. When assembling of all groups is completed, total number of rats in each group must be same. Assign not >3 rats from 1 litter to assay group unless equal number of rats from same litter is assigned to reference group. There must be enough animals in each group to meet requirements specified in **936.14N**.

K. Assay Period

Rat is suitable for assay period provided depletion period is >18 days but ≤25 days, and provided rat shows evidence of rickets characterized by distinctive wobbly rachitic gait and enlarged joints. Presence of rickets may also be established by examination of leg bone of one member of litter by "line test,"

936.14L, or by X-ray examination of animals selected for assay. Keep each rat in individual cage, provided with rachitogenic diet and H_2O *ad libitum*. On any calendar day of assay period, assay and reference groups must receive rachitogenic diet compounded from same lots of ingredients.

Following optional methods of feeding reference oil solution and sample solution are permissible, but both reference oil solution and sample solution must be fed according to same method in any 1 assay. Supplements may be fed on first day of assay period, or in equal portions on first, third, and fifth days, or on first and third days, or on first and fourth days of 7 day or 10 day assay period, or on first 6 days of 7 day assay period, or on first 8 days of 10 day assay period; supplements may be fed admixed with amount of basal ration that will be consumed within first 5 days of 7 day assay period or within first 8 days of 10 day assay period. In each case make unsupplemented ration available during remainder of assay period.

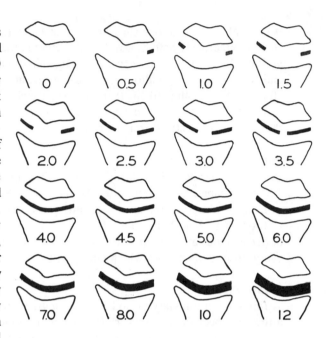

Figure 936.14A.—Line test chart.

Feed amount of reference oil found by experience to cause extent and degree of calcification of rachitic metaphysis equivalent to 4 on line test chart. Feed that volume of sample solution which is calculated to contain, on basis of claimed or assumed potency, same number of units of vitamin D as contained in amount of reference oil fed.

After assay period, kill each rat and examine ≥ 1 leg bone for healing of rachitic metaphysis according to "line test," **936.14L**.

Reference oil may be diluted with edible vegetable oil free from vitamins A and D before being fed. Diluted oil must be stored in dark at temperature $\leq 10°$ for ≤ 30 days. Do not feed > 0.2 mL of diluted oil as daily dose. During assay period, keep all conditions of environment (particularly physiologically active radiations) as uniform as possible with respect to assay and reference groups.

L. Line Test

Make line test on proximal end of tibia or distal end of radius or ulna. Remove end of desired bone from animal and clean off adhering tissue. Make longitudinal median section through end of bone with clean, sharp blade to expose plane surface through junction of epiphysis and diaphysis. In any one assay use same bone of all animals and section through same plane. Rinse both sections of bone in H_2O and immerse in 2% $AgNO_3$ solution 1 min. Then rinse sections in H_2O and expose sectioned surfaces in H_2O to daylight or other source of actinic light until calcified areas have developed clearly defined stains without marked discoloration of uncalcified areas. Immediately record extent and degree of calcification of rachitic metaphysis of every section.

Staining procedure may be modified to differentiate more clearly between calcified and uncalcified areas. Suitable alternative procedure is to take freshly sectioned bone and proceed as follows: (*1*) Soak in ether-acetone mixture (3 + 1) ≥ 5 min (at this stage, after bone sections are dry, they may be mounted for convenience and ease of handling on standard microscope slides with aid of rubber cement and remainder of procedure performed in Coplin staining jars); (*2*) soak in alcohol 10 min; (*3*) soak in acetone 10 min; (*4*) soak 40 min in H_2O which is completely changed after 1, 10, 20, and 30 min; (*5*) stain with 2% $AgNO_3$ solution 60 s; and (*6*) wash 40 min with H_2O in dark with complete changes after 1, 10, 20, and 30 min. Expose stained sections in H_2O to daylight or other source of actinic light until stains have developed.

Score degree of calcification of rachitic metaphysis in each rat according to scale shown in Fig. **936.14A**. Because lines pictured in chart differ somewhat from line of healing being scored, it is necessary to visualize calcification as if it were compact and continuous in comparing it with appropriate figure in chart. Use of chart is illustrated by accompanying photographs of actual sections of radii, Fig. **936.14B**.

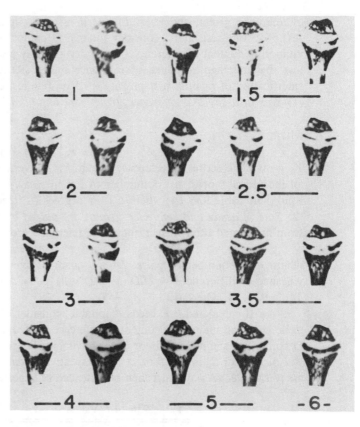

Figure 936.14B.—Photographs of radii sections scored according to line test chart. For illustrative purposes only; should not be used as scoring scale.

M. Recording of Data

On day beginning assay period and on seventh or tenth day thereafter, depending on duration of assay period, record body weight of each rat. Keep record of amount of rachitogenic diet consumed/rat during assay period. Assign numerical values to extent and degree of calcification of rachitic metaphyses of bones examined by line test by comparison with line test chart so that it is possible to average performance of each group.

N. Potency of Assay Sample

Consider data from rat valid for establishing vitamin D potency of assay sample only when weight of rat at termination of assay period equals or exceeds weight of rat on beginning day of assay period, and only when rat has consumed each prescribed dose of assay sample within 24 h from time it was fed.

Consider data from reference group valid for establishing vitamin D potency of assay sample when ≥⅔ but not <7 rats in reference groups that meet weight criteria show degree of calcification of rachitic metaphysis ≥0.5 and ≤8.0 on line test chart.

Consider data from assay group valid for establishing vitamin D potency of assay sample when ≥7 rats in assay group meet weight criteria.

When average response of assay group equals or exceeds average response of reference group, consider that vitamin D content of sample fed during assay period equals or exceeds vitamin D content of reference oil fed during assay period. When average response of assay group is less than average response of reference group, and $<1/2$ of rats in assay group show degree of calcification of rachitic metaphysis ≥ 0.5 on line test chart, consider vitamin D content of sample fed during assay period to be less than vitamin D content of reference oil fed during assay period. When average response of assay group (A) is less than average response of reference group (R) and if $\geq 1/2$ rats in assay group show degree of calcification of rachitic metaphysis ≥ 0.5 on line test chart, and:

(1) *Rats in assay and reference groups are unpaired by litter mates, then:*

$$t^2 = C_u(\bar{Y}_R - \bar{Y}_A)^2/S_u^2$$

where:
$$C_u = n_A n_R/(n_A + n_R)$$
$$S_u^2 = (\Sigma Y^2 - n_R \bar{Y}_R^2 - n_A \bar{Y}_A^2)/(n_A + n - 2)$$

$\bar{Y}_R$ = average score for reference group, $\bar{Y}_A$ = average score for assay group, ΣY^2 = sum of squares of all individual scores, n_A = number of rats in assay group, and n_R = number of rats in reference group. Find t^2 in Table **936.14**, where d.f. = degrees of freedom = $n_A + n_R - 2$. Or:

(2) *Rats in assay and reference groups are paired by litter mates,* subtract each response in assay group from associated litter mate response in reference group. Maintain sign of difference. Then:

$$t^2 = n_P D^2/S_D^2$$

where n_P = number of pairs, D^2 = square of average difference, D = average of differences, S_D^2 = variance of differences = $(\Sigma D^2 - n_P D^2)/(n_P - 1)$, and ΣD^2 = sum of squares of differences. Find t^2 in Table **936.14**, where d.f. = $n_P - 1$.

If calculated t^2 exceeds t^2 in table, consider vitamin D content of sample fed during assay period to be less than vitamin D content of reference oil fed during assay period; otherwise consider that vitamin D content of sample equals or exceeds vitamin D content of reference oil, provided S_u^2 is <1.5, or S_D^2 is <2.5. If S_u^2 or S_D^2 is >1.5 or >2.5, respectively, data of this assay are inadequate to establish potency of assay sample. (Assay must then be extended or repeated.)

Table 936.14 t^2 Values

d.f.	t^2	d.f.	t^2	d.f.	t^2
6	3.775	14	3.101	22	2.948
7	3.591	15	3.073	23	2.938
8	3.460	16	3.049	24	2.928
9	3.360	17	3.028	25	2.917
10	3.283	18	3.007	26	2.910
11	3.226	19	2.989	27	2.900
12	3.176	20	2.976	28	2.893
13	3.136	21	2.962	29	2.887
				30	2.880

Calculation of t^2 and S^2 is illustrated as follows:

(1) *For unpaired data:*

	Healing Scores	
	Reference	Assay
	3.62	4.00
	3.12	4.37
	6.00	2.37
	5.50	2.00
	4.25	3.75
	5.50	2.50
	4.75	4.00
Average = $\bar{Y}$	4.68	3.28

$$\Sigma Y^2 = 240.9901$$
$$C_u = (n_A \times n_R)/(n_A + n_R)$$
$$= (7 \times 7)/(7 + 7) = 3.5$$
$$S_u^2 = (\Sigma Y^2 - n_R \bar{Y}_A^2 - n_A \bar{Y}_A^2)/(n_A + n_R - 2)$$
$$= [240.9901 - 7(4.68)^2 - 7(3.28)^2]/12$$
$$= 1.0304$$
$$t^2 = (C_u/S_u^2)(\bar{Y}_R - \bar{Y}_A)^2$$
$$= (3.5/1.0304)(4.68 - 3.28)^2 = 6.658$$
$$\text{d.f.} = n_R + n_A - 2 = 12$$

Tabular t^2 for d.f. = 12 is 3.176.

Calculated t^2 (6.658) exceeds value in table for d.f. = 12 (3.176); therefore, vitamin D content of assay sample is less than vitamin D content of reference oil. Since S_u^2 (1.0304) is < 1.50, assay is valid.

(2) *For paired data:*

	Healing Scores		
Litter	Reference	Assay	Difference
1	4.02	4.40	- 0.38
2	3.52	4.77	- 1.25
3	6.40	2.77	+ 3.63
4	5.90	2.40	+ 3.50
5	4.65	4.15	+ 0.50
6	5.90	2.90	+ 3.00
7	5.15	4.40	+ 0.75
Average = $\bar{D}$			1.39
ΣD^2			36.9463

$$S_D^2 = (\Sigma D^2 - n_P \bar{D}^2)/(n_P - 1)$$
$$= [36.9463 - 7(1.39)^2]/6 = 3.9036$$

$$t^2 = (n_p \bar{D})/(S_D^2)$$
$$= 7(1.39)^2/3.9036 = 3.4647$$
$$\text{d.f.} = n_p - 1 = 6$$

Tabular t^2 for d.f. = 6 is 3.775.

Although calculated value of t^2, 3.4647, is less than tabular value for d.f. = 6 of 3.775, indicating that vitamin D content of assay sample equals or exceeds vitamin D content of reference oil, *assay must be repeated* since value for S_D^2 of 3.9036 is >2.5. Available data are inadequate to establish potency of sample.

(If desired, potency of vitamin D_2 may be calculated from multiple level assays by statistical procedure of USP XXI.)

References: JAOAC **19**, 248(1936); **20**, 213(1937); **21**, 243(1938); **22**, 468(1939); **23**, 341(1940); **32**, 480, 801(1949); **38**, 165(1955); **39**, 141(1956); **41**, 588(1958); **43**, 59(1960); **46**, 160(1963). Anal. Chem. **24**, 1841(1952).
CAS-67-97-0 (cholecalciferol; vitamin D_3)
CAS-50-14-6 (ergocalciferol; vitamin D_2)

38.3　　　　981.17—Vitamin D in Fortified Milk and Milkpowder
Liquid Chromatographic Method
First Action 1981
Final Action 1982

(Applicable to fluid milk and milkpowder containing ≥1 IU vitamin D/g)
(*Caution: See Appendix* for safety notes on flammable solvents.)

A. Principle

Samples are saponified and extracted. Vitamin D and isomers are separated from interfering substances on cleanup column. Second column separations vitamin D from impurities. Vitamin D is corrected for amount previtamin D formed during saponification. Vitamin D is sum of vitamin D and previtamin D.

B. Apparatus

(a) *Liquid chromatograph.*—Hewlett Packard 1010A, or equivalent, with 254 nm UV detector with 2 columns: cleanup and analytical.

(b) *Cleanup column.*—Stainless steel, 250 × 4.6 mm id, packed with 10 μm particle size Sil-60D-10CN. Typical operating conditions: chart speed, 1 cm/min; eluant flow rate, 1 mL/min; detector sensitivity, 0.128 AUFS; temperature, ambient; valve injection volume, 200 μL; mobile phase, *n*-hexane containing 0.35% *n*-amyl alcohol.

(c) *Analytical column.*—Stainless steel, 250 × 4.6 mm id, packed with 5 μm particle size Partisil, passing system suitability test. Typical operating conditions: chart speed, 1 cm/min; eluant flow rate, 2.5 mL/min; detector sensitivity, 0.008 AUFS; temperature, ambient; valve injection volume, 500 μL; mobile phase, *n*-hexane containing 0.35% *n*-amyl alcohol.

C. *Reagents*

    (a) *n-Hexane.—See* **979.24C(a)**.

        979.24C(a)

        (a) *n-Hexane.*—Spectroquality. Dry by passing through column 60 × 8 cm diameter containing 500 g 50–250 μm silica dried 4 hr at 150°.

    (b) *Antioxidant solution.*—0.1% butylated hydroxytoluene (BHT) in *n*-hexane.

    (c) *Vitamin D standard solution.*—USP Reference Standard Ergocalciferol (if sample labeled as containing vitamin D_2) or Cholecalciferol (if labeled as containing vitamin D or D_3). Accurately weigh ca 12.5 mg vitamin D standard in 100 mL amber volumetric flask. Dissolve without heat in toluene and dilute to volume with toluene. Dilute 10 mL of this solution to 100 mL with mobile phase. Dilute 25 mL of this solution to 100 mL with toluene-mobile phase (5 + 95) for vitamin D standard (3.125 μg/mL, 125 IU/mL). Prepare fresh daily.

    (d) *System suitability standard solution.*—Prepare solution containing 2 mg vitamin D_3 and 0.2 mg trans-vitamin D_3/g in vegetable oil. Peaks of trans-vitamin D_3 and previtamin D_3 must have ca same peak heights. If necessary, increase previtamin D_3 content by warming oil solution at 90° ca 45 min. Store solution at 5°.

D. *System Suitability Test for Analytical Column*

    Dissolve 0.1 g system suitability standard solution in 100 mL toluene-mobile phase (5 + 95) and chromatograph 200 μL. Determine peak resolution between previtamin D_3 and trans-vitamin D_3 as: $R = 2D/(B + C)$, where D = distance between peak maximum of previtamin D_3 and trans-vitamin D_3, B = peak width of previtamin D_3, and C = peak width of trans-vitamin D_3. Performance is satisfactory if $R \geq 1.0$.

E. *Calibration*

    Inject 200 μL vitamin D standard solution onto cleanup column through sampling valve, and proceed as in *Determination,* ". . . adjust operating conditions. . . ." Determine retention time of vitamin D on analytical and cleanup columns and peak height of vitamin D on analytical column. Retention time of vitamin D on cleanup column should be between 10 and 20 min; adjust amyl alcohol content of mobile phase, if necessary, to achieve this situation.

F. *Preparation of Sample*

    (a) *Isolation of unsaponifiable matter from powder.*—Accurately weigh ca 50 g milkpowder into saponification flask. Add 100 mL alcohol, 25 mL 25% aqueous Na ascorbate solution, and 25 mL 50% (weight/volume) aqueous KOH solution. Reflux 45 min on steam bath. Cool rapidly under running H_2O. Transfer liquid to separator with two 75 mL portions H_2O, two 25 mL portions alcohol, and two 100 mL portions ether. Shake vigorously 30 s and let stand until both layers are clear. Transfer aqueous phase to second separator and shake with mixture of 25 mL alcohol and 100 mL pentane. Let separate, and transfer aqueous phase to third separator and pentane phase to first separator, washing second separator with two 10 mL portions pentane, adding washings to first separator. Shake aqueous phase with 100 mL pentane and 25 mL alcohol and add pentane to first separator. Wash combined pentane extracts with three 100 mL portions freshly prepared 3% solution of KOH in 10% alcohol, shaking vigorously. Then wash with 100 mL portions H_2O until last washing is neutral to phenolphthalein. Drain last few drops of H_2O, add 4 sheets 9 cm filter paper in strips to separator, and shake.

Transfer dried pentane extract to 500 mL round-bottom flask, rinsing separator and paper with pentane, and add 1 mL antioxidant solution. Evaporate to dryness under vacuum by swirling in H_2O bath at $\leq 40°$. Cool under running H_2O and restore atmospheric pressure with N. Dissolve residue immediately in 2–3 mL toluene-mobile phase (5 + 95).

Transfer extract to 10 mL round-bottom flask, rinsing 500 mL round-bottom flask with pentane. Evaporate under N stream at room temperature. Dissolve residue immediately in 2.0 mL toluene-mobile phase (5 + 95). Use this solution as working sample solution for injection.

(b) *Isolation of unsaponifiable matter from fluid milk.*—Pipet 200 mL milk into 1 L saponification flask. Add 300 mL alcohol, 5 g Na ascorbate, and 50 mL 50% aqueous KOH. Proceed as in (a), beginning, "Reflux 45 min. ... "

G. Determination

(a) *Cleanup.*—Inject 200 μL working sample solution onto cleanup column through sampling valve and adjust operating conditions of detector to give largest possible on-scale peaks for vitamin D. Collect fraction between 2 min before and 2 min after vitamin D peak, in 10 mL volumetric flask. Add 1 mL antioxidant solution and evaporate to dryness under N stream. Dissolve residue immediately in 2 mL toluene-*n*-hexane (5 + 95). Use this solution for injection onto analytical column.

Note: To regenerate cleanup column, wash with amyl alcohol-*n*-hexane (10 + 90) at 6 mL/min until detector response returns to 0 (ca 15 min). Switch to mobile phase, hexane containing 0.35% amyl alcohol. Column is ready for reuse.

(b) *Assay.*—Inject 500 μL solution, (a), onto analytical column through sampling valve, and adjust operating conditions of detector to give largest possible on-scale peaks of vitamin D. Repeat injections of sample and standards to verify that response remains constant. Measure peak height of vitamin D in sample and external standard solutions.

(c) *Calculation.*—Vitamin D potency, IU/g = $(1.25 \times P \times W' \times V \times 40\ 000)/(P' \times W \times V')$ where 1.25 = correction factor for previtamin D formed during refluxing for saponification; P and P' = peak height of vitamin D in sample and reference standard, respectively; W and W' = g sample and mg reference standard, respectively; V and V' = total mL sample and reference standard solutions, respectively; 40 000 = IU vitamin D/mg USP Reference Standard.

Reference: JAOAC **65,** 1228(1982).
CAS-67-97-0 (cholecalciferol; vitamin D_3)
CAS-50-14-6 (ergocalciferol; vitamin D_2)

Chapter 39
Vitamin E

39.1   971.30—α-Tocopherol and α-Tocopheryl Acetate in Foods and Feeds
Colorimetric Method
First Action 1971
Final Action 1972

(Caution: See Appendix for safety notes on hazardous radiations, distillation, petroleum ether, ethanol, diethyl ether, monitoring equipment, spraying chromatograms.)

A. Principle

The following methods are designed to determine vitamin E in foods and feeds in the several forms in which it may occur. Unsupplemented food or feed will contain *natural* α-tocopherol associated with many other reducing substances. This type of sample is extracted, lipid residue saponified, and α-tocopherol isolated by TLC and determined colorimetrically. Foods or feeds may be supplemented with α-tocopheryl acetate added either as oil or in various dry forms. Assay for *total* α-tocopherol (natural plus supplemental) follows same operations described above. To specifically determine α-tocopheryl acetate, sample is extracted, reducing substances, including natural α-tocopherol, are removed by oxidative chromatography, α-tocopheryl acetate is saponified, and resulting α-tocopherol is determined colorimetrically.

Calculation of assay results for supplemented foods and feeds in terms of International Units (IU) is complicated by fact that natural and synthetic α-tocopheryl acetates have different weight-activity factors. α-Tocopherol occurring naturally is in *RRR*-form. With samples supplemented with *RRR*-α-tocopheryl acetate (natural), resulting total α-tocopherol is all in *RRR*-form and IU potency of sample can readily be determined by using appropriate factor. With samples supplemented with *all-rac*-α-tocopheryl acetate (synthetic), resulting total α-tocopherol is mixture of *RRR*- and *all-rac*-forms. To convert to IU, level of supplementation with *all-rac*-α-tocopheryl acetate must be determined specifically and natural α-tocopherol is determined by difference. Appropriate factors are then separately applied to determined levels of *RRR*- and *all-rac*-forms and results are added to determine IU potency of sample. If isomeric nature of supplement is not known, it must be determined separately, **975.43** (*Official Methods of Analysis* [1990] 15th ed.), before IU potency of supplemented samples can be determined.

Precautions.—Evaporate tocopherol solutions with N stream or under vacuum. Do not use air stream. Do not let solution of tocopherol evaporate to dryness for >2–3 s because tocopherol in thin film is subject to oxidation. Perform TLC, including detection step (except for UV light), in darkness or very subdued light. Complete all steps as promptly as possible. If analysis cannot be completed in 1 day, store solutions at −20°.

B. Apparatus

(a) *Spectrophotometric colorimeter.*—Bausch & Lomb Spectronic 20 colorimeter with matched 13 mm test tubes (Milton Roy Co., Analytical Products Div., 820 Linden Ave, Rochester, NY 14625, or equivalent).

(b) *Spectrophotometer.*—Beckman Model DU (replacement Model DU-70) with incandescent light source and matched cells (1 cm light path; 4.5 or 1.6 mL capacity), or equivalent. (If cell holder does not elevate larger cells so liquid is in light path, use small plugs [usually 1 cm] in bottom of holder.)

(c) *Extractor.*—Hot alcohol extraction apparatus (*Anal. Chem.* **20**, 1221[1948]), Goldfisch extractor (Labconco Corp.), or equivalent.

(d) *Chromagram® sheet.*—Type X6062. Alumina adsorbent without fluorescent indicator, for AOAC vitamin E assay. If activation is necessary, heat 30 min at 105° in air oven.

(e) *Pipets.*—Ultra-micro, measuring pipets, 50 μL capacity (VWR Scientific, No. 53477-089, or equivalent).

(f) *Developing chamber.*—Corning Glass Works Pyrex 6944, or equivalent.

(g) *Sprayer.*—Aerosol propellant (VWR Scientific No. 21434-086, or equivalent).

(h) *Vials.*—Glass 1.8 mL (1/2 dram) with inert lining (e.g., polyethylene ot Teflon caps) and 25 mL (7 dram) with polyethylene stoppes (Kimble Glass No. 60975-L, or equivalent).

(i) *Ultraviolet lamps.*—366 nm wavelength (longwave) (Blak-Ray UVL-21, Ultra-Violet Products, Inc.) or 254 nm wavelength (shortwave) (Spectronics Corp, 956 Brush Hollow Rd, Westbury, NY 11590, Model R-51, or equivalent).

(j) *Chromatographic tubes.*—18 (id) $\times$ 270 mm.

C. Reagents

(a) *Petroleum ether.*—(*1*) *Purified.*—Boiling range 35–60° (Skellysolve F, Getty Refining and Marketing Co, or equivalent). Redistil from KOH pellets and Zn granules or dust, discarding first and last 5%. (*2*) *High boiling.*—Boiling range 60–71° (Skellysolve B, or equivalent).

(b) *Alcohol.*—Absolute or SDA 3-A (absolute). If significant reducing substances are present, redistil from Al and KOH.

(c) *Petroleum ether-absolute alcohol mixture.*—Dilute 600 mL petroleum ether, (a)(*2*), to 1 L with absolute alcohol.

(d) *RRR-α-Tocopherol.*—Eastman Kodak grade or equivalent purity. Prepare 1 mg/mL standard solution in absolute alcohol and store at 5°.

(e) *2′,7′-Dichlorofluorescein solution.*—Dissolve 4 mg dye (Eastman Kodak No. 373) in 100 mL absolute alcohol.

(f) *Anhydrous ether.*—Redistil from KOH pellets and Al granules or dust, discarding first and last 5%.

(g) *Bathophenanthroline solution.*—0.003M. Dissolve 100 mg 4,7-diphenyl-1,10-phenanthroline (bathophenanthroline, G. Frederick Smith Chem. Co.) in 100 mL absolute alcohol. Store in amber or opaque glassware at 5°. Prepare fresh solution every 3 weeks.

(h) *Ferric chloride solution.*—0.002M. Dissolve 55 mg $FeCl_3 \cdot 6H_2O$ in 100 mL absolute alcohol. Store in amber or opaque glassware at 5°.

(i) *Orthophosphoric acid.*—0.172M. Dilute 1.1 mL 86% H_3PO_4 to 100 mL with absolute alcohol.

(j) *Anhydrous sodium sulfate.*—Granular and powdered.

(k) *Concentrated potassium hydroxide solution.*—Dissolve 80 g KOH pellets in 50 mL H_2O.

(l) *Phenolphthalein solution.*—Dissolve 1 g phenolphthalein in 100 mL absolute alcohol.

(m) *Isopropyl ether.*—Eastman Kodak No. 1193, or equivalent.

(n) *Water-saturated n-butanol.*—Mix 800 mL *n*-BuOH with 160 mL H_2O.

(o) *Ascorbic acid.*—Eastman Kodak No. 4640, or equivalent.

(p) *Cyclohexane.*—Eastman Kodak No. 702, or equivalent.

(q) *Fuller's earth.*—Florex AA-RVM grade, 60–100 mesh (Floridin Co.).

(**r**) *Ceric sulfate-treated fuller's earth.*—To 4.8 g $Ce(HSO_4)_4$ (G. Frederick Smith Chemical Co.) add mixture of 0.5 mL H_2SO_4 and ca 5 mL H_2O, and stir. Dilute to 100 mL with H_2O. Warm in hot H_2O bath and shake until almost all $Ce(HSO_4)_4$ is dissolved. Cool to ca 35–40° and use promptly ($Ce(HSO_4)_4$ precipitates on standing at room temperature). Spread 200 g fuller's earth in large glazed porcelain dish. Distribute 100 mL $Ce(HSO_4)_4$ solution on fuller's earth, stir gently but thoroughly, and dry 48 h in 60° oven. Store in tightly capped bottle.

(**s**) *Diatomaceous earth.*—Celite 501, or equivalent inert filter-aid.

(**t**) *Benzene.*—Aldrich Chemical Co., Inc., No. 27, 070-9, or product of equivalent purity without additional purification.

(**u**) *Olive oil.*—USP, containing 1.5 mg total reducing substances/g, or equivalent oil.

D. Preparation of Sample and Extraction

(Use for determination of natural α-tocopherol, total α-tocopherol [natural α-tocopherol + supplemental α-tocopheryl acetate], or supplemental α-tocopheryl acetate.)

Sample size of 10 g is convenient for most foods and feeds. Use 40 g with dry feeds and foods supplemented with high potency preparations at low levels (1 IU/100 g). Minimum weight is 1 g, containing 0.1 IU of total α-tocopherol or supplemental α-tocopheryl acetate; if assay for both is performed on same initial sample, minimum amount is 0.2 IU for each component.

(**a**) *Fat or oil.*—Gently warm solid fat to liquefy, mix thoroughly, and weigh. To determine total α-tocopherol, place sample in ℉ 125 mL round-bottom flask for saponification as in **971.30E**. To determine supplemental α-tocopheryl acetate, proceed directly as in **948.26B** (*see* 39.2).

(**b**) *Milk and milk products.*—Measure exactly 60 mL milk or reconstituted powdered or concentrated milk product, add equal volume absolute alcohol, and shake to mix. Add 150 mL ether, shake 30 s, add 150 mL petroleum ether, (**a**)(*1*), and shake 30 s. Let layers separate and remove ether layer. Repeat extraction ≥2 times, using 25 mL absolute alcohol, 100 mL ether, and 100 mL petroleum ether each time. Combine ether layers and evaporate to 50 mL. Take 10 mL aliquot, evaporate solvent, and weigh lipid. Transfer remaining 40 mL or aliquot containing ca 1 g lipid and ≥0.1 IU vitamin E to ℉ 125 mL round-bottom flask. Evaporate solvent under N on steam bath. To determine total α-tocopherol, proceed immediately to saponification as in **971.30E**. To determine supplemental α-tocopheryl acetate, proceed as in **948.26B**.

(**c**) *Wet products.*—Place accurately weighed sample in large mortar and grind thoroughly with 2–3 times its weight of anhydrous powdered Na_2SO_4 until dry mixture is obtained. Quantitatively transfer mixture to ≥1 Soxhlet thimbles, using absolute alcohol as rinsing liquid, and proceed as in (**d**).

(**d**) *Dry products.*—(Applicable to products such as premixes, feed concentrates, and feeds which may or may not be supplemented with α-tocopheryl acetate, either in dry carrier or added directly to product, but not in gelatin, vegetable gum, or dextrin matrix.) If coarse particles are present, grind sample. Place accurately weighed sample into Soxhlet thimble. Place 100 mL absolute alcohol and boiling chip in flask and either mark liquid level or weigh flask and contents. Assemble hot ethanol extraction apparatus, attach condenser, and extract over steam bath 16 h (overnight). (Use 4 h extraction with Goldfisch extractor.) Stopper flask, cool extract to room temperature, and add absolute alcohol, if necessary, to restore to ca original volume.

Transfer extract to separator, rinse flask with 100 mL H_2O followed by 50 mL petroleum ether, (**a**)(*2*), and ca 0.5 g granular anhydrous Na_2SO_4, and add rinses to separator. Shake separator 10 min, let layers separate, and drain and discard aqueous layer. Dilute petroleum ether extract to 50 mL; take 10 mL aliquot, evaporate solvent, and weigh lipid. Continue as in (**b**), beginning "Transfer remaining 40 mL or …''

(e) *Dry products supplemented with α-tocopheryl acetate in gelatin, vegetable gum, or dextrin matrix.*—Proceed as in (d), through ". . . discard aqueous layer." Retain petroleum ether extract. Quantitatively transfer contents of Soxhlet extraction thimble to ⍦ round-bottom flask, with total of 50 mL 2.5N H_2SO_4. Attach reflux condenser and reflux 30 min on hot plate. Cool to room temperature and transfer to separator, rinsing flask with 50 mL absolute alcohol. Extract with two 75 mL and one 50 mL portions petroleum ether, (a)(2). Combine petroleum ether extracts and petroleum ether extract obtained from hot alcohol extraction. Evaporate under N to <50 mL and dilute to 50 mL. Take 10 mL aliquot, evaporate solvent, and weigh lipid. Continue as in (b), beginning "Transfer remaining 40 mL or . . ." except that **948.26B** is not applicable to determine supplemental α-tocopheryl acetate.

(f) *Expanded dog foods and baked dog biscuits supplemented before expansion, processing, or baking.*—Grind sample. Place accurately weighed portion in ⍦ 250 mL round-bottom flask connected to H_2O condenser. Add 25 mL H_2O-saturated *n*-BuOH. Insert condenser, heat solution to bp over steam bath, and reflux 1 h, swirling every 10 min. Cool, and evaporate to absolute dryness under vacuum at 60°. Quantitatively transfer dried sample to ≥1 Soxhlet extraction thimbles, using absolute alcohol as rinsing liquid, and proceed as in (d).

E. Saponification and Re-extraction

Prepare sample as in **971.30D** or **948.26C**. For each gram (or fraction of gram) of lipid residue in ⍦ 125 mL round-bottom flask, add 4 mL absolute alcohol and 0.3 g ascorbic acid. Attach reflux condenser and heat to bp in boiling H_2O bath. Raise condenser and add 1 mL concentrated KOH solution for each gram (or fraction of gram) of lipid residue, replace condenser, and reflux 15 min. (*Note:* Exclusion of air is essential, since tocopherols in alkaline solutions are easily oxidized.)

Stopper and cool rapidly under cold running H_2O. Transfer solution to separator, using 20 mL H_2O/g (or fraction of gram) of lipid residue. Extract unsaponifiable matter by rinsing saponification flask and shaking with each of three 25 mL portions ether for each gram (or fraction of gram) of lipid residue. (*Caution:* Emulsions may form; add salt to break.) Combine ether extracts and wash with equal volumes H_2O until solution is neutral to phenolphthalein. Filter washed ether extract through anhydrous granular Na_2SO_4 into erlenmeyer, rinsing with ether. Concentrate ether solution to ca 5 mL under N with gentle warming. Transfer solution to 10 mL volumetric flask, rinse, and dilute to volume with ether. Use one aliquot of this ether solution for TLC, **971.30F**, and another aliquot for determination of total reducing substances, **971.30G**.

(*Note:* If samples contain ethoxyquin or BHA, wash ether unsaponifiable extract [before H_2O wash] twice with equal volume H_2SO_4 [1 + 1]. Then proceed with H_2O wash of ether. *Caution:* If ether is visible in the H_2SO_4 [1 + 1], wash the H_2SO_4 [1 + 1] once with ether and combine this ether with original ether.)

F. Thin-Layer Chromatography of Unsaponifiable Matter and Elution of α-Tocopherol

Perform TLC of α-tocopherol in darkness or subdued light.

(a) *Establishment of recovery factor.*—(TLC method is sensitive to ambient humidity.) Based on ambient relative humidity, treat alumina sheet and select solvent systems as given in Table **971.30** to obtain R_f for α-tocopherol of 0.5–0.7.

Table 971.30.—Humidity Conditions for TLC of α-Tocopherol

Relative Humidity, %	Activation of Sheet	Solvent Systems	
		1st Dimension Benzene-Ether	2nd Dimension Pet Ether, (a)(1)-IsoPr Ether
<20	No	$60+40+1\%$ H_2O	$50+50+1\%$ H_2O
20	No	$60+40$	$50+50$
40	No	$90+10$	$80+20$
60	No	$100+0$	$90+10$
>60	Yes	cyclohexane-benzene, $20+80$	$100+0$

Using micropipet, quantitatively transfer 10 μL standard solution (10 μg α-tocopherol) slowly to form small spot ca 2 cm from lower and left-hand edges of alumina sheet. Use small amount of ether to rinse micropipet and add to spot. Dry spot with N jet during spotting.

Immediately place sheet in chamber and develop in first dimension, using predetermined first dimension solvent system (Table **971.30**). Develop chromatogram until solvent front has moved ca 15–16 cm from bottom of sheet, remove sheet from chamber, and dry with N. Turn sheet 90° counterclockwise, immediately place in second chamber, and develop with predetermined second dimension solvent system until solvent front is ca 15–16 cm from bottom of sheet.

Remove sheet from chamber and dry with N. Spray sheet lightly with alcoholic dichlorofluorescein solution. When sheet is completely dry (ca 5 min), locate tocopherol spots under UV light. (*Warning:* Excessive use of UV light can destroy tocopherol.)

Circle tocopherol spot (allowing safety margin of ca 5 mm around spot) and also circle spot of comparable size from unused but sprayed portion of sheet for blank. Cut out both spots and place in separate 25 mL vials containing 1.4 mL bathophenanthroline solution, (**g**), replace cap, swirl, and let stand 15 min for elution. Proceed as in **971.30G(a)** for colorimetry.

Recovery factor(s) = μg α-tocopherol recovered from sheet/μg-tocopherol taken as sample. (Recovery factors should be constant within a laboratory but may range from ca 75 to 85%.)

(**b**) *TLC of sample.*—Pipet aliquot of ether solution of unsaponifiable matter, containing ca 10–20 μg α-tocopherol, into 1.8 mL screw-cap vial. Evaporate ether with N until 0.1–0.2 mL remains. Using micropipet, transfer entire contents of vial slowly to form small spot ca 2 cm from lower and left-hand edges of alumina sheet. Use few drops ether to rinse vial and transfer this solution to same spot. Dry spot with jet of N during spotting.

Immediately place sheet in chamber and develop as in (**a**). (If ethoxyquin has not been completely removed in **971.30E**, it will be very bright blue fluorescent spot located ca 1 cm above α-tocopherol spot [dark purple with no fluorescence].)

Elute α-tocopherol spot as in (**a**). (Most desirable way to identify α-tocopherol spot correctly is to chromatograph α-tocopherol standard with extract aliquot. In first dimension, spot standard ca 2 cm from lower and right-hand edges of sheet. In second dimension, spot standard ca 2 cm from lower and left-hand edges of sheet *after* sheet has been turned 90° counterclockwise.)

G. Colorimetry of α-Tocopherol

Method (**a**) is applicable only to Beckman spectrophotometer and samples low in fat; (**b**) is applicable to any spectrophotometer using working volume of ≤ 6 mL in colorimeter tube and sample may contain considerable fat.

(**a**) *Colorimetry after TLC.*—Take 1.0 mL from 1.4 mL bathophenanthroline solution from each vial. Place in 15 mL centrifuge tube, add 0.3 mL $FeCl_3$ solution, (**h**), dropwise, and swirl. Exactly 15 s after addition of last drop, add 0.3 mL H_3PO_4 solution, (**i**), and swirl. After 3 min, color formed is stable 90 min.

If necessary, centrifuge to settle adsorbent particles. Add supernate to separate cells and measure A in Beckman spectrophotometer at 534 nm against A of blank spot.

Determine amounts of α-tocopherol in circled spot, using response factor or calibration curve prepared by colorimetry above and recovery factor determined in **971.30F(a)**.

(**b**) *Colorimetry of α-tocopherol or total reducing material.*—Select colorimeter tubes matched with 6 mL petroleum ether, (**a**)(*2*)-absolute alcohol (3 + 2). Maintain constant subdued lighting conditions throughout colorimetry.

(*1*) *Calibration curve.*—Place exactly 4 mL petroleum ether, (**a**)(*2*)-absolute alcohol (3 + 2) containing 5 μg pure α-tocopherol in 25 mL vial. Add exactly 1.0 mL bathophenanthroline solution, swirl, add exactly 0.5 mL $FeCl_3$ solution dropwise, and swirl. Exactly 15 s after addition of last drop of $FeCl_3$ solution, add exactly 0.5 mL H_3PO_4 solution and swirl. After 3 min, color formed is stable 90 min.

Transfer solution to matched colorimeter tube and measure A in spectrophotometer at 534 nm against reagent blank prepared in same manner but without addition of α-tocopherol.

Repeat steps 5 times, using 5–50 μg α-tocopherol; plot A against μg α-tocopherol/6 mL on linear graph paper. Draw best fitting smooth curve through 6 points and origin. Check calibration curve daily and prepare new curve when new reagent solutions are prepared.

(*2*) *Colorimetric determination.*—Accurately transfer sample or aliquot containing ca 20 μg α-tocopherol or equivalent amount of reducing substances to 25 mL vial. Evaporate to dryness under N, immediately add exactly 4 mL petroleum ether, (**a**)(*2*)-absolute alcohol (3 + 2), and swirl until sample is dissolved. Proceed as in (*1*), beginning "Add exactly 1.0 mL bathophenanthroline solution. . . ."

If sample contains appreciable amounts (>100 mg) of lipid or unsaponifiable matter, transfer solution to colorimeter or centrifuge tube and centrifuge ca 10 min at ca 2500 rpm before colorimetric determination. If color formed is too great for accurate A determination, dilute solution with reagent blank solution and read A again.

Determine α-tocopherol or α-tocopherol equivalent of reducing substances from previously established standard curve in μg α-tocopherol/6 mL.

H. Calculations

(**a**) *For TLC.*—mg α-Tocopherol/sample = μg α-tocopherol measured × (1.4/1.0) × (*x*/*y*) × (*v*/*w*) × (1/1000), where 1.4 and 1.0 = mL bathophenanthroline used for elution and taken from eluate, respectively; x = total mL extract before saponification; y = mL of x used for saponification; v = total mL unsaponifiable extract; w = mL of v used for spotting on TLC, 1/1000 = factor to convert μg to mg.

(**b**) *For total reducing material.*—mg α-Tocopherol equivalent/sample = μg α-tocopherol measured × (*x*/*y*) × (*d*/*e*) × (1/1000), where symbols are defined in (**a**), d = total mL unsaponifiable extract, and e = mL of d used for colorimeter reading.

I. Calculation of IU Potency

(**a**) *For products not containing added α-tocopheryl acetate.*—IU/g sample = (mg α-tocopherol in sample/weight sample in grams) × 1.49.

(**b**) *For products supplemented with RRR-α-tocopheryl acetate (natural).*—Calculate as in (**a**).

(**c**) *For products supplemented with all-rac-α-tocopheryl acetate (synthetic).*—mg *all-rac*-α-Tocopherol/g sample = (mg *all-rac*-α-tocopherol in sample [**948.26E(c)**]/weight sample in grams).

mg *RRR*-α-Tocopherol/g sample = (mg α-tocopherol in sample (**971.30H**)/weight sample in grams)
− (mg *all-rac*-α-tocopherol/weight sample in grams).

IU/g sample = (mg *RRR*-α-tocopherol/weight sample in grams) × 1.49
+ (mg *all-rac*-α-tocopherol/weight sample in grams) × 1.10.

References: Anal. Chem. **20**, 1221(1948); **28**, 376(1956); **33**, 849(1961). Analyst **84**, 356(1959). J. Chromatogr. **30**, 502(1967). JAOAC **45**, 425(1962); **49**, 1060(1966); **54**, 1(1971).
CAS-59-02-5 (α-tocopherol)
CAS-7695-91-2 (α-tocopheryl acetate)

39.2   948.26—α-Tocopheryl Acetate (Supplemental) in Foods and Feeds
Colorimetric Method
Final Action 1980

(*Caution*: *See Appendix* for safety notes on distillation, vacuum, flammable solvents, and petroleum ether.)

A. Modified Extraction for Supplemental α-Tocopheryl Acetate Only

(Methods for sample preparation and extraction described in **971.30D** (*see* 39.1), are usually sufficient. Following modified extraction techniques may be used for special cases.)

(**a**) *Wet products.*—Place accurately weighed sample in large mortar and grind thoroughly with 2–3 times its weight anhydrous powdered Na_2SO_4 until dry mixture is obtained. Quantitatively transfer mixture to glass-stoppered flask, add 50 mL purified ether, shake thoroughly 15 min, and let solids settle. Take 10 mL aliquot of clear extract, evaporate solvent, and weigh lipid. Transfer ≤30 mL aliquot containing ca 1 g lipid and ca 0.1 IU supplemental vitamin E to ℑ 125 mL round-bottom flask, evaporate solvent under N on steam bath, and proceed as in **948.26B**.

(**b**) *Expanded dog foods and baked dog biscuits supplemented before expansion, processing, or baking.*—Proceed as in **971.30D(f)**, except after refluxing, cool solution and let solids settle. Assume that volume liquid present equals volume H_2O-saturated *n*-BuOH added plus H_2O content of sample extracted. Take aliquot of H_2O-saturated *n*-BuOH extract containing ca 0.1 IU supplemental vitamin E and evaporate to dryness under vacuum in 60° H_2O bath. Quantitatively transfer dried aliquot to Soxhlet extraction thimble, using purified petroleum ether, (**a**)(*1*), as rinsing liquid. Re-extract residue in Soxhlet 45 min with 50 mL purified petroleum ether, (**a**)(*1*). Evaporate under N to <50 mL and dilute to 50 mL. Take 10 mL aliquot, evaporate solvent, and weigh lipid. Transfer remaining 40 mL or aliquot containing ca 1 g lipid and 0.1 IU supplemental vitamin E to ℑ 125 mL round-bottom flask, evaporate solvent under N on steam bath, and proceed as in **948.26B**.

B. Oxidative Chromatography

(**a**) *Preparation of column.*—See **975.43D(c)(1)**.

975.43D (Identification of *RRR*- or *all-rac*-α-Tocopherol in Drugs and Food or Feed Supplements, Polarimetric Method)

> *D. Preparation of Sample and Extraction*
>
> (*Caution: See Appendix* for safety notes on distillation, vacuum, flammable solvents, benzene, diethyl ether, ethanol, and petroleum ether.)
>
> *See* **971.30D** (*see* 39.1) and following:
>
> (**c**) *Soft-shelled multivitamin capsules.*—(*1*) *Preparation of column.*—Place in order, on top of small glass wool plug in chromatographic tube: 3 g fuller's earth, 3 g Ce(HSO$_4$)$_4$-treated fuller's earth, 3 mm layer fuller's earth, 3 g Ce(HSO$_4$)$_4$-treated fuller's earth, 4 g fuller's earth, and 5 mm layer diatomaceous earth on top. Tap gently after addition of each portion of adsorbent to ensure even packing. Wash column under suction with ca 200 mL petroleum ether, **971.30C(a)(*1*)**. Keep layer of solvent above top of adsorbent at all times. Use new column for each assay.

(**b**) *Elution of α-tocopheryl acetate.*—Quantitatively transfer test sample or aliquot containing ca 0.1 IU supplemental α-tocopheryl acetate from **971.30D** or **948.26A** in 4 mL petroleum ether, (a)(*1*) (aliquot may be evaporated just to dryness under N and residue then dissolved in petroleum ether, (a)(*1*)) to top of chromatographic column, using elongated dropper. If aliquot contains <500 mg lipid, add olive oil as necessary to give this minimum amount of lipid. Use ca five 1.0 mL portions petroleum ether, (a)(*1*), as rinses for quantitative transfer. To prevent column from running dry, do not use vacuum during sample transfer. Elute column with 100 mL benzene. Evaporate benzene eluate to ca 4 mL on steam bath under N stream and then to dryness under N with reduced heat. Dissolve residue and dilute to 10 mL with petroleum ether, (a)(*2*)-absolute alcohol (3 + 2). Use ≤5 mL to determine reducing substances before saponification as in **948.26D(a)**. Use ≤4 mL for saponification in **948.26C**.

C. Saponification

Accurately transfer ≤4 mL aliquot of petroleum ether, (a)(*2*)-absolute alcohol (3 + 2) containing ca 20 μg α-tocopherol to T 125 mL round-bottom flask. Evaporate to dryness under N and saponify as in **971.30E**, except that entire dry ether extract should be concentrated to small volume in 25 mL vial. Proceed as in **948.26D(b)**.

D. Colorimetry

(**a**) *Before saponification.*—Using ≤5 mL petroleum ether, (a)(*2*)-absolute alcohol solution from **948.26B**, determine α-tocopherol equivalent of extraneous reducing substances not removed in oxidative chromatography by colorimetry as in **971.30G(b)**.

> (*Note:* If α-tocopherol equivalent of reducing substances before saponification [μg/g sample] exceeds 15% of α-tocopherol after saponification [μg/g sample], repeat assay, using ≥2 oxidative chromatographic columns, or equivalent. With unusually high levels of antioxidants, solvent partition or other purification steps may be necessary.)

(**b**) *After saponification.*—Assay concentrated ether extracts in 25 mL vial from **948.26C** for α-tocopherol as in **971.30G(b)**.

> (*Note:* If excessive amounts of non-α-tocopheryl acetate [>15%] are present in feed supplement or supplemented feed, determine α-tocopherol as follows: After oxidative chromatography as in **948.26B** and saponification as in **971.30E**, use aliquot of ether extract for TLC, **971.30F**. Apply ratio of α-tocopherol in **971.30G[a]** to total tocopherols as determined in **948.26D[b]** as correction factor to mg α-tocopherol/g sample in **948.26E[c]**.)

E. Calculations

(a) mg Reducing substances before saponification/sample = μg substances measured $\times$ (x/y) $\times$ ($10/w$) $\times$ (1/1000), where x = total mL extract from **971.30D**; y = mL extract used for chromatography, **948.26B**; 10 = mL solution after chromatography; w = mL taken for colorimetry; and 1/1000 = factor to convert μg to mg.

(b) mg α-Tocopherol after saponification/sample = μg α-tocopherol measured $\times$ (x/y) $\times$ ($10/v$) $\times$ (1/1000), where symbols are defined in (a), 10 = mL solution after chromatography, and v = mL taken for saponification.

(c) mg α-Tocopherol/sample = (mg α-tocopherol/sample, after saponification) − (mg reducing substances/sample, before saponification).

(d) mg α-Tocopheryl acetate/g sample = (mg α-tocopherol in sample/weight sample in grams) $\times$ 1.098.

(e) Determine IU added vitamin E/g sample as follows:

If *RRR*-α-tocopheryl acetate is present: IU vitamin E/g sample = (mg α-tocopheryl acetate/weight sample in grams) $\times$ 1.36.

If *all-rac*-α-tocopheryl acetate is present: IU vitamin E/g sample = (mg α-tocopheryl acetate/weight sample in grams) $\times$ 1.00.

References: Anal. Chem. **20**, 1221(1948); **28**, 376(1956); **32**, 849(1961). Analyst **84**, 356(1959). J. Chromatogr. **30**, 502(1967). JAOAC **45**, 425(1962); **49**, 1060(1966); **54**, 1(1971).
CAS-7695-91-2 (α-tocopheryl acetate)

39.3   992.03—Vitamin E Activity (*All-rac*-α-Tocopherol) in Milk-Based Infant Formula
Liquid Chromatographic Method
First Action 1992

(Applicable to determination of vitamin E activity in milk-based infant formula.)

Method Performance (milk-based liquid, ready-to-feed):
Mean recovery = 24.14 IU vitamin E/L infant formula
s_r = 2.04; s_R = 2.82; RSD_r = 8.46%; RSD_R = 11.69%

A. Principle

Vitamin E activity in samples of infant formula is determined by saponification of all-rac-α-tocopherol, partitioning with organic solvent, separation from sample matrix, and quantification by liquid chromatography.

B. Apparatus

(a) *Liquid chromatograph (LC).*—Capable of pressures up to 3000 psi with injector capable of 100 μL injections. Operating conditions: eluent flow rate 2.0 $\pm$ 0.2 mL/min; temperature ambient.

(b) *Detector.*—Capable of measuring absorbance at 280 nm, with sensitivity 0.02 AUFS.

(c) *Precolumn.*—2 mm id × 2 cm stainless steel, packed with 40 μm pellicular reversed-phase C18 (Alltech 28551 is suitable).

(d) *Column.*—4.6 mm id × 25 cm stainless steel, packed with 5 μm silica (Hypersil Silica is suitable).

(e) *Shaking water bath.*—Capable of maintaining 70 ± 2°, with variable speed capable of 60 oscillations/min, ca 11 × 14" sample area (Precision Scientific model 25 is suitable).

(f) *Glassware.*—*(1)* 125 mL separatory funnels. *(2)* 5 mL volumetric flasks. *(3)* 100 mL low-actinic volumetric flasks.

C. Reagents

(a) *Mobile phase solution.*—Hexane–isopropyl alcohol (99.92 + 0.08, v/v), HPLC grade solvents. Degas 2–5 min under vacuum.

(b) *Wash solution.*—H_2O–absolute ethanol (3 + 2, v/v).

(c) *Extraction solution.*—Hexane–methylene chloride (3 + 1, v/v), HPLC grade solvents.

(d) *Saponification solution.*—10.5N potassium hydroxide (KOH). Dissolve 673 g KOH in 1 L H_2O.

(e) *Antioxidant solution.*—1% pyrogallol. Dissolve 5.0 g pyrogallol (1,3,5-trihydroxybenzene, 98%, Aldrich is suitable source) in 500 mL absolute ethanol.

(f) *Standard solutions.*—*(1) Stock standard solution.*—0.5 mg/mL *all-rac*-α-tocopheryl acetate in hexane. Accurately weigh ca 50 mg *all-rac*-α-tocopheryl acetate (USP Reference Standard) into 100 mL low-actinic volumetric flask and dilute to volume with hexane (HPLC grade). Shake well to dissolve. Make fresh every 3 weeks. Store at –20° in explosion-proof freezer when not in use. *(2) Working standard solution.*—10 μg/mL *all-rac*-α-tocopheryl acetate. Pipet 2 mL stock standard solution, *(1)*, into 100 mL low-actinic volumetric flask. Evaporate to dryness under nitrogen. Dissolve residue in antioxidant solution, C(e), and dilute to volume. Prepare fresh daily.

(g) *Suitability test solution.*—Approximately 15 μg/mL *all-rac*-α-tocopherol (USP Reference Standard) and *all-rac*-α-tocopheryl acetate (USP Reference Standard) in hexane (HPLC grade).

D. Extraction of Standard and Samples

Pipet 10.0 mL working standard solution, C(f)*(2)*, or sample volume containing ca 0.095 IU vitamin E activity (10 mL for ready-to-feed formulas) into 150 mL centrifuge tube. Bring sample volume to 10 mL with H_2O, if necessary. To standard tubes, add 10 mL H_2O, 20 mL antioxidant solution, C(e), and 5 mL saponification solution, C(d). To sample tubes, add 30 mL antioxidant solution and 5 mL saponification solution. Cap tubes and swirl briefly to mix. Place tubes in 70° shaking H_2O bath (ca 60 oscillations/min) for 25 min. Remove tubes and place in ice 5 min, or until contents cool to room temperature.

Quantitatively transfer contents to separate 125 mL separatory funnels. Wash remaining sample or standard from tube into funnel with 30 mL H_2O. Pipet 30.0 mL extraction solvent, C(c), into funnel and shake ca 2 min. When layers separate, discard aqueous (lower) layer. Add 30 mL wash solution, C(b), to funnel and shake very gently 30 s, venting frequently. Let phases separate and discard aqueous layer. Repeat wash step 3×. Pipet 20.0 mL portion from funnel into 50 mL tube and evaporate to dryness under nitrogen. Transfer residues quantitatively to separate 5 mL volumetric flasks and dilute to volume with mobile phase solution, C(a). Inject 100 μL standard or sample into LC.

E. System Suitability Test

Inject 100 μL test solution, C(g), into LC. Typical peak retention times for tocopherol and tocopheryl acetate are 6.0 and 5.0 min, respectively. Calculate resolution (R) factor between tocopherol and tocopheryl acetate as follows:

$$R = 2(t_2 - t_1)/(W_1 + W_2)$$

where t_1 and t_2 = retention time measured from injection time to elution time of peak maximum of tocopherol and tocopheryl acetate, respectively, and W_1 and W_2 = width of peak measured by extrapolating relatively straight sides to baseline of alcohol and acetate, respectively.

If R factor is >1.0, proceed with sample analysis; if R factor is <1.0, decrease amount of isopropyl alcohol added per liter (mobile phase solution, **C[a]**) by ca 0.01%. Inject working standard solution, **C(f)**(2), 5×. Calculate reproducibility of replicate injections in terms of standard deviations (per USP), which should be ≤2%. Typical relative standard deviation values for peak height are ±1.5%.

F. Liquid Chromatography

Inject 100 μL standard or sample into LC.

G. Calculations

Measure peak heights or peak areas of *all-rac*-α-tocopherol in both sample and standard chromatograms. Calculate IU per reconstituted quart of vitamin E activity (A) as follows:

$$A = H_{sam}/H_{std} \times C_{std} \times 0.001 \text{ IU}/\mu g \times 946.33 \text{ mL/quart}$$

where H_{sam} = peak height of sample; H_{std} = peak height of standard; C_{std} = concentration of standard, μg/mL.

Ref.: J. AOAC Int. **76**, 398(1993).
CAS-59-02-9 (α-tocopherol)
CAS-7695-91-2 (α-tocopheryl acetate)

Chapter 40
Zinc

40.1

968.08—Minerals in Animal Feed
Atomic Absorption Spectrophotometric Method
First Action 1968
Final Action 1969

See Chapter 12.1.

40.2

975.03—Metals in Plants
Atomic Absorption Spectrophotometric Method
First Action 1975
Final Action 1988

See Chapter 12.2.

40.3

980.03—Metals in Plants
Direct Reading Spectrographic Method
Final Action 1988

See Chapter 12.3.

40.4

965.09—Nutrients (Minor) in Fertilizers
Atomic Absorption Spectrophotometric Method
First Action 1965
Final Action 1969

See Chapter 12.4.

40.5   986.15—Arsenic, Cadmium, Lead, Selenium, and Zinc in Food
Multielement Method
First Action 1986
Final Action 1988

A. Principle

Sample is digested with HNO_3 in closed system. Cd and Pb are determined by anodic stripping voltammetry (ASV). As, Se, and Zn are determined by atomic absorption spectrophotometry (AAS) after generation of metal hydrides (for As and Se).

(*Caution: See Appendix* for safety notes on pipets, nitric acid, perchloric acid, sodium hydroxide, and arsenic trioxide.)

B. Apparatus

(a) *Polarograph.*—With anodic stripping accessories. Typical operating parameters for Model 174 with hanging drop Hg electrode are: Scan rate, 5 mv/s; scan direction, + ; scan range, 1.5 v; initial potential, −0.7 v; modulation amplitude, 25 mv; operation mode, differential pulse; display direction, "−"; drop time, 0.5 s; low pass filter, off; selector, off; pushbutton, initial; output offset, off; and current range, 5–10 μamp, or as needed.

Other instruments and electrodes such as wax impregnated graphite may be used according to manufacturer's directions.

(b) *Atomic absorption spectrophotometer.*—Perkin-Elmer Corp. Model 403, or equivalent, with Zn, As, and Se hollow cathode lamps or As and Se electrodeless discharge lamps, 3 slot, 10 cm Bolling burner head, air-C_2H_2 and H-N-entrained air flames, and deuterium arc background corrector.

(c) *Decomposition vessel.*—70 mL. See **974.14A**.

> **974.14** (Mercury in Fish, Alternative Digestion Method)
>
> *A. Apparatus*
>
> *Digestion vessel.*—*See* Fig. **974.14**. Stainless steel body supporting Teflon crucible and screw-on cap with Teflon liner to provide Teflon sealing surface. Teflon spout is snapped on outside rim to permit quantitative transfer of contents without contact with metal parts. (Available from Uni-Seal Decomposition Vessels, PO Box 9463, Haifa, Israel.)

(d) *Hydride generator.*—*See* Fig. **986.15A** (Key to figure: 1, polyethylene tubing; 2, rubber stopper; 3, flame sealed polyethylene tubing with holes punched at one end; 4, reagent cup; 5, sodium borohydride solution; 6, sample solution; 7, nitrogen inlet from "auxiliary" line of AAS). Constructed from following: (*1*) *Flat-bottom flask.*—Borosilicate glass, 50 mL (Corning No. 5160, or equivalent). (*2*) *Stopper fittings.*—Two-hole (1 through center) No. 9 rubber stopper, fitted with gas outlet tube of 100 mm × ⅛″ (3 mm) id polyethylene tubing through center hole. Place bottom of gas outlet tube through cut off bottom 1″ segment of ⅝″ polyethylene test tube with hole in bottom so that 3 mm of tube protrudes through test tube. Insert through second hole 75 mm × ⅛″ (3 mm) id polyethylene tubing as N inlet tube. Seal bottom end of tube with burner and then punch several holes at sealed end with 21 gage needle. Alternatively, prepare similarly 500 mm × 1/16″ (1.5 mm) id polyethylene tubing and hold in place in stopper with hole-through septum. Connect other end of tubing to AA spectrophotometer with 500 mm Tygon tubing by cutting auxiliary line at ca 75 mm from mixing chamber and attaching tubing. (*3*) *Generator mount.*—(Optional) 64 mm × 0.5″ id pipe secured to laboratory ring stand by means of clamp holder. Insert extension clamp into pipe and attach another clamp to back of clamp to hold clamp in place and to

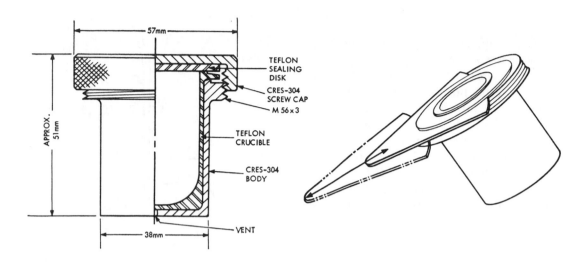

Figure 974.14.—Digestion vessel.

serve as handle; clamp is now free to rotate ca 180°. Attach rubber stopper of hydride generator to extension clamp with stiff wire and position just at level of clamp jaws. In operation, place flask of generator between jaws of extension clamp, insert stopper firmly into neck of flask, then tighten clamp jaws around neck of flask. Unit can be rapidly and uniformly inverted by rotating handle on extention clamp, thus allowing sample and sodium borohydride to mix rapidly and reproducibly.

(**e**) *Pipets.*—50 and 100 μL Eppendorf micropipets, or equivalent.

C. Reagents

(Use double distilled H_2O. Rinse all glassware with HNO_3 (1 + 1) followed by thorough H_2O rinse. Decontaminate digestion vessels by digesting with reagents to be used in digestion. Rinse thoroughly with the H_2O. Decontamination is necessary to reduce blanks, especially for Pb, to acceptable level.)

(**a**) *Acids.*—(*1*) *Nitric acid.*—Redistilled. (*2*) *Perchloric acid.*—70%, double vacuum distilled (G. Fredrick Smith Chemical Co., or equivalent). (*3*) *Hydrochloric acid.*—8M. Dilute 66 mL HCl to 100 mL with H_2O.

(**b**) *Nitrate solution.*—*Equimolar solution of KNO_3 and $NaNO_3$.* Dissolve 54.3 g KNO_3 and 45.7 g $NaNO_3$ (available as Suprapur®, Nos 5065 and 6546, respectively, EM Science) in H_2O in 200 mL volumetric flask, dilute to volume, and mix. To further purify, add 1–2 drops NH_4OH to 25 mL aliquot and extract with 2 mL 10 μg dithizone/mL CCl_4 until lower solvent layer is colorless.

(**c**) *Magnesium solutions.*—(*1*) *Magnesium chloride solution.*—37.5 mg/mL. Dissolve total of 3.75 g MgO, USP, by adding small amounts at time to 100 mL 8M HCl. (*2*) *Magnesium nitrate solution.*—75 mg/mL. Mix 3.75 g MgO, USP, with ca 30 mL H_2O, slowly add HNO_3 to dissolve (ca 10 mL), cool, and dilute to 50 mL with H_2O.

(**d**) *Sodium borohydride solution.*—4.0 g $NaBH_4$/100 mL 4% NaOH.

(**e**) *Potassium iodide solution.*—Dissolve 20 g KI in H_2O and dilute to 100 mL. Prepare just before use.

(**f**) *Metal powders.*—Purity: 99.99+% Cd, Pb, Zn; 99.99% Se. Alfa Products, Morton Thiokol, Inc., 152 Andover St, Danvers, MA 01923.

(**g**) *Cadmium standard solutions.*—(*1*) *Stock solution.*—1 mg/mL. Dissolve 1.000 g Cd powder in 20 mL HNO_3 (1 + 1) in 1 L volumetric flask, and dilute to volume with H_2O. (*2*) *Working solution.*—2 μg/mL. Pipet 10 mL stock solution into 100 mL volumetric flask, and dilute to volume with H_2O. Pipet 2 mL diluted solution into 100 mL volumetric flask and dilute to volume with H_2O.

(**h**) *Lead standard solutions.—(1) Stock solution.*—1 mg/mL. Dissolve 1.000 g Pb powder in 20 mL HNO_3 (1 + 1) in 1 L volumetric flask, and dilute to volume with H_2O. (*2*) *Working solution.*—5 μg/mL. Pipet 1 mL stock solution into 200 mL volumetric flask and dilute to volume with H_2O.

(**i**) *Zinc standard solutions.—(1) Stock solution.*—1 mg/mL. Dissolve 1.000 g Zn powder in 20 mL HCl (1 + 1) in 1 L volumetric flask, and dilute to volume with H_2O. (*2*) *Working solutions.*—0.2, 0.5, 1.0, and 1.5 μg/mL. Pipet 1 mL stock solution into 100 mL volumetric flask and dilute to volume with H_2O. Pipet 2, 5, 10, and 15 mL diluted solution into separate 100 mL volumetric flasks, each containing 1 mL $HClO_4$, and dilute to volume with H_2O.

(**j**) *Arsenic standard solutions.—(1) Stock*

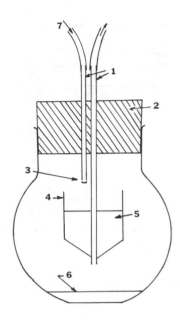

Figure 986.15A.—Hydride generator.

solution.—Dissolve 1.320 g As_2O_3 in minimum volume 20% NaOH in 1 L volumetric flask, acidify with HCl (1 + 1), and dilute to volume with H_2O. (*2*) *Working solutions.*—1, 2, 3, 4, and 5 μg/mL. Pipet 10 mL stock solution into 100 mL volumetric flask, and dilute to volume with H_2O. Pipet 1, 2, 3, 4, and 5 mL diluted solution into separate 100 mL volumetric flasks, and dilute to volume with H_2O.

(**k**) *Selenium standard solutions.—(1) Stock solution.*—1 mg/mL. Dissolve 1.000 g Se powder in minimum volume HNO_3 in 200 mL beaker and evaporate to dryness. Add 2 mL H_2O and evaporate to dryness. Repeat addition of H_2O and evaporation to dryness twice. Dissolve in minimum volume HCl (1 + 9) in 1 L volumetric flask, and dilute to volume with HCl (1 + 9). (*2*) *Working solutions.*—1, 2, 3, 4, and 5 μg/mL. Pipet 10 mL stock solution into 100 mL volumetric flask and dilute to volume with H_2O. Pipet 1, 2, 3, 4, and 5 mL diluted solution into separate 100 mL volumetric flasks and dilute to volume with H_2O.

D. Closed System Digestion

(Do not exceed manufacturer's specifications of 0.3 g solids with 70 mL vessel. Proceed cautiously with new or untried uses. Let such samples stand with HNO_3 overnight or heat on hot plate cautiously until any vigorous reaction subsides. Then proceed with closed vessel digestion. Open vessel in hood since N oxides are released.)

Weigh 0.3 g sample (dry basis) into decontaminated decomposition vessel, add 5 mL HNO_3, close vessel with lid, and heat in 150° oven 2 h. Cool in hood, remove vessel from jacket, and transfer contents to 10 mL volumetric flask. Add 4 mL H_2O to vessel, cover with lid, and while holding lid tightly against rim, invert several times, and add rinse to flask. Dilute to volume with H_2O and mix.

E. Anodic Stripping Voltammetry

(For Cd and Pb)

Pipet aliquot of digested sample solution into decontaminated 50 mL Vycor crucible and add 2 mL nitrate solution, (**b**). Conduct reagent blank simultaneously. Heat on hot plate at low heat to dryness; then increase heat to maximum (ca 375°). Nitrate salts will melt and digest organic matter in 15–20 min. Place crucibles in 450° furnace to oxidize any remaining carbonaceous matter (10–20 min). Digestion is complete when melt is clear. Let cool, add 1 mL HNO_3 (1 + 1) to solidified melt, and heat on hot plate to dryness to expel carbonates and nitrites and to control acidity. Dissolve in 5.0 mL HNO_3 (0.5 mL/L), warming on hot plate to speed solution. Transfer to polarographic cell with 5.0 mL H_2O. Bubble O-free N through solution 5 min; then direct N over solution.

Set dial for Hg drops at 4 μm divisions. Stir solution with magnetic stirrer at constant and reproducible rate so Hg drop is not disturbed. Slide selector switch to "Ext. Cell" and measure time for 120 s with stopwatch. Turn off stirrer and let stand 30 s. Press "Scan" button to obtain peaks corresponding to Cd and Pb at ca −0.57 and −0.43 v, respectively, against saturated calomel electrode.

Add known volumes of each standard to sample solution in cell from Eppendorf pipet. Amounts added should be ca 1×, 2×, etc., of amount metal present initially in cell, and each addition should not change original volume significantly. After each addition, bubble N through solution briefly and perform deposition and stripping operations exactly as for original solution. Plot μg metal added on x-axis against peak height on y-axis. Extrapolate linear line to x-axis to obtain μg metal in cell.

$$\mu\text{g metal/g sample} = [(M - M')/\text{g sample}] \times (10/\text{mL aliquot taken})$$

where M and $M' = \mu$g metal from standard curve for sample and blank, respectively.

F. Atomic Absorption Spectrophotometry

(For As, Se, and Zn)

(a) *Arsenic.*—Pipet aliquot digested sample solution into decontaminated 50 mL round, flat-bottom borosilicate flask, and add 1 mL $Mg(NO_3)_2$ solution, (c) (2). Heat on hot plate at low heat to dryness; then increase heat to maximum (ca 375°). Place flask in 450° furnace to oxidize any carbonaceous matter and to decompose excess $Mg(NO_3)_2$ ($\geq$30 min). Cool, dissolve residue in 2.0 mL 8M HCl, add 0.1 mL 20% KI to reduce As^{5+} to As^{3+}, and let stand $\geq$2 min. Conduct reagent blank with sample.

Prepare standards as follows: To six 50 mL flasks (same type as used for sample) add 2.0 mL $MgCl_2$ solution, (c) (1), and to 5 flasks add 50 μL aliquots of respective working standard solutions so that series will contain 0, 0.05, 0.1, 0.15, 0.20, and 0.25 μg As. (Other amounts may be used depending on sensitivity of system.) Add 0.1 mL 20% KI to each flask, mix, and let stand $\geq$2 min.

Connect generator to instrument as shown in Fig. **986.15B** and adjust pressures and flows as in Table **986.15**. Operate instrument according to manufacturer's instructions, with lamp in place and recorder set for 20 mm/min.

Table 986.15.—Flow Rates and Pressures for Arsenic and Selenium Determinations

Gas	Tank, psi	AA Control Box, psi	Perkin-Elmer Model 403 Flowmeter, divisions
H	20	10	20 (4 L/min)
N	40	30	25 (10 L/min)

Add 2.0 mL 4% NaBH₄ solution to reagent dispenser of generator, and insert rubber stopper tightly into neck of flask containing sample or standard. With single rapid, smooth motion, invert flask, letting solution mix with sample or standard. (This operation must be performed reproducibly.) Sharp, narrow A peak will appear immediately. When recorder pen returns to baseline, remove stopper from flask, and rinse reagent dispenser with H_2O from squeeze bottle; then suck out H_2O. Proceed with next sample or standard. When series is complete, rinse glassware thoroughly.

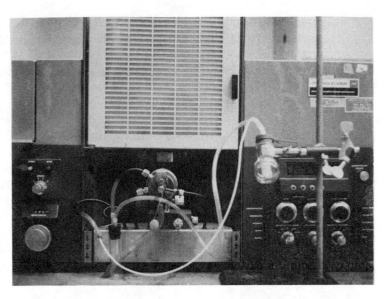

Plot calibration curve of μg As against A, and obtain μg As in sample aliquot from this curve. Correct for reagent blank.

Figure 986.15B.—Hydride generator and mount connected to auxiliary line of spectrophotometer. Test tube acid trap connected between generator and instrument is not included in method.

(b) *Selenium.*—Proceed as in **(a)**, using Se lamp and standards, but omit addition of KI solution. KI will reduce Se to elemental state and cause loss of signal. Instead, cover flask with small watch glass and place on steam bath 10 min, and cool to room temperature.

(c) *Zinc.*—Pipet 1 mL aliquot digested sample solution into decontaminated 25 mL Erlenmeyer, and add 0.1 mL HClO₄. Heat on hot plate to white fumes of HClO₄. Sample should be completely digested as indicated by clear, practically colorless solution. If sample chars, add 0.5 mL portions HNO₃ and again heat to white fumes. Finally, heat just to dryness but do not bake. Cool, and dissolve residue in 3.0 mL HClO₄ (1 + 99).

Operate instrument in accordance with manufacturer's instructions, using air-C₂H₂ flame, and measure A of sample and standards, **(i)(2)**. Dilute sample solution with HClO₄ (1 + 99), if solution is too concentrated. Plot calibration curve of μg Zn against A, and obtain μg Zn in sample aliquot from this curve. Correct for reagent blank.

Reference: JAOAC **63,** 485(1980).
CAS-7440-38-2 (arsenic)
CAS-7440-43-9 (cadmium)
CAS-7439-92-1 (lead)
CAS-7782-49-2 (selenium)
CAS-7440-66-6 (zinc)

40.6   **944.09—Zinc in Food**
Colorimetric Method
Final Action 1976

A. Principle

Method involves wet oxidation of sample; elimination of Pb, Cu, Cd, Bi, Sb, Sn, Hg, and Ag as sulfides with added Cu as scavenger agent; simultaneous elimination of Co and Ni by extracting metal complexes of α-nitroso-β-naphthol and dimethylglyoxime, respectively, with $CHCl_3$; extraction of Zn dithizonate with CCl_4; transfer of Zn to dilute HCl; and final extraction of Zn dithizonate for color measurement.

B. Reagents

(All H_2O must be redistilled from glass. Pyrex glassware should be used exclusively and must be scrupulously cleaned with hot HNO_3. Purify HNO_3 (usually unnecessary) and NH_4OH by distillation in Pyrex if appreciably contaminated. Test H_2SO_4 if Zn contamination is suspected.)

(a) *Copper sulfate solution.*—2 mg Cu/mL. Dissolve 8 g $CuSO_4 \cdot 5H_2O$ in H_2O and dilute to 1 L.

(b) *Ammonium citrate solution.*—Dissolve 225 g $(NH_4)_2HC_6H_5O_7$ in H_2O, make alkaline to phenol red with NH_4OH (pH 7.4, first distinct color change), and add 75 mL in excess. Dilute to 2 L. Extract this solution immediately before use as follows: Add slight excess of dithizone and extract with CCl_4 until solvent layer is clear bright green. Remove excess dithizone by repeated extraction with $CHCl_3$, and finally extract once more with CCl_4. (It is essential that excess dithizone be entirely removed, otherwise Zn will be lost during elimination of Co and Ni.)

(c) *Dimethylglyoxime solution.*—Dissolve 2 g reagent in 10 mL NH_4OH and 200–300 mL H_2O, filter, and dilute to 1 L.

(d) *Alpha-nitroso-beta-naphthol solution.*—Dissolve 0.25 g in $CHCl_3$ and dilute to 500 mL.

(e) *Chloroform.*—Redistilled.

(f) *Diphenylthiocarbazone (dithizone) solution.*—Dissolve 0.05 g dithizone in 2 mL NH_4OH and 100 mL H_2O, and extract repeatedly with CCl_4 until solvent layer is clear bright green. Discard solvent layer and filter aqueous portion through washed ashless paper. (This solution is best prepared as needed, since it is only moderately stable, even when kept in dark and under refrigeration.)

(g) *Carbon tetrachloride.*—Redistilled.

(h) *Dilute hydrochloric acid.*—0.04N. Dilute required amount of HCl with H_2O (redistilled acid may be used although usually unnecessary).

(i) *Zinc standard solutions.*—(1) *Stock solution.*—500 μg/mL. Dissolve 0.500 g pure granulated Zn in slight excess of dilute HCl and dilute to 1 L. (2) *Working solution.*—5 μg/mL. Dilute 10 mL stock solution to 1 L with 0.04N HCl.

C. Preparation of Sample

(*Caution: See Appendix* for safety notes on wet oxidation, nitric acid, perchloric acid, and sulfuric acid.)

Weigh, into suitable size Erlenmeyer, representative sample $\leq$25 g, estimated to contain 25–100 μg Zn. If sample is liquid, evaporate to small volume. Add HNO_3 and heat cautiously until first vigorous reaction subsides somewhat; then add 2–5 mL H_2SO_4. Continue heating, adding more HNO_3 in small portions as needed to prevent charring, until fumes of SO_3 evolve and solution remains clear and almost colorless. Add 0.5 mL $HClO_4$ and continue heating until it is almost completely removed. Cool, and dilute to ca 40 mL. (Wet digestion and subsequent sulfide separation may also be advantageously performed in small Kjeldahl flask.)

D. Separation of Sulfide Group

(*Caution: See Appendix* for safety notes on bromine and hydrogen sulfide.)

To H_2SO_4 solution add 2 drops methyl red and 1 mL $CuSO_4$ solution, and neutralize with NH_4OH. Add enough HCl to make solution ca $0.15N$ with respect to this acid (ca 0.5 mL excess in 50 mL solution is satisfactory); pH of solution as measured with glass electrode is 1.9–2.1. Pass stream of H_2S into solution until precipitation is complete. Filter through fine paper (Whatman No. 42, or equivalent, previously fitted to funnel and washed with HCl (1 + 6), then with redistilled H_2O). Receive filtrate in 250 mL beaker, and wash flask and filter with 3 or 4 small portions H_2O. Gently boil filtrate until odor of H_2S can no longer be detected; then add 5 mL saturated Br-H_2O and continue boiling until Br-free. Cool, neutralize to phenol red with NH_4OH, and make slightly acid with HCl (excess of 0.2 mL 1 + 1 HCl). Dilute resultant solution to definite volume. For optimum conditions of measurement, solution should contain 0.2–1.0 μg Zn/mL.

E. Elimination of Nickel and Cobalt

Transfer 20 mL aliquot of prepared solution to 125 mL separator; add 5 mL ammonium citrate solution, 2 mL dimethylglyoxime solution, and 10 mL α-nitroso-β-naphthol solution; and shake 2 min. Discard solvent layer and extract with 10 mL $CHCl_3$ to remove residual α-nitroso-β-naphthol. Discard solvent layer.

F. Isolation and Estimation of Zinc

To aqueous phase following removal of Ni and Co, which at this point has pH of 8.0–8.2, add 2.0 mL dithizone solution and 10 mL CCl_4, and shake 2 min. Let phases separate and remove aqueous layer as completely as possible, withdrawing liquid with pipet attached to vacuum line. Wash down sides of separator with ca 25 mL H_2O and without shaking again draw off aqueous layer. Add 25 mL $0.04N$ HCl and shake 1 min to transfer Zn to acid-aqueous layer. Drain and discard solvent, being careful to dislodge and remove drop that usually floats on surface. To acid solution add 5.0 mL ammonium citrate solution and 10.0 mL CCl_4 (pH of solution at this point is 8.8–9.0).

Determine volume dithizone to be added as follows: To separator containing 4.0 mL working Zn standard (20 μg), diluted to 25 mL with $0.04N$ HCl, 5.0 mL citrate buffer, and 10.0 mL CCl_4, add dithizone reagent in 0.1 mL increments, shaking briefly after each addition until faint yellow in aqueous phase indicates bare excess of reagent. Multiply volume dithizone solution required by 1.5 and add this volume (to nearest 0.05 mL) to all samples. Shake 2 min. Pipet exactly 5.0 mL solvent layer into clean, dry test tube, dilute with 10.0 mL CCl_4, mix, and determine T (or A) at 540 nm.

G. Preparation of Standard Curves

Prepare series of separators containing 0, 5, 10, 15, and 20 μg Zn diluted to 25 mL with $0.04N$ HCl; add 5.0 mL citrate buffer, and proceed as with final extraction of Zn, **944.09F**.

Plot T in logarithmic scale (or A on linear scale) against concentration and draw smooth curve through points. (Intercept of this curve may vary slightly from day to day, depending on actual concentration of dithizone used in final extraction, but slope should remain essentially same.)

References: JAOAC **27**, 325(1944); **28**, 271(1945).
CAS-7440-66-6 (zinc)

40.7

969.32—Zinc in Food
Atomic Absorption Spectrophotometric Method
First Action 1969
Final Action 1971

(*Caution: See Appendix* for safety notes on AAS, wet oxidation, nitric acid, and sulfuric acid.)

A. Principle

Representative sample is dry or wet ashed. Residue is taken up in acid and diluted to optimum working range. A of this solution as determined by AA spectrophotometry at 213.8 nm is converted to Zn concentration through calibration curve.

B. Reagents

(Use Pyrex glassware exclusively; clean thoroughly before use with hot HNO_3. If glass beads are used to prevent bumping, clean first with strong alkali followed by hot HNO_3. Since Pt used in laboratory may contain significant traces of metals, clean Pt dishes by $KHSO_4$ fusion followed by 10% HCl leach.)

(**a**) *Zinc standard solutions.*—(*1*) *Stock solution.*—500 µg/mL. Dissolve 0.500 g pure Zn metal in 5–10 mL HCl. Evaporate almost to dryness and dilute to 1 L with H_2O. Solution is stable indefinitely. (*2*) *Working solution.*—Dilute aliquots of stock solution with H_2SO_4 (1 + 49) or 0.1N HCl (depending on method of ashing) to obtain ≥5 solutions within range of instrument. Prepare standards in 0–10 µg/mL range daily. (Do not use <2 mL pipets or <25 mL volumetric flasks.)

(**b**) *Acids.*—Reagent grade HNO_3, HCl, and H_2SO_4. Test acids for freedom from Zn by AA measurement of appropriately diluted sample. If contaminated, purify HNO_3 and HCl by distillation. Further test purity of reagents and efficiency of cleaning by conducting blank determinations by appropriate ashing method.

C. Preparation of Sample Solution

Prepare representative sample by mixing, blending, or grinding.

(**a**) *Wet ashing.*—Accurately weigh, into 300 or 500 mL Kjeldahl flask, representative sample ≤10 g, estimated to contain 25–100 µg Zn. (If sample is liquid, evaporate to small volume.) Add ca 5 mL HNO_3 and cautiously heat until first vigorous reaction subsides. Add 2.0 mL H_2SO_4 and continue heating, maintaining oxidizing conditions by adding HNO_3 in *small* increments (large amounts may introduce Zn) until solution is colorless. Continue heating until dense fumes of H_2SO_4 are evolved and all HNO_3 has been removed. Cool, dilute with ca 20 mL H_2O, filter through fast paper (pre-washed) into 100 mL volumetric flask, and dilute to volume with H_2O. Dilute further, if necessary, with H_2SO_4 (1 + 49) to attain working range of spectrophotometer.

(**b**) *Dry ashing.*—Accurately weigh, into clean Pt dish, representative sample estimated to contain 25–100 µg Zn. Char under IR lamp and ash at temperature ≤525° until C-free. (Raise temperature of furnace slowly to 525° to avoid ignition.) Dissolve ash under watch glass in minimum volume HCl (1 + 1). Add ca 20 mL H_2O and evaporate to near dryness on steam bath. Add 20 mL 0.1N HCl and continue heating ca 5 min. Filter through fast paper into 100 mL volumetric flask. Wash dish and filter with several 5–10 mL portions of 0.1N HCl, cool, and dilute to volume with 0.1N HCl. Dilute further, if necessary, with 0.1N HCl to attain working range of instrument.

D. Determination

Set instrument to previously established optimum conditions or according to manufacturer's instructions. Determine A of ashed solution or dilution, and ≥5 standards within optimum working range, taking ≥2 readings (before and after sample readings). Flush burner with H_2O and check 0 point between readings. Determine Zn content from standard curve obtained by plotting A against μg Zn/mL:

ppm Zn = [(μg Zn/mL from curve) × (dilution factor, mL)]/g sample

Reference: JAOAC **51,** 1042(1968).
CAS-7440-66-6 (zinc)

40.8   953.01—Metals in Plants
General Recommendations
for Emission Spectrographic Methods
First Action 1988

See Chapter 12.5.

40.9   985.01—Metals and Other Elements in Plants
Inductively Coupled Plasma Spectroscopic Method
First Action 1985
Final Action 1988

See Chapter 12.6.

40.10   941.03—Zinc in Plants
Mixed Color Method
Final Action

A. Reagents

(Redistil all H_2O from Pyrex. Treat all glassware with HNO_3 (1 + 1) or fresh chromic acid cleaning solution. Rinse repeatedly with ordinary distilled H_2O and finally with Zn-free H_2O.)

(a) *Carbon tetrachloride.*—Use ACS grade without purification. If technical grade is used, dry with anhydrous $CaCl_2$ and redistil in presence of small amount CaO. (Used CCl_4 may be reclaimed by distillation in presence of NaOH (1 + 100) containing small amounts of $Na_2S_2O_3$, followed by drying with anhydrous $CaCl_2$ and fractional distillation in presence of small amounts of CaO.) (*Caution: See Appendix* for safety notes on distillation and carbon tetrachloride.)

(b) *Zinc standard solutions.*—(*1*) *Stock solution.*—1 mg/mL. Place 0.25 g pure Zn in 250 mL volumetric flask. Add ca 50 mL H_2O and 1 mL H_2SO_4; heat on steam bath until all Zn dissolves. Dilute to volume and store in Pyrex vessel. (2) *Working solution.*—10 μg/mL. Dilute 10 mL stock solution to 1 L. Store in Pyrex vessel.

(c) *Ammonium hydroxide solution.*—1N. With all-Pyrex apparatus distil NH_4OH into H_2O, stopping distillation when half has distilled. Dilute distillate to proper concentration. Store in glass-stoppered Pyrex vessel.

(d) *Hydrochloric acid.*—1N. Displace HCl gas from HCl in glass flask by slowly adding equal volume H_2SO_4 from dropping funnel that extends below surface of the HCl. Conduct displaced HCl gas through delivery tube to surface of H_2O in receiving flask (no heat is necessary). Dilute to proper concentration. Use of 150 mL each of HCl and H_2SO_4 will yield 1 L purified HCl solution of concentration $> 1N$.

(e) *Diphenylthiocarbazone (dithizone) solution.*—Dissolve 0.20 g dithizone in 500 mL CCl_4, and filter to remove insoluble matter. Place solution in glass-stoppered bottle or large separator, add 2 L 0.02N NH_4OH (40 mL 1N NH_4OH diluted to 2 L), and shake to extract dithizone into aqueous phase. Separate phases, discard CCl_4, and extract ammoniacal solution of dithizone with 100 mL portions CCl_4 until CCl_4 extract is pure green. Discard CCl_4 after each extraction. Add 500 mL CCl_4 and 45 mL 1N HCl, and shake to extract dithizone into CCl_4. Separate phases and discard aqueous phase. Dilute CCl_4 solution of dithizone to 2 L with CCl_4. Store in brown bottle in dark, cool place.

(f) *Ammonium citrate solution.*—0.5M. Dissolve 226 g $(NH_4)_2HC_6H_5O_7$ in 2 L H_2O. Add NH_4OH (80–85 mL) to pH of 8.5–8.7. Add excess dithizone solution (aqueous phase is orange-yellow after phases have been shaken and separated), and extract with 100 mL portions CCl_4 until extract is full green. Add more dithizone if necessary. Separate aqueous phase from CCl_4 and store in Pyrex vessel.

(g) *Carbamate solution.*—Dissolve 0.25 g sodium diethyldithiocarbamate in H_2O and dilute to 100 mL with H_2O. Store in refrigerator in Pyrex bottle. Prepare fresh after 2 weeks.

(h) *Dilute hydrochloric acid.*—0.02N. Dilute 100 mL 1N HCl to 5 L.

B. Preparation of Solutions

To reduce measuring out reagents and minimize errors due to variations in composition, prepare 3 solutions in appropriate amounts from reagents and store in Pyrex vessels, taking care to avoid loss of NH_3 from *Solutions 1* and *2*. Discard solutions after 6–8 weeks because Zn increases slowly with storage. Determine standard curve for each new set of reagents. Following amounts of *Solutions 1* and *2* and 2 L dithizone solution are enough for 100 determinations:

(1) *Solution 1.*—Dilute 1 L 0.5M ammonium citrate and 140 mL 1N NH_4OH to 4 L.

(2) *Solution 2.*—Dilute 1 L 0.5M ammonium citrate and 300 mL 1N NH_4OH to 4.5 L. Just before using, add 1 volume carbamate solution to 9 volumes NH_3-ammonium citrate solution to obtain volume of *Solution 2* immediately required.

Note: If Zn-free reagents have been prepared, they can be used to test chemicals for Zn. Certain lots of NH_4OH and HCl are sufficiently free of Zn to be used without purification.

C. Ashing

Ash 5 g finely ground, air-dried plant material in Pt dish in furnace at 500–550°. Include blank determination. Moisten ash with little H_2O; then add 10 mL 1N HCl (more if necessary) and heat on steam bath until all substances soluble in HCl are dissolved. Add 5–10 mL hot H_2O. Filter off insoluble matter on 7 cm paper (Whatman No. 42, or equivalent, previously washed with two 5 mL portions hot 1N HCl, then washed with hot H_2O until HCl-free), and collect filtrate in 100 mL volumetric flask. Wash filter with hot H_2O until washings are not acid to methyl red. Add 1 drop methyl red (dissolve 1 g methyl red in 200 mL alcohol) to filtrate in 100 mL flask; neutralize with $1N$ NH_4OH and add 4 mL $1N$ HCl. Cool, and dilute to volume with H_2O.

D. First Extraction

(Separation of dithizone complex-forming metals from ash solution)

Pipet aliquot of ash solution containing ≤ 30 μg Zn into 125 mL Squibb separator. Add 1 mL $0.2N$ HCl for each 5 mL ash solution < 10 mL taken, or 1 mL $0.2N$ NH_4OH for each 5 mL > 10 mL taken. (10 mL aliquot is usually satisfactory in analysis of plant materials.) Add 40 mL *Solution 1* and 10 mL dithizone reagent. Shake vigorously 30 s to extract from aqueous phase the Zn and other dithizone complex-forming metals that may be present; then let layers separate. At this point excess dithizone (indicated by orange or yellow-orange aqueous phase) must be present. If excess dithizone is not present, add more reagent until, after shaking, excess is indicated. Shake down the drop of CCl_4 extract from surface, and drain CCl_4 extract into second separator as completely as possible without letting any aqueous layer enter stopcock bore. Rinse down CCl_4 extract from surface of aqueous layer with 1–2 mL clear CCl_4; then drain this CCl_4 into second separator without letting aqueous phase enter stopcock bore. Repeat rinsing process as often as necessary to flush extract completely into second separator. Add 5 mL clear CCl_4 to first separator, shake 30 s, and let layers separate (CCl_4 layer at this point will appear clear green if metals that form dithizone complexes have been completely extracted from aqueous phase by previous extraction.) Drain CCl_4 layer into second separator and flush extract down from surface and out of separator as directed previously. If last extract does not possess distinct clear color, repeat extraction with 5 mL clear CCl_4 and flushing-out process until complete extraction of dithizone complex-forming metals is assured; then discard aqueous phase.

E. Second Extraction

(Separation of Cu by extraction of Zn into $0.02N$ HCl)

Pipet 50 mL $0.02N$ HCl into separator containing CCl_4 solution of metal dithizonates. Shake vigorously 1.5 min, and let layers separate. Shake down drop from surface of aqueous phase, and as completely as possible drain CCl_4 phase containing all Cu as dithizonate, without letting any aqueous phase, which contains all the Zn, enter stopcock bore. Rinse down CCl_4 extract from surface of aqueous phase, and rinse out stopcock bore with 1–2 mL portions clear CCl_4 (same as in first extraction) until all traces of green dithizone have been washed out of separator. Shake down drop of CCl_4 from surface of aqueous phase, and drain CCl_4 as completely as possible without letting any aqueous phase enter stopcock bore. Remove stopper from separator and lay it across neck until small amount of CCl_4 on surface of aqueous phase evaporates.

F. Final Extraction

(Extraction of Zn in presence of carbamate reagent)

Pipet 50 mL *Solution 2* and 10 mL dithizone solution into 50 mL $0.02N$ HCl solution containing the Zn. Shake 1 min and let phases separate. Flush out stopcock and stem of separator with ca 1 mL CCl_4 extract; then collect remainder in test tube. Pipet 5 mL extract into 25 mL volumetric flask, dilute to volume with clear CCl_4, and measure A with spectrophotometer set at absorption maximum, ca 525 nm. (*Caution:* Protect final extract from sunlight as much as possible and read within 2 h.)

Determine Zn present in aliquot from curve relating A and concentration, correct for Zn in blank, and calculate % Zn in sample.

G. Standard Curve

Place 0, 5, 10, 15, 20, 25, 30, and 35 mL Zn working standard solution in 100 mL volumetric flasks. To each flask add 1 drop methyl red and neutralize with $1N$ NH$_4$OH; then add 4 mL $1N$ HCl and dilute to volume. Proceed exactly as for ash solutions, beginning with first extraction, and using 10 mL aliquots of each of the Zn solutions (0, 5, 10, 15, 20, 25, 30, and 35 μg Zn, respectively). Construct standard curve by plotting μg Zn against A.

References: Ind. Eng. Chem. Anal. Ed. **13**, 145(1941). JAOAC **24**, 520(1941).
CAS-7440-66-6 (zinc)

40.11 953.04—Zinc in Plants
Single Color Method
Final Action 1965

A. Reagents

See **941.03A** and **B** (*see* 40.10), plus following:

(**a**) *Dilute dithizone solution.*—Dilute 1 volume dithizone solution, **941.03A(e)**, with 4 volumes CCl$_4$.

(**b**) *Carbamate solution.*—Dissolve 1.25 g sodium diethyldithiocarbamate in H$_2$O and dilute to 1 L. Store in refrigerator and prepare fresh after long periods of storage.

(**c**) *Dilute ammonium hydroxide.*—Dilute 20 mL $1N$ NH$_4$OH, **941.03A(c)**, to 2 L.

B. Ashing

Weigh 2 g sample finely ground plant material into well-glazed porcelain, Vycor, or Pt crucible, include crucible for blank determination, and heat in furnace at 500–550° until ashing is complete. Cool, moisten ash with little H$_2$O, add 10 mL $1N$ HCl (more if necessary to ensure excess of acid), and heat on steam bath until all soluble material dissolves. Add few mL hot H$_2$O and filter through quantitative paper into 200 mL volumetric flask. Wash paper with hot H$_2$O until washings are not acid to methyl red. Add 2 drops methyl red solution to filtrate, neutralize with $1N$ NH$_4$OH, add exactly 3.2 mL $1N$ HCl, dilute to volume with H$_2$O, and mix.

C. Formation of Zinc Dithizonate

(Removal of interferences and separation of excess dithizone.)

Pipet aliquot of ash solution containing ≤ 15 μg Zn into 125 mL amber glass separator. (25 mL aliquot is usually satisfactory.) If necessary to use different volume, add 0.4 mL 0.2N HCl for each 5 mL less, or 0.4 mL 0.2N NH$_4$OH for each 5 mL more, than 25 mL taken. If <25 mL of the solution is taken, add H$_2$O to 25 mL.

Add 10 mL dithizone reagent, **941.03A(e)**, to aliquot in separator and shake vigorously 1 min. Let layers separate and discard CCl$_4$ layer. Add 2 mL CCl$_4$ to aqueous solution, let layers separate, and discard CCl$_4$. Repeat this rinsing once. Then add 5 mL CCl$_4$, shake vigorously 15 s, let layers separate, and discard CCl$_4$. Rinse once more with 2 mL CCl$_4$ as above. Discard CCl$_4$ layer and let CCl$_4$ remaining on surface of solution in funnel evaporate before proceeding.

Add 40 mL ammonium citrate *Solution 1*, **941.03B(I)**, 5 mL carbamate solution, **953.04A(b)**, and 25 mL dilute dithizone reagent, **953.04A(a)**. Accurately add carbamate and dithizone reagents from pipet or buret. Shake vigorously 1 min. Let layers separate and draw off aqueous layer through fine tip glass tube connected to aspirator with rubber tubing. To remove excess dithizone from CCl_4 layer, add 50 mL $0.01N$ NH_4OH and shake vigorously 30 s.

D. Determination

Dry funnel stem with pipestem cleaner and flush out with ca 2 mL of the zinc dithizonate solution. Collect adequate portion of remaining solution in 25 mL Erlenmeyer, or other suitable container, and stopper tightly. (Amber glass containers are convenient, but colorless glassware will suffice if solutions are kept in dark until A readings are made.)

Measure A of each solution against CCl_4 with spectrophotometer set at absorption maximum, ca 535 nm. Correct for Zn in blank determinations. Calculate amount Zn present in solution from curve relating concentration and A.

E. Standard Curve

Into 200 mL volumetric flasks place 0, 2, 4, 6, 8, 10, 12, and 14 mL, respectively, Zn working standard solution. To each flask add 2 drops methyl red solution, neutralize with $1N$ NH_4OH, add 3.2 mL $1N$ HCl, and dilute to volume with H_2O. Pipet 25 mL aliquots of each of these solutions, containing 0, 2.5, 5, 7.5, 10, 12.5, 15, and 17.5 μg Zn, respectively, into amber glass separators, and proceed as for ash solutions, **953.04C**, beginning with second paragraph. Determine A of each solution and plot values against corresponding amounts Zn.

Reference: JAOAC **36,** 397(1953).
CAS-7440-66-6 (zinc)

40.12   984.27—Calcium, Copper, Iron, Magnesium,
Manganese, Phosphorus, Potassium, Sodium, and Zinc in Infant Formula
Inductively Coupled Plasma Emission Spectroscopic Method
First Action 1984
Final Action 1986

See Chapter 12.13.

40.13   985.35—Minerals in Ready-to-Feed Milk-Based Infant Formula
Atomic Absorption Spectrophotometric Method
First Action 1985
Final Action 1988

See Chapter 12.14.

Appendix: Laboratory Safety

Eugene C. Cole, *Associate Chapter Editor*
University of North Carolina

Introduction

This chapter is not intended to be an exhaustive treatise on laboratory safety. These precautionary notes serve only as a reminder of possible hazards involved in the use of particular operations or substances. Refer to recommended texts at end of chapter for fuller treatment of subject. Follow safety requirements of your organization and state, provincial, or federal government. Consult guidelines issued by professional associations and government agencies.

Cautionary Statements

Nature and amount of each chemical and its prescribed use were criteria used in determining if cautionary statement for method was indicated.

Safety hazard was considered to exist when nature, amount, and use of chemical or equipment specified in method appeared likely to produce any of following:

(**a**) Concentration of vapors from flammable liquid exceeding 25% of lower flammability limit of that liquid described by National Fire Protection Association, Boston, MA.

(**b**) Contact between analyst and amounts of material highly active physiologically or toxic to humans in excess of Threshold Limit Values published by American Conference of Governmental Industrial Hygienists, P.O. Box 1937, Cincinnati, OH 45201.

(**c**) Contact between analyst and amounts of highly corrosive material sufficient to produce serious injury.

(**d**) Contact between analyst and radiations which could be harmful.

(**e**) Explosion or violent reaction.

(**f**) Injury to analyst by hazards in equipment or processes which are not readily detectable by analyst.

When in doubt about possible hazards not covered in this chapter, consult references at end of chapter or other sources of information such as hazard warnings on labels and manufacturers' data sheets.

Potential Hazards of Equipment

Refrigerators

Refrigerators should be explosion proof or explosion resistant when used for storage of ether and other highly volatile, flammable liquids. Ordinary refrigerators can be made explosion resistant by removal of light switch, receptacle, and associated wiring and placing thermoregulation controls on outside of refrigerator.

Glass

Dispose of chipped or broken glassware in special containers; minor chips may be fire-polished and glassware retained. If glassware is to be repaired, mark defective area plainly and store in special location until repairs are completed.

Use heat-resistant glassware for preparation of solutions that generate heat (e.g., not bottles or graduates).

Fire Extinguishers

Class B and C dry chemical fire extinguishers (for flammable liquid and electric fires) should be conveniently available to each laboratory room. Carbon dioxide fire extinguishers should be used on fires in electronic equipment.

Become familiar with the location of all fire extinguishers and the appropriate methods for their effective use.

Blenders

Motor on high-speed blenders used to mix flammable solvent with other materials should be explosion proof. Blend toxic or flammable liquids in effective fume removal device.

Centrifuges

Adjust all tubes to equal weight before loading them into centrifuge. Make certain that stoppers of tubes placed in pivot-type head will clear center when tubes swing to horizontal. Do not open centrifuge cover until machine stops completely. Before removing tubes, turn electric switch to "off." Do not rely on zero-set rheostat. Use only tubes specially designed for centrifuging. Do not exceed safe speed for various tube materials (glass, cellulose nitrate, polyethylene, etc.) recommended by tube manufacturer. Cellulose nitrate tubes may explode if autoclaved. Heating cellulose nitrate tubes $>60°$ may cause them to produce harmful nitrogen oxide fumes.

Atomic Absorption Spectrophotometer

Follow all manufacturer's instructions for installation, operation, safety, and maintenance. Use only hose/tubing to conduct gases approved by manufacturer and supplier. Use effective fume removal device to remove gaseous effluents from burner. Use only C_2H_2 which is dissolved in solvent recommended by manufacturer. Open C_2H_2 tank stem valve only ¼ turn. Change tank when C_2H_2 pressure shows 75-100 lb. If instrument has a drain trap, ensure that it is filled with H_2O before igniting burner. Following repair to C_2H_2 supply line, check for gas tightness at all connections with soap solution or combustible gas detection system. Whenever solutions are aspirated which contain high concentrations of Cu, Ag, or Hg, spray chamber should be rinsed with 50-100 mL H_2O before shutting down to clean these metals from chamber. See safety notes on compressed gas cylinders.

Flame Photometer

Use effective fume removal device to remove gaseous burner effluents.

Photofluorometer

Considerable amounts of O_3 are formed by UV light radiated by quartz lamp. Ozone is toxic even in low concentrations; remove through effective fume removal device placed near quartz lamp.

Monitoring Equipment

Monitor unattended operations with equipment that will automatically shut down process if unsafe condition develops.

Reference: N. V. Steere, "Handbook of Laboratory Safety" (1971); CRC Press, Inc., 2255 Palm Beach Lakes Blvd, West Palm Beach, FL 33409.

Compressed Gas Cylinders

Identify by name(s) of gas(es) contents of compressed gas cylinders on attached decal, stencil, or tag, instead of by color codes. Move cylinders (with protective cap) upright secured to cart. Secure cylinders in upright position by means of strap, chain, or non-tip base. Let contents of C_2H_2 cylinders settle and let all cylinders come to room temperature prior to opening. Use only correct pressure gages, pressure regulator, flow regulator, and hose/tubing, for each size of gas cylinder and type of gas as specified by supplier. Use soap solution or combustible gas detection system to check all connections, especially when system is pressurized and gas is not flowing, to check for slow leak. Use special heater on N_2O gas line. Close gas tank valve and diaphragm on regulator (turn counter-clockwise) when gas is not in use. Service regulator at least yearly. Use toxic gases only in effective fume removal device. When burning gas, use flashback prevention device in gas line on output side of regulator to prevent flame being sucked into cylinder.

Reference: Handbook of Compressed Gases (1981). Compressed Gas Association, Van Nostrand Reinhold Co., New York, NY.

Distillation, Extraction, and Evaporations

(a) *Flammable liquids.*—Perform operations behind safety barrier with hot H_2O, steam, or electric mantle heating. Use effective fume removal device to remove flammable vapors as produced. Set up apparatus on firm supports and secure all connections. Leave ample headroom in flask and add boiling chips *before* heating is begun. All controls, unless vapor sealed, should be located outside vapor area. Dispose of waste flammable solvents by evaporation as above unless other provisions for safe disposal are available.

(b) *Toxic liquids.*—Use effective fume removal device to remove toxic vapors as produced. Avoid contact with skin. Set up apparatus on firm supports and secure all connections. Dispose of waste toxic solvents by evaporation, using effective fume removal device unless other provisions for safe disposal are available.

Electrical Equipment

Accidents involving electric equipment may result in *mechanical injury,* e.g., fingers being caught in chopping mill knives; *electric shock,* which may be due to lack of or improper grounding, defective equipment, exposed wiring, or inadequate maintenance; and *fire* through ignition of flammable vapors by electrically produced spark. Ground all electric equipment to avoid accidental shock. Installation, maintenance, and repair operations should be performed by qualified electricians.

Parr Bomb

Follow manufacturer's directions closely to avoid explosion.

Pressure

Do not conduct pressure operations with standard glassware. In certain circumstances, glassware specifically designed to withstand pressure may be used. Observe manufacturer's recommended safeguards when using pressure apparatus such as calorimeter bomb, hydrogenator, etc.

Vacuum

Tape or shield with safety barrier containers and apparatus to be used under vacuum to minimize effects of possible implosion. Vacuum pump drive belts must have effective guards.

Hazardous Radiations

UV radiation is encountered in AA spectrophotometry, fluorometry, UV spectrophotometry, germicidal lamps, and both long- and shortwave UV lamps used to monitor chromatographic separations. Never expose unprotected eyes to UV light from any source either direct or reflected (e.g., flames in flame photometer, lamps, electric arcs, etc.). Always wear appropriate eye protection such as goggles having uranium oxide lenses, welder's goggles, etc., when such radiations are present and unshielded. Keep skin exposure to UV radiations to minimum.

Safety Techniques and Practices

Spraying Chromatograms

When strong corrosive and toxic reagents are sprayed on chromatograms, use gloves, face shield, respiratory protection, and appropriate fume removal device to protect skin, eyes, and respiratory tract against mists or fumes generated by spraying device.

Pipets

Do not pipet hazardous liquids by using mouth suction to fill pipet. Use pipet fillers or rubber tubing connected through trap to vacuum line for this purpose.

Wet Oxidation

This technique is among most hazardous uses of acids but can be performed safely. Observe precautions in this chapter for particular acids used and rigorously follow directions given in specific method being used.

Hazardous or After Hours Work

Anyone working alone after hours or on hazardous procedures should arrange to be contacted periodically as a safety measure.

Glass Tubing

Protect hands with heavy towel or gloves when inserting glass tubing into cork or rubber stopper. Fire polish all raw glass cuts.

Open ampules in fume removal device over tray large enough to hold contents if ampule should break. If contents are volatile, cool before opening.

Safe Handling of Acids

Use effective *acid-resistant* fume removal device whenever heating acids or performing reactions which liberate acid fumes. In diluting, always add acid to H_2O unless otherwise directed in method. Keep acids off skin and protect eyes from spattering. If acids are spilled on skin, wash immediately with large amounts of H_2O.

Acetic Acid and Acetic Anhydride

React vigorously or explosively with CrO_3 and other strong oxidizers. Wear face shield and heavy rubber gloves when using.
CAS-108-24-7 (acetic anhydride)

Chromic and Perchromic Acids

Can react explosively with acetic anhydride, acetic acid, ethyl acetate, isoamyl alcohol, and benzaldehyde. Less hazardous with ethylene glycol, furfural, glycerol, and methanol. Conduct reactions behind safety barrier. Wear face shield and heavy rubber gloves.

Formic and Performic Acids

Strong reducing agents; react vigorously or explosively with oxidizing agents. Irritating to skin, forming blisters. Performic acid (formyl hydroperoxide) has detonated for no apparent reason while being poured. Wear face shield and heavy rubber gloves when using.
CAS-64-18-6 (formic acid)

Hydrofluoric Acid

Very hazardous with NH_3. It can cause painful sores on skin and is extremely irritating to eyes. Use effective removal device. Wear goggles and acid-resistant gloves.
CAS-7664-39-3 (hydrofluoric acid)

Nitric Acid

Reacts vigorously or explosively with aniline, H_2S, flammable solvents, hydrazine, and metal powders (especially Zn, Al, and Mg). Gaseous nitrogen oxides from HNO_3 can cause severe lung damage. Copious fumes are evolved when concentrated HNO_3 and concentrated HCl are mixed. Avoid premixing. Use effective fume removal device when fumes are generated. Handle with disposable polyvinyl chloride, not rubber, gloves.

Oxalic Acid

Forms explosive compound with Ag and Hg. Oxalates are toxic. Avoid skin contact and ingestion.
CAS-144-62-7 (oxalic acid)

Perchloric Acid

Contact with oxidizable or combustible materials or with dehydrating or reducing agents may result in fire or explosion. Persons using this acid should be thoroughly familiar with its hazards. Safety practices should include following:

(a) Remove spilled $HClO_4$ by immediate and thorough washing with large amounts of H_2O.

(b) Hoods, ducts, and other devices for removing $HClO_4$ vapor should be made of chemically inert materials and so designed that they can be thoroughly washed with H_2O. Exhaust systems should discharge in safe location and fan should be accessible for cleaning.

(c) Avoid use of organic chemicals in hoods or other fume removal devices used for $HClO_4$ digestions.

(d) Use goggles, barrier shields, and other devices as necessary for personal protection; use polyvinyl chloride, not rubber, gloves.

(e) In wet combustions with $HClO_4$, treat sample first with HNO_3 to destroy easily oxidizable org. matter unless otherwise specified. *Do not evaporate to dryness.*

(f) Contact of $HClO_4$ solution with strong dehydrating agents such as P_2O_5 or concentrated H_2SO_4 may result in formation of anhydrous $HClO_4$ which reacts explosively with organic matter and with reducing agents. Exercise special care in performing analyses requiring use of $HClO_4$ with such agents. Extremely sensitive to shock and heat when concentration is $>72\%$.

(g) Also observe precautions outlined in (1) ''Perchloric Acid Solution,'' Chemical Safety Data Sheet SD-11 (1965), Manufacturing Chemists Association of the US, 1825 Connecticut Ave, NW, Washington, DC 20009; (2) ''Applied Inorganic Analysis,'' W. F. Hillebrand, G. E. F. Lundell, H. A. Bright, and J. I. Hoffman, 2nd ed. (1953), pp. 39–40, John Wiley and Sons, Inc., New York, NY; (3) ''Notes on Perchloric Acid and Its Handling in Analytical Work,'' Analyst **84**, 214–216(1959); (4) ''Perchlorates,'' ACS Monograph No. 146, J. C. Schumacher, ed., Reinhold (1960). See references at end of chapter.

Picric Acid

Highly sensitive to shock when in dry state. In contact with metals and NH_3, it produces picrates which are more sensitive to shock than picric acid. Readily absorbed through skin and irritating to eyes. Wear heavy rubber gloves and eye protection.
CAS-88-89-1 (picric acid)

Sulfuric Acid

Always add H_2SO_4 to H_2O. Wear face shield and heavy rubber gloves to protect against splashes.
CAS-7664-93-9 (sulfuric acid)

Fuming Acids

Prepare and use with effective fume removal device. Wear acid-resistant gloves and eye protection.

Safe Handling of Alkalies

Alkalies can burn skin, eyes, and respiratory tract severely. Wear heavy rubber gloves and face shield to protect against concentrated alkali liquids. Use effective fume removal device or gas mask to protect respiratory tract against alkali dusts or vapors.

Ammonia

Extremely caustic liquid and gas. Wear skin, eye, and respiratory protection when handling in anhydrous liquid or gaseous state. NH_3 vapors are flammable. Reacts violently with strong oxidizing agents, halogens, and strong acids.

Ammonium Hydroxide

Caustic liquid. Forms explosive compounds with many heavy metals such as Ag, Pb, Zn, and their salts, especially halide salts.
CAS-1336-21-6 (ammonium hydroxide)

Sodium, Potassium, Lithium, and Calcium Metals

Violently reactive with H_2O or moisture, CO_2, halogens, strong acids, and chlorinated hydrocarbons. Emit corrosive fumes when burned. Can cause severe burns. Wear skin and eye protection when handling. Use only dry alcohol when preparing sodium alcoholate and add metal directly to alcohol, one small piece at a time. Avoid adding metallic Na to reaction through condenser.
CAS-7440-23-5 (sodium)

Sodium Peroxide

Less caustic than sodium and potassium hydroxides but reacts violently with H_2O, organic matter, charcoal, glycerol, diethyl ether, or P. Wear skin, eye, and respiratory protection when handling multigram amounts.
CAS-1313-60-6 (sodium peroxide)

Calcium Oxide (Burnt Lime)

Strongly caustic! Reacts violently with H_2O. Protect skin, eyes, and respiratory tract against contact with dust.
CAS-1305-78-8 (calcium oxide)

Sodium and Potassium Hydroxides

Extremely caustic. Can cause severe burns. Protect skin and eyes when working with these alkalies as solids or concentrated solutions. Add pellets to H_2O, not vice versa.
CAS-1310-58-3 (potassium hydroxide)
CAS-1310-73-2 (sodium hydroxide)

Sodium Biphenyl, Sodium Methylate, and Sodium Ethylate

Less caustic than NaOH but can be injurious. React vigorously with H_2O. Protect skin and eyes when handling.

Safe Handling of Organic Solvents
(Do not mix waste solvents.)

Flammable Solvents

Do not let vapors concentrate to flammable level in work area, since it is nearly impossible to eliminate all chance of sparks from static electricity even though electric equipment is grounded. Use effective fume removal device to remove these vapors when released.

Toxic Solvents

Vapors from some volatile solvents are highly toxic. Several of these solvs are readily absorbed through skin. Use effective fume removal device to remove vapors of these solvents as they are liberated.

References:

Gosselin, Smith, and Hodge, "Clinical Toxicology of Commercial Products (Home and Farm)," 5th ed. (1976); The Williams & Wilkins Co., 428 E Preston St, Baltimore, MD 21202.

American Conference of Governmental Industrial Hygienists, "Threshold Limit Values"; PO Box 1937, Cincinnati, OH 45201.

Sax, "Dangerous Properties of Industrial Materials," 7th ed. (1988); Van Nostrand Reinhold Publishing Corp., New York, NY 10022.

N. V. Steere, "Handbook of Laboratory Safety" (1971); CRC Press, Inc., 2255 Palm Beach Lakes Blvd, West Palm Beach, FL 33409.

Journal of the American Society of Safety Engineers **7,** Feb. 1964.

See references at end of chapter.

Safe Handling of Special Chemical Hazards

Pesticides

Many pesticide chemicals are extremely toxic by various routes of exposure, especially in concentrated form. These chemicals include organic Cl, carbamate, and organic P insecticides, mercurials, arsenicals, nicotine, and other chemicals. As an example, organic P family of pesticides is consistently highly toxic, not only by oral ingestion, but dermally and by inhalation as well. Observe following minimum precautions at all times. Consult safety data sheets or labels for additional information.

(**a**) Do all laboratory sampling, mixing, weighing, etc., under effective fume removal device in area having good forced ventilation of nonrecirculated air, or wear gas mask of proper type. If mask is used, replace cartridges as recommended, since using contaminated mask may be worse than no mask.

(**b**) Keep off skin. Wear clean protective clothing and nonpermeable gloves (such as polyethylene gloves) as necessary. Wash thoroughly with soap and water to avoid contaminating food and smoking materials.

(**c**) Label all sample containers with name and approximate content of all pesticides.

(**d**) Have readily available and study information on symptoms of poisoning and first aid treatment for each type of pesticide being handled.

(**e**) Consult physician about preventive measures and antidotes for use in emergencies when pesticide poisoning is suspected.

(**f**) Follow your organization's procedures when disposing of waste pesticides. The manufacturer can be contacted for advice on disposal problems.

(g) Do not enter pesticide *residue* or other laboratories after handling pesticide formulations until protective clothing and gloves have been removed and face and hands thoroughly washed with soap and water.

U.S. Environmental Protection Agency operates "hotline" staffed to handle pesticide questions, called National Pesticide Telecommunications Network (NPTN). To reach this hotline, dial: 800-858-7378.

References:

Gosselin, Smith, and Hodge, "Clinical Toxicology of Commercial Products (Home and Farm)," 5th ed. (1984); The   Williams and Wilkens Co., Baltimore, MD 21202.

Farm Chemicals Handbook, 75th ed. (1989), Meister Publishing Company, 37841 Euclid Ave, Willoughby, OH 44094.

Morgan, D.P., Recognition and Management of Pesticide Poisonings, 4th ed. (1989), U.S. Environmental Protection Agency, Office of Pesticide Programs, Washington, DC.

Citizens Guide to Pesticides (1987), U.S. Environmental Protection Agency, Office of Pesticides and Toxic Substances, Washington, DC.

Aniline

Toxic. Avoid contact with skin and eyes. Use effective fume removal device. Highly toxic when heated to decomposition. Flammable. May react vigorously with oxidizing agents. Ignites in presence of fuming HNO_3. May react violently with O_3.

CAS-62-53-3 (aniline)

Acetonitrile

Toxic. Avoid contact with skin and eyes. Use effective fume removal device.

Ammoniacal Silver Nitrate

Use soon after preparation and do not allow to stand for long periods of time.

Benzene

Toxic. Highly flammable. Avoid contact with skin. Do not breathe vapors. Use effective fume removal device. Decomposes violently in presence of strong oxidizing agents. Reacts violently with Cl. Considered to be tumor producing agent.

CAS-71-43-0 (benzene)

Acetone

Highly flammable. Forms explosive peroxides with oxidizing agents. Use effective fume removal device. Do not mix with $CHCl_3$.

CAS-67-64-1 (acetone)

Bromine and Chlorine

Hazardous with NH_3, H, petroleum gases, turpentine, benzene, and metal powders. Extremely corrosive. Use effective fume removal device. Protect skin against exposure.

Carbon Disulfide

Extremely flammable with low ignition temperature. Toxic. Use effective fume removal device. Can react vigorously to violently with strong oxidizing agents, azides, and Zn. Avoid static electricity.

CAS-75-15-0 (carbon disulfide)

Carbon Tetrachloride

Reacts violently with alkali metals. Toxic. Fumes may decompose to phosgene when heated strongly. Use effective fume removal device.

CAS-56-23-5 (carbon tetrachloride)

Cyanides

React with acids to form highly toxic and rapid acting HCN gas. Use only in effective fume removal device. Destroy residues with alkaline NaOCl solution.

Cyclohexane

Highly flammable. Use effective fume removal device. Can react vigorously with strong oxidizing agents.

CAS-110-82-7 (cyclohexane)

Di- and Triethylamine

Flammable. Toxic. Corrosive to skin and eyes. Use effective fume removal device. Can react vigorously with oxidizing materials.

Dimethylformamide

Toxic. Flammable. Avoid contact with skin and eyes. Use effective fume removal device. Can react vigorously with oxidizing agents, halogenated hydrocarbons, and inorganic nitrates.

Diethyl Ether

Store protected from light. Extremely flammable. Unstable peroxides can form upon long standing or exposure to sunlight in bottles. Can react explosively when in contact with Cl, O_3, $LiAlH_4$, or strong oxidizing agents. Use effective fume removal device. Avoid static electricity. *See* safety notes on peroxides.

CAS-60-29-7 (ether)

Ethanol

Flammable. Use effective fume removal device when heating or evaporating.

Chloroform

Can be harmful if inhaled. Forms phosgene when heated to decomposition. Use effective fume removal device. Can react explosively with Al, Li, Mg, Na, K, disilane, N_2O_4, and NaOH plus methanol. Considered to be tumor producing agent.

CAS-67-66-3 (chloroform)

Ethyl Acetate

Flammable, especially when being evaporated. Irritating to eyes and respiratory tract. Use effective fume removal device.

CAS-141-78-6 (ethyl acetate)

Formaldehyde

A suspect human carcinogen. Exposure to high concentrations may cause skin irritation and inflammation of mucous membranes, eyes, and respiratory tract. Use skin protection and effective fume removal device.

CAS-50-00-0 (formaldehyde)

Hydrogen Sulfide

Hazardous with oxidizing gases, fuming HNO_3, and Na_2O_2. Forms explosive mixtures with air. Toxic. Use effective fume removal device.

CAS-7783-06-4 (hydrogen sulfide)

Hypophosphorus Acid

Reacts violently with oxidizing agents. On decomposition, emits highly toxic fumes (phosphine) and may explode. Use effective fume removal device.

Hexane

Highly flammable. Use effective fume removal device.

CAS-110-54-3 (hexane)

Isooctane

Highly flammable. Use effective fume removal device.

CAS-26635-64-3 (isooctane)

Magnesium

When finely divided, liberates H in contact with H_2O. Burns in air when exposed to flame. Can be explosive in contact with $CHCl_3$ or CH_3Cl.

Magnesium Perchlorate

Explodes on contact with acids and reducing materials. Use as drying agent on inorganic gases and materials only.

CAS-10034-81-8 (magnesium perchlorate)

Mercury

Hazardous in contact with NH_3, halogens, and alkali. Vapors are extremely toxic and cumulative. Regard spills on hot surfaces as extremely hazardous and clean up promptly. Powdered S sprinkled over spilled Hg can assist in cleaning up spills. High degree of personal cleanliness is necessary for persons who use Hg. Handle only in locations where any spill can be readily and thoroughly cleaned up. When Hg evaporation is necessary, use effective fume removal device.

To avoid environmental contamination, dilute liquid remaining in Kjeldahl distillation flask to ca 300 mL with H_2O, cool to room temperature, and add 50 mL 30% H_2O_2. (If Raney powder method is used, 6 mL is enough.) Warm gently to initiate reaction, let reaction go to completion in warm flask, and separate precipitated HgS. Reserve precipitate in closed labeled container for recovery of Hg or disposal appropriate for Hg.

See safety notes on mercury salts.

Methanol

Flammable. Toxic. Avoid contact with eyes. Avoid breathing vapors. Use effective fume removal device. Can react vigorously with NaOH plus $CHCl_3$, and KOH plus $CHCl_3$ or $HClO_4$.

CAS-67-56-1 (methanol)

Methyl Cellosolve

Vapors can be harmful. Use effective fume removal device.

CAS-109-86-4 (methyl cellosolve)

Nitrobenzene and Other Nitroaromatics

Readily absorbed through skin. Symptoms of intoxication are sense of well-being and bluish tint on tongue, lips, and fingernails. Wear resistant rubber gloves when handling. Heat or evaporate in effective fume removal device.

CAS-98-95-3 (nitrobenzene)

Oxidizers

(Perchlorates, peroxides, permanganates, persulfates, perborates, nitrates, chlorates, chlorites, bromates, iodates, concentrated H_2SO_4, concentrated HNO_3, CrO_3)

Can react violently with most metal powders, NH_3, and ammonium salts, P, many finely divided organic compounds, flammable liquids, acids, and S. Use exactly as specified in method. Handle in effective fume removal device from behind explosion-resistant barrier. Use face shield.

Peroxides

(a) *Hydrogen peroxide.*—30% strength is hazardous; can cause severe burns. Drying H_2O_2 on organic material such as paper or cloth can lead to spontaneous combustion. Cu, Fe, Cr, other metals, and their salts cause rapid catalytic decomposition of H_2O_2. Hazardous with flammable liquids, aniline, and nitrobenzene. Since it slowly decomposes with evolution of O, provide stored H_2O_2 with vent caps. Wear gloves and eye protection when handling.

(b) *Ether peroxides.*—These peroxides form in diethyl ether, dioxane, and other ethers during storage. They are explosive and must be destroyed chemically before distillation or evaporation. Exposure to light influences peroxide formation in ethers. Filtration through activated alumina is reported to be effective in removing peroxides. Store over sodium ribbon to retard peroxide formation.

CAS-7722-84-1 (hydrogen peroxide)

Phosphotungstic Acid

Emits highly toxic fumes when heated to decomposition or in strong alkali.

Pyridine

Toxic. Flammable. Use effective fume removal device. Releases toxic cyanides when heated to decomposition.

CAS-110-86-1 (pyridine)

Petroleum Ether

Extremely flammable. Use effective fume removal device. Avoid static electricity.

CAS-8030-30-6 (petroleum ether)

Pentane

Extremely flammable. Use effective fume removal device. Avoid static electricity.

CAS-109-66-0 (pentane)

Radioactive Chemicals

Consult NBS Handbook No. 92, "Safe Handling of Radioactive Materials" (available as NCRP Report No. 30 from National Council on Radiation Protection, Publications Dept., 4201 Conn. Ave. NW, Washington, DC 20008) and NCRP Report No. 39 "Basic Radiation Protection Criteria," before handling these materials.

Silver Nitrate

Powerful oxidizing agent; strongly corrosive. Dust or solid form is hazardous to eyes. Handle as noted for oxidizers.

Silver Iodate

Powerful oxidizing agent. Can initiate combustion in contact with organic material (e.g., paper or cloth). Can react vigorously with reducing agents. Handle as noted for oxidizers.

Arsenic Trioxide

Toxic. Forms toxic volatile halides in contact with halide acids. Forms volatile, highly toxic arsine when reduced in acid solution. Protect skin and respiratory tract when handling. Use effective fume removal device when arsine or arsenic trihalide is formed.
CAS-1327-53-3 (arsenic trioxide)

Mercury Salts

Mercuric salts are quite toxic and mostly H_2O-soluble. Use skin and respiratory protection when dry mercuric salts are to be used. Use skin protection when concentrated aqueous solutions of mercuric salts are used. Mercurous salts are generally less toxic than mercuric salts. Use of personal protection is advisable when handling these salts and their concentrated solutions.
See safety notes on mercury.

Permanganates

Moderately toxic. Readily soluble in H_2O. Strong oxidizing agent. May form explosive mixture with H_2SO_4 or $HClO_4$. When using with strong acids to destroy organic matter, perform reaction behind safety barrier.

Sulfur Dioxide

Toxic gas. Forms H_2SO_3 in contact with moisture. Use effective fume removal device to remove SO_2 vapors released by reaction or from gas cylinder. Avoid contact with skin, eyes, and respiratory tract.
CAS-7446-09-5 (sulfur dioxide)

Di- and Trichloroacetic and Trifluoroacetic Acids

Protein precipitants. Can cause severe burns to skin and respiratory tract. Use rubber gloves, eye protection, and effective fume removal device to remove vapors generated.

Uranyl Acetate

Highly toxic. Avoid skin contact and breathing dusts.

Toxic Dusts

Use gloves and goggles to avoid contact with skin and eyes. Use effective fume removal device or other respiratory protection.

Carcinogens

Regulations of U.S. Department of Labor require special precautions to avoid exposure of persons to carcinogenic chemicals. Consult 29CFR1910.93c (U.S. Government Printing Office, Washington, DC 20402) and guidelines for the Laboratory Use of Chemical Substances Posing a Potential Occupational Carcinogenic Risk, USDHEW, 1978.

Asbestos

Dry asbestos fibers are hazardous when inhaled. Wet fibers form a mat which does not constitute a hazard. Transfer dry fibers in hood to container of distilled H_2O and store under H_2O until needed, e.g., for preparation of mats in Gooch crucibles. Do not dry asbestos in forced draft oven, only in convection oven. Open oven doors slowly to avoid developing convection currents that will make fibers airborne. Reuse of filtering mats is often possible by washing, drying, and ignition, as appropriate.

CAS-8012-01-9 (asbestos)

SPECIAL REFERENCES

Chemical Safety

Safe Storage of Laboratory Chemicals, D. A. Pipitone (ed.) (1984), John Wiley & Sons, Inc., New York, NY 10158.

Dangerous Properties of Industrial Materials, 7th ed., N.I. Sax (1988), Van Nostrand Reinhold, New York, NY 10001.

Prudent Practices for Disposal of Chemicals from Laboratories, National Academy of Sciences (1983), National Academy Press, Washington, DC.

Flammable and Combustible Liquids Code Handbook, 2nd ed. (1984), National Fire Protection Association, Boston, MA 02110.

Guidelines for Selection of Chemical Protective Clothing, A.D. Schwope, P.P. Costas, J.O. Jackson, and D.J. Weitzman (1983), American Conference of Governmental Industrial Hygienists, Inc., Cincinnati, OH.

Health and Safety for Toxicity Testing, D.B. Walters and C.W. Jameson (1984), Butterworth Publishers, Stoneham, MA.

Compendium of Safety Data Sheets for Research and Industrial Chemicals, Parts 1, 2, and 3, L.H. Keith and D.B. Walters (1985), VCH Publishers, Inc., Deerfield Beach, FL.

Health Risks to Female Workers in Occupational Exposure to Chemical Agents, R.L. Zielhuis, A. Stijkel, M.M. Verberk, and M. Vande Poel-Bot (1984), Springer-Verlag, Berlin, FRG.

Guide to Safe Practices in Chemical Laboratories (1986), Royal Society of Chemistry, Letchworth, Herts SG6 1HN, UK.

Hazards in the Chemical Laboratory, L. Bretherick (1986), Royal Society of Chemistry, Letchworth, Herts SG6 1HN, UK.

Solvents in Common Use: Health Risks to Workers (1986), Royal Society of Chemistry, Letchworth, Herts SG6 1HN, UK.

Sichere Arbeit im Chemischen Laboratorium; Ein Lernprogram (1977), 2 Volumes, Berufsgenossenschaft der Chemischen Industrie, Heidelberg, FRG.

Onderzoek Kwaliteit Zuurkasten, G. Bolkesteijn (1985), Technical University Twente, Enschede, The Netherlands.

Handboek Bedrijfsveiligheid (1986), 4 Volumes, Kluwer, Deventer, The Netherlands.

La Securite dans les Laboratoires Utilisant des Substances Chimiques: Guide Practique (1983), p. 305, Centre National de Prevention et de Protection (CPP), Paris, France.

Zuurkasten In Laboratoria: Hoe zijn ze, Hoe blijven ze en hoe moeten we er mee werken, A.G. Kroes (1982), pp. 68, Cursus Hogere Veiligheidskunde, Royal Shell Laboratory Safety, Environment and Security, Amsterdam, The Netherlands.

Biological Safety

Laboratory Biosafety Manual, World Heath Organization (1983), WHO Publications Center USA, 49 Sheridan Ave, Albany, NY 12210.

Biohazards Reference Manual, AIHA Biohazards Committee (1985), American Industrial Hygiene Association, Akron, OH 44331-1087.

Biosafety in Microbiological and Biomedical Laboratories, 2nd ed., Centers for Disease Control and National Institutes of Health (1988), HHS No. (NIH) 88-8395, Superintendent of Documents, U.S. Government Printing Office, Washington, DC 20402.

EPA Guide for Infectious Waste Management (1986), Stock No. PB86-199130, National Technical Information Service, Springfield, VA 22161.

Laboratory Safety

CRC Handbook of Laboratory Safety, 2nd ed., N.V. Steere (1971), CRC Press, Inc., Boca Raton FL 33431.

Prudent Practices for Handling Hazardous Chemicals in Laboratories, National Academy of Sciences (1981), National Academy Press, Washington, DC.

Handbook of Laboratory Waste Disposal, M.J. Pitt and E. Pitt (1985), Ellis Horwood Ltd, Halstead Press-John Wiley & Sons, New York, NY.

Handling Radioactivity—A Practical Approach for Scientists and Engineers, D.C. Stewart (1981), John Wiley & Sons, New York, NY.

Radionucleotiden-Laboratoria; Richtlijnen voor Inrichting van en Werken in Radio-Nucleotiden-Laboratoria (1983), Ministerie van Volkshuisvesting, Ruimtelijke Ordening, en Milieubeheer, 44 pp., Publication 83-02, The Hague, The Netherlands.

Index of Method Numbers